B & T

STO

ACPL ITEM
DISCARDED

Y0-BVR-692

616.89 P9533   7065798

PSYCHIATRY IN THE PRACTICE
OF MEDICINE

CIRCULATING WITH THE LISTED PROBLEM(S):

Water Damage

12-1-03 DCB

DO NOT REMOVE
CARDS FROM POCKET

ALLEN COUNTY PUBLIC LIBRARY

FORT WAYNE, INDIANA 46802

You may return this book to any agency, branch,
or bookmobile of the Allen County Public Library.

DEMCO

Psychiatry in the Practice of Medicine

Edited by
Hoyle Leigh, M.D.

Professor of Psychiatry
Director, Psychiatric Consultation-Liaison Service
and Yale Behavioral Medicine Clinic
Yale University School of Medicine and Yale-New Haven
Hospital

With forewords by **Morton Reiscr**, M.D.
Professor and Chairman, Department of Psychiatry

and **Samuel O. Thier**, M.D.
Professor and Chairman, Department of Internal Medicine
Yale University School of Medicine

ADDISON-WESLEY PUBLISHING COMPANY

Medical/Nursing Division • Menlo Park, California
Reading, Massachusetts • London • Amsterdam
Don Mills, Ontario • Sydney

Dedication:
To Vinnie

Sponsoring Editor: *Richard W. Mixter*
Production Coordinators: *Betty Duncan-Todd and Fannie Gray Toldi*
Copyeditor: *Adrienne Mayor*
Interior Design: *John Edeen*
Cover Design: *Lisa Mirski*

The symbol used on the cover and throughout the book was designed by John Edeen to represent the Patient Evaluation Grid, developed by Hoyle Leigh, M.D.

Allen County Public Library
Ft. Wayne, Indiana

Copyright © 1983 by Addison-Wesley Publishing Company, Inc.

All rights reserved. No part of this publication may be reproduced, stored in a retrieval system, or transmitted, in any form or by any means, electronic, mechanical, photocopying, recording, or otherwise, without the prior permission of the publisher. Printed in the United States of America. Published simultaneously in Canada.

Library of Congress Cataloging in Publication Data

Main entry under title:
Psychiatry in the practice of medicine.
Includes bibliographical references and index.
1. Psychiatry—Handbooks, manuals, etc.
I. Leigh, Hoyle. [DNLM: 1. Family practice.
2. Mental disorders. WM 100 P974]
RC456.P79   1983   616.89   83-2522
ISBN 0-201-05456-6

ABCDEFGHIJ-MA-89876543

ADDISON-WESLEY PUBLISHING COMPANY
Medical/Nursing Division
2725 Sand Hill Road
Menlo Park, California 94025

7065798

List of Contributors

Robert L. Arnstein, M.D.
Clinical Professor of Psychiatry
Yale University School of Medicine
Psychiatrist-in-Chief, Yale University
  Health Services Center
New Haven, Connecticut

Henry Black, M.D.
Associate Professor of Medicine
Yale University School of Medicine
Director, Primary Care Center,
  Yale-New Haven Hospital
New Haven, Connecticut

Malcolm B. Bowers, Jr., M.D.
Professor of Psychiatry
Yale University School of Medicine
Chief of Psychiatry, Yale-New Haven Hospital
New Haven, Connecticut

Donald J. Cohen, M.D.
Professor of Pediatrics, Psychiatry, and
  Psychology
Yale University School of Medicine
New Haven, Connecticut

Alvan R. Feinstein, M.D.
Professor of Medicine and
  Epidemiology
Director, Robert Wood Johnson Clinical
  Scholar Program and Clinical
  Epidemiology Unit
Yale University School of Medicine
New Haven, Connecticut

Stephen Fleck, M.D.
Professor of Psychiatry and Public
  Health

Yale University School of Medicine
New Haven, Connecticut

Richard J. Goldberg, M.D.
Assistant Professor of Psychiatry
Brown University School of Medicine
Associate Chief of Psychiatry
The Rhode Island Hospital
Providence, Rhode Island

Robert D. Hunt, M.D.
Assistant Professor of Psychiatry
  (Child Study Center)
Yale University School of Medicine
New Haven, Connecticut

Herbert D. Kleber, M.D.
Professor of Psychiatry
Yale University School of Medicine
Director, Substance Abuse Treatment Unit
Connecticut Mental Health Center
New Haven, Connecticut

Hoyle Leigh, M.D.
Professor of Psychiatry
Yale University School of Medicine
Assistant Chief of Psychiatry, Yale-New
  Haven Hospital
Director, Psychiatric Consultation-Liaison
  Service and Yale Behavioral Medicine
  Clinic
New Haven, Connecticut

Vincenta Leigh, R.N., M.S.N.
Lecturer, Department of Psychiatry
Yale University School of Medicine
Clinical Specialist, The Institute
  of Living
Hartford, Connecticut

Richard Loewenstein, M.D.
  (formerly) Assistant Professor of Psychiatry
  Yale University School of Medicine
  Assistant Director, Psychiatric
    Consultation-Liaison Service
  Yale-New Haven Hospital
  New Haven, Connecticut

Daniel C. Moore, M.D.
  Assistant Professor of Psychiatry
  Yale University School of Medicine
  Chief, Dana Psychiatric Clinic, Yale-New
    Haven Hospital
  New Haven, Connecticut

Morton F. Reiser, M.D.
  Charles G. Murphy Professor of Psychiatry
    and Chairman, Department of Psychiatry
  Yale University School of Medicine
  New Haven, Connecticut

David R. Rubinow, M.D.
  Staff Psychiatrist
  National Institute of Mental Health
  Bethesda, Maryland

Lorna J. Sarrel, M.S.W.
  Assistant Clinical Professor of Social Work in
    Obstetrics and Gynecology and Psychiatry
  Yale University School of Medicine
  Yale University Health Services Center
  New Haven, Connecticut

Philip M. Sarrel, M.D.
  Associate Professor of Obstetrics and
    Gynecology and Psychiatry
  Yale University School of Medicine
  Yale University Health Services Center
  New Haven, Connecticut

Andrew E. Slaby, M.D., M.P.H., Ph.D.
  Professor of Psychiatry and Human Behavior
  Brown University School of Medicine

Chief of Psychiatry, The Rhode Island
    Hospital
  Providence, Rhode Island

Jon Streltzer, M.D.
  Associate Professor of Psychiatry
  Director, Psychiatric Consultation-Liaison
    Service
  University of Hawaii at Manoa
  John A. Burns School of Medicine
  Honolulu, Hawaii

Jane Sturges, M.S.W.
  Assistant Clinical Professor of Social Work in
    Psychiatry
  Yale University School of Medicine
  New Haven, Connecticut

Mary E. Swigar, M.D.
  Associate Professor of Psychiatry
  Yale University School of Medicine
  Director, In-patient Services and
    Neuropsychiatric Evaluation Unit
  Yale-New Haven Hospital
  New Haven, Connecticut

Samuel O. Thier, M.D.
  Sterling Professor of Medicine and
    Chairman, Department of Internal
    Medicine
  Yale University School of Medicine
  New Haven, Connecticut

Craig Van Dyke, M.D.
  Associate Professor of Psychiatry
  Chief, Psychiatric Consultation-Liaison
    Service
  University of California at San Francisco
  San Francisco, California

Foreword

It is generally agreed that an increasingly significant part of the primary physician's task consists of evaluating and managing psychological and psychosocial aspects of the problems that bring patients to them. Furthermore, primary physicians clearly can and should carry a major share of responsibility for administering to the population's (general health-related) mental health needs. Needless to say, this responsibility imposes a considerable burden on the primary physician because responsible discharge of these functions requires not only a broad knowledge of disease, psychology, and medical sociology, but also the special intellectual and interpersonal skills required to work effectively with these problems in everyday practice.

No wonder, then, that there is a pressing demand for books and articles to meet the special reading needs of the busy primary physician who is continually confronted by a rapidly expanding knowledge base and by a burgeoning technical repertoire in this field as well as in all other aspects of clinical practice. This volume is one of many that have been generated in response to this challenge. Like most of them, it is multi-authored. Dr. Leigh, fully cognizant of the limitations inherent in a book written by multiple authors, has taken special pains to minimize limitations by careful selection and integration of the contributors. First, they have been selected from within a single departmental structure and each of them has worked with Dr. Leigh in clinical situations and in educational programs focused on consultation-liaison psychiatry and primary care. This selection of contributors ensures a considerable degree of shared philosophy, approach, and style. Each of the contributors, in addition to being expert in his/her

topic, has also worked intensively and extensively with non-psychiatric physicians and health care professionals, and so is acquainted with the kinds of questions they generate and with the difficulties of getting help from readings that contain a great deal of unfamiliar terminology and theoretical concepts. The book has been written, then, with special respect for the primary physician as reader. Chapter content is supplemented by selected annotated reference lists and bibliographies for those who wish to pursue further study of sources from the psychiatric and behavioral science literature.

Topical coverage is broad and comprehensive, beginning with chapters on patient evaluation (part 1), evaluation and management of major psychiatric syndromes and disorders in adults (part 2), and evaluation of psychiatric syndromes and disorders of childhood (part 3). Chapters are organized to be convenient for the clinician to find answers to questions as they arise in the course of daily work. For example, there are separate chapters on suicidal potential and attempts, psychophysiologic symptoms, alcoholism, drug dependency, violence, etc. The volume contains a wealth of important, useful, and well-organized information—rendering it useful both as an immediate reference for problem solving and as an introductory text that can be studied at leisure. If the book is as successful in its aims as I think it should be, a great many physicians will find a place for it within in easy reach in their consultation rooms and/or studies.

Morton F. Reiser, M.D., F.A.P.A
Charles B. Murphy Professor of Psychiatry
and Chairman, Department of Psychiatry
Yale University School of Medicine

Foreword

"The most common criticism made at present by older
practitioners is that young graduates have been taught a great
deal about the mechanism of disease, but very little about the
practice of medicine—or, to put it more bluntly, they are too
'scientific' and do not know how to take care of patients."

(Francis Peabody, J. Amer. Med. Assoc., March 19, 1927)

The assertion that physicians are simultaneously
becoming too scientific and less caring is not
new, and will continue to be made as long as
medical knowledge and technology advance.
Each new generation of physicians is called
upon to master increasingly complex concepts
of pathophysiology and treatment as well as
more complicated technology. This mastery is
obtained at a price. The price is that older
physicians threatened with becoming outdated
seek to identify weakness in the training and
performance of their better-informed succes-
sors. Patients find that they are less able to share
common knowledge about health with their
physicians and feel a greater distance between
themselves and their doctors. Many physicians
and patients yearn for a simpler era, while few
perceive that the present time is the simpler era
of the next generation.

It is a fact that many diseases can be treated
more effectively than ever before. Yet the perceived widening of the gulf between patient and
doctor has permitted the success of therapy to
be greeted with as much resentment as relief.
The problem is important enough to merit
thoughtful consideration. Among physicians, is
there a loss of humanism due to an inability to
adjust to change in medicine; and, if so, is such a
loss an unnecessary byproduct of that change?

There is little evidence that those entering the
study of medicine are inherently less caring than
their predecessors. Even if the advance of medical science has detracted from the development
of humanistic qualities in physicians, slowing
medical progress is not a reasonable solution
unless we are prepared to withhold the benefits
of progress. Rather, a bit of perspective and
common sense may be in order. Viewed in
proper perspective, some of the current changes
are inevitable. When physicians could do little
but comfort patients, the skills related to providing comfort through personal attention and contact were honored. As treatment directed at the
cause of illness became possible on a broad
scale, the knowledge required to apply such
treatment grew rapidly. Physicians needed to
know more in order to do more. The time and
effort required to obtain and use new knowledge was taken from time for personal interaction with the patient. Time spent comforting
with little ability to heal was exchanged for less
time comforting and more time providing successful therapy. Physicians became secure in
their ability to diagnose and treat well-defined
pathophysiologic entities and were nearly mes-
merized by the explosion of technology.

The previous division of illness into organic
and functional has become a division into

diseases explicable on the basis of pathophysiology and therefore real (organic), versus "unreal" (functional) illnesses. Nevertheless, sophisticated clinicians have always recognized that pathophysiology may define a disease process without defining the clinical presentation or the success of treatment. They recognize that the patient's personality, behavior, family setting, and work environment might dramatically affect the clinical picture. Furthermore, aspects of psychological response translated through neuroendocrine events might well merge functional with pathophysiologic components in producing a clinical illness. Finally, they knew that primary psychiatric illness can modify physiology or mimic organic pathology.

Given the importance of a knowledge of psychiatry to the practice of medicine, the question is how to provide that knowledge during the education of physicians and how to update what is already known by the practicing doctor. Courses in psychiatry have always struck me as adequate for teaching the discipline from the perspective of its practitioners. However, what is needed most is the use of principles and concepts of psychiatry in the everyday practice of medicine. The Department of Psychiatry at Yale has a long tradition of teaching psychiatry to other services through its Liaison Psychiatric Service. In such teaching, the tenets of psychiatry are not isolated issues for discussion but useful tools in caring for medical, surgical, and pediatric patients. The strength of this approach is that focus on what is useful in the general care as opposed to the psychiatric care of patients. Dr. Leigh has called upon a group of authors skilled in interacting with non-psychiatric physicians and has produced an easily-read, well-organized book to which physicians in the primary care of patients can refer easily. In addition to a practical, straightforward presentation of progressively more complex issues, the book provides excellent reference sections with key references annotated for ease of use.

This book stresses the recognition that attention to the patient's personality and environment is as critical as the measurement of blood chemistries in providing the best medical care. There is no debate about one focus of attention being more valuable than the other, simply the underlying belief that all information about the patient including that which can be quantified and that which can be assessed but not quantified is necessary for the best care. This book should be ideal for those physicians committed to providing comprehensive care.

Samuel O. Thier, M.D., F.A.C.P.
Sterling Professor of Medicine and
Chairman, Department of Internal
Medicine
Yale University School of Medicine

Preface

Approximately 50 to 80 per cent of general medical patients suffer from some psychiatric disorder[1]. Many of the psychiatric disorders can be managed effectively by the primary physician, often in consultation with a psychiatrist, if the presence of these disorders is recognized.

The purpose of this book is to convey to the physician and the medical student who will be engaged in patient care, the necessary practical information concerning psychiatric syndromes commonly seen in general medical practice. This book provides, especially for the medical student, a core body of knowledge concerning psychiatry that is useful regardless of future specialization.

We present throughout this book, *a comprehensive approach* based on the Patient Evaluation Grid (PEG)[2]; this approach takes into account the biological, personal, and environmental dimensions of the patient. Whenever possible, vignettes concerning the specific syndromes are analyzed with the use of the PEG.

This is intended to be a practical book. We emphasize the recognition, evaluation, and management of psychiatric disorders by the nonpsychiatric physician. Specific diagnostic criteria and treatment regimes are given whenever possible, and indications for referral to the psychiatrist are also discussed. Psychiatric jargon and technical terms are kept to a minimum. Each chapter provides a section on recommended reading for further information.

This book follows the *DSM-III*[3] *diagnostic nomenclature and criteria* whenever feasible. A complete list of psychiatric diagnoses and their code numbers according to DSM-III is given as an Appendix.

Psychiatry in the Practice of Medicine may be used in conjunction with a basic medical behavioral science text (for example, Leigh and Reiser's *The Patient*[2]) to provide the medical student and physician with a broad overview of psychiatric principles in patient evaluation and management of specific psychiatric syndromes.

This is a Yale book—all the contributors are either current faculty members or were in the past associated with the Yale Department of Psychiatry. Many contributors have a special affiliation with the Psychiatric Consultation-Liaison Service at Yale-New Haven Hospital. The diversity of expertise of the Yale psychiatry department is represented in this volume, as well as, importantly, a share perspective—that of comprehensive and nondogmatic care of patients.

Much impetus for this volume came from the editor's clinical work in the Psychiatric Consultation-Liaison Service at Yale-New Haven Hospital. Many medical and surgical house staff and students on clinical clerkships expressed a desire for a book that contained the kinds of information that the liaison psychiatrists were teaching them: practical information about recognition,

1. Lipowski, ZJ. 1967. Review of consultation psychiatry and psychosomatic medicine II. Clinical aspects. *Psychosom Med* 29:201–224.
2. Leigh, H. and Reiser, M.F. 1980. *The Patient, Biological, Psychological and Social Dimensions of Medical Practice.* Plenum Medical Publishing Co. New York.
3. *Diagnostic and Statistical Manual of Mental Disorders, 3rd Edition.* 1980. American Psychiatric Association, Washington D.C.

diagnosis, differential diagnosis, and management.

The ultimate aim of this book is to help the student of medicine not only to recognize psychiatric syndromes in their patients, but to develop a collaborative relationship with the psychiatrist for comprehensive care of the patient.

Hoyle Leigh, M.D., F.A.P.A.
Professor of Psychiatry
Director, Psychiatric Consultation-liaison
Service and
Yale Behavioral Medicine Clinic
Yale University School of Medicine and
Yale-New Haven Hospital
New Haven, Connecticut

Contents

PART I

Comprehensive Evaluation of Patients   1

CHAPTER 1
Systematic Approach to Comprehensive Care: The Patient Evaluation Grid   3

Hoyle Leigh, M.D.
Alvan R. Feinstein, M.D.
Morton F. Reiser, M.D.

Patient Evaluation Grid   4
PEG Information   5
    Column A—Current Context   5
    Column B—Recent Context   6
    Column C—Background Context   6
Using the PEG   7
Summary   9
Appendix: Case History—The Sick Tarzan 11

CHAPTER 2
Mental Status Examination: Systematic Observation of the Patient   15

Hoyle Leigh, M.D.

Appearance   16
Level of Consciousness   16
Speech and Movement   16
Cognitive Processes   17
    Orientation   17
    Memory, Attention, Concentration, and Comprehension   17
    Abstraction   18
    Judgment   18
    Perceptions   18
    Content of Thought   18
Affect and Mood   18
Conclusion   19

CHAPTER 3
Evaluation of the Family in General Medical Care   21

Stephen Fleck, M.D.

Family Systems   23
    Leadership   23
    Boundaries   23
    Affectivity   24
    Communication   24
    Evolutionary Family Tasks   24
Families and Aging   26
Families and Illness   26
    Psychosomatic Conditions   26
    Family Pathology   27
Family Health   30
Family Health Care   31
Summary   32

PART II

Evaluation and Management of Psychiatric Syndromes and Disorders in Adults   35

CHAPTER 4
Personality Types and Personality Disorders   37

Richard J. Goldberg, M.D.

Formation of Personality   38
    Psychobiological Drives and Society: Conflict and Personality Development   38
    Constitutional Endowment: Precursers of Personality   38
Recognition and Diagnosis   39
    Observation   39
    Listening   40
    Asking Questions   40

Family, Friends, and Staff as Observers   41
Psychological Testing   41
Personality Disorders   42
Dependent Personality Disorder   43
Compulsive Personality Disorder   44
Histrionic Personality Disorder   45
Paranoid Personality Disorder   47
Narcissistic Personality Disorder   48
Schizoid Personality Disorder   48
Antisocial Personality Disorder   49
Borderline Personality Disorder   51
Long-Suffering, Self-Sacrificing
Personality Type   52
General Management Considerations   53
Summary   54

CHAPTER 5
Recognition, Evaluation, and Differential Diagnosis of Psychiatric and Somatic Conditions   57

Richard J. Loewenstein, M.D.
Henry Black, M.D.

Relationships Between Physical and Mental
Disorders   58
Psychiatric Disorders That Present with Somatic
Complaints   59
Depression and Anxiety   59
Differential Diagnosis   61
Medical Illnesses That Present with Psychiatric
Symptoms   65
Hysteria and Medical Disease   65
Catatonia and Paranoia   66
Other Psychiatric Symptoms   66
Differential Diagnosis   67
Depression and Mood Changes   67
Anxiety   71
Confusion, Psychosis, and Disordered
Thinking   73
Conclusion   78

CHAPTER 6
Evaluation and Management of Confusion—Organic Brain Syndromes   83

Daniel C. Moore, M.D.

Symptoms of Organic Brain Syndrome   85
Diagnosis   87
Differential Diagnosis   89
Measuring Intellectual Function   93
Specific Diagnosis   94
Treatment   95
Management   98
Criteria for Referral   99
Conclusion   99
Appendix: Case History—The Confused
Prisoner   99

CHAPTER 7
Evaluation and Management of Psychosis   103

Malcolm B. Bowers, M.D.

Clinical Evaluation of Psychotic Patients   104
Etiology of Acute Psychosis   105
Psychosis Related to Drug Use   105
Psychosis Associated with General Metabolic
Illness   106
Functional Psychosis   107
Management of Psychosis   107
Referral   107
Chronic Psychosis   109
Summary   109
Appendix: Case History—The Little Green
Men   110

CHAPTER 8
Schizophrenia   113

Hoyle Leigh, M.D.

Etiologic Theories   114
Biological Theories   114
Psychosocial Theories   116
Conclusion   116
Management   116
Biological Dimension   117
Personal Dimension   117
Environmental Dimension   118
Referral   118
Summary   118
Appendix: Case History—Religious Delusion
and Somatic Hallucinations   119

CHAPTER 9
Evaluation and Management of Depression and Affective Disorders   123

Hoyle Leigh, M.D.

Depressive Syndrome   124
Etiologic Theories   125
    Psychological Theories   125
    Biological Theories   125
    Integrated Models   126
Evaluation   126
Management of Depression   129
    Hospitalization Options   129
    Grief and Situational Adjustment Reaction with Depressive Features   129
    Depression Secondary to Medical Disease, Toxins, or Drugs   130
    Depression in Major Affective Disorders   130
Psychotherapy   130
Antidepressant Drug Therapy   131
    Tricyclic Antidepressants   131
    Lithium   133
    Electroconvulsive Therapy   134
Environmental Therapy   134
Referral   134
Summary   135
Appendix: Case History—The Hypertensive Insomniac   135

CHAPTER 10
Evaluation and Management of Suicidal Potential and Attempts   139

Andrew E. Slaby, M.D., Ph.D., M.P.H.

Epidemiology   140
    Suicide and Depression   141
Theories on Suicidal Behavior   141
Evaluation of Suicide Potential   143
    Age   143
    Sex   144
    Marital Status   144
    Race and Ethnic Group   145
    Occupation   146
    Family History   146
    Location   146
    Method   146
    Education   147

    Psychiatric Illness   147
    Religion   147
    Socioeconomic Factors   148
    Season and Day of the Week   148
    Pregnancy, Abortion, Surgery, and Physical Illness   148
    Previous Attempts   149
    Psychological Correlates   149
    Other Correlates of Suicidal Behavior   149
Management   151
Summary   153
Appendix: Case History—The Suicidal Complainer   154

CHAPTER 11
Evaluation and Management of Anxiety   159

Hoyle Leigh, M.D.

Evaluation of Anxiety   161
Differential Diagnosis   161
    Classification of Anxiety Disorders   162
Management of Anxiety   164
    Biological Dimension   164
    Personal Dimension   165
    Environmental Dimension   166
Referral   166
Summary   166
Appendix: Case History—The Choking Type A   167

CHAPTER 12
Psychophysiologic Symptoms—Headache   171

David R. Rubinow, M.D.

Psychosomatic Relationships   172
    Stress, Defense Mechanisms, and the Endocrine System   173
    Personality and Sick Role   173
Evaluation   174
    Current Emotional State   174
    Why Seek Help Now?   175
    How Do Symptoms Affect Ability to Function?   176
    Object of Complaint   176

Personal Meaning of Symptoms   176
Does the Patient Know of Someone Else with
    the Same Symptoms?   176
Nature of the Stress Response   176
Physician's Emotional Response   177
Headache   177
    Pain   177
Headache Classification   178
    Vascular Migraine   179
    Muscle Contraction Headache   181
Conclusion   184
Appendix: Case History—The Persistent
    Headaches   185

CHAPTER 13
Hysteria and Hypochondriasis   189

Craig Van Dyke, M.D.

Historical Note   190
Recognition and Diagnosis   192
    Conversion Disorder   192
    Psychogenic Pain Disorder   194
    Histrionic Personality   195
    Somatization Disorder   196
    Hypochondriasis   198
    Factitious Illness   199
    Malingering   200
    Compensation Neurosis   200
Management and Referral   201
Summary   202
Appendix: Case History—The Aphonic
    Student   203

CHAPTER 14
Problems of Everyday Living   207

Vincenta Leigh, R.N., M.S.N.
Jane S. Sturges, M.S.W.

Diagnosis   208
Recognition   208
    Practical Suggestions for Identifying
        Patients   211
Management   212
Referral   213
Summary   215
Appendix: Case History—Anxiety, Depression,
    and Lower Back Pain   217

CHAPTER 15
Evaluation and Management of Alcoholism   221

Mary E. Swiger, M.D.

Definition and Classification   223
    National Council on Alcoholism
        Classification   223
    International Statistical Classification of
        Diseases   223
    Diagnostic and Statistical Classification of
        Diseases   223
    Jellinek's Phases of Alcoholism   226
Epidemiologic and Social Problems and
Alcoholism   228
Predisposition to Alcoholism   229
    Genetics   229
    Gender and Alcoholism   230
    Personality Factors and Alcoholism   230
Evaluation and Management   231
    Acute Stages of Alcoholism   231
    Alcohol Abstinence Syndromes   232
    Subacute Stage   236
Suicide and Alcoholism   240
Alcoholism and Aggression   240
Treating Alcoholism As An Ongoing
Condition   248
    Psychological Therapies   249
    Self-Help Systems Support   249
    Aversion and Conditioning Therapies   249
    Deterrent Drug Therapy   249
    Lithium Therapy and Alcoholism   250
Chronic Stage of Alcoholism—Neurologic
Deficits   251
    Alcoholic Dementia   251
    Wernicke–Korsakoff Syndrome   251
    Peripheral Neuropathy   252
    Cerebellar Degeneration   252
    Treatment   252
Alcoholism and the Family   252
    Parental Drinking   252
    Spouses of Alcoholics   253
    Adolescent Alcoholism   253
    Fetal Alcohol Syndrome   253
Referral   254
Legal Issues   255
    Tests for Intoxication   255
    Informed Consent   256
    Danger to Self or Others   256
Appendix: Case History—The Postoperative
    Monsters

CHAPTER 16
Drug Dependence   265

Herbert D. Kleber, M.D.

Introduction   266
    Definitions   266
    Theories of Etiology   267
Evaluation   269
    Interview   269
    Physical Examination   270
    Narcotics   271
    Sedatives   273
    Stimulants   275
    Hallucinogens   275
    Phencyclidine   276
    Marijuana   278
    Laboratory Tests   279
    Managing Physical Aspects   280
Management and Referral   280
    Roles of the Family   280
    Role of Drugs in the Family   280
    Referral   281
    Specialized Treatment Approaches   283
    Pain Management in Narcotic-Dependent
        Patients   285
Summary   286
Appendix A: Technique of Narcotic Withdrawal
    through Methadone Substitution   286
Appendix B: Technique of Rapid Withdrawal
    from Opiates with Clonidine Hydrochloride
    289
Appendix C: Technique of Barbiturate–Sedative
    Withdrawal   290
Appendix D: Case History—The Woman with
    Tracks   292

CHAPTER 17
Violence   295

Daniel C. Moore, M.D.

Safety Precautions   297
    Use of Restraints   298
    Medication of Violent Patients   299
Evaluation of Violence   299
Differential Diagnosis of Violence   301
    Intoxicants   301
    Psychiatric Disorders   303
    Organic Conditions   306

Emergency Certification   308
Summary   308

CHAPTER 18
Sexual Dysfunctions   311

Phillip M. Sarrel, M.D.
Lorna J. Sarrel, M.S.W.

Introduction   312
Diagnosis   314
    Classification   315
    Female Desire Phase Dysfunctions   316
    Male Desire Phase Dysfunctions   318
    Excitement Phase Dysfunctions   320
    Orgasmic Phase Dysfunctions   322
    Vaginismus   326
Treatment   327
    Clarifying the Problem   327
    Treating Physical Causes   328
    Impact of Contraception   328
    Sex Education and Counseling   328
    Appropriate Reading   329
    Self-Help   329
    Encouraging Communication   329
    Changing Attitudes   329
    Behavior Modification   330
    Referral   330
Prevention   331
Summary   332
Appendix: Case History—The Frustrated
    Wife   333

PART III
General Considerations in Management   337

CHAPTER 19
Chronically Ill Patients—Hemodialysis, Diabetes, and Cancer   339

Jon Streltzer, M.D.

Psychiatric Issues   340
    Caregiver–Patient Interactions   340
    Behavioral Responses to Chronic Illness   341

Specific Illnesses   346
    Hemodialysis   346
    Diabetes   354
    Cancer   357
Summary   362

CHAPTER 20
Psychotherapy   367

Robert L. Arnstein, M.D.

Evaluation   368
    Indications   368
    Referral Conditions   370
    Discussion with Patients   370
Psychotropic Medication Trial or Immediate
    Referral?   372
Timing of Referral   373
Types of Psychotherapy   374
    Analytically Oriented Psychotherapy   375
    Supportive Therapy   375
    Behavior Modification   375
    Psychoanalysis   375
    Biofeedback   376
    Group Therapies   376
Choosing a Psychotherapist   376
Making a Referral   377
    Patient Reaction   379
    Other Referral Considerations   379
Summary   380

CHAPTER 21
Psychotropic Drugs and Their Interactions   383

Craig Van Dyke, M.D.

Antipsychotic Medication   384
    Phenothiazines   385
    Butyrophenone   385
    Dosage   385
Antidepressant Medication   387
    Tricyclic Antidepressants   388
    Monoamine Oxidase Inhibitors   389
    Lithium Carbonate   390
Antianxiety Medication   391
    Benzodiazepines   392

Sedative Medication   392
    Benzodiazepines   393
    Barbiturates   393
Alternative Sedatives   394

PART IV
Evaluation of Psychiatric Syndromes and Disorders in Children   397

CHAPTER 22
Psychiatric Problems of Childhood   399

Robert D. Hunt, M.D.
Donald J. Cohen, M.D.

Recognizing Psychiatric Problems   401
Evaluation   402
    Talking with Parents   402
    Talking with School Personnel   404
    Interviewing the Child   404
    Family Sessions   405
    Psychological Testing   405
Formulation   406
    Diagnosis   409
Developmental Context   410
    Prenatal   410
    Infancy   411
    The Toddler   412
    Preschoolers   413
    Sexuality   414
Psychiatric Problems in Preschool
    Children   417
    Pandevelopment Delay and Organicity   417
    Childhood Autism   417
    Childhood Schizophrenia   418
    Evaluation and Treatment   418
    Aphasia   419
    Stuttering   421
Middle Childhood   421
    Physical Abuse   422
    Psychosomatic Interaction   423
    Hospitalization   424
    Chronic Illness   425
    Enuresis   426
    Encopresis   428
    School Avoidance   428
    Learning Disabilities   429

Attention Deficit Disorder with
Hyperactivity   430
Tourette Syndrome   434
Appendix: Case History—The Sad, Bad
Boy   436

CHAPTER 23
Psychiatric Problems of Adolescence

Robert O. Hunt, M.D.
Donald J. Cohen, M.D.

Early Adolescence and Puberty   450
Family Changes   451
Midadolescence   451
Social Changes   451
Cognitive Development   452
Self-examination   453
Values   453
Late Adolescence   454
Counseling the Adolescent   455
Sexual Problems of Adolescence   456
Contraception   457
Venereal Disease   458
Abortion   458
Rape   459
Incest   459
Homosexuality   460

Medical Illness in Adolescence   461
The Self-Starving Adolescent: Anorexia
Nervosa   461
Treatment   462
The Substance Abuser   462
Treatment   463
Depression   464
Bipolar Illness   465
The Anxious Adolescent   466
Separation Anxiety   467
Extreme Shyness   467
Emancipation Disorder   468
The Passive Loner: Unsocialized, Unaggressive
Conduct Disorder   468
Academic or Work Inhibition   469
Violence and Aggression   469
Unsocialized Aggressive Conduct
Disorder   469
Socialized Aggressive Conduct Disorder   470
Identity Disorders   470
The Negativistic, Defiant Teenager: Oppositional
Disorder   471
Summary   471
Referral   472
Appendix: Case History—The Youthful
Burglar   473

Index   481

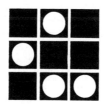

PART I

Comprehensive Evaluation of Patients

CHAPTER 1

Systematic Approach to Comprehensive Care: The Patient Evaluation Grid

Hoyle Leigh, M.D.
Alvan R. Feinstein, M.D.
Morton F. Reiser, M.D.

Patient care cannot be comprehensive unless the physician is aware of those elements essential to comprehensive evaluation. Psychosocial information about the patient is essential not only for diagnosis and treatment of psychiatric syndromes but also for effective care of all medical patients. This chapter presents an operational method of systematically obtaining psychosocial and biological information on all patients.

CASE HISTORY 1–1

A 59-year-old white, married male was admitted to the Intensive Care Unit with the chief complaints of nausea and chest pain radiating to the left arm, which developed suddenly this morning following a hot bath. There was no previous history of chest pain, nausea, or vomiting. The admission record contained the following information: *Personal History*—the patient smokes one pack of cigarettes per day and reports social drinking; *Family History*—father died of myocardial infarction at age 72 years, mother died of pulmonary edema at age 75 years. Two younger siblings are alive and well. (See appendix at the end of this chapter for further discussion and PEG.)

Although the approach to *disease* in modern medicine is orderly and systematized, comprehensive *patient* care often suffers because of lack of a systematic method for integrating psychosocial with biological information about the individual patient. In psychiatry, on the other hand, analogous problems may exist because of lack of a system for organizing biological and psychosocial information within an integrated framework. As a result the psychiatrist frequently is confronted with missing but relevant information in attempting to bridge the gap between medicine and psychiatry. The method of conceptualizing and organizing clinical information about patients described in this chapter takes into account the biological, personal, and environmental spheres in the contexts of the present, recent past, and background of each patient.

PATIENT EVALUATION GRID

The Patient Evaluation Grid (PEG) method organizes information about patients in three dimensions or levels. They are: (a) *biological components* (tissues, organs, chemicals) of the

☐ Part of this chapter is a modified version of an article entitled "The patient evaluation grid: A systematic approach to comprehensive care," which appeared in *General Hospital Psychiatry* 2:3–9, 1980. Reprinted with permission.

patient, including any diseased organ(s); (b) *personal attributes*, including the psychological and behavioral characteristics; and (c) *environmental interaction* between the patient and the outside world, which includes other people. To be useful, these three kinds of information are related meaningfully to the patient's current problem, which may be the chief complaint or other reasons for seeking help.

A format for these relationships is achieved by conceptualizing current, recent, and background *contexts* in time. These three time contexts expand in scope and complexity as one goes from consideration of the present to the remote past. The *current context* refers to the present state of each PEG dimension at the time of the patient's initial evaluation. The *recent context* takes into account changes and events that have occurred lately, including symptoms and experience of illness, as well as events such as bereavement or recent hospitalization. The *background context* embraces a patient's character traits and cultural and environmental influences. The three dimensions of information intersected by the three time contexts produces nine squares in which systematic information about the patient can be organized. This configuration is the Patient Evaluation Grid shown in Table 1–1. (A blank PEG, which may be photocopied, is on p. 10.)

TABLE 1–1
Patient Evaluation Grid (PEG)

DIMENSIONS	CONTEXTS		
	CURRENT (CURRENT STATES)	RECENT (RECENT EVENTS AND CHANGES)	BACKGROUND (CULTURE, TRAITS, CONSTITUTION)
BIOLOGICAL	Physical symptoms Physical examination Vital signs Status of related organs Medications Disease	Recent bodily changes Injuries, operations Disease Drugs	Heredity Early nutrition Constitution Predisposition Early disease
PERSONAL	Chief complaint Mental status Expectations about illness and treatment	Recent illness, occurrence of symptoms Personality change Mood, thinking, behavior Adaptation-defenses	Developmental factors Early experience Personality type Attitude to illness
ENVIRONMENTAL	Immediate physical and interpersonal environment Supportive figure, next of kin Effect of help-seeking	Recent physical and interpersonal environment Life changes Family, work, others Contact with ill persons Contact with doctor or hospital	Early physical environment Cultural and family environment Early relations Cultural sick-role expectation

Demographic data: age, sex, ethnic group, marital status, occupation.

During the patient's initial evaluation, the PEG is helpful as a "review of systems" for the three dimensions that summarize the information contained in the traditional history and physical examination. To elicit relevant information in the outline, the physician should ask questions of the patient and/or family about cultural and family expectations about the sick role, the meaning of illness, personality style, and other pertinent data.

PEG INFORMATION

Column A—Current Context

The first column, which concerns the current state of the patient, has most immediacy for both patient and physician since the information indicates the pressing needs of the patient as well as any constraints in therapeutic plans.

Biological Dimension. The biological dimension square contains data about the patient's physical state, vital signs, and the signs and symptoms of the present illness, including physical symptoms, laboratory data, and so on. This information forms the basis of clinical diagnosis and of many therapeutic decisions.

Personal Dimension. Data concerning chief complaint, appearance, current psychological state, and anxiety level are contained in the personal dimension square. Note that the chief complaint relating to physical state belongs in the biological *and* personal dimensions to the extent that the patient is complaining or suffering because of it. This square also contains answers to questions such as: Is the patient coherent, confused, frightened, or depressed? What does the patient think about the symptoms? Does the patient expect hospitalization, a "shot," an operation and so on?

Personal information is valuable in assessing the patient's experience of illness and motivation for seeking help. Prompt recognition of the patient's immediate need for help consolidates the doctor–patient relationship and increases patient compliance.

Environmental Dimension. Examples of environmental data are revealed in answers to questions such as: Who accompanied the patient? Who lives with the patient? What is his or her marital status? Who suggested seeing a doctor? What are the effects of the patient's illness on his or her family and occupation? Who are the patient's significant others? At a very practical level, a patient's next of kin, family, or friends are important sources of information, support, and occasionally, consent.

Column B—Recent Context

The recent context column reflects *changes and events* in the recent past, including symptoms, illness, disease processes, and their effects on the patient's life and family as well as changes in long-standing patterns such as habits. This column also displays information about possible contributing, complicating, or precipitating factors of illness and help-seeking behavior. All entries here should include the *date* or approximate *duration* of the event.

Biological   Dimension. Recent   physical changes, such as weight gain or loss, injuries, discovery of hypertension or other conditions, recent surgery, prescribed medications, and so on, are examples of data to be included in the biological dimension. Data in this square provide information concerning early signs of current disease, and possible contributing or antecedent factors, as well as physical effects of recent environmental and behavioral changes.

Personal Dimension. The recent context of personal data concerns any personality change, change in habits (for example, increased drinking), mood change (for example, depression), preoccupation with disease (for example, the conviction that one has cancer), and so on.

Mood and life-style changes may contribute to disease (depression may cause self-neglect, malnutrition, and susceptibility to infection) or they may be symptoms of a disease process (for example, personality changes may accompany frontal lobe tumors).

Environmental Dimension. The section that denotes possible environmental stressors causing disease or illness behavior (Mechanic, 1962; Rahe, 1972; McWhinney, 1972), shows data such as change in residence or job, marriage, separation, divorce, bereavement, recent travel, exposure to doctors or hospitals, recent illness in the family, and the like.

Column C—Background Context

Background factors indicate previous illnesses, medical experiences, and predispositions to disease. This column's data set the tone and disclose the attitude of the patient towards illness and help-seeking behavior and may predict response or adaptation to the sick role through personality, constitution, predisposition, and cultural experiences. The items appearing here represent relatively long-standing, stable characteristics of the patient. Since these elements are resistant to change, background information is vital for setting realistic goals for care as well as understanding the patient's needs.

Biological Dimension. The biological dimension of a patient's background highlights constitutional vulnerability, predisposition to disease, genetic endowment, and acquired tendency for specific diseases. A history of hereditary disease, early injuries, diseases, and deformities also belong here, along with answers to questions about past functional disorders under stress, allergies, and so on.

Personal Dimension. Data such as the patient's personality type (Kahana and Bibring, 1964; Leigh and Reiser, 1980), habitual psychological defenses, and coping styles belong in the personal dimension square. Answers to such questions as: Does the patient tend to deny the presence of symptoms and signs? Has there been habitual complaining of minor symptoms? Is there a tendency to be exacting and somewhat obsessive, or to become overly dependent? The patient's habits (alcohol use, smoking), hobbies, ambitions, educational and intelligence level, and so forth, are pertinent here. The way new information is processed and interpreted by the patient and what current illness means to the patient becomes evident in this square, which in turn may suggest how the patient will respond to planned therapeutic approaches.

Environmental Dimension. A patient's cultural background, early physical environment, ethnic origin, and religion are examples of data to be entered into the environmental square. Asking whether there has been early exposure to

illness, doctors, or hospitals may uncover unrealistic or irrational attitudes toward medical care. Questions about cultural sick-role expectations, cultural myths about illness and treatment, or religious qualms about medical procedures may provide clues to the patient's attitudes and expectations about illness.

USING THE PEG

By organizing longitudinal data into current, recent, and background contexts, the immediacy, novelty, or degree of habituation to a particular phenomenon becomes clear. For example, chest pain appearing in the recent context *de novo* has greater immediacy for the patient than chest pain that took place in the past. Although one is dealing with chronologic material along a time continuum, the information is seen from the vantage point of the patient's help-seeking behavior. Thus, the background, recent, and current contexts may affect one another bidirectionally. For example, a presently confused patient may not be able to give a complete or accurate past history.

The need for intervention or treatment and its accomplishment are determined by the combination of background, recent, and current contexts. Although the background context information is usually limited in degree of potential change, certain phenomena are amenable to modification. For example, the patient's fantasies about a medical procedure may be altered if the specific expectations are elicited and discussed realistically.

In formulating a comprehensive patient management plan, the interrelationship among the nine PEG zones is acknowledged. Although illness and disease usually occur together, they do not always have a one-to-one correlation (Feinstein, 1967; Barondess, 1974). Accordingly, suffering may be present despite the absence of disease, as in the case of bereavement, or may be due to the treatment of a disease rather than to the disease itself, for example, when pain is caused by surgical operation for an asymptomatic tumor. Conversely, someone may have myocardial infarction without any symptoms. Another example is provided by a patient who has physical symptoms, but whose real difficulties may arise from problems of living (McWhinney, 1972).

A PEG will show, in each instance, precipitating and contributing factors in one of the squares in the recent or current contexts. Events such as bereavement, unemployment, psychological depression, and so on, may be found in conjunction with biological events leading to a disease, creating a pattern that suggests avenues for psychosocial management. When the cause of the illness and suffering is not clear after studying the person and environmental dimensions, one may need to look further into possible unidentified or incompletely understood diseases (biological dimension).

Management plans for the whole patient that emerge from the PEG process will again be three-dimensional, with priorities determined by the context and gravity of the illness. Priority is a matter of clinical judgment. Even when etiologic treatment in the biological dimension is indicated, its priority may be secondary to intervention in the personal dimension. For example, a patient may need relief from anxiety before hospitalization for etiologic treatment for the disease can take place.

On the other hand, treatment of a grave disease may take priority over possible job loss due to prolonged hospitalization for a patient. For a patient with a congenital heart disease (background context, biological dimension) who comes to the physician with vague symptoms, depressive affect (recent context, personal dimension), and recent loss of a spouse (recent context, environmental dimension), the first priority may be relief from depression, which in turn may relieve the vague symptoms; second, interpersonal support; and third, treatment of the congenital heart disease.

To apply the PEG to patient care planning, the following steps are taken:

1. Underline the factors that appear important in the patient's current suffering, to the pathogenesis of the disease, to the patient's attitude and fantasies concerning the illness, and in his or her perception and attitudes concerning the health care system.

2. Underline major limiting factors in possible intervention and care, such as constitution, personality style, nature and quality of interpersonal relationships (supportive persons), occupation, and so on.

3. On the basis of the PEG and especially the underlined factors, make a three-dimensional plan of problems and diagnoses, and then assign priorities.

Although the PEG is a method of summarizing relevant data, it is not a substitute for traditional medical history, which is an effective tool leading to diagnosis and treatment in the biological dimension. The PEG is intended to complement the medical history by drawing the physician's attention to psychosocial and environmental factors and their interaction with the biological dimension of the patient.

The approach and the kind of information described here are not new. In fact, good clinicians have always collected this type of information (Feinstein, 1967). The PEG is a formal, operational classification scheme for gathering comprehensive information. Its practical aim is to stimulate the clinician to think in terms of the three dimensions and the three contexts in which the patient's illness and disease must be understood (Engel, 1960, 1977; Menninger, 1963; Leigh and Reiser, 1977). It also helps the physician organize and assign priorities to management plans in each of the three dimensions. Moreover, it may allow the physician to assess a patient's readiness to enter into the sick role or to anticipate possible problems arising out of the interaction between the patient and the hospital staff on the basis of the patient's past contact with the hospital (Leigh and Reiser, 1980).

Although constructing a PEG for every patient in day-to-day medical practice does mean additional work, the effort is amply compensated by a reduction in number of problems that may have to be entered into the medical record in the course of treatment and hospitalization. Problems of "management," "noncompliance," and so on, arising from miscommunication and neglect of the personality and coping styles of the patient and the family may be avoided (see Appendix for a case example). In psychiatric practice, the tendency to neglect existing or developing medical disease and/or predispositions will be reduced as well.

The PEG makes the clinician aware of areas where further research is needed in our patients. For example, what combinations of disease, interpersonal tension, and specific environmental changes result in the experience of illness and help-seeking behavior? What combination of diseases and personalities results in silent progression of disease without awareness of symptoms?

SUMMARY

Comprehensive approach to patients requires a systematic method which complements the clinical approach to disease. We describe a method entitled the *Patient Evaluation Grid* (PEG) that takes into account the biological, personal, and environmental dimensions of the patient and the current, recent, and background contexts of illness. This allows the clinician to anticipate problems relating to patient care and to assign priorities in management plans, and further may also facilitate research into the interrelationships among the multiple determinants of illness. This approach may bridge the gap between psychiatry and medicine by providing an integrated conceptual framework for organizing information.

PATIENT EVALUATION GRID (PEG)			
	CONTEXTS		
DIMENSIONS	CURRENT (Current States)	RECENT (Recent Events and Changes)	BACKGROUND (Culture, Traits, Constitution)
BIOLOGICAL			
PERSONAL			
ENVIRONMENTAL			

Demographic data: age, sex, ethnic group, marital status, occupation.

APPENDIX: CASE HISTORY—THE SICK TARZAN

The history is a typical medical history found in many charts. This man seemed to be a relatively typical coronary patient and the diagnosis of massive anterior wall infarction was confirmed upon admission. His hospital course, however, turned out to be quite stormy.

On the first day of admission, he posed no problems. On the second day, he was found sitting up in a chair beside the bed, in spite of the physician's orders to stay in bed. The nurse wrote, "Patient is very arrogant and uncooperative, but easily subdued with firmness." On the fourth day of hospitalization, he refused to have his blood taken for tests and appeared quite agitated. He screamed to the nurses that he wanted to sign out. On the same day, he was found exerting himself trying to lift up his bed. He refused to cooperate in measuring his fluid intake and output and poured urine on the floor. He said, "You think I had a heart attack. All I need is to get my strength back, which I lost from staying in bed too long." He told nurses that he wanted to exercise by lifting up his bed 40 times a day. He was flushed and diaphoretic, and multiple paroxysmal ventricular contractions occurred. A psychiatric consultation was requested.

So far the hospital course of this patient clearly indicated that his medical treatment could not proceed smoothly because of a conflict between his psychological needs and the regimen. A PEG constructed from the data in the admission record is shown in the box.

DIMENSIONS	CONTEXTS		
	CURRENT	RECENT	BACKGROUND
BIOLOGICAL	Nausea Chest pain after hot bath Relevant physical data		
PERSONAL	Nausea		Smokes one pack per day; social drinking
ENVIRONMENTAL	Married		Two siblings alive and well

The information concerning his parents' deaths could not be entered into the PEG because we do not know when they occurred—should they be considered in the recent or background context? When one compares this man's PEG with Table 1–1, it becomes immediately clear that information about a number of items is missing, for example, mental status, expectations about illness, supportive persons, life changes, personality, defense mechanisms, and so forth. When the psychiatric consultant assigned to interview the patient directed attention to such matters, additional information was elicited. The PEG that emerged appears on p. 12.

In fact, a psychiatric consultant may not have been needed had the primary clinician specifically asked about and obtained information such as the underlined items in the PEG. Then it would have been obvious that this man's active, "take charge"

	CONTEXTS		
PATIENT EVALUATION GRID			
DIMENSIONS	**CURRENT** (Current States)	**RECENT** (Recent Events and Changes)	**BACKGROUND** (Culture, Traits, Constitution)

BIOLOGICAL	Chest pain
	Nausea
	Relevant physical data
	  Diagnosis
	  Myocardial
	    infarction (MI)
	  Diazepam,
	    procainamide
	  Meperidine
		Borderline
		  hypertension (7–8
		  yr,
		  no medications)
			History of heart disease
			  and cancer in family

PERSONAL	Nausea
	Pain
	Thinks pain due to
	  indigestion
	Believes exercise
	  essential for survival
		Increased smoking
		  (3–4 yr)
		Increased drinking
		  (3–4 yr)
			No previous
			  hospitalization
			Has a "strong man"
			  image
			Uses denial as a
			  defense
			History of "nerves"—
			  thought he had
			  cancer, decided to
			  deny—"nothing
			  bothers me"
			Active, "take charge"
			  type of personality
			  boastful, dramatic
			Believes in exercise

ENVIRONMENTAL	ICU
	Bed rest
	Nurses
	Wife
	Very attached to wife;
	  will "do anything for
	  her"
	Being in hospital
	  means
	  business associates
	  will be in charge
		Father d. of MI 6 yr ago
		Mother d. of
		  pulmonary edema
		  (3 yr ago)
		Two daughters
		  married within
		  last 4 yr, live in
		  another state
		Sex immediately
		  before MI
		  hospitalization
			Middle class
			Italian, Catholic
			  background
			High school education
			Many relatives died of
			  cancer
			Father was very
			  authoritarian
			  executive of a small
			  company for 25 yr

Demographic data: 59-year-old male, married, two daughters (ages 26 and 24 years), president of a small company.

personality would become problematic when he had to assume a dependent, "sick role" in which bed rest is prescribed. Personality style, being an item in the background context, is not amenable to change, meaning that his sick role expectations probably need to be modified while in the hospital. The clinician would also have seen that the patient's "strong man" self-image may have been threatened by the deaths of his parents and the marriage and moving away of two of his daughters in the recent past. The subsequent increase in anxiety level may, in turn, have resulted in his increased drinking and smoking.

The patient's immediate belief that his pain was due to indigestion and that exercise was essential for survival would also have to be dealt with when the patient was informed of his medical condition and bed rest was prescribed. Noticing that the importance he attributes to exercise is of long duration, the clinician should be aware that some token form of limited exercise (for example, toe-wiggling, ankle-bending) should be permitted so that the patient's anxiety does not rise to an intolerable level.

Possible management plans that take PEG data into account include the following:

1. **Biological dimension:** Bed rest, pain medications, and other necessary therapy.
2. **Personal dimension:** Educate the patient that pain is due to a heart problem, but also recognize that the patient's image of himself as a strong man should not be attacked. In prescribing bed rest, the patient's active personality style and need for exercise need to be recognized. For example, the physician may say, "You had a mild heart attack, which causes pain like indigestion. Since you have always been a strong man, and are in good shape physically, I anticipate that you should recover smoothly. To let your heart recover, though, you should rest in bed for a week or so. This is not going to be easy for you, because you are such a strong and active man—but you should apply your strength of character to ensure that your heart can heal and build up your strength." In long-term management, the clinician may consider teaching relaxation techniques to control his anxiety, which may have accelerated the drinking and smoking behavior and perhaps contributed to hypertension.
3. **Environmental dimension:** The ICU environment with its implicit aura of danger might be very threatening to the patient; thus, a speedy transfer is in order when feasible. In view of his positive relationship with his wife, allowing her to visit as much as possible, and enlisting her help in ensuring compliance with the treatment regimen would be beneficial. The wife could say, "I know it's hard for you to stay in bed and I know that you feel strong enough to be up and around. But, I worry so much because the doctors have not yet told you to get up—so, please stay in bed, for me, until the doctors say you should be getting up." Allowing the patient to have some contact with business associates may alleviate anxiety that he may be losing control of his business.

If the type of comprehensive management plan outlined above had been mobilized, the crisis in the ICU might never have occurred.

RECOMMENDED READINGS

Leigh, H., and Reiser, M.F. 1980. *The patient: Biological, psychological, and social dimensions of medical practice.* New York: Plenum Medical Book Co. This introductory textbook on the integration of biological and psychosocial factors in understanding and managing patients uses the Patient Evaluation Grid as the basic organizing principle. It presents basic concepts in behavioral sciences concerning patienthood, as well as discussions on such phenomena as depression, anxiety, defense mechanisms, pain, and sleep and dreaming. Colorful vignettes illustrating basic concepts are included. This book is highly recommended as a companion volume to any psychiatric textbook.
companion volume to any psychiatric textbook.

Feinstein, A.R. 1967. *Clinical judgment.* Huntington, N.Y.: Robert E. Krieger Publishing Co. This is a classic and scholarly book that deals with the concepts of disease, illness, and general clinical taxonomy as well as with the science and art of medicine.

REFERENCES

Barondness, J.A. 1974. Science in medicine, some negative feedbacks. *Arch Intern. Med.* 134: 152–57.

Engel, G.L. 1960. A unified concept of health and disease. *Perspect. Biol. Med.* 3:459–85.

———. 1977. The need for a new medical model: A challenge to biomedicine. *Science* 196:129–36.

Feinstein, A.R. 1967. *Clinical judgment.* Huntington, N.Y.: Robert E. Krieger Publishing Co.

Kahana, R.J., and Bibring, G.L. 1964. Personality types in medical management. In N. Zinberg, ed., *Psychiatry and medical practice in a general hospital,* pp. 108–23. New York: International Universities Press.

Leigh, H., and Reiser, M.F. 1977. Major trends in psychosomatic medicine: The psychiatrist's evolving role in medicine. *Ann. Intern. Med.* 83: 233–39.

———. 1980. *The patient: Biological, psychological, and social dimensions of medical practice.* New York: Plenum Publishing Co.

McWhinney, J.R. 1972. Beyond diagnosis—An approach to the integration of behavioral science and clinical medicine. *N. Engl. J. Med.* 287: 384–87.

Mechanic, D. 1962. The concept of illness behavior. *J. Chronic Dis.* 15:189–94.

Menninger, K. 1963. *The vital balance.* New York: Viking.

Rahe, R.H. 1972. Subjects' recent life changes and their near future illness susceptibility. *Adv. Psychosom. Med.* 8:2–19.

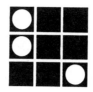

CHAPTER 2

Mental Status Examination: Systematic Observation of the Patient

Hoyle Leigh, M.D.

Systematic observation of the patient's behavior and psychological state constitutes the mental status examination. Mental status is a cross-sectional current state information. Mental status forms an important part of the *current context personal dimension* in the PEG. With data obtained by physical examination and laboratory findings (current context biological dimension), the patient's mental status is an essential part of information leading to, or ruling out, many diagnostic possibilities. Combined with the patient's social, occupational, and family environment the mental status of the patient is a major consideration in developing management plans (see Chapter 3).

A systemic observation of the patient's behavior is as important as physical examination or comprehensive history-taking in understanding the patient as a person. Mental status examination is a method of systematizing this observation. Although mental status may be formally tested according to a format, what is important is not the format but the systematic approach in documenting the patient's behavior.

Mental status consists of the following components: (a) appearance, (b) level of consciousness, (c) speech and movement, (d) cognitive processes (orientation, attention, comprehension, memory, perception, logical thoughts, abstraction, judgment), and (e) affect. Generally, a thorough history-taking and physical examination will provide enough data for the clinician to document a fairly thorough mental status, without formally testing it. For example, being able to answer questions concerning history of present illness accurately and lucidly indicates good levels of consciousness, orientation, and memory. In discussing possible diagnostic tests and therapeutic plans, the physician obtains a reliable impression of the patient's comprehension, logical thinking, and judgment. By observing the patient's facial expression and speech, the clinician forms an idea of the patient's affect (feeling tone) and determines whether it is stable or labile.

APPEARANCE

Appearance is an excellent indicator of the sum total of a patient's mental status. Disheveled, sloppy appearance may indicate self-neglect due to depression, psychosis, or dementia. Disorganized behavior with flushed facies and alcohol on the breath is practically diagnostic of alcohol intoxication. Bizarre gestures, dress, and behavior often reflect psychosis or dementia.

LEVEL OF CONSCIOUSNESS

Level of consciousness (arousal) denotes awareness of the self and environment. Arousal level is measured on a continuum from *hyperalert* to *clouded* to *confusional*, and on through *delirious, stuporous* states to *coma*. The level of arousal probably reflects the activity of the reticular activating system.

SPEECH AND MOVEMENT

Speech and movement should be observed closely since they represent the communicative facilities of the patient. In evaluating speech and movement, the physician should first determine if the apparatuses concerned are in good working order in conjunction with physical examination. Pareses of certain muscles may produce dysarthria and unusual expressions or gestures.

Patterns, speed, and content of speech should be considered carefully. Pressured, rapid speech is characteristic of mania and hypomania while slow, "retarded" speech is indicative of depression or stupor. Bizarre or incomprehensible speech may signal a psychosis, but may also occur in aphasia. Explosive speech, often filled with foul language, accompanied by multiple tics and compulsive behaviors are diagnostic of Tourette syndrome (see Chapter 22). Explosive speech in the absence of associated movements and gesturing may indicate Parkinsonism in some patients.

Content of speech, or what the patient says, of course, is usually the most important part of the communication process. Content may alert the physician to the most pressing need for intervention (for example, suffering), and also may suggest possible psychopathology (delusions, bizarre ideas, and so on). The physician should attempt to understand the underlying *meaning* of the patient's communication whenever the overt part of the communication seems to be somewhat unusual or emotionally charged. For example, the patient who asks, "Is there a cure for congenital syphilis?" may be motivated by much more than simple intellectual curiosity.

COGNITIVE PROCESSES

Testing for *cognitive processes* is crucial in evaluating organic brain syndromes. The nine cognitive processes are: orientation, memory, attention, concentration, comprehension, abstraction, judgment, perception, and content of thought. The status of these processes is determined by various factors including native intelligence, educational level, functional level and training, and the effects of illness. When informal observation in the course of history-taking and physical examination warrants suspicion concerning possible abnormalities, then formal testing may be in order. The following is a simplified testing method; for comprehensive documentation, neuropsychological testing may be in order.

Orientation

Orientation refers to the person's consciousness of his or her current position in relation to time, place, person (self and others), and situation. Impairment of orientation results in confusion. When there is some evidence that the patient is confused or bewildered, asking specific questions will reveal disturbed orientation:

1. What day is today?

2. What is the month and year?

3. What is the name of this place?

4. In what city and state are we?

5. What is your full name?

Impairment of orientation is common in organic brain syndromes (Chapter 6). Typically orientation problems occur in this order: time, place, and finally, person. Disorientation to time is relatively frequent among hospital patients even without severe organic brain syndrome. Only in severe dementia is orientation to self impaired.

Memory, Attention, Concentration, and Comprehension

Formal testing for **recent memory** may be accomplished by asking questions such as: Who is the president of the United States now? Who was president before him? Can you name four presidents before him? (Ability to name four or five is normal.) When did you come into the hospital? **Remote memory** may be tested by asking Where were you born? and What is your birth date? **Immediate memory** may be tested by requesting the patient to repeat immediately certain words or numbers. In organic brain syndrome, recent memory is especially likely to be impaired. Immediate memory may be impaired in delirious states; remote memory may be impaired in certain dissociative and amnestic states.

Attention and concentration as well as memory and comprehension may be assessed by certain tests of calculation, such as "serial sevens" and simple additions and multiplications. In serial sevens, the patient is asked to subtract 7 from 100 and keep on subtracting sevens from the resulting number. If serial sevens are too difficult, serial threes or twos may be used. Other calculations may be requested, such as: $15 + 16$, 4×3, and so on (note that simple multiplications, such as 4×5, are more a test of remote memory than of concentration). By asking the patient to repeat a series of random digits in the same order (such as 3–7–9–7–2) or to repeat certain numbers in reverse order ("If I say, 1–2–3, say 3–2–1"), the physician may measure short-term memory and concentration. Most patients without brain dysfunction can repeat at least six digits forward and four digits backwards (digit span). Difficulty with concentration, attention, and comprehension may be exhibited by patients with major affective disorders (depression and mania), psychoses, or severe anxiety.

Abstraction

Abstraction is a part of higher intellectual function susceptible to deterioration by brain dysfunction, as with recent memory. Abstraction may also be impaired in psychotic states, especially in schizophrenia. Low intelligence level and lack of education may also result in low levels of abstract thinking. The ability to do abstract thinking may be measured by use of similarities and proverbs. The patient is asked to state the similarities of such pairs of objects as table and chair (furniture), dog and cat (animals), or apple and banana (fruits). A patient's grasp of the abstract meaning of proverbs may be tested by asking, "If someone said to another person, 'you know, Rome was not built in a day', what is he trying to tell him?" or "What does it mean to be told not to cry over spilt milk?" or "Why is it said that people who live in glass houses should not throw stones?" In using proverbs, the clinician should be aware that patients from other cultural backgrounds may have difficulty in understanding so-called standard proverbs. Idiosyncratic, bizarre, and paranoid responses to questions about similarities and meanings of proverbs may indicate the presence of a psychosis, or they may reflect creativity in some cases.

Judgment

Good *judgment* entails the ability to act appropriately in social and emergency situations. Good judgment requires logical thinking. Asking "If you were in a crowded theater, and happened to see smoke and flames on the ceiling, what should you do?" or "What would you do if you found an envelope with a stamp and address lying on the street?" can provide an assessment of this ability. Judgment may be impaired in

organic brain syndromes, personality disorders, psychoses, or mental retardation. In psychoses and personality disorders, answers may range from bizarre to antisocial.

Perceptions

The presence of *illusions* and *hallucinations* is best shown by observing the patient's behavior (for example, does he or she seem to be conversing with a nonexistent person or responding to voices?) and then, by asking direct questions such as: Have you ever had the experience of seeing things or hearing voices that other people couldn't see or hear? Have you had any experience of things changing shape or becoming distorted?

Content of Thought

Abnormal *contents of thought* include delusions (convictions not based on reality), which may be grandiose, persecutory, or bizarre. Delusions may be indicative of various psychoses (schizophrenia, mania, drug-induced states, psychosis due to organic brain syndrome, and so on). On occasion, a misunderstanding about medical terminology or procedure may give rise to suspiciousness, delusions, and general breakdown in doctor-patient relationship.

AFFECT AND MOOD

Affect refers to the patient's feeling, and is synonymous with emotion (although emotion is sometimes used to denote the physiologic aspects of affect). *Mood* is the prevailing and relatively enduring affective tone.

Observation of the patient will usually reveal the formal aspects of affect, that is, whether it is labile or stable, appropriate or inappropriate to the occasion or content of thought. For example, if the patient smiles broadly while narrating how she discovered a lump in her breast, her affect may be considered inappropriate. The clinician can also surmise the dominant affect by observation of the content of speech and facial expression (euphoric, sad, angry). Direct questioning, however, is often necessary, especially if the patient is not an emotionally expressive person. Do you feel anxious? or It must be very upsetting to you, or Do you sometimes feel downhearted and blue? are some comments and questions that might elicit patient's affect. Persistent feelings of anxiety, sadness, anger, or elation may be indicative of a number of psychiatric disorders discussed in other chapters.

CONCLUSION

Just as the physical examination is essential in determining the state of the patient's biologic dimension, so is the mental status examination in evaluating the patient's personal or psychological dimension, which in turn reflects the status of the central nervous system and the personality system.

Mental status usually can be analyzed on the basis of ordinary history-taking and physical examination. In case abnormality is suspected, a formal mental status examination may be performed. It is essential that the physician *observe* the patient's behavior systematically and thoroughly report any findings. The PEG is useful in this documentation.

RECOMMENDED READINGS

Leigh, H., and Reiser, M.F. 1980. The Current Context of Help-Seeking Behavior in *The patient: Biological, psychological, and social dimensions of medical practice,* Ch. 10. New York: Plenum Medical Book Co. This chapter includes a somewhat more extensive discussion of the mental status and its relationship with other current context factors.

CHAPTER 3

Evaluation of the Family in General Medical Care

Stephen Fleck, M.D.

The family is a dynamic component in the environmental dimension of the patient (see Chapter 1); it exerts a pervasive influence in current, recent, and background contexts. Family relationships are important factors in the patient's personality development, and changes in family relationships in the recent past (including marriage, divorce, bereavement) may contribute to current illness. Evaluation of the family is crucial in understanding the patient's present and future support systems. This chapter examines in detail the functions of the family, and its role in health and illness. It is of note that this chapter is written by Dr. Stephen Fleck, one of the pioneers in family research in schizophrenia. (See Chapter 8 for further discussion of schizophrenia).

In addressing the examination and evaluation of families, this chapter emphasizes normative and adaptive family functions and processes. The family as a human institution is presented through a general systems approach, employing five variables that may be studied separately despite their interdependence.

The role of the family in illness and the impact of illnesses on families is discussed, but specific *family* dysfunctions related to certain illnesses will not be considered here because they are the concern of specialists other than the primary care physician or team. Prevention and health education are stressed because they are not only part of primary health care, but also are important family responsibilities. So is patient care, which more often takes place in the home than in the hospital, a fact often overlooked in medical education (Richardson, 1948; Rakel and Conn, 1978).

No evaluation of patients is comprehensive without evaluation of their immediate contexts, in particular the significant other persons in their lives. As Richardson (1948) stated it over 30 years ago, "to treat a patient as if he had no family is to treat the liver as if there was no patient." Unfortunately scientific medicine has, at times, treated organs as if there were no patient, a reductionistic caricature of scientific medicine, sometimes paradoxically referred to as "the medical model" (Dubos, 1965; Engel, 1977). Scientific attention to the patient as a person and to patients' families, however, has become possible only in recent decades, although general practitioners have considered themselves "family physicians" because they likely treated all members of a family and often brought, and still bring, an empirical and intuitive awareness of family processes to their work (Osler, 1932; Engel, 1962; Aldrich, 1975).

Primary care, and particularly the preventive efforts in primary care, cannot be accomplished without attention to the context in which patients live and interact with others; indeed, any form of treatment requires appreciation of this context, whether it is a ward environment in a hospital, a nursing home, the patient's own home, or other domicile. Both the clinical approach to and the evaluation of the interpersonal matrix in which a patient lives imply questions about the role of environment in the pathogenesis of the illness and its treatment. Usually this environment is the family—either family of origin, or family of procreation, or both in a three-generational household. In medical practice, therefore, an understanding of the family as the shaping system of people's personalities, and as the basic social institution in any society is essential. The family can be defined minimally as a two-generational system in which people are related either biologically or through legal sanction (marriage or adoption). However, other persons living in the same household may function as family members depending on the relationships among them and especially for our consideration, their relationships to the patient.

The role of family members in response to an illness in their midst must be considered in three different respects. One is the possible causal contribution of the family to the illness on either a biological or a psychosocial level, or both. The second question concerns the family's willingness and ability to assume the care and treatment the patient needs. The answer requires an estimation of the family's tangible and psychosocial resources to accommodate the patient and his or her needs. Finally, one must recognize the impact of the sick person, the illness, and the treatment needs upon the family system. Thus, primary care is based on knowledge of the clinical condition per se, on knowledge of the patient as a person, and on knowledge of that person's family and an appreciation of the dynamic interactions among all these systems. It is useful to employ a general systems approach in the clinical assessment of families' strengths, needs, and deficiencies in establishing indications for supportive and therapeutic measures (Jackson, 1966; Meissner, 1966; Fleck, 1975; Minuchin et al., 1978).

The general systems approach involves five system functions and is two-dimensional in that it provides a longitudinal or historic dimension and a horizontal or cross-sectional examination for data collection and evaluation. The five sectors to be considered in assessing family functioning, coping capacity, or deficiencies are: (a) leadership or governance; (b) boundary management; (c) affectivity; (d) communication; and (e) the evolutionary task and goal performance. Specific and tangible family task performance is also examined, especially in connection with caring for a diseased member.

These five system functions are evaluated in terms of competence or deficiency through reviewing the family history and in family interviews. Quantitative system assessment of the family is also feasible, but is more important in instances of psychiatric illnesses and family treatment indications than in primary care practice. It is important, however, that in addition to their experience and skill as consultants and teachers in the primary care setting, psychiatrists also be versed in the assessment of families and indications for family treatment, and be able to undertake the latter if indicated. In general, this chapter is predicated on a primary care team model where the psychiatrist and other mental health care clinicians are integral members of the primary care staff (Luban-Piozza, 1972; Coleman, 1975; GAP 105, 1980).

FAMILY SYSTEMS

The family is a human group consisting minimally of one parent and a child, that is, a two-generational system.* The five variables used to evaluate the family system are discussed in the following sections; more detailed informa-

---

* Childless couples may call themselves "a family," but by our definition they are not because the marital system is not the same as a family system. Childless couples are part of family systems—those of their families of origin and of collaterals' families in extended family structures.

tion is available in the references listed at the end of the chapter.

Leadership

Leadership, normally and modally, especially in the nuclear, two-generational family is provided by the parents, but if leadership appears to reside outside this system, such outsiders ought to be included in the family analysis. This may involve separate contacts with a grandparent, collateral relative, or significant other, or he or she may be included in family unit interviews, or both. However, leadership, and therefore power, is usually vested in the parents; their effectiveness depends upon their personalities *and* their dual relationship conceived as the parental coalition. This coalition, also a subsystem of the family, ought to be earmarked by mutual respect, emotional closeness, rapport, and the ability to communicate with and about each other as well as about family issues. If one of a couple is the identified patient, the other parent's or spouse's capacity for caring and nursing is of major consequence. In families with children who have not yet reached adulthood, the parents' leadership role is essential, whether they are well or sick. Death of a parent or other reasons for one-parent families usually constitute a handicap in leadership functions. Children remain dependent on being provided some imagery from and about both parents. Even if the absent parent, whether deceased or separated, is represented through the live parent, the latter's attitude toward the absent parent is important.

In primary care practice, therefore, one-parent families should be considered families at risk for emotional disturbance and stress-related illnesses. Also to be considered at risk are children in reconstituted families; that is, where a divorced parent has remarried and one or both of them become stepparents.

Boundaries

Family *boundaries* are difficult to define and are best thought of as selectively permeable structures. Three types of boundaries must be considered. First, parents must inculcate ego boundaries in children, fostering their sense of self; the process involves age-appropriate forms of independence and self-direction (Winnicott, 1965; Fleck, 1972). Next, the parental coalition also must effect a generation boundary dividing the family into a leader-teacher-provider group, and a follower-learner generation. This boundary is rigid with regard to sexual activity in the family, constituting the incest taboo. The most tangible boundary is the family-community interface. For very young children or infants it is rather impermeable, but eventually it becomes increasingly flexible. Yet the boundary should not become so loose that children seek parental caring and guidance at random outside the home because of insufficient boundary control by their parents. Management of this boundary can be appraised in terms of children's duration of absences and distances allowed.

Affectivity

Affectivity, or the feeling, tone and intimacy level in the family, can best be assessed by meeting with the family as a group. It is obviously important that the family atmosphere is one of caring for each other even in the presence of conflicts or difficulties, and that a sick member in particular feels a welcome part of the family despite his or her handicap. Affectivity is also involved in how power is wielded in the family; the source of power should rest with the parents and in the parental coalition rather than in any other dyad, a situation that signals family malfunction. Decision-making and discipline methods are good indicators of how power is managed, for example, whether punishment is meted out commensurate with a child's misbehavior, age, and underlying needs, or instead matches the anger and hostility experienced by a parent for whatever reasons. In the modern rather isolated nuclear family, affects constitute the major cohesive force in the system in contrast to earlier times when survival

needs and ritualistic constraints might have been overriding bonds. Unwanted or scapegoated children fail to thrive and the family itself also suffers from their disturbed and disturbing behavior. Child abuse is the extreme result of distorted family affectivity and power misuse (Gil, 1971; Ackerman, 1977). Parent-child incest is one form of child abuse and like all child abuse, a reportable condition in most states.

Communication

Communication is evaluated in family unit meetings, although certain handicaps, such as a member suffering aphasia, may affect communication. Clarity, mutual responsivity, whether or not members speak for themselves or for others, congruence of verbal and nonverbal behavior, evidence of appropriate abstraction and syntax, and whether or not speakers come to closure in what they say, are major factors in assessing communication.

Evolutionary Family Tasks

Performance of *evolutionary family tasks* are of substantial import with regard to clinical management. Unlike other human systems, the family has a threefold mission no matter what its composition or surrounding culture. As a system the family must tend to its own survival tasks; moreover, the family must adapt to the changing needs and capacities of all members because of inevitable growing and aging processes; lastly, it should provide society with adults who can function and participate in that society's traditions and values. Knowledge and comprehension of the family life cycle and the biopsychosocial givens under which the system operates are prerequisites for the examination and assessment of family function and dysfunction (Fleck, 1980).

From Dyad to Triad. Family functions begin with the establishment of a marital and eventually parental coalition already described. If children are present or are expected, it is important to determine whether a decision to reproduce was made by the couple, whether or not pregnancy and parenthood are or were welcome, planned or unplanned. The dyad then becomes a triad, and each child lives to some extent in his or her particular triangular subsystem. The triangle is the basic family structure and like all triangular relationships tends to be unstable, especially because there are two leaders in contrast to most human systems where leadership is vested in one person. Effecting a workable triangle or triangles therefore depends, as already emphasized, on the nature of the marital and interparental bond. Pregnancy is not only a time for child-birth preparation but also an opportunity to educate about parental responsibilities and to anticipate possible stresses in early parenthood (Fleck, 1974).

Nurturance and Separation. The family's next life-cycle task is the stage of nurturance, which is the overriding need of infants. Weaning of the beginning toddler and the inculcation of body mastery, including sphincter control and locomotion, are part of this stage. These are the first and therefore prototypical separation experiences in the young child's subsequent psychosocial separation mastery in the process of individuation. Clinicians must be aware that the mother may experience the toddler stage as a loss, so that even this earliest separation can be a two-way crisis (Winnicott, 1965; Goldberg, 1977).

Socialization. The family with toddlers moves to the phase of teaching language and relationships, crucial tasks in the humanization of the child. The goal at this stage is that the child find a comfortable relationship with both parents and begin to develop peer relationships, especially after entering school. Although children's communication will remain concrete as defined by Piaget until puberty, the child's grasp of basic syntax and the idea that communication serves to express oneself as well as evoke re-

sponses from and reactions in others is learned within the family context (Lidz, 1963; Piaget, 1968).

Integration. Following the socialization phase the family ideally enters a period of harmony and togetherness—a period essential for establishing a sense of family cohesiveness and rapport. The sense of family-belonging cemented during this phase can be likened to the establishment of object constancy in the toddler—the ability to maintain a relationship and trust therein even when the "object" is not perceivable through one's sense organs. At this stage the family can move as a unit and master crises as an integrated group, although children and parents also have their own relationships outside the home—at work, in school and on the playground. Role and task assignments within the system can be shared and interchanged to some degree, especially during crisis periods such as illness. Thus, primary care personnel can get a good impression of a family's coping capacity, their emotional state, and ability to give incident to an illness, whether the patient is treated at home or elsewhere. During this stage children can also assume responsibilities for others in the family at least temporarily, and sharing and caring can be quite reciprocal.

Independence. Children's puberty ushers in adolescence; the family with teenagers is not a peaceful unit, and ought not to be in the service of youngsters' experimentation with independence. That experimentation often begins with hostile, negativistic stances toward parental values and direction. All the same, this disharmony is essential to adolescents' individuation and maturation, at least in Western societies. The stage provides an opportunity for primary care professionals to render preventive services in family counseling and also to provide alternative adult models for adolescents eager to differentiate themselves as persons from their parents. The period of youngsters' emotional emancipation from the family of origin, begins the last stage of the family life cycle as such maturing young adults eventually can seek their own mates and begin new families.

FAMILIES AND AGING

The life cycle of the family is never closed entirely. As parents become grandparents, their renewed status as a dyad may constitute a crisis for them with attendant symptoms, if not illness. If their relationship and coalition has not grown and changed since early marriage, and if parental functions have preempted their life together, they may find "the empty nest" a very unrewarding and frustrating life stage. Others may welcome living as a couple again and even experience a second honeymoon. Yet marital counseling or therapy may be needed at this stage and should be available through a comprehensive primary care agency. In addition, personal and social crises may emerge in late-middle life—for example, women may wish to resume work or professional lives only to find that their earlier skills are no longer needed or that middle-aged job-seekers are not welcome. Pain and grief of rejection may result in symptoms of actual illness. Men and women may realize that they have achieved what they will in the productive world or may even find themselves unemployed, either of which can result in depression and/or physical complaints. Retirement may entail the same risks (Mechanic, 1966; Rahe et al., 1967; Kasl et al., 1975; Jacobs, 1979).

Eventually the couple must prepare for aging and death, both chief issues in clinical practice and for families, especially if infirmities necessitate support from children or from other sources. In this connection one can recognize that the attitudes of middle-aged persons toward their aging parents and their readiness for possible role reversals if aging parents become dependent hinge primarily on the feelings over time between the two generations during ear-

lier family life stages. Unresolved conflicts and ambivalence may lead to neglect of and distance from aging parents, or guilt may result in over-solicitous, excessive care for the parents. Such issues may require clinicians' attention and intervention (Nat. Acad. Med., 1978; Weisman and Brettell, 1978).

FAMILIES AND ILLNESS

An essentially normative process of the family system with some indications for preventive intervention or opportunities was presented in the preceding sections; next, the role of the family in the etiology and the course of illness is considered. Etiologic familial factors are manifold and range from the cellular level to the interactional plane. The foregoing overview of the family as a system addresses primarily the psychosocial aspects of intergenerational transmission. It should be emphasized that transmission of attitudes, behaviors, coping patterns, and pathology extends over more than two generations. Every person has a familial heritage that resides not only in the genes, but also in one's personality, attitudes, ambitions, and goals (Winnicott, 1965; Lidz, 1976).

Psychosomatic Conditions

Aside from hereditary conditions, causative familial contributions to illness may be most dominant in so-called psychosomatic illnesses. The search for psychogenic causes of disease has been going on for several decades and was first undertaken with great optimism. More sophisticated concepts of the complex coaction of pathogenic forces was first established in a paradigm by Mirsky (1958), Reiser (1957), and others. Other research focused on social stress and its connection with illness, symptoms, and disease incidence (Hinkle, 1968; Halliday, 1948; Morris, 1964). More recently, Holmes and Rahe (1967), Cobb (1973), Kasl et al. (1975), and Mechanic (1966) among others have employed epidemiologic methods to explore connections between life stresses and illness. Although the majority of the most stressful life events are familial in nature, relatively little objective research with regard to the familial role as such in the genesis of disease has been reported, despite the fact that in 1940 Hilde Bruch pointed to the "family frame" of obese children as being etiologically relevant to their condition (Bruch, 1973). Jackson (1966) explored familial conditions connected with ulcerative colitis, and recently Minuchin and his colleagues (1978) painstakingly demonstrated the familial influences on metabolic systems and the control of diabetes in children and young people. These and other studies are not detailed here, but it can be stated that in addition to the concept of psychosomatic and somatopsychic factors in illness, we must add familio-psychosomatic and somatopsycho-familial dimensions in pathologic developments. Osler's (1932) dictum that it is more important to know what kind of patient has the disease than what kind of disease the patient has, might be amended to say: it is as important to know *what kind of family is to cope with the disease* as it is to know with what kind of illness the family must cope. However, the main point is to avoid conceptualizing data demonstrating connections of this type in linear cause-and-effect fashion. We are dealing with complex interrelated mechanisms and conditions—systems and subsystems—which affect one another in circular or cybernetic fashion (Engel, 1977; Leigh and Reiser, 1977; Weiner, 1978).

Family Pathology

Malfunctioning families can contribute significantly to the development of illness, and families influence the course and outcome of disease. Babies who fail to thrive are often found to have mothers—often single mothers—whose nursing and nurturance capacities need to be developed or who are significantly disturbed persons themselves. Conditions like asthma or colic sometimes may be related to maternal anxiety or insecurity (Freedman and

Thornton, 1979; Goldberg, 1977). In general, pediatricians, primary care physicians, and visiting nurses are aware of and used to dealing constructively with the many uncertainties of young parents with regard to child care (Engel, 1962; Beloff et al., 1970; Dykman et al., 1970). Ignorance or uncertainties can lead to unwholesome behavior and practices and to illness, or even to neglect. Child abuse, as already mentioned, is a manifestation of family pathology and should be treated as such (Gil, 1971).

As the family gets older other forms of family dysfunction or deficiencies may present themselves in the form of disturbance or illness in one member. The role of family system deficiencies on severe psychosomatic or psychiatric illnesses such as anorexia nervosa, psychoses, or delinquent behavior is listed in Table 3–1. These disorders are not discussed here in detail since familial disturbances as well as profound, rather fixed individual psychopathology, require care and treatment by specialists (Meissner, 1966; Grolnick, 1972; Minuchin et al., 1978).

Other degrees of family dysfunction come to the attention of primary care staffs when schools or other agencies make referrals. The symptoms of a family member may reflect family deficiencies. This is particularly common in children having problems with school adjustment (for example, a hyperactive child). Both school officials and primary care personnel should be alert to the possibility that maladjustment or misbehavior in school may be the expression of conflicts and disturbance at home in addition to, or because of, minimal brain dysfunctions in a child. For instance, so-called school phobias and their attending truancy must always be considered a joint problem for the child and at least one parent or parent-figure in the context of shared anxiety about separation. If not treated as a family problem, symptoms may indeed subside under external pressure of the authorities, but incomplete separation mastery, submerged for a number of years, probably will reappear as a problem in adolescence and handicap the

TABLE 3–1
Some family system deficiencies in disease

	NEUROSES	CHRONIC MEDICAL DISEASE	PSYCHOPHYSIOLOGIC DISORDERS	AFFECTIVE DISORDERS	PSYCHOPATHY	SCHIZOPHRENIA
CELLULAR	—	Possible inheritance, e.g., diabetes	Specific organ or system vulnerability	Undefined inheritance factor	Possible pre- or parianatal embarrassment	Undefined inheritance factor
PSYCHOBIOLOGICAL ORGANIZATION	Nurturance weaning may be disturbed	Undernurturance in nonthriving infants	Overemphasis on particular body-function and/or deficient autonomic nervous system stabilization	Rigid emphasis on developmental achievement	Perfunctory nurturance and affectivity	Nurturance/weaning disturbed
PERSONALITY DEVELOPMENTS	Selective repression of conflicts; identification with neurotic parent	"A" personality in coronary disease using treatment in interpersonal issues	Bodily expression of stress and conflict; body image disturbances	Intolerance for conscious hostility and sadness. Inculcation of guilt and shame	Overemphasis on appearance; disregard for feelings of self and others	Handicapped by inadequate parental models and aberrant communication
FAMILY ORGANIZATION	Clinically nonsignificant pathology	May be disturbed by illness	Illness may lead to or be function of special mother-child dyad	Patients with unipolar disease often the "stoic" one	Inconsistent discipline; lack of family unity sense	All parameters disturbed or deficient
SOCIALIZATION	Phobias, sexual inhibitions	May be handicapped, e.g., sensory defects, diets, joint or neurologic diseases	Disease may interfere	—	Loose family community boundary. Manipulative communication modes	Emancipation handicapped by previous deficiencies, especially communication and thought disorders

child's full emancipation from the family (Dykman et al., 1970; Fleck, 1975).

Delinquent children likewise bespeak family pathology; referral for family and individual treatment is usually indicated, but may in itself require considerable skill and tact by the primary care staff. Families with such problems tend to understate or deny the gravity of the situation and may not accept treatment recommendations unless exterior pressure such as probation is exerted.

In general, referrals to specialists, psychiatrists in particular, are facilitated if the psychiatrist is already part of the primary care team, or at least in regular contact as a consultant and therapist with the primary care physician or staff (Coleman et al., 1976; Borus, 1976; GAP, 1980).

Family Response to Illness. The impact of a member's illness on the family system is always a vital factor. In particular, primary care personnel need to determine whether chronic patient care in the family home is adequate and whether the family resources are overly taxed by the burden. Caring for a chronically ill spouse may inhibit the other spouse's career. A sick family member may preempt energies essential for the normative development and even existence of the rest of the family. Sickness may interfere with experiences such as family excursions or may tie an adolescent to the home in a way that hinders his or her progressive emancipation from the family.

Thus, once illness has occurred, no matter what its origin, the role of the family, especially in the primary care context, is paramount. Nursing and even nurturance in instances of acute illness are important, but in a stable family this does not often cause significant difficulties, despite temporary interference with the family's comfort and income. If there are indications or hope that the problem is time-limited, most families will rally to provide the additional care necessary and to make necessary role adjustments, and some relatively disturbed families

may even find such a crisis an impetus to function more adequately. This crisis phenomenon, however, may cause difficulties in chronic illness because the rallying impulse may become a homeostabilizing element in the life and equilibrium of a disturbed family. Prolongation of a disability, therefore, may be due to the family's or some family member's need to have the sick person in their midst. The same or similar issues can operate in intermittent or chronic illnesses, such as diabetes, where family problems can be diverted or sidestepped by decompensation of the diabetic member, or by similar recrudescence in other illnesses such as arthritis or cardiac disease (Minuchin et al., 1978). For instance, a spouse who must become the sole wage-earner in the family because of chronic disability of the other spouse, and finds this role too onerous, may decide that the sick spouse needs more and more nursing care, thereby making the patient more of an invalid than he or she might be with encouragement and expectation of self-care. In such a family one may also find that medication that requires a family member's help to administer may be forgotten or that there was "no time" to prepare the prescribed diet.

The family's role is even more critical if the chronic illness is a psychiatric one, because such patients are particularly sensitive and vulnerable to events or changes in their environments. Often in such instances medication supervision is also required, and can become a source of conflict and stress for all concerned. Increasingly, chronic psychiatric patients are expected to live in the community, so that their medication and other management will also become increasingly the responsibility of primary care physicians or teams and the families involved (Brown and Wing, 1972; Borus, 1976; Rakel and Conn, 1978).

If the patient is a spouse, the issue of reproduction must be considered. In serious illness, conception should probably be prevented unless the psychiatrist and primary care physician can determine that the patient is able to undertake new parenthood (Grunebaum et al., 1971). If the patient is already a parent the effect of his or her patienthood on the family must be monitored, and children's growth and progress should be observed, perhaps a few times a year during home visits and through informal conversations with the family as a unit. Visiting nurses are ideally prepared for this kind of scrutiny. When the patient is a child, the impact of illness may be deleterious for the family as a whole, in which case a specialist should be consulted and involved in planning and treatment.

If chronic patients receive disability payments, this may form a significant part of the family income. Sometimes motivation towards continued rehabilitation and improvement is compromised, because disability payments may be a more reliable source of income than the wages of a rehabilitating patient.

Aging and Death. Geriatric medicine is a constant aspect of primary care. Elderly people have special problems and more illness than any other age group, yet most of their ailments are chronic and do not require hospitalization and technically sophisticated care which, if needed, is provided for through Medicare (Part A). Outpatient care, nursing home care, and rehabilitative or prosthetic measures, which constitute the bulk of care needs of the aging population, are often not covered adequately by public or private insurance systems (President's Commission, 1978). Financial provisions for nonhospital care vary from state to state, and even where the federal government has assumed some responsibility through Medicare (Part B) or categorical stipends, for conditions such as blindness, bureaucratic encumbrances are obstacles for the handicapped and frustrate their families (Nat. Acad. Med., 1978). Lack of public transportation often makes health care for the elderly difficult and may also burden their families. Primary care therefore must include administrative assistance

for such patients so that they and their families can secure available reimbursements without which the family may not be able to provide the care for an aging and infirm member. Families that assume the care of elderly parents and grandparents may need not only support from visiting nurses and home visits by the primary physician if transporting the patient is difficult, but also require and deserve the opportunity for a respite from such care. Here volunteers can help if a patient is in need of constant attendance or if the family plans a vacation. In such instances a limited stay in a nursing home, or for certain terminal illnesses in a hospice, may be beneficial to all concerned (Lack, 1979; Jacobs, 1979).

Terminal illness in any family member is a crisis for the whole family, whether the patient is cared for at home or in a nursing home or hospice. Primary care staffs should be familiar with processes of anticipatory mourning, grief reactions, predictable phases of denial, unrealistic hopes and plans, anger, frustration, and gradual adaptation following either the announcement of a hopeless prognosis or sudden death. Mourning and mutual support and consolation are family tasks, but they often need professional support and guidance in this crisis especially if it is the first death in the family (Weisman, 1972).

FAMILY HEALTH

Primary health care should be not only reactive to illness, but also preventive. Although specific prevention and health promotion have been an integral part of pediatric and general practice, including well-baby clinics, and in both contexts mothers have usually been helped with advice and guidance about children's wholesome development, these practices have not usually been family-focused. Yet health and healthful behavior and habits are tangible family tasks, and wholesome personality development is a function of the integrity of the family system.

Healthful habits and behaviors are learned

and established in the family. Health education in the schools is helpful but one or two lectures about alcoholism or smoking, or eating or exercise patterns will not significantly counteract parental examples of drinking, smoking, eating, or exercising. In all these respects primary care professionals are in a strategic position to promote health (Belof et al., 1970; Luban-Piozza, 1972; Morris, 1973). Furthermore, if they are knowledgeable about the family life cycle and family functions, staff members can detect lags or deficiencies before they attain symptomatic expression. For instance, even before a child reaches puberty, it may be discovered that the family cannot converse about sex openly and comfortably; or that the parents cannot discuss their sexual wishes and needs together. It should be routine in primary care practice that along with premarital examination or even when young people happen to be sick the opportunity to discuss sexual and reproductive behavior can be utilized. In particular, family planning and family formation are part of primary care, and need not be left until the time to see an obstetrician has arrived. Of course the obstetrician can fulfill this primary care task just as he or she should include preparation for parenthood in the prenatal care and education for delivery. Many issues of family health and its promotion can and should be discussed with expectant couples (Fleck, 1974; Freedman and Thornton, 1979).

Health screening is often devalued because of the statistically meager harvest of pathologic findings through physical examinations and laboratory tests. If such screening, however, is oriented toward family health and psychosocial functioning within the context of reviewing the family as a system, as is done at the Kaiser-Permanente Clinic in Santa Clara, California, then such screening can be cost-effective by promoting sound health and improved family functioning even if no specific treatable or preventable conditions are found (Garfield et al., 1976).

FAMILY HEALTH CARE

A family focus in primary care is obviously in order, lest health or illness is considered out of context. The revolution in medical education early in this century, the subsequent surge in biological knowledge, its attendant specialization, and the increments in medical technology and therapeutic application have not been matched by an increase in physicians' practical knowledge about the family. If we want modern family physicians who provide medical care to members of a family, they should be able to attend to family health problems with a thorough understanding of the roles and involvement of the family in health and disease. Through the ages from Hippocrates to the recent establishment of the Academy of Family Practice in 1948, physicians have viewed the patient's family as a necessary appendage of the patient, sometimes helpful and often a burden. Yet we must now recognize in practice that, besides genes and integral physiologic and metabolic development, family patterns and organization have significant impact on health and disease (Table 3–2). Indeed, thanks to modern psychosocial research in the behavioral sciences, amplified by family therapy experiences, a clinically relevant body of knowledge about the family as a system now exists (Ackerman, 1977; Rakel and Conn, 1978).

Family health care is best rendered early in the life of the nuclear family and not delayed until reactive care is needed, or when an illness occurs. The first pregnancy may occur rather late in the life of the family but the fact that 40% of pregnancies are conceived premaritally demonstrates the inadequate family life education and insufficient parenthood preparation in our nation (Langton, 1970). However, it may also represent lack of access to preventive medical care, in that most people are "illness insured" if insured at all—rather than having continuous access to health care in the strict sense. Such care is theoretically available through various

TABLE 3-2
Levels of intergenerational transmission

A. Cellular and subcellular
1. Fixed chromosomal defects
2. Accidental one-generational aberrations of genes

B. Prenatal environment
1. Mechanical
2. Metabolic-nutritional

C. Biopsychological
1. Transmission through maternal behavior (e.g., anxiety, unresponsiveness, abuse)
a. Autonomic stabilization and integration
b. Special foci-loci of least resistance or specific overattention
2. Body image and self-boundary conceptualization
a. Attachment behaviors (e.g., symbiosis vs individuation) and separation mastery
b. Identifying and labeling feelings
c. Helping child develop self-sense (toddling vs engulfment)
d. Culture-typical gender identity
3. Language and thought-ordering
a. Content
b. Form
c. Categorization and symbol formation
4. Habit formation—healthful vs unhealthy behaviors

D. Relational
1. Modeling-gender identity, affectivity and its expression
2. Culture-appropriate repression—incest taboo and psychosexual moratorium
3. Sense of family unity and group belonging
4. Provisions, guidance for and control of peer relationships

E. Socialization
1. Communication competence regarding linguistic and interactional symbols and abstract thinking
2. Tolerance for identity and independence experimentation in adolescence
3. Emancipation from family of origin according to cultural modes

prepaid medical plans, such as Health Maintenance Organizations, some private health care plans, or Neighborhood Health Centers (GAP, 1973, 1980). Community hospitals, teaching centers included, also operate primary care centers effectively and bring a family orientation to bear (Lidz and Fleck, 1950; GAP, 1980; Leigh and Reiser, 1977). But these programs are often hampered in preventive care because of the stringent cost-accounting rules under which they must operate. For instance, some of these plans apparently exclude birth control measures, even premarital examinations or routine health checks. Solo practitioners also find it difficult to find time to consider psychosocial issues related to health and disease and may limit preventive measures to specific technical ones.

As already stated, family-oriented primary care is better rendered through a primary care team with easy access to a psychiatrist or other mental health professional; ideally these professionals should be integral members of the team or organization. As stated recently, instead of aiming at producing more primary care physicians, it may be wiser to encourage more specialists to participate in primary care (Aiken et al., 1979).

SUMMARY

A scheme for evaluation of family dynamics and structure as it is particularly relevant to general medicine was presented in this chapter. The family is conceptualized and examined as a system having five major variables that may be analyzed along historic and cross-sectional interactional axes. The five elements are leadership, boundaries, affectivity, communication, and the evolutionary task and goal performance. The role of the family in illness along with the impact of illness on the family is of primary significance. The family should be considered an important agent for good health of its members. Certainly primary medical care must include professional attention to patients' families to understand the context of both patient and illness and to prevent any related problems from creating additional ill health for any part of the family unit.

RECOMMENDED READINGS

Engel, G. 1962. *Psychological development in health and disease.* Philadelphia: W.B. Saunders. This volume was written primarily for the medical student and blends development under average and stressful conditions.

Erikson, E.H. 1950. *Childhood and society.* New York: W.W. Norton & Co. A classic monograph, this is the first documented study in social psychiatry.

Glick, I.D., and Kessler, D.R. 1974. *Marital and family therapy.* New York: Grune & Stratton. Here is a concise presentation of the clinician's task and work in marriage and family evaluation and treatment decisions.

Lidz, T. 1976. *The person.* Rev. ed. New York: Basic Books. The most up-to-date compendium on personal development and life-cycle changes is offered in this edition.

Sze, W.C. 1975. *Human life cycle.* New York: Jason Aronson, Inc. This is a collection of treatises on the stages of the human condition.

Worby, C., and Gerard, R. 1978. Family dynamics. In *Family practice*, eds. R.E. Rakel and H.F. Conn, pp. 32–46. Philadelphia: W.B. Saunders. This chapter is geared to the ambience of family physicians and their practices.

REFERENCES

Ackerman, N.W. 1977. Family diagnosis and clinical process. In *American handbook of psychiatry*, vol. 11, ed. G. Caplan, pp. 37–50. New York: Basic Books.

Aiken, L.H.; Lewis, C.E.; Craig, J., et al. 1979. The contribution of specialists to the delivery of primary care: A new perspective. *N. Engl. J. Med.* 300:1363–70.

Aldrich, C. 1975. Office psychotherapy for the primary care physician. In *American handbook of psychiatry*, vol. 5, eds. D.X. Freedman and J.E. Dyrud, pp. 739–55. New York: Basic Books.

Belof, J.S.; Korper, M.; and Weinerman, E.R. 1970. Medical student response to a program for teaching comprehensive care. *J. Med. Educ.* 45:1047–59.

Borus, J.F. 1976. Neighborhood health centers as providers of primary mental health care. *N. Engl. J. Med.* 295:140–45.

Brown, G.W., and Wing, J.K. 1972. Influence of family life on the course of schizophrenic disorders: A replication. *Br. J. Psychiatry* 121:241–58.

Bruch, H. 1973. *Eating disorders.* New York: Basic Books.

Cobb, S., and Rose, R.M. 1973. Hypertension, peptic ulcer and diabetes in air traffic controllers. *J.A.M.A.* 224:489.

Coleman, J.V., and Patrick, D.L. 1976. Integrating mental health services into primary medical care. *Med. Care* 14:654–61.

Dubos, R. 1965. *Man adapting.* New Haven: Yale University Press.

Dykman, A.; Walls, R.C.; Tetsuko, S., et al. 1970. Children with learning disabilities: Conditioning, differentiation and the effect of distraction. *Am. J. Orthopsychiatry* 40:766–82.

Engel, G. 1962. *Psychological development in health and disease.* Philadelphia: W.B. Saunders.

———. 1977. The need for a new medical model: A challenge for biomedicine. *Science* 196:129–36.

Fleck, S. 1980. The family and psychiatry. In *Comprehensive Textbook of Psychiatry-III*, third edition. Eds. A.M. Freedman, H. Kaplan, and B. Sadock, pp. 513–30. Baltimore: Williams and Wilkins.

———. 1974. Some psychosocial aspects of fertility regulation and preparation for parenthood. In *Social psychiatry*, vol. 1, eds. J.H. Masserman and J.J. Schwab. New York: Grune & Stratton.

———. 1975. Unified health services and family-focused primary care. *Int. J. Psychiatry Med.* 6:501–15.

Freedman, D.S., and Thornton, A. 1979. The long-term impact of pregnancy at marriage on the family's economic circumstances. *Fam. Plann. Perspect.* 11:6–21.

GAP-Group for the Advancement of Psychiatry. 1973. *Humane reproduction.* vol. 8, report. no. 86, formulated by the Committee on Preventive Psychiatry.

GAP-Group for the Advancement of Psychiatry. 1980. Mental health and primary medical care, vol. 10, report no. 105, formulated by the Committee on Preventive Psychiatry.

Garfield, S.R.; Collen, M.F.; Feldman, R., et al. 1976.

Evaluation of an ambulatory medical-care delivery system. *N. Engl. J. Med.* 294:426–31.

Gil, D.G. 1971. Violence against children. *J. Marriage & Fam.* 33:637–48.

Goldberg, S. 1977. Social competence in infancy: A model of parent-infant interaction. *Merrill-Palmer Q.* 23:163–77.

Grolnick, L. 1972. A family perspective of psychosomatic factors in illness: A review of the literature. *Family Process* 11:457–86.

Grunebaum, H.U.; Abernethy, V.D.; Rofman, E.S., et al. 1971. The family planning attitudes, practices and motivations of mental patients. *Am. J. Psychiatry* 128:740–43.

Halliday, J.L. 1948. *Psychosocial medicine: A study of the sick society.* New York: Norton.

Hinkle, L.E. 1968. Relating biochemical, physiological, and psychological disorders to the social environment. *Arch. Environ. Health* 16:77–82.

Hinkle, L.E., and Wolf, S. 1952. A summary of experimental evidence relating life stress to diabetes mellitus. *J. Mt. Sinai Hosp.* 19:537–70.

Holmes, T.H., and Rahe, R.H. 1967. The social readjustment rating scale. *J. Psychosom. Res.* 11:213–18.

Jackson, D.D. 1966. Family practice: A comprehensive medical approach. *Compr. Psychiat.* 7:338–48.

Jacobs, S., and Douglas, L. 1979. A mediating process between a loss and illness. *Compr. Psychiatry* 20:165–76.

Kasl, S.F.; Gore, S.; and Cobb, S. 1975. The experience of losing a job: Reported changes in health, symptoms and illness behavior. *Psychosom. Med.* 37:106–22.

Lack, S. 1979. Hospice—A concept of care in the final stages of life. *Conn. Med.* 43:367–72.

Langton, M.R. 1970. Connecticut Out-of-Wedlock Study, 1966, Connecticut Health Bulletin, no. 84,2, pp. 31–40.

Leigh, H., and Reiser, M. 1977. Major trends in psychosomatic medicine: The psychiatrist's evolving role in medicine. *Ann. Intern Med.* 87:233–39.

Lidz, T. 1976. *The person.* Rev. ed. New York: Basic Books.

Lidz, T., and Fleck, S. 1950. Integration of medical and psychiatric methods and objectives on a medical service. *Psychosom. Med.* 12:103–7.

Luban-Piozza, B. 1972. Preventive medical and psychosocial aspects of family practice. *Int. J. Psychiatry Med.* 3:327–32.

Mechanic, D. 1966. Response factors in illness: The study of illness behavior. *Soc. Psychiatry* 1:11–20.

Meissner, W.W. 1966. Family dynamics and psychosomatic processes. *Fam. Process* 5:142–61.

Minuchin, S.; Rosman, B.; and Baker, L. 1978. Psychosomatic families: Anorexia nervosa in context. Cambridge, Mass.: Harvard University Press.

Mirsky, I.A. 1958. Physiologic, psychologic and social determinants in the etiology of duodenal ulcer. *Am. J. Dig. Dis.* 3:285–314.

Morris, J.N. 1964. *The uses of epidemiology.* 2nd ed. Baltimore: Williams & Wilkins.

———. 1973. Four cheers for prevention. *Proc. R. Soc. Med.* 66:225–32.

National Academy of Sciences. 1978. Aging and medical education. A report of a study by a Commission of the Institute of Medicine, National Academy of Sciences, Washington, D.C., Sept., 1978.

Osler, W. 1932. *Aequanimitas, with other addresses.* 3rd ed. Philadelphia: Blakiston Co.

Piaget, J. 1968. *Six psychological studies.* New York: Vintage Books.

President's Commission on Mental Health. 1978. Vol. 1. Washington, D.C.: U.S. Government Printing Office.

Rahe, R.H.; McKean, J.D.; and Ransom, J.A. 1967. A longitudinal study of life-change and illness patterns. *J. Psychosom. Res.* 10:355–66.

Rakel, R.E., and Conn, H.F., eds. 1978. *Family practice.* 2nd ed. Philadelphia: W.B. Saunders.

Reiser, M.F.; Thaler, M.; and Weiner, H. 1957. Patterns of object relationships and cardiovascular responsiveness in healthy young adults and patients with peptic ulcer and hypertension. *Psychosom. Med.* 19:498.

Richardson, H.B. 1948. *Patients have families.* New York: Commonwealth Fund.

Weiner, H. 1978. The illusions of simplicity: The medical model revisited. *Am. J. Psychiatry* (Suppl.) 135:27–33.

Weisman, A.D. 1972. *On death and dying: A psychiatric study of terminality.* New York: Behavioral Publications.

Weisman, A.D., and Brettell, H.R. 1978. The dying patient. In *Family practice,* ed. R.E. Rakel and H.F. Conn, pp. 249–57. Philadelphia: W.B. Saunders.

Winnicott, D.W. 1965. *The family and individual development.* London: Tavistock Publications.

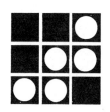

PART II

Evaluation and Management of Psychiatric Syndromes and Disorders in Adults

CHAPTER 4

Personality Types and Personality Disorders

Richard J. Goldberg, M.D.

Effective medical care is often frustrated either because of problems in patient management or signing out of the hospital against medical advice. Underlying these events are often conflicts in personality between physician and patient, or the physician's neglect to take into account special needs of the patient's personality. This chapter discusses the salient aspects of personality development, special needs of certain personalities, and personality disorders.

Why is it important for the physician to know anything about personality disorders? Every person has a generally consistent way of perceiving, thinking about, and relating to his or her environment. The term "personality" refers to such pervasive tendencies, which are exhibited in a wide range of personal and social contexts including the medical care setting. Since personality is a significant determinant of the way a person values health, experiences symptoms, and interacts with health care providers, an understanding of such inherent characteristics should be a fundamental skill of the primary physician.

"Personality" sometimes seems to be such an amorphous term and so subjective and difficult to characterize that it is assumed to have little clinical utility. This impression is overcome with knowledge of the basic personality disorders and of the intervention strategies pertaining to personality factors in medical care. Every clinician is familiar with the frustration engendered by personality problems, for example, the patient who continuously challenges the physician's recommendations, the demanding complainer who never seems to be satisfied, or the patient who seems to replace one symptom with another in a seemingly endless series. The key to management of such problems lies in understanding personality factors and using skill and compassion to intervene in a rational and effective way.

FORMATION OF PERSONALITY

The process of personality formation is an area of research traditionally belonging to the psychoanalyst. Personality, as a fixed collection of tendencies to perceive, think, and behave in certain ways, must be viewed as the outcome of a complex developmental process. Therefore, it is probably an error to attempt an assessment of personality before late adolescence, even though certain tendencies may be evident before that time.

In brief, personality development may be thought of as an outcome of the interaction of the following factors: The unfolding of an individual's innate drives in relation to the demands of society, and the inherent cognitive and regulatory tendencies of the central nervous system (CNS)

Psychobiological Drives and Society: Conflict and Personality Development

Psychological development of the individual involves a struggle between the unfolding of personal drives and the boundaries of social realities (Erikson, 1950). At each stage of development, the child engages in conflict between his or her demands for individual satisfaction and the realities of the environment. According to the concepts of early psychoanalytic work, a personality trait was thought to emerge as an outcome of exaggerated difficulties encountered in a particular developmental stage. However, early attempts to "explain" an obsessive-compulsive personality solely on the basis of problems encountered in toilet training, for example, now seem oversimplified. Of course, the clinical observations used to formulate such a theory cannot simply be discarded. It is becoming clearer that childhood developmental and nurturant experiences, whether deficient or excessive, play a significant though not necessarily causal role in later personality disorder. In addition, psychoanalytic theory has gradually broadened its theoretical scope with the recognition that an individual's development may be modified by modes of nervous system functioning that are independent of developmental conflicts.

Constitutional Endowment: Precursors of Personality

Even before engaging in the conflicts of psychological development, the infant is endowed with a unique nervous system with particular neuroregulatory processes. The foundations of perception, thought, and behavior (the three activities that constitute personality) lie in individual peculiarities of these constitutional neuroregulatory processes. There is evidence that the neurologic competency of the newborn (which includes factors such as calmness, attention, and ability to modulate physiologic arousal) clearly influences personality characteristics evident is later childhood (Cohen, 1974). While definitive studies have not been done yet, it seems warranted to conclude that constitutional neuroregulatory functions partly determine subsequent adult behavioral characteristics such as impulsiveness, ability to tolerate stress, and degrees of dependence and organization.

Cognitive as well as behavioral characteristics have a foundation in CNS modes of function. Most physicians with a classic psychiatric education have learned that personality characteristics (such as obsessiveness, hysteria, or passivity) emerge as residua of stages of psychosexual development. However, it should be noted that the CNS, as an information-processing system, is a cognitive apparatus with a variety of possible modes of functioning. It is generally agreed that in typical right-handed people, language processes and arithmetic (the verbal-digital-analytic mode) depend primarily on the brain's left hemisphere, while the right hemisphere is particularly specialized for spatial relations and some musical functions (nonverbal-analogue-synthetic mode) (Galin, 1974). For reasons not yet understood, it seems that individuals may use predominately one or the other mode as the basis for a cognitive style. Each mode may comprise a particular cognitive style which, in turn, may predispose one to certain personality traits independent of instinctual conflict (Shapiro, 1965). As a simple example, those who inherently process information in a verbal mode are more likely to develop the trait of intellectualism than those who process data using im-

ages rather than words. Or, those whose mode of processing information leads abruptly to action-outflow are more likely than others to develop impulsive personality features. While work in this area is in its early stages, it is clear that psychosexual conflict or social environment alone do not shape the personality, but that so-called autonomous CNS characteristics are also influential.

RECOGNITION AND DIAGNOSIS

It is no simple task to observe and describe the complex processes of another human being. If knowledge of personality factors is to fulfill its potential, the physician must acquire a practical ability to elicit and recognize personality features, along with a vocabulary to describe them.

To begin with, everyone has a personality, which for our purposes may be considered identical to another frequently used term, "character." Personality is not a pathologic phenomenon, nor is its assessment a diagnosis in the traditional sense. Identifying someone's personality is a process of describing certain observed traits. Generally speaking, there is no need for technical jargon in talking about personality. It is important to keep in mind that most people have a very complex variety of features that make up their personalities. It is usually impossible and counterproductive to describe a personality with a single term.

Accordingly, no single question can elicit a patient's personality traits. The following suggestions may facilitate evaluation by drawing out critical areas of personality functions.

Observation

In observing the patient's dress, manner of approach, and overall way of dealing with the interview, the physician may note such features as excessive orderliness of appearance, disorganization, a guarded manner, or lack of sociability. Experienced clinicians make such observations continuously and automatically take note if a patient seems unaccustomed to or uncomfortable about the initial handshake. As an example, some tentative inferences may be drawn about a patient's personality if he or she prefers being seen while lying on a stretcher although physically able to sit in a chair for the interview.

Listening

Listen to the way the patient lets current needs be known.

The universal question, Why are you here to see me? is often sufficient to elicit a vast amount of personality data. For example, does the patient relate his or her story in a demanding, overly dramatic, or excessively complaining manner? Does the patient go out of the way to impress with self-importance? After listening to the patient for a while, is the physician still unable to identify the main point of the patient's discourse? Is such confusion indicative of the patient's general way of dealing with information? Is there an identifiable style of communication? Examples given in Case History 4–1 contrast two cognitive-communicative styles. Information gained by observing language may provide important clues to personality.

Asking Questions

The clinician's task is to *elicit* information on a number of critical topics. Some suggestions for

---

CASE HISTORY 4–1

Mr. Restricted visits his physician for chest pain. He reports: "I've been having pain for one week; it is exactly here [points out the spot]. It starts all of a sudden one-half hour following meals and lasts for 15 minutes. I tried taking antacids but they haven't worked for the last few days so I made an appointment. Can you tell me what's causing it?"

Mr. Diffuse visits his physician for chest pain. He reports: "The pain is awful, it's all over my chest, and it seems like it never goes away. I can't remember when I last felt OK. It's just terrible, doctor, like little devils with sharp forks are pricking me, do something for me! Oh yes, my feet hurt me too. It wasn't easy getting here."

Mr. Diffuse provides dramatic information on the quality of the pain that Mr. Restricted omits; however, his elaboration is less accurate for the clinician and his added concern for his feet detracts from the central concern. Mr. Diffuse is more insistent on getting a solution while Mr. Restricted seems to be asking for intellectual answers. Mr. Restricted's language reveals an "obsessional" cognitive style; Mr. Diffuse's language reveals a "hysterical" cognitive style. Mr. Diffuse tends to annoy clinicians and is often considered overdramatic, vague, and therefore unreliable. His complaints tend to seem less credible. However, what may actually most interfere with effective treatment is not so much that his disorder seems vague, as his personality and the manner in which he describes his disorder to clinicians.

questions are discussed in the following paragraphs.

How has the patient interacted with significant people in his or her life? It is not easy to ask one specific question to get a patient to characterize the nature of close relationships. At first it is helpful to find out whether the patient feels close to or confides in anyone, or whether he or she is isolated. If the patient is isolated, has this isolation always been present, and is this by choice, fear, or some other reason? Asking, "How is your current problem affecting your closest relationships?" often reveals what the patient expects from relationships. For example, is there any sense that relationships are characterized by manipulation, exploitiveness, or overdependence? Contrariwise, is there evidence that the patient has an experience of mutual warmth and tenderness with another person?

What sort of illness behavior has the patient shown in the past? Asking, "Could you tell me about previous times in the hospital and what it was like for you?" is a good starting point, because the stress of illness often throws the main features of the personality into sharp relief. The patient may answer, "The worst thing about it was the feeling of being so helpless," or, "Of course, I was grateful for the medical help but it was one argument after another when the doctors tried to get me to do things their way." In these answers, each patient is describing a personality characteristic in which a different sort of situational control is an important aspect of the personality. Listen especially for complaints about previous medical care since they may reveal the underlying emotional needs of the patient. Naturally, it is also noteworthy if the patient does not complain at all. Finally, comments about previous physicians may provide insights into personality features relevant to current care.

Certain other information that contributes to assessment of personality belongs to a *general data base* for each patient. This includes any history of antisocial behavior (such as childhood truancy, delinquency, lying, vandalism,

adult problems with the law, assaults, illegal occupations, unstable job record, or multiple marriages); episodes of severe identity crises; suicidal gestures or acts; brief psychotic episodes; or unrealistic thinking. These data form basic criteria for a number of personality disorders discussed later.

It is useful to ask, "What sort of interests do you have and what do you do to enjoy yourself?" This question summons up a multitude of personality features including general mood states, levels of social involvement, and degree of maturity.

Family, Friends, and Staff as Observers

Seek out and listen to what family, friends, and staff have to say about the patient. For example, it is important to hear a patient's son state, "Father never really trusts anyone. No one ever gets to know what is really on his mind. He may tell you otherwise but he probably isn't taking any of the medication you give him." Or, someone may say, "Please don't get discouraged, doctor, mother has always been a complainer like this. No matter what we've done for her, we get no thanks." It is necessary to pay attention to such informants to find out if the patient's presentation is uncharacteristic, since evidence of personality change may be a clue to an underlying organic mental disorder. Observe medical care staff reactions to the patient, since they often provide a key to some facet of the patient they are dealing with.

Psychological Testing

A variety of standard instruments are available to assess personality. Most psychological tests are time-consuming, some require skilled administration, and the benefit for the primary physician is often questionable. Nevertheless, it is worth mentioning that vast amounts of information have been collected on medical patients by the Minnesota Multiphasic Personality Inventory (MMPI), which is probably the best known and most widely used of the personality tests available. This test is self-administered and for a small fee can be rapidly scored by computer (a service now offered by several companies). Though the test takes a few hours to complete, it does not require the physician to be present. In cases where the physician feels unable to assess the personality in question or feels uncertain even after following the interview recommendations discussed in this section, the MMPI may give some insight into a complex clinical relationship. It may be especially useful in evaluating personality assets that can be utilized in the rehabilitation of chronic physically disabled patients (Freeman et al., 1976). The MMPI has been used in attempting to sort out the contribution of personality factors in complex pain syndromes, such as low back pain, where the presence of certain personality factors may influence response to back surgery (Wiltse and Rocchio, 1975).

PERSONALITY DISORDERS

Because the study of personality disorders depends so much on observations that are difficult to standardize and validate, there have been obstacles in organizing a systematic, generally accepted, classification system. The prevalence of personality disorders is not known; it would be interesting to know how often patients with these disorders appear in the general medical setting, how they utilize health care services, and whether medical conditions are any more frequent in this population. Systematic studies of the relationship between personality disorders and medical symptoms is a fairly new area of research. This chapter uses a classification based on the third edition of the *Diagnostic and statistical manual (DSM-III)* of the American Psychiatric Association.

Primary care physicians do not see patients with personality disorders *primarily* because of their personality problems. However, when individuals with personality disorders do get sick, they raise two types of special management considerations.

For some, the medical-surgical disorder is an *inherent* part of the personality disorder. For example, substance abuse is often present in antisocial or borderline personalities. In these cases, recognition of personality disorder becomes relevant since the overall treatment of the presenting problem (substance abuse) requires consideration of the other personality or behavior features likely to complicate therapy (such as impulsiveness, unreliability, drug dealing, manipulativeness, or recidivism).

The second management consideration involves patients with *coincidental* medical-surgical disorders whose treatment runs afoul because of the effect of personality disorder on the doctor-patient interaction. For instance, there are special difficulties in the management of a patient who is excessively paranoid, histrionic, or withdrawn. In such situations (and others to be discussed) it is important for the primary physician to have several skills, among them ability to recognize salient personality features, understanding of how personality factors influence the clinical management of the patient, and knowledge of rational intervention strategies.

In the following section, several personality disorders are discussed along with current *DSM-III* criteria. It is helpful to keep in mind that the general definition of a personality disorder involves *deeply ingrained, inflexible, maladaptive patterns of sufficient severity to cause either significant impairment in adaptive functioning or subjective distress.* The diagnosis of the personality disorders that follow should only be made when such patterns are typical of the individual's long-term functioning, and not limited to discrete episodes of illness. Such guidelines, while important for the development of a more rigorous understanding of these disorders, often appear to force the clinician into making an all-or-none diagnosis. In daily practice, patients exhibit personality *traits* that are clinically relevant even though they may not meet the rigorous criteria of a diagnostic complex. For those individuals characterized by a specific trait, it makes sense to introduce the category of personality *type* instead of disorder.

What makes the consideration of personality types both practical as well as meaningful is this general principle: *The basic elements of personality are thrown into sharper relief under conditions of stress and illness.* Under such conditions, the complex personality which may flourish in routine living conditions is often reduced to one or two basic, relatively immature, and easily observed traits. One sees this phenomenon whenever one observes a mature adult becoming more "childlike" under the duress of hospitalization. A similar pattern occurs following brain damage (Goldstein, 1952). Such *temporary*, *stressed*, and *less mature* conditions of the personality should *not* be considered disorders, but should be thought of as time-limited shifts in function that are induced by stress. These shifts represent coping attempts by the individual and should be recognized as serving an important defensive function for the patient. Unfortunately, this defensive function may be so extreme as to interfere with positive response to therapy and may even be maladaptive.

Remembering that personality "types" are not intended as scientific terms or diagnoses, the clinician is aware that types are not disorders or character assessments based on an in-depth knowledge of the developmental history and psychodynamics of an individual—a type of evaluation that usually involves a trained psychiatric interviewer anyway. Instead, personality types are best viewed as operational categories based on clinical impressions and observations of patient behavior along with whatever information can be gathered from friends, family, or old records. Therefore, the category of a personality type must remain as a working hypothesis that is open to revision as more information is obtained.

The next section lists the criteria for personality disorders. When a patient is characterized by some of the signs and symptoms but does not meet the complete criteria for a personality disorder, he or she may be considered as a personality type. The use of the category "personality type" allows consideration of many more clinical problems than would be possible by limiting discussion to the stricter criteria of personality disorders. It seems, in any case, that similar clinical approaches and management considerations apply to the type as well as the full-blown disorder. Personality disorders and associated personality types are discussed together in this section.

Management considerations are included here instead of in a separate section because they emerge so directly from the clinical material as it is presented. Each subsection will describe: (a) criteria for diagnosis of personality disorder; (b) an example of a clinical presentation of such a patient; (c) a description of how each personality experiences illness; (d) behavioral outcomes of such experience; and (e) intervention strategies that logically follow to facilitate management.

Dependent Personality Disorder

Recognition. Often from an emotionally deprived background, the dependent person behaves in a very needy fashion. Such individuals seek out relationships in which they get others to assume significant responsibility. There is little evidence of self-sufficiency or interest in acquiring it. There is often strong attachment and involvement with one provider, or a series of providers. A dependent person is intensely uncomfortable when separated from the provider: they see themselves as helpless. Patients with such traits have also been called "dependent clingers" or "dependent, overdemanding types" (Kahana and Bibring, 1964).

The Problem.   One might conceive of a dependent patient saying to himself (if he were aware of his 'motivations), "I'm the kind of person that needs to be taken care of. Now that I'm sick, I somehow feel more needy than ever, and wonder if I can ever get as much care as I require. Well, I'll do what I can to assure myself of getting as much as possible; or, if it seems that my needs are overwhelming, I might just give up altogether." Problems typically arise when frequent, seemingly unnecessary, office visits or evening phone calls become intolerable to the physician, who views the patient's behavior as a series of unwarranted requests for special attention. The patient insists on having everything done for him or her and is incessantly calling the physician to renew a prescription that has been lost, reschedule an office visit for yet another nonspecific symptom, make a phone call on the patient's behalf, and so on. At first, the physician may be willing to comply; however, tolerance is inevitably exceeded when the physician rightly perceives that the patient's requests and demands are reaching unrealistic proportions. In a *dysfunctional response*, the physician may suddenly "draw the line." Authoritatively telling such a patient to stop calling, or scheduling appointments on a less frequent basis only serves to increase the fears of a dependent patient.

Intervention.   Recognition of the "dependence" characteristic leads to several possible interventions. First, the physician should inquire about the nature of currently perceived stresses that are contributing to the patient's desperate coping attempts. If such behavior occurs in the context of recent or current illness, the physician might say, "I know that your recent illness has you very worried. I know that your many visits and attempts to call me must be because you're frightened in some way and feel somewhat helpless. We've had some difficulty getting together a few times, and this may have made you feel less secure. To help deal with these

issues let's set up brief weekly meetings. In addition, on Wednesday afternoon I'll be available if you want to reach me by phone. Of course, you can call me any time if you feel there is a real emergency." Drawing reasonable boundaries and setting up compromises with the patient must be done in such a way that the patient does not experience punishment or withdrawal. Generally, explicit definition of the care-giving relationship significantly reduces the patient's uncontrolled attempts to assure contact.

Of course, not all complaining and demanding patients are the dependent, overdemanding personality type. Such behavior may be the outcome of other personality types to be discussed. Therefore, as a general principle, intervention decisions cannot be made on the basis of immediate behavior without understanding such behavior in the context of the patient's personality type (Leigh and Reiser, 1980).

Compulsive Personality Disorder

Recognition.   The behavior of the compulsive personality type reflects the need for organization and the urge for control and self-discipline. The issue of control and the value of logic are often paramount in interpersonal relationships. The ability to express warmth or spontaneity is lacking. Compulsive types are preoccupied with procedure and detail to the extent of losing perspective of the overall picture. Decision-making is often impaired by excessive preoccupation with details and undue fear of making an error. Such a patient has been called the "orderly, controlling type" (Kahana and Bibring, 1964; Leigh and Reiser, 1980) and is related to the so-called Type A personality (Keith et al., 1965).

The Problem.   One might conceive of the compulsive patient saying to himself or herself (if he/she were aware of his/her motivations), "As much as possible I need to feel that things are under my control. I need to understand things to help me do this. Now that I'm sick, I feel frightened that things I don't know about are happening to me totally out of my control. The illness, the treatment, decisions about appointments and medications are a mountain of detail I must know about, but which all seem beyond me. What I must do is redouble my efforts to remain on top of things. At worst, I'll simply not go along with anything, as a way of keeping control." Case History 4–2 is an example of compulsive personality disorder.

Intervention. By recognizing the controlling personality type, the primary physician may realize that such a patient is not comfortable simply being told what to do. This patient needs to be given some sense of participation in treatment. Ways to return some control to the patient might include asking the patient to monitor and record his own blood pressure, or to initiate an exercise program. Appropriate amounts of information must be provided so he can participate in decisions about management in a meaningful way. Since the patient is most likely missing appointments as a way of reinstituting control over the treatment situation, the

physician may want to work out a schedule of appointments with the patient in a collaborative way that takes the patient's needs more into account. Time spent on such a collaboration is a worthwhile investment, since it is an important step in helping to ensure regularity and continuity of treatment. Such collaboration allows the patient to participate in the treatment without feeling more threatened than he already does by virtue of having a significant cardiovascular problems. Central nervous system depressants, like diazepam, are to be avoided if possible since this type of patient usually experiences sedative medication as a further interference with his sense of autonomy. The physician must be responsive to adjusting prescriptions and providing a reasonable amount of information, but must be careful not to get embroiled in excessively detailed descriptions of insignificant side effects.

Histrionic Personality Disorder

Recognition. The histrionic type of patient is often described as "hysterical" (Chodoff and Lyons, 1958) or the "dramatizing captivating

---

CASE HISTORY 4–2

A middle-aged business executive is being treated for angina pectoris and hypertension. His behavior with the physician is obstinate. He questions every medication, takes some and does not take others with no apparent rhyme or reason. He misses some appointments altogether, and then calls up demanding that he be seen immediately. He presents lists of questions asking for details, technical reasons, and explanations for everything that is being done and that is not

being done. In a *dysfunctional response*, the physician takes a firm stand. He or she orders the patient to take his medication as directed. Because of his or her sense that the patient only seems to get more upset knowing the technical details of his illness, the physician abandons his or her early attempts to provide reasonable explanations of the disorders. Finally, since the patient is clearly becoming more agitated, diazepam (Valium) is added to the treatment regimen.

type" (Kahana and Bibring, 1964; Leigh and Reiser, 1980). From a descriptive point of view, the features that make up the so-called hysterical personality include behavior that is self-centered and histrionic, and an impression on others as emotionally shallow, capricious, and coquettish. Interpersonally, these people may come across as dependent, helpless, and in need of constant reassurance. Their responses are generally exaggerated, dramatic, and out of proportion to the stimulus; for example, this personality type may exude signs of intense affection to a casual acquaintance.

The Problem.   Clinical problems arise with histrionic patients not so much from the disorders they present, as from the way they present their disorders. This personality type is usually characterized by a vague, nonfactual,

cognitive style as described in an earlier section of the chapter. They pay more attention to impressions and feelings than to logic and detail. At first, such patients often have a certain seductive appeal to the physician. An example of histrionic personality disorder is illustrated in Case History 4–3.

Intervention.   The physician must be aware of the personality and cognitive style of histrionic patients and resist automatically discounting their credibility on the basis of apparently inappropriate behavior. Instead, the physician should appreciate the special threat that illness poses to a person to whom attractiveness is so important. The patient's seductive behavior is not directed to the physician as an individual; rather, it is a response style utilized in coping with situations of distress. Calmly and objectively

---

CASE HISTORY 4–3

A 35-year-old woman is being evaluated for joint pains. As the physician listens to and observes her, he begins to notice some discrepancy. Despite her requests for increased pain medication and claims of being poorly treated, this patient is at the same time paying a great deal of attention to her makeup, dress, and appearance. The physician is confused because the suffering this patient claims to have seems inconsistent with the impression conveyed by her behavior. Her presentation is incongruously mixed with overly dramatic accounts of her disability and seductive teasing of the physician with what seem to be sexually provocative remarks. In a *dysfunctional response*, the physician begins to discount her complaints of pain. In his eyes, she is

an exaggerator whose credibility is questionable. The physician may even tend to decrease or withhold medication because of his doubts concerning the "reality" of her symptoms. With such a shift of attention, the patient becomes even more dramatic in presenting her symptoms and needs. One might conceive this patient saying to herself (if she were aware of her motivations), "I've learned that my appearance and attractiveness are important in keeping others close to me. Now that my illness has impaired my attractiveness, how can I assure myself that anyone will be interested enough to treat me? What I can do is to become more insistently dramatic or in some way seduce other people to be interested in me."

reassuring the patient that the physician is interested in taking care of the illness is paramount. If the patient is especially seductive, the physican might tell the patient that such behavior makes it more difficult for clinical treatment to take place, and that a "special" relationship with the patient is not necessary for the clinician to be interested in providing the best medical treatment of the disorder. The physician must be especially scrupulous in maintaining a professional stance in this situation despite any temptation to collude with the patient in a flirtatious and misleading way. Above all, the physician must try to separate the style of presentation from the disorder itself.

Paranoid Personality Disorder

Recognition. The paranoid personality has also been called the "guarded, querulous type" (Kahana and Bibring, 1964) or the "guarded, suspicious" type (Leigh and Reiser, 1980). Such people are continually vigilant about others and are always suspicious of the motives of those around them. Tensely guarding against some threat from the outside world, they continually question reasons for events that relate to them as

if there were an expectation of harm. Though these patients may not admit it, they frequently blame other people for their illness. In reviewing the social and work history of such a person, it quickly becomes evident that this type has difficulty establishing close relationships. They usually work alone, are cold and unemotional, and often readily admit that they never share with other people what's really on their mind. Such patients also have a litigious strain, easily take offense, and may recount a series of incidents that they feel justify legal action of some sort.

The problem. An example of paranoid personality disorder is demonstrated in Case History 4–4.

Intervention. Suspicious by nature, the paranoid patient feels especially vulnerable and concerned about what will happen to him or her in a weakened condition. When they find themselves in the passive position of a patient, they become especially sensitive to the intrusions of history-taking and the ambiguities of the diagnostic process. In this context of uncertainty, unable to protect herself or himself, the patient

---

CASE HISTORY 4–4

A 27-year-old man seeks help for vague gastrointestinal complaints of several months' duration. He is generally tight-lipped and volunteers little information about himself or his symptoms. He makes the physician feel that any questions about his life are an intrusion and he answers them grudgingly. The physician hears that treatment has not gone well with previous doctors but details are

not forthcoming. The patient accepts prescriptions for medication, but never takes any of them because of his suspicions and concerns about what they might do to him. Suddenly without warning, after several visits the patient does not return. A month later he returns with the same complaints but no explanation of his disappearance.

suddenly flees because suspicion and fear become intolerable within the treatment system. In order to counteract apprehension, such a patient requires careful, straightforward explanations of all tests and procedures, including history-taking. It is useful to give warnings about possible effects of treatment, to explain new directions in treatment strategies, and to offer reasons for any delays or uncertainty. A written schedule of treatment protocol, given to the patient in advance, may be helpful in enlisting cooperation. Sympathetically recognizing that the circumstances of medical treatment are uncomfortable and an appeal for tolerance are often effective when dealing with a paranoid personality.

Narcissistic Personality Disorder

Recognition.   The narcissistic person, actively engaged in establishing superiority over others, has been called the "superior type" (Kahana and Bibring, 1964; Leigh and Reiser, 1980), as well as the "entitled demander" (Groves, 1978). In health, he or she may secure this "exalted" position through accomplishments or claimed accomplishments and a general attitude of arrogance. They are overly sensitive to criticism, which may provoke either rage or humiliation or both. Narcissists have difficulties feeling dependent on others, since this would imply that others are superior to them. Interpersonal relationships may show a history of being disrupted because of the inability to accept criticism or interdependence, or else the narcissist may settle into relationships that serve to reinforce a sense of power, brilliance, or success.

The Problem.   During illnesses, the narcissistic patient may bolster a damaged sense of superiority by disparaging others. They may actively question the competence of physicians or any member of the treatment team, or may feel that only an eminent physician is appropriate to deal with his or her illness. Remarks that directly or indirectly demean the physician may be made, for example, the patient might spend a lot of time talking about how good a previous physician was. Such a patient is especially astute at noticing any weakness of the caretakers. Unfortunately, such a strategy results in an effect opposite of what the patient hopes for, since criticism may make people perform less well than they usually do. A narcissistic patient is apt to make an issue out of demanding a referral to a specialist instead of accepting treatment by a primary physician. As a **dysfunctional response**, the physician may begin to engage in some sort of argument or power struggle with the patient.

Intervention.   By definition, the sick role involves being placed in an inferior position. Despite this, physicians must do what they can to avoid threatening or challenging narcissistic patients by highlighting their vulnerable position. The physician must walk a fine line in the dilemma: On one hand, if the physician appears too controlling or powerful, the patient cannot tolerate his or her relative inferiority and weakness; on the other hand, if the patient feels that the physician is in some way not a powerful and special figure, he or she feels devalued and worries that the clinician is incapable of providing special treatment. Giving a sense of competence and unassuming self-confidence on the part of the physician is usually reassuring to the narcissistic patient.

Schizoid Personality Disorder

Recognition.   The very introverted patient is rarely thought to be a problem. Quiet or withdrawn patients are generally considered to be "good" patients, while the agitated or more active personality types draw attention to themselves quite readily. The introverted personality prefers to live apart from others, and describes him or herself as a "loner." Their occupations often involve areas that require little interpersonal contact. This patient has been called the "uninvolved, seclusive, aloof type" (Kahana and Bibring, 1964; Leigh and Reiser, 1980). If there are additional features of eccentricities in communication or behavior, the patient may be classified as having a schizotypal personality disorder according to the *DSM-III*. Such eccentricities may include magical thinking (telepathy or clairvoyance), referential thinking ("everything going on somehow pertains to me personally"), or odd communication (wandering or metaphorical speech). In the introverted personality, the paucity of personal relationships may be due to lack of desire for or indifference to social involvement. If, on the other hand, the lack is due to a hypersensitivity to rejection and there is actually an underlying desire for acceptance, the individual may be thought of as an *avoidant personality* according to the *DSM-III*.

The Problem. During illness, extremely introverted patients deal with the anxiety of health care contacts by withdrawing. Recognition of essential clinical problems may, therefore, be difficult. This patient simply has trouble sharing his or her feelings. Significant emotional or physical disorders may go unreported. As a *dysfunctional response*, the physician may overlook such withdrawal and fail to uncover symptoms that patients are keeping to themselves. In another dysfunctional response, the physician might attempt to "draw out" such a person. Case History 4–5 illustrates such an example.

Intervention. Recognition of the introverted personality type leads the physician to "scale down" efforts at resocialization. Realistic, lowered expectations of social rehabilitation avoid otherwise inevitable frustration. At the same time, the physician must rely more on diagnostic thoroughness and acumen so as not to overlook disorders that the patient does not volunteer.

Antisocial Personality Disorder

Recognition. The antisocial personality category does not pertain to the individual who exhibits isolated antisocial acts. The full criteria include an extended period of multiple antisocial behaviors beginning before age 15 years and continuing on into adulthood. Before age 15

CASE HISTORY 4–5

A 70-year-old widow seeks relief from severe arthritis and stasis ulcers of her feet. With increasing incapacity, she spends more and more time at home. After thoroughly evaluating her metabolic status, eliminating all sedative drugs, and ruling out depression, the physician feels convinced that the patient would improve if only she were to get out and spend more time with people. He helps make daily transportation arrangements for this patient to attend large group socializing activities. In ensuing visits, the patient becomes even quieter and less communicative. Such a problem highlights the point of this section. While the dictates of common sense and of social support theory suggest that socialization should help this isolated, elderly patient, those assumptions simply cannot hold true as a general guideline for all patients. Being forced into an unwanted social setting is incompatible with the adaptive capacities of the introverted personality.

years, such individuals are characterized by several of the following attributes: truancy, expulsion from school, delinquency, running away from home, persistent lying, vandalism, very early sexual behavior, or substance abuse. After age 15 years, this personality type demostrates a number of the following behavioral features: arrests, assaults, thefts, debt defaulting, illegal occupations, itinerancy, or poor occupational performance. Such personalities have previously been classified as "sociopaths" or "psychopaths." Frequent complications include functional illiteracy and substance abuse. There does appear to be a strong familial pattern to this disorder (Hutchings and Mednick, 1974). Several subgroups of antisocial behavior have been described, such as emotionally unstable character disorder (Rifkin et al., 1972) and episodic dyscontrol syndrome (Maletzky, 1973), which may be responsive to lithium and diphenylhydantoin (Dilantin), respectively.

The Problem. Dealing with antisocial individuals can be very frustrating. They may be highly sophisticated (or simply persistent) in making inappropriate demands. Case History 4–6 shows such an example.

Intervention. Several guidelines must be kept in mind in dealing with the antisocial type of patient. Because these patients tend to evoke a variety of frustrated, angry, or rejecting responses, it is important to document objective physical signs in the management of clinical problems. For example, the patient just described should be examined for signs of barbiturate withdrawal (see Chapter 14). With evidence of an impending withdrawal, treatment becomes a medical rather than a moral question. If the barbiturate blood level is significantly elevated without signs of intoxication, one can infer that tolerance is present, and a serious withdrawal syndrome is possible. In this case, the physician is in a position to offer the patient admission to a substance abuse program where detoxification, most likely as an inpatient, could be undertaken. The sine qua non of effectve treatment for antisocial patients is effective behavioral control. Instead of the temptation to dismiss the patient as untreatable, a straightforward confrontation with an effective and reasonable treatment plan is important. Of course, it is probable that the patient will reject the plan and try to make the physician feel guilty in some way for not providing help.

It is generally not the business of the primary physician to treat a personality disorder per se. Dealing with the antisocial personality will most likely be in the context of associated substance abuse, or due to a coincidental medical condition. Treatment of substance abuse in these patients is best handled by well-organized, comprehensive, peer-oriented treatment systems, such as methadone programs. An individual therapy approach is never enough. In regard to substance abuse problems, the primary physi-

---

CASE HISTORY 4–6

A man in his mid-twenties comes to the physician's office requesting pentobarbital sodium (Nembutal), relating a complex story to rationalize his request. As a *dysfunctional response*, the physician simply dismisses this patient as a barbiturate addict. The patient leaves the office angrily stating that if he has to rob someone for these drugs, the physician will be at fault.

cian can only function successfully as an entry way into another treatment system. In general, the treatment of antisocial personalities requires clear limits and behavioral controls. Such a patient should not be allowed to disrupt inpatient medical settings, the primary physician may need to call on a psychiatric consultant to provide behavioral guidelines.

Borderline Personality Disorder

Recognition. The term "borderline" has been loosely applied to a variety of patients. Use of such a nonspecific label serves little purpose in understanding and simply relegates the patient to some ambiguous category. Recently, there has been increasing interest in standardizing the diagnostic criteria for this disorder (Gunderson and Kolb, 1978) along with clarification of both its precursors (Zetzel, 1971) and management considerations (Groves, 1981). Clinicians should apply the term "borderline" only when the patient exhibits instability in a variety of areas including interpersonal relationships, behavior, mood, and self-image. At least five of the following eight characteristics of the patient's long-term functioning are required to make the diagnosis of borderline personality.

1. A pattern of *unstable and intense interpersonal relationships* marked by sharp shifts between idealization, manipulation, and devaluation of other people. The relationship with the physician often fits this pattern. Such patients may become intensely dependent and may manipulate the relationship using the implications of suicidal behavior along with other threats.

2. Impulsive behaviour that is potentially self-damaging in such areas as substantive abuse, eating, spending, or physical acts.

3. Physically self-damaging acts, including suicidal gestures, fights, accidents or acts such as wrist-slashing or overdosing, in an attempt to manipulate someone else is a frequent reason for hospital contact.

4. Inappropriately intense and unstable affects with outbursts of brief but intense anger, depression, or anxiety.

5. Identity disturbance in several areas such as self-image, gender identity, values, and loyalties.

6. Mild psychotic experiences, which may take any form but most commonly involve paranoid ideation or feelings of unreality not induced by drug use.

7. Problems tolerating being alone.

8. Chronic feelings of emptiness or boredom, with a relative absence of self-satisfaction.

The Problem. The borderline patient creates specific, repetitive, and somewhat predictable problems in any treatment setting. For an example, see Case History 4–7.

Intervention. As a general principle, successful treatment of the borderline personality requires that a single clinician be in charge of all phases of therapy. The primary physician will face certain predictable problems in attempting to coordinate treatment. Since the borderline personality creates complications when participating in a relationship and is exquisitely sensitive to feelings of rejection, the physician must pay special attention to relationship nuances which in other cases would seem insignificant.

To minimize potential misunderstandings, all communication with the patient should be simple and straightforward. From the outset, the physician should avoid giving in to the patient's implicit or stated demands, but must reassure the patient that he or she deserves the best possible treatment and that the physician has every intention of providing it. Calmly and firmly, over and over again, the physician should reiterate therapeutic goals and methods of treatment. Unfortunately, the patient may not be able to tolerate such limit-setting, and may express anger and dissatisfaction in a number of ways, including new complaints, noncompliance, outright hostility, a suicide attempt, or termination from treatment. The physician should learn to interpret such intensifications as a reflection of some obstacle in the therapeutic relationship.

Some borderline patients respond well in the context of a reliable, consistent treatment relationship. However, when extreme turbulence arises that necessitates psychiatric consultation, the primary physician and the psychiatrist must communicate carefully and completely; they must avoid being played off against one another by a patient who is expert at fostering disagreement and conflict among potential caretakers. The limits and tasks of each treatment relationship must be agreed upon, clearly explained to the patient, and reclarified at intervals.

Joint management of borderline patients who have significant medical and psychiatric illness has not been well studied. As the physician-patient relationship deepens, the greater the difficulty in referral, since borderline personalities are keenly sensitive to shifts in relationships and are prone to intensification of pathologic

behaviour at any suggestion of rejection or termination. Repeated catastrophes in the treatment histories of these patients often can be traced to naively or clumsily managed terminations or transfers. It is essential to prepare the patient for referral early on and to continually define the current therapeutic role in a clear and undistorted manner.

Long-Suffering, Self-Sacrificing Personality Type

Recognition. While a corresponding personality disorder is not included in the *DSM-III*, the long-suffering, self-sacrificing personality type warrants consideration since it frequently presents clinical problems. Groves (1978) has called these individuals "manipulative help rejectors," they resemble Lipsitt's "crock" (Lipsitt, 1970), and they have features central to Engel's pain-prone patient (Engel, 1959). This type of personality regards sacrifice as the necessary burden of

---

CASE HISTORY 4–7

Mrs. W., a 38-year-old woman, is being treated for impaired renal function secondary to phenacetin abuse. In addition, she has multiple somatic complaints including joint pains, myalgias, headaches, sleeplessness, and anxiety. Her marriage is in crisis and she receives no emotional support from her spouse. The patient phones the physician at all hours with relatively insignificant complaints, insisting on immediate attention and implying that otherwise some catastrophe might ensue. During office visits it seems difficult to pin down or follow through on any specific problems because the patient

is so upset and disorganized. She has been in psychiatric treatment many times, has had several overdoses, and sees her most recent therapist irregularly. Even the physician who is usually vigilant about unnecessary medication somehow compromises and provides a series of medications for the cascading complaints of hopelessness. Despite himself, the physician is lured into an untenable position in which trying to "draw the line" becomes equated with abandonment, something the patient hints might lead to a suicide attempt.

life, and little is done for personal pleasure. Very often, those who are supposed to "benefit" from their sacrifices feel guilty and frustrated.

The problem. An example of the long-suffering, self-sacrificing personality type is illustrated in Case History 4–8.

Intervention. In fact, there is no easy way to alter this self-pitying behavior. The physician may gain some solace by recognizing the problem as a continuation of the patient's lifelong style of dealing with others. At times it may be worthwhile to confront the patient in a non-rejecting way by pointing out the negative behavior. However, several other interventions are logical ploys if one keeps in mind the general principle that it is best to support or accommodate personality tendencies of the individual patient rather than try to replace them. Suggesting to the patient discussed previously that she view her recovery as yet another burden to be undertaken allows her to continue her moaning and complaining while she does other things along the way to assist her recovery. One might say, "It seems that in a life of trials, you have one more burden to take on." Another approach requires suggesting to a self-sacrificing patient that he or she work on recovery for the sake of someone else, (the children, for example) rather than for the patient's own sake.

GENERAL MANAGEMENT CONSIDERATIONS

The primary physician ought not to be treating personality disorder per se. If one recognizes a personality disorder as the primary problem, one should refer the patient to a psychotherapist. The therapist may be a psychiatrist; an alternative referral source is a psychologist, psychiatric social worker or psychiatric nurse-clinician if the therapist is adequately trained, experienced, and has had appropriate supervision for the management of such patients. Referral should always be discussed openly with the patient. One suggested format is to tell the patient, "We have been working together to resolve your current problems. At this point, I believe that there is a significant emotional component to your difficulties and I would like to refer you to a psychiatrist." The manner of making the referral is important and is discussed in Chapter 20.

CASE HISTORY 4–8

A 65-year-old woman is being treated for recently discovered diabetes. Each visit is characterized by her constant complaining. Everything is too much for her. At first, she mobilizes the physician's sympathy, who redoubles efforts to comfort, reassure, and assist her. However, eventually the clinician is worn down by the constant stream of moaning. This patient never returns any thanks or recognition for the efforts that others are making on her behalf. The physician becomes frustrated and as a *dysfunctional response* first may take an authoritarian stance and insist that the patient change her attitudes. When this command fails, the usual remaining strategy seems to be to increasingly ignore the patient. It is not only the complaining, but the apparent lack of initiative and motivation towards recovery that demoralizes the physician.

When disruptive personality factors are concurrent with medical-surgical problems, it is important for the primary clinician to be aware of the appropriate management considerations. Referral is not often necessary since the goal of treatment is resolution of the medical-surgical problem and not reorganization of the patient's personality. In inpatient settings, nursing and social work staff can be educated to participate in a consistently therapeutic behavioral approach to the patient. Only in certain cases is referral preferred; namely, in dealing with substance abuse in an antisocial or borderline personality where manipulative behavior defeats treatment, and where suicide threats are used as a means of controlling the therapeutic relationship. Of course, at any time, an informal consultation with a psychiatrist may help clarify a management strategy most helpful for the primary physician and tailored to the patient's personality type.

While some forms of therapy attempt to change personality, the goal of the primary physician should be to "support" the existing personality and help it to function more adaptively. To support the personality, the physician must identify the unique needs of the patient that are being bolstered by the particular exaggerated personality function. The physician must decide, "How can I assist the patient with coping in a way consistent with his or her personality, so the patient can feel less strained and thereby recover a more mature way of interacting?" The priority of management is to develop rapport and maintain a working alliance with the patient.

Behavior is a final pathway and cannot be treated as a primary symptom. Consider the hostile patient. As the previous section demonstrates, hostility can emerge for a number of reasons: for example, the paranoid patient who is fending off a presumed threat, the narcissistic patient who feels he or she is not getting adequate recognition, the borderline patient whose behavior is characterized by rage, the dependent

patient who feels angry that deeply felt needs are not being met, or the compulsive personality who feels self-control is challenged in the medical setting. Naive or simplistic management of hostility is not effective; the physician must attempt to glean information about the patient's personality and adroitly match intervention to the individual personality type. For some, firm limit-setting will be successful, for others, forms of accommodation, acquiescence, and compromise are in order.

SUMMARY

Since primary care physicians deal with patients as people rather than as isolated disease entities, knowledge of personality factors is essential. Personality refers to a generally consistent way of relating to environment and is the outcome of a complex developmental process which includes constitutional characteristics of the central nervous system as well as social and psychological factors.

Useful information about a patient's personality is gathered by perceptive observation, listening, and elicitation of specific information regarding the patient's interpersonal interactions and past illness behavior. Friends, family, and other observers may also offer relevant information. If personality features seem problematic, the MMPI may be a useful diagnostic adjunct.

The primary physician does not deal with personality issues per se, but confronts them when a patient with a personality disorder has a concurrent medical problem, or when the stress of illness brings out a disorder in the patient's personality that interferes with clinical management. This chapter classifies personality disorders according to the most recent American Psychiatric Association criteria and includes clinical examples and discussion of paranoid, introverted, histrionic, narcissistic, antisocial, borderline, dependent, and compulsive personality disorders. In addition, there is discussion of the "long-suffering, self-sacrificing" type of personality not included in the *DSM-III* classification. Each section discusses identification, typical clinical problems, and management strategies. A final section provides an overview of management issues and covers questions of referral and goals of management.

RECOMMENDED READINGS

American Psychiatric Association. 1980. *Diagnostic and statistical manual of mental disorders.* 3rd ed. Prepared by the APA Task Force on Nomenclature and Statistics. Washington, D.C.: American Psychiatric Association. It may seem somewhat unusual to refer the general medical reader to a diagnostic and statistical manual written for the subspeciality of psychiatry. However, the *DSM-III* is a clearly written and very instructive text. It avoids jargon and attempts to clarify psychological terminology. Clarifying terms, which often clarifies thinking, is especially important in an area as amorphous as personality. The clinician who reads this section will acquire a language to speak about patients with personality problems in a constructive way and thereby is able to deal with them more effectively.

Kahana, R.J., and Bibring, G.L. 1964. Personality types in medical management. In *Psychiatry and medical practice in a general hospital,* ed. N. Zinberg, pp. 108–23. New York: International Universities Press. Kahana and Bibring should receive credit for the presentation of a model that applies an understanding of personality factors to practical patient management problems in the hospital setting. If the reader can overlook objections to the stereotyping of patients, which is inevitable in any attempt of classification, these authors provide a foundation for further developments in this important area.

Shapiro, D. 1965. *Neurotic styles.* New York: Basic Books. This monograph is consequential insofar as it provides a connection between three conceptual systems: the neurophysiologic, the cognitive, and the behavioral. Since this material is intended to be consistent with a larger body of psychoanalytic personality theory, some of its terminology may seem difficult to the general medical reader. However, the basic argument is clear and offers a creative perspective for the understanding of personality. Basically, the author sees that different styles of interacting with the world (in other words, personality styles) reflect underlying differences in information processing determined by factors in brain function. This thesis provides the clinician with a means of understanding some difficult patients and dealing with them more objectively and effectively.

REFERENCES

American Psychiatric Association. 1980. *Diagnostic and statistical manual of mental disorders.* 3rd ed. Prepared by the Task Force on Nomenclature and Statistics. Washington, D.C.: American Psychiatric Association.

Chodoff, P., and Lyons H. 1958. Hysteria, the hysterical personality and "hysterical conversion." *Am. J. Psychiatry* 114:734–40.

Cohen, D.J. 1974. Competence and biology: Methodology in studies of infants, twins, psychosomatic disease, and psychosis. In *The child in his family—Children at psychiatric risk*, vol. 3, pp. 361–94. New York: John Wiley & Sons Inc.

Engel, G.L. 1959. "Psychogenic" pain and the pain-prone patient. *Am. J. Med.* 26:899–18.

Erikson, E. 1950. *Childhood and society.* New York: W.W. Norton & Co.

Freeman, C.; Calsyn, D.; and Louks, J. 1976. The use of the Minnesota Multiphasic Personality inventory with low back pain patients. *J. Clin. Psychol.* 32:294–98.

Galin, D. 1974. Implications for psychiatry of left and right cerebral specialization. *Arch. Gen. Psychiatry* 31:572–83.

Goldstein, K. 1952. The effect of brain damage on the personality. *Psychiatry* 15:245–60.

Groves, J.E. 1978. Taking care of the hateful patient. N. *Engl. J. Med.* 298:883–87.

——— 1981. Borderline personality disorder. *N. Engl. J. Med.* 305:259–62.

Gunderson, J.G., and Kolb, J. 1978. Discriminating features of borderline patients. *Am. J. Psychiatry* 135:792–96.

Hutchings, B., and Mednick, S.A. 1974. Registered criminality in the adoptive and biological parents of registered male adoptees. In *Genetic research in psychiatry*, eds. R.R. Fieve; H. Bill; and D. Rosenthal. New York: University Press.

Kahana, R.J., and Bibring, G.L. 1964. Personality types in medical management. In *Psychiatry and medical practice in a general hospital*, ed. N. Zinberg., pp. 108–23. New York: International Universities Press.

Keith, R.A.; Lown, B.; and Stare, F.J. 1965. Coronary heart disease and behavior patterns: An examination of method. *Psychosom. Med.* 27:424–34.

Leigh, H., and Reiser, M.F. 1980. *The patient: Biological, psychological and social dimensions of medical practice.* New York: Plenum Medical Book Co.

Lipsitt, D.R. 1970. Medical and psychological characteristics of "crocks." *Psychol. Med.* 1:15–25.

Maletzky, B.M. 1973. The episodic dyscontrol syndrome. *Dis. Nerv. Syst.* 34:178–85.

Rifkin, A.; Quitkin, E.; Carillo, C., et al. 1972. Lithium carbonate in emotionally unstable character disorder. *Arch. Gen. Psychiatry* 24:519–23.

Shapiro, D. 1965. *Neurotic styles.* New York: Basic Books.

Wiltse, L.L., and Rocchio, P.D. 1975. Predicting success to low back surgery by use of preoperative psychological tests. *J. Bone Joint Surg.* (Am.) 57:478–83.

Zetzel, E. 1971. A developmental approach to the borderline patient. *Am. J. Psychiatry* 128:867–71.

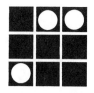

CHAPTER 5

Recognition, Evaluation, and Differential Diagnosis of Psychiatric and Somatic Conditions

Richard J. Loewenstein, M.D.
Henry R. Black, M.D.

In previous chapters we discussed the elements of comprehensive evaluation of patients in the biological, personal, and environmental dimensions. Implicit in this approach is the recognition that factors in these dimensions interact with each other in disease and health. In this chapter, we will examine more closely the interaction between physical and psychiatric conditions, or the somatopsychosomatic relationships. A most important task for the physician is the differential diagnostic process that *includes* physical disorders in patients who have psychiatric symptoms and psychiatric disorders in patients who have physical symptoms.

RELATIONSHIPS BETWEEN PHYSICAL AND MENTAL DISORDERS

Physicians have traditionally been taught that disease is either "organic" or "functional." This dichotomy has its roots in nineteenth-and early twentieth-century anatomic-pathologic studies which failed to find gross changes in the brains of patients with mental illness except for those suffering from general paresis of the insane (tertiary neurosyphilis). (See Mayer-Gross, 1969; Akiskal and McKinney, 1973; and Geschwind, 1975; for historical and theoretical discussion.) Eventually, clinical thinking about disease evolved so that illness was classified as functional if symptoms were thought only to have a psychologic etiology, and organic if grossly detectable disturbances were present in brain tissue. Logically, this dichotomy is specious since all "mental" activity is on some level reducible to organic terms. Although clinically useful in many ways, a rigid distinction between functional and organic means that clinicians often view symptoms as *either* functional or organic and fail to recognize the complex interplay between psychologic and physical factors in determining the nature of a patient's symptoms, complaints, and behavior.

The goal of this chapter is to establish a method of differential diagnosis of medical and psychiatric illnesses that exhibit overlapping and, often, nonspecific symptoms. This task is one of the most difficult and challenging in medicine and one that most often falls to the primary physician. The possibility of misdiagnosis is serious; errors may result in long, unnecessary delays in discovering grave, treatable illness. Unfortunately, using terms like "medical illness" and "psychiatric illness" may seem to perpetuate the organic/functional split discussed above. It is regrettable that current medical vocabulary is unable to account adequately for these complex disease entities without perpetuating aspects of terminological dualism, but our use of such terms here does not imply that one group of disorders is any more or less organic—or for that matter any more or less "psychosocial" than the other. Rather, we use these terms almost sociologically, in that the internist who makes the diagnosis of depressive illness may wish to consult with a psychiatric colleague or a psychiatrist who finds evidence that his or her psychotic patient suffers from Wilson's disease would probably seek counsel from medical associates.

Consideration of psychiatric illness in the differential diagnosis of physical complaints should be an *active* and *routine* process. Clinicians are aware of the consequences of failing to recognize medical illness and falsely labeling a patient as "psychiatric." On the other hand, failure to make the appropriate psychiatric diagnosis may have equally grave consequences. The absence of a usual medical explanation for a patient's complaint certainly does not mean that nothing is wrong. The primary care physician must be cognizant of the complexity of ambiguous situations or seemingly unclassifiable problems. The physician should be especially careful to avoid premature categorization of a patient's difficulties as having *either* a medical or psychiatric origin.

Psychiatrically ill patients may first show symptoms of behavioral, or emotional dysfunction by their exaggerated reaction to minor physical problems. They may also compromise their health by maladaptive behavior, such as failure to comply with medical regimen, denial of the existence of illness, or avoidance of appropriate healthy activity. These maladaptive patterns of response to illness or to medical care may be revealing signs of disturbance best understood in psychiatric terms, and not necessarily evidence of consciously "bad" behavior, inexplicable ingratitude, or stupidity. The alert physician is attuned to the possible meanings behind these often frustrating behavior patterns. Notable clues to psychiatric disturbance may be discovered by meticulous evaluation of the patterns of response to illness. Even physicians' reactions to these patients may be of use in evaluating them (see Chapter 4; and Groves, 1978).

On the other hand, many patients who come to a physician, or are brought by their families have disturbances *they* already believe to have a psychological cause. In this case the historical data will be slanted in that direction. If the possibility of a medical etiology is not entertained at the outset, referral to psychiatrists may be premature and the potential for missing serious disease is increased (Koranyi, 1972). The psychiatrist may feel a false sense of security when a patient is referred by a medical colleague, since the psychiatrist may assume that the possibility of organic disease has been excluded. This situation may be particularly dangerous when referral is made to a nonmedical mental health care professional (Hall et al., 1979).

The primary physician has to make critical determinations about the origin of a patient's disturbance to undertake appropriate medical strategy and referral. Thus, he or she must be aware of the presenting patterns of important psychiatric disorders as well as those of the usual medical problems. Delineation of the underlying cause of symptoms may be slow and frustrating, especially in cases in which both types of illness coexist. The next section describes a general framework to simplify the task of differential diagnosis and points out areas of ambiguity where errors are most easily made.

PSYCHIATRIC DISORDERS THAT PRESENT WITH SOMATIC COMPLAINTS

Primary physicians spend a considerable portion of their time—estimates range up to about 50%—in treating patients who suffer primarily from psychiatric disturbance, particularly anxiety

disorder and depression. Many of these patients see only the primary physician for their treatment (Kline, 1976). Such patients may be particularly confusing since they may have physical complaints with little or no obvious medical explanation. They frequently resist vigorously the suggestion that their difficulties lie in the psychiatric realm. To further complicate the clinician's predicament, many patients with chronic medical illness will tolerate symptoms for long periods of time, but only complain of them at times of emotional stress (Shulman, 1977). For these reasons, the clinician in the primary care setting must be especially adept at evaluating perplexing or atypical patients.

Depression and Anxiety

One diagnostic issue is important to clarify: psychiatrists distinguish "depressive illness" and "anxiety disorder" from the temporary moods of depression and anxiety normally experienced by all human beings from time to time. The former are thought of as complex states characterized by specific symptoms in addition to depressed or anxious moods (see Chapters 9 & 11). This differentiation may be difficult in patients with chronic medical illnesses with symptoms which overlap with those of depressive and anxiety disorders. Furthermore, some patients may show "masked depressions" in which the main symptoms are persistent physical complaints. One such patient was described by Kline (1976). He was a young man who was seen by over 40 different physicians, had two abdominal operations, and spent 21 weeks in the hospital before the diagnosis of depression was entertained!

The primary clinician should *routinely* consider depressive illness in the differential diagnosis especially when a patient's symptoms are atypical or seem not to respond to usual treatments. Often fruitful historical inquiry can be made by asking questions that help relate the somatic complaint to a depressive syndrome. For example, if asking, "Does the pain keep you awake at night?" evokes an affirmative answer, the primary clinician then can pursue the exact nature of the sleep problem. Then it may be easier to distinguish a sleep disturbance typical of depression from one with a pattern more typical of a medical illness (such as, paroxysmal nocturnal dyspnea or sleep interrupted by pain). If depression is considered early in the evaluation of the complicated patient, many patients will be spared painful, expensive, and, even mutilating diagnostic procedures.

Some patients in fact may have an awareness that they are anxious, depressed, or suffering acute emotional stress. They may prefer, however, to focus initially on a physical complaint as a reason for seeking medical help. A physical problem is a socially acceptable reason to see the doctor while a stigma remains about psychiatric illness. The patient who comes with a minor complaint may need much more than simple reassurance. The symptom, however trivial, may be a clue to much turmoil below the surface. The importance of further pursuit of

symptoms that seem to be without apparent organic etiology is illustrated in Case History 5–1.

The case history shows that the failure to recognize depressive illness is not only costly and fraught with risk, but *it can be life-threatening!* Capstick (1960) found that of 889 reported suicides in Wales in the years 1951 to 1955, 78% had been treated by a physician (usually a nonpsychiatrist) in the month prior to death *for symptoms related to their psychiatric disturbance*. Some 9% had "*openly wished for death or had said they intended to kill themselves*" (italics ours). Only 18% of these future suicides were referred for psychiatric evaluation. In more recent studies in America, Murphy (1977) found that of 60 suicides, 10 had seen a physician in the 48 hours prior to death. More than two thirds of his sample had seen a physician during the 3 months before death.

The best approach to avoid missing serious depressive illness is to *routinely* inquire about a

---

CASE HISTORY 5–1

A hard-working woman in her mid-twenties consulted her family doctor because of 'arm heaviness.' She had become pregnant some months ago despite severe marital difficulties. Her husband insisted that the patient have an abortion. Despite a strong desire for children and a strict religious upbringing, she acquiesced to her husband in the hope of saving the marriage. After the abortion, the husband withdrew even further and soon appeared to be having an affair. The patient suffered from severely depressed mood, guilty ruminations about the abortion, crying spells, difficulties with sleep, loss of appetite, and lack of concentration

and energy. She continued to work with considerable difficulty. She began to have paranoid ideas that people were calling her a 'murderess.' She began to wonder what it would feel like to hold a baby. This gave rise to a sensation of 'heaviness' in her arms. She was a shy and constricted woman who was deeply ashamed of the abortion. Thus she volunteered only the information about her arms to her physician. After a brief physical exam, the doctor told her, 'It's nothing to worry about, it's just nerves.' The next day she ingested a lethal dose of medication and was hospitalized.

patient's mood, sleep, appetite, weight change, concentration ability, energy level, sexual function, and ability to perform daily tasks. The assessment of these areas will often be extremely productive in evaluating symptoms acutely as well as in establishing the vital baseline data about a patient's life style. If depressive symptoms are elicited, the patient should be questioned *routinely* about suicidal ideas, plans, and intent (see Chapters 9 and 10).

In addition to inquiry about symptoms suggestive of mood disorder, a routine history should contain information about significant relationships in the patient's life: spouse, children, parents, friends, relatives. It is particularly important to have information about deceased relatives: what they died of, at what age, as well as how old the patient was when parents or other important relatives died. These data are useful in assessing reactions that patients may have to illness. For example, if a patient contracts the same disorder as a family member, the patient may assume that he or she will suffer exactly as the relative did. Clarification of an issue like this may greatly simplify treatment.

The clinician should be aware of the phenomena of "anniversary reactions." The time of year that a close relative or spouse passed away may occasion depressed feelings—and sometimes a full-blown depressive episode. Anniversary reaction may also occur when a person reaches the age at which a parent died. The patient may worry that his or her time has come. The physician who routinely obtains such information is in a much better position to evaluate future change in the status of a patient's complaints. It is also important to determine the patient's usual reaction to stress. Some people become angry, others anxious; some develop diarrhea, others headaches. Understanding the patient's usual repertoire of psychic and somatic reactions is important since the development of a new uncharacteristic symptom solely in response to stress is an unusual event. One should assess carefully patients with chronic somatic complaints or those suffering from chronic anxious or depressive disorders who change their usual pattern of symptoms or exhibit new ones. The first task in this situation is to rule out a new medical illness. Another possible cause for such a change would be an acute psychiatric decompensation with a marked exacerbation of symptoms.

Differential Diagnosis

Other historical data may be quite revealing in sorting out the cause of a patient's complaints. *Ask the patient* what he or she thinks is wrong. In the extreme case, the symptom may represent a delusional preoccupation which may go unrecognized unless the patient's own interpretation of the symptom is solicited. An example is illustrated in Case History 5–2.

Other revealing information may be obtained by questioning the patient about any changes in his or her life. "Good" events may actually be quite stressful. A promotion, an impending marriage, a move to a new city are generally pleasurable and satisfying but may have frightening or worrisome aspects for many people. Such life events may mean worries over loss of friends, changes in routine, or anxiety over sexual matters. Even in our liberated age considerable ignorance and fear about sex abounds—even among those with considerable sexual experience. A good rule of thumb is to assume that all patients are in need of accurate information concerning sexual matters. Even if the patient is not in need of such information, inquiries concerning sexual matters will not be wasted. The patient will remember the physician as one with whom he or she can discuss such matters in the future. As long as the questioning is respectful and tactful, even if the patient denies any difficulty, the patient will be appreciative of the knowledge that sex is an area that can be discussed with the physician.

How, then, does the harried and hurried clinician decide which patients have primarily medical illness, or primarily psychiatric illness, or both? Hall and colleagues (1979) describe a number of patient characteristics that may help to discriminate those with psychiatric illness from those with medical illness. The time frame may be helpful. *Psychiatric* symptoms of *medical* etiology are likely to begin suddenly, whereas similar symptoms caused by psychiatric disturbance often begin insidiously, have a vague onset and continue for long periods of time. Thus, development of a notable change in behavior, mood, or thinking in a previously healthy person with a seemingly adequate work, family, social, and personal adjustment is presumptive evidence of a medical disorder. Caution is necessary, however, even on this point, since disorders such as carcinoma or chronic renal or hepatic disease may exhibit vague symptoms such as depression, fatigue, and weight loss which develop slowly and insidiously. On the other hand, some psychiatric disorders such as mania or depression may begin quite suddenly with little apparent prodrome.

Other characteristics cited by Hall and associates (1979) that suggest underlying psychiatric disturbance include:

1. Long history of social and emotional problems

2. Numerous somatic complaints, which involve multiple organ systems and correspond to no known physical disease

3. Bizarre symptoms

4. Conventional treatment failure

5. Exaggerated, minimized, or distorted concern about a particular symptom

6. History of "doctor shopping"

7. Multiple social or psychological stresses

8. Drug abuse.

None of the characteristics cited, however, exclude the presence of a medical disorder. Eastwood (1975) presents data to suggest that patients with many of these characteristics may in fact have the greatest risk of concurrent medical illness. Hall and associates (1979) feel that if only one or a few of these characteristics are present, they may be more misleading than helpful. Focusing on the psychosocial difficulties may lead to neglect of the possible medical problems. Using standard tests Eastwood (1975)

CASE HISTORY 5–2

A 24-year-old single unemployed male came to an outpatient medical clinic of a university hospital. His complaint was of crampy abdominal pain, localized in the mid-epigastrium. He was monosyllabic and seemed guarded and expressionless during history-taking. The patient denied history of alcohol or drug abuse. He felt the pain was improved by eating. He assented when asked if the pain awakened him from sleep. Physical findings were equivocal. The patient underwent gallbladder series, upper GI studies and endoscopy, the results of all of which were normal. The patient was finally told that there was 'nothing wrong' with his stomach. Referral to psychiatry was obtained. During a psychiatric interview the patient confided that he was particularly upset at his medical doctor's statement that 'nothing was wrong.' The patient state that something definitely *was* wrong: He was dead and in Hell. Devils and demons were eating his stomach, causing him pain.

generated results that imply that there is a "positive and significant association" between psychiatric and medical morbidity. He suggests that the results are consistent with the notion that "either . . . individuals with long-standing psychiatric disorder are subject to all forms of physical morbidity or that in the community there are people who are vulnerable to all types of illness."

Differential diagnosis becomes even more obscure when medical and psychiatric disorders coexist. Depressive and anxious states are frequently seen in patients with medical illness and clearly affect the symptoms and the treatment of clinical illness.

It has been found that 30%–60% of medical inpatients and 50%–80% of medical outpatients suffer from some type of emotional difficulties (Lipowski, 1975; Glass et al., 1978; Lancet; 1979). Medical patients manifesting a depressive syndrome are more likely to suffer from multiple or severe medical disorders. They are more likely to have stress at home, to be in pain, to be confined to bed, and to have diminished alertness (Moffic and Paykel, 1975).

These studies confirm the intuitive clinical observation that it is frightening and upsetting to suffer a serious medical illness, especially where long hospitalization, chronic disability, and major disruption of life is involved. Even the hospital environment itself can be stressful.

Reactions to Illness. Illness can *mean* many things to patients and a patient's reactions to illness can be colored as much by those perceptions as by the actual fact of illness. Illness may mean loss of income; change in relationship between family members; reduction in feelings of pride in one's body or control over its fate; or fear of death or disablement.

What an illness actually means to a patient may significantly affect his or her behavior. Some reactions to illness may show themselves in indirect and often self-destructive ways. Patients who fail to comply with medical regimens

are often struggling with problems involved with the meaning of being ill. Medication, for example, becomes the *tangible* symbol of illness. Not taking it means that there is no sickness. All medical people have had experience with the hard-driving coronary patient who flagrantly violates restrictions on physical activity, weight, and stress. At the other extreme, one finds the "cardiac neurotic" who is terror-stricken lest any activity should cause chest discomfort.

The above-mentioned patients are more likely to be reacting to the *meaning* of being ill in general, or the meaning of having the specific illness in question. Because of this, strategies such as shame, exhortation, condemnation, blanket reassurance, and threats rarely help. Careful inquiry into what the patient understands of his or her condition, what causes it, where it is located, how long it will last, how it will affect the quality of life, how long the treatment will last, and whether it will interfere with sexuality often reveal glaring factual distortions which compromise the patient's abilities to cope with the illness. Clarification of factual information may be sufficient to improve maladaptive emotional reactions, but often psychiatric consultation may be warranted for more specialized assessment. Case History 5–3 illustrates how a very demanding and difficult patient showed much improvement after clarification of the nature of the illness.

This case illustrates the complex interrelation between medical illness and psychological functioning. Among the reasons that this patient had difficulty understanding his situation was that the encephalitis had directly affected cognitive functioning. He was an anxious man at baseline. Fever, fear, and CNS dysfunction all combined to make it difficult for him to comprehend the initial explanations offered him when the nature of illness was first diagnosed.

It is wise to reassess the patient's level of understanding of a condition as the course of a hospitalization or episode of illness progresses. Many patients with illnesses that affect oxygenation, metabolism, CNS functioning, endocrine function, or temperature regulation even if only mildly, may have transient decreases in ability to process new information and deal with it constructively. This is especially true if these patients are anxious, sedated, or have mild underlying dementia. The physician should expect patients to misconstrue, misunderstand, and forget information when they are acutely ill. Instead of an angry or indignant response, understanding the need to frequently reeducate the patient about his or her problem is the best strategy. One way to begin this process is to ask the patient what he or she understands is wrong. In this way, the physician can quickly correct distortions and reinforce what is accurate.

The provision of accurate information may at times be stressful; for the cancer patient who finds out that the illness is terminal; for the paraplegic who must hear that movement will no longer return to his legs. The reactions to grave or profoundly disabling illness are quite complex but predictable and the clinician should be aware of what may occur. Patients often go through a *series* of responses to a severe chronic illness beginning with denial and progressing through anger and despair to acceptance. Not all patients exhibit all stages or go through them in the same order. Recognition of this phasic process may help in reassuring staff and family in their interactions with the patient. The physician who can anticipate problems and assist the patient in resolving his or her feelings is creating an alliance with the patient that will help with treatment and improve the quality of life for the patient and his or her family (see for example, Kubler-Ross, 1969; Weller and Miller, 1977a and 1977b).

CASE HISTORY 5–3

An automobile mechanic in his twenties was admitted to the hospital with the sudden onset of weakness in his lower extremities. Neurologic exam indicated abnormal reflexes and a fluctuating sensory deficit in the lower extremities, as well as weakness. The patient had recently undergone an extensive workup for symptoms of weakness, malaise, fatigue, and adenopathy. A lymphoma had been suspected. The test results had been normal and a diagnosis of mononucleosis was entertained. On admission, the staff was concerned that the patient had a spinal cord tumor. Further tests, however, suggested a viral myelitis and encephalitis. Conservative treatment was instituted. The patient became anxious, demanding, agitated, and complaining. He suffered from back pain unrelieved by large amounts of analgesics. Asking the patient about his understanding of the current medical situation revealed that he was terrified that he had a malignancy. He was ruminating over one doctor's statement that since this was a viral problem, 'there was nothing one could do.' The patient had seen several family members die of cancer and lymphoma. The patient was certain his case was 'hopeless.' He was anxious about the effect his sickness would have on his young wife. Clarification of the nature of the patient's illness by the attending physician was of immense relief to the patient—and to his wife in whom the patient had been confiding his worst fears. After this, the demands for medication and the other maladaptive behaviors decreased markedly, although they did not cease altogether.

MEDICAL ILLNESSES THAT PRESENT WITH PSYCHIATRIC SYMPTOMS

Many medical illnesses are known to cause dysfunction in thinking, emotions, or behavior. Medical illnesses can present with a depressive syndrome, anxiety symptoms, confusional states, paranoid reactions, schizophreniform psychoses, manic behavior, and even personality disorder, as well as the more classical organic brain syndromes (see Chapters 6–12). Systemic lupus erythematosus (SLE), acute intermittent porphyria (AIP), Wilson's disease, intracranial neoplasm, and complex-partial seizures (temporal lobe epilepsy), among other diseases, may mimic a variety of psychiatric disorders— sometimes before the more typical physical symptoms and signs are evident.

Recent studies from psychiatric outpatient facilities suggest that a great many more medical diseases may present with psychiatric symptoms than had been suspected (Koranyi, 1972, 1977a, 1977b, 1979; Hall et al., 1978). Koranyi (1979) found that 43% of 2070 patients referred to a psychiatric clinic had significant medical illness. In about half of these patients the medical illness was undiagnosed by referral sources at the time of intake at his clinic. Of the medically ill patients, 18% had an illness producing the symptoms for which psychiatric referral had been sought. In another 51%, the physical illness was thought to aggravate an already existent psychiatric problem. In the remainder, the medical and psychiatric disorders coexisted. In addition, in the total group of patients, death rates from all causes—accident, suicide, and "natural"—were found to be twice as high as in the general population. Even the patients who died of accidents or suicide had more intercurrent medical illness than suspected (Koranyi, 1977a).

Koranyi's work (1972, 1977a, 1979) and that of others (Lipowski, 1975; Hall et al., 1978) imply that underdiagnosis of medical problems is common in a variety of psychiatric populations. In particular, these studies suggest that diabetes mellitus is frequently overlooked as a cause or exacerbating factor in psychiatric disturbance. Anxiety, depressive illness, and disturbance due to the effects of this illness—such as marital conflict in reaction to impotence—are thought to be extremely common. Illnesses commonly producing or exacerbating psychiatric dysfunction were:

1. Endocrine disorders (such as thyroid disease)

2. Cardiovascular disease (such as coronary artery disease, rheumatic heart disease, congestive heart failure)

3. Infectious diseases (especially venereal diseases, hepatitis, and mononucleosis)

4. Blood disorders (especially anemia and hemoglobinopathies)

5. Pulmonary disorders (such as pneumonia, asthma, and chronic obstructive pulmonary disease)

6. Cerebrovascular disease, seizure disorders, encephalopathies, and demyelinating disorders.

Koranyi (1979) found that infectious, endocrine, and hemotologic disorders were the most likely to be missed at the time of psychiatric referral. In addition, toxic drug reactions were often overlooked at the time of referral (Koranyi, 1979).

Hysteria and Medical Disease*

The classic study of Slater and Glithero (1965) presents another aspect of the problem of medical illnesses with so-called psychiatric presentations. They followed up 99 patients who had received the diagnosis of "hysteria" after an inpatient workup at a large teaching hospital. After 7–9 years, they found that 4 patients had committed suicide, and 8 patients had died of disorders such as vascular diseases and neoplasia which *"must have been present at the time*

---

* See also Chapter 13.

the diagnosis of 'hysteria' was made" (italics added). Some 22 patients had significant organic illness which explained the presenting complaints but had remained undiagnosed at the time the diagnosis of hysteria was made. Included were gallbladder disease, meningitis, Takayashu's syndrome, and presenile dementia. Only 32 patients showed no physical illness at the time of follow-up studies. Of these, however 11 patients had developed symptoms of a major psychiatric disorder such as schizophrenia or major depressive disorder. Thus, *only about 20% of the original sample were diagnosed as hysterical when follow-up studies were completed.*

The implications of these studies are clear. Careful baseline physical and laboratory screening of patients who have alterations in behavior, mood, and thinking is mandatory. Furthermore, one must always maintain an index of suspicion that *at a later time* a medical etiology may declare itself. Thus, longitudinal evaluation of such patients is paramount.

Catatonia and Paranoia*

The initial difficulty in labeling a patient as having psychiatric or medical disease is that the behavioral syndromes or symptoms are often "final common pathways" of diverse etiologic forces. Although there are some data which may be suggestive of a medical etiology or a behavioral disorder, none is absolutely diagnostic. For example, recent reviews of catatonic (Gelenberg, 1976), and paranoid syndromes (Manshreck and Petri, 1978), suggest multiple etiologies for these symptoms previously thought to be monolithically diagnostic of schizophrenia. To be sure, catatonic symptoms are found in schizophrenia, although this is not as common as it used to be. Catatonic symptoms are also found, however, in unipolar depressions, manic-depressive illness, conversion disorder, and dissociative states. Catatonia can be found in neurologic diseases, especially

* See also Chapters 7, 8, and 13.

those involving the basal ganglia, limbic system, diencephalon, and frontal lobes, as well as in diffuse processes such as viral encephalitis. Catatonic symptoms have been seen in hypercalcemia from parathyroid adenoma, diabetic ketoacidosis, pellagra, AIP, and hepatic encephalopathy. Toxic and pharmacologic agents such as mescaline, phencyclidine (PCP), phenothiazines, and steroids have been described as causing catatonic symptoms (Gelenberg, 1976).

Paranoia can be seen not only in schizophrenia but also mania, depression, personality disorders, and classically in acute delirium. Neurologic disorders such as presenile and senile dementia, temporal lobe epilepsy, Huntington's chorea, brain tumor, subarachnoid hemorrhage, subdural hematoma, and postencephalitic Parkinsonism have frequently been reported as having associated paranoid features. Endocrine, metabolic, and infectious conditions also have shown paranoid symptomatology. Abnormalities of sex chromatin, especially Klinefelter's syndrome, have also been associated with paranoid symptoms. Alcohol, cocaine, marijuana, amphetamines, bromides, barbiturates, hallucinogens, PCP, anticholinergics, exogenous steroids, levodopa, phenytoin, tricyclic antidepressants, and monoamine-oxidase (MAO) inhibitors, *among others* are drugs which have been associated with paranoid symptoms in acute or chronic use (Slater and Beard, 1963; Swanson and Stipes, 1969; Mayer-Gross, 1969; Glass and Bowers, 1970; Bowers, 1972; Sorensen and Nielsen, 1977; Freedman and Schwab, 1978; Kristensen and Sindrup, 1978a and 1978b; Manschrek and Petri, 1978).

Other Psychiatric Symptoms

Symptoms such as depressed mood, anxiety, anorexia, weight loss, fatigue, decreased energy, interference with libido, pain, and gastrointestinal dysfunction may be the presenting manifestations of metabolic, infectious, toxic, endocrine, and malignant, as well as psychiatric, disorders (Mayer-Gross, 1969; Kiev, 1974; Post, 1975). The importance of accurate diagnosis is even crucial because institution of psychiatric therapy with behavior-altering drugs or electroconvulsive therapy (ECT) may considerably cloud the diagnostic picture.

A complicating factor in the evaluation of mental changes associated with many organic disorders with psychiatric symptoms is the reaction of people to the stress of having the disorder itself. Changes in appearance, life-threatening complications, disability, loss of limbs or organs, and difficulty with activities of daily living all may cause profound psychological reactions. As emphasized before, these psychological reactions may interact with or contribute to symptoms caused more directly by pathologic derangements of metabolism or structure of brain tissue (Sachar, 1975).

The current view is that many mental disturbances like manic-depression and schizophrenia ultimately will be found to have a major contribution from organic factors—although derangements will be observed in *pathophysiology* not pathoanatomy (see for example, Lipton et al., 1977). Data continues to support a significant role for environmental factors in the etiology of these disorders, as well (Baldessarini, 1977; Kidd and Matthysee, 1978).

The version just given of "mental illness" is not so different from current views of the etiologic factors in such diseases as diabetes mellitus or coronary artery disease. Current concepts of these diseases take into account genetic factors (family history), environmental factors (such as smoking, obesity, diet), immediate stressors (for example, physical exertion, strong emotion, infection), and even personality variables (Type A or Type B personality) in a complex interplay that may result in an episode of illness. In addition, once an illness is established as an autonomous condition, aspects of the disease process itself or side effects of treatment may cause problems quite apart from the initial etiologic factors. Thus diabetics may develop renal failure or difficulties secondary to insulin

reactions. Schizophrenics may suffer from the effects of chronic psychosis on personality function or become afflicted with tardive dyskinesia secondary to use of neuroleptic medication.

Since there are no absolutely reliable criteria for differential diagnosis of medical illness that present with psychiatric dysfunction, the clinician must maintain a high index of suspicion in both directions—that somatic symptoms may have psychiatric causes and that behavioral disturbances may have somatic etiology.

DIFFERENTIAL DIAGNOSIS

Depression and Mood Changes*

It seems that diagnosis of depression is often the most problematic in medical patients with medical illness, or in patients with physical symptoms without easily explicable organic cause. Thyroid disease, carcinoma, renal failure, heart failure, hepatic failure, and early senile dementia, as well as viral infections and anemias of all types can be associated with syndromes of dysphoric mood, poor appetite, weight loss, sleep disturbances, decreased libido, and changes in energy and ability to concentrate Table 5–1. The clinician can usually exclude most of these conditions with simple laboratory tests although it may be difficult to exclude an occult malignancy.

One helpful differential diagnostic strategy is to pursue the subjective perception of the patient concerning his or her condition. Depressed patients are more likely to experience guilty ruminations, to blame themselves for their predicament, to feel sad, tearful, unhappy, and suicidal. They may appear to be *unrealistically* pessimistic about treatment, chance for recovery, and future restoration of function. Depressed patients may be preoccupied exclusively and unshakably with personal concerns such as contamination, cancer, or venereal disease.

---

* See also Chapter 9.

TABLE 5–1
Medical illnesses presenting with alterations in mood

ENDOCRINE	SUBSTANCE ABUSE	OTHER DRUGS	INFECTIOUS DISEASES	SYSTEMIC DISEASES	HEMATOLOGIC DISORDERS
Thyroid disease	Alcohol	Reserpine	Syphilis	Carcinoma	Anemias
Disorders of pituitary-adrenal function	Sedative-hypnotics	Methyl-dopa	Influenza	End-organ failure (renal, cardiac, hepatic)	
Cushing's disease	Narcotic analgesics	Propran-olol	Common cold	Wilson's disease	
Cushing's syndrome	Cocaine, ampheta-mines	Diuretics	Hepatitis	Systemic lupus erythema-tosus	
Exogenous ACTH			St. Louis encephalitis	Acute intermittent por-phyria	
Exogenous corticoster-oids			Rabies		
Addison's disease			Typhus		
Hypo/hyperparathyroidism			Typhoid		
Klinefelter's syndrome					
Pituitary/hypothalamic syn-dromes					
Diabetes mellitus					

Although these subjective perceptions of the patient may represent evidence for the presence of depressive illness, their presence alone is not sufficient for the diagnosis of the psychiatric disorder. Fras and his coworkers (1967) showed that carcinoma of the pancreas was frequently associated with psychiatric symptoms, especially those of a depressive nature, and that these symptoms often occurred before other physical manifestations of the cancer. A substantial percentage of those patients complained of "loss of ambition" or "loss of initiative" in the absence of fatigue or weakness. Many of these patients also felt inexplicably sad, low, "down in the dumps" and described premonitions of impending disaster. In this study other neoplastic disorders such as colonic carcinoma or lymphoma were found to be far less likely to produce a depressive syndrome, although it still occurred in a number of cases.

Another complicating variable may be a depressive disorder *superimposed* upon a terminal or chronic medical illness such as carcinoma or renal failure. Such situations are extremely hard to sort out. It may be difficult to distinguish a patient's realistic resignation and pessimism from inappropriate nihilism. Since the physical concomitants of depressive illness, such as sleep, appetite, and energy disturbance, can be produced by such diseases, these physical signs become less useful in diagnosis. In such a situation consultation with the family to uncover any noticeable mood or behavior change may be of help. Knowledge of the cultural, religious, or philosophic background of the patient and family may also help in assessing appropriateness of response to a chronic or terminal illness.

Endocrine Disorders.   Other medical illnesses may show symptoms of depression. Patients with endocrine disturbances frequently manifest changes in mood. *Thyroid disease* is one of the most well-known examples. Authorities agree that the vast majority of patients with mental changes due to hypothyroidism will show sub-

stantial recovery with treatment. Diagnosis and treatment are critical, however, because the degree of recovery is inversely proportional to the duration of illness in most cases—complete recovery generally occurs if duration of illness is less than two years (Smith et al., 1972; Sachar, 1975; Hall et al., 1979).

Despite the commonly held association between hypothyroidism and psychosis ("myxedema madness"), this presentation of hypothyroidism is relatively rare (see Davidoff and Gill, 1977). The most important and common mental changes that accompany hypothyroidism may lead to an erroneous diagnosis of depressive illness. The patient exhibits psychomotor retardation, decreased interest, slowed thinking, easy fatiguability, insomnia, self-blame, and poor concentration. Activities of daily living may become too difficult to perform. Signs of intellectual and cognitive impairment appear with deficits in attention, abstraction, and comprehension. Psychotic features may be present with depressive or persecutory delusions, hallucinations, anxiety, agitation, and hypochondriasis. Epidemiologic considerations may actually add to the difficulty in diagnosis since both depression and hypothyroidism occur most frequently in women between the ages of 30–60 years (Weissman and Meyers, 1978; Hall et al., 1979). The more characteristic physical findings of hypothyroidism may not be present. Since laboratory diagnosis of thyroid function is relatively cheap and simple, and since this is one of the few completely reversible mental illnesses, one should never hesitate to order thyroid function tests for depressed patients. Although it is rare, apathetic hyperthyroidism may be manifested as a depressive syndrome, often complicated by psychotic and paranoid features as well as suicidal behavior (Taylor, 1975; Brenner, 1978).

Mood disorder has been frequently described in conjunction with disorders of the pituitary-adrenal axis. Reports of "moderate to severe" mental changes in disorders of pituitary-adrenal function have ranged from 40%–60% in some series (Smith et al., 1972). Psychiatric syndromes have been described in Cushing's disease (arising from intracranial pathology), Cushing's syndrome (based on an extracranial primary lesion), and in situations where exogenous steroids or adrenocorticotropic hormones (ACTH) are administered. Elated states, manic excitement, depressed states, psychotic depression, and mixed dysphoric-euphoric or rapidly alternating states have been described. In addition, paranoid and hallucinatory states similar to schizophrenia are seen. Symptoms such as agitation, irritability, insomnia, anxiety, and poor concentration have been described. Confusional states and other typical organic brain syndromes with disorientation are thought to be less frequent. Organic features may color the mood disorder, however (Mayer-Gross, 1969; Smith et al., 1972; Sachar, 1975; Carroll, 1977).

Sachar (1975) and Carroll (1977) compiled data to suggest that depression may be more common in conditions with high ACTH production such as Cushing's disease, Addison's disease or in situations where exogenous ACTH has been used in treatment. Exogenous corticosteroids seem more likely to produce elation.

Mental syndromes due to administration of exogenous corticosteroids or ACTH are of increasing importance since these agents are widely used therapeutically. Differentiation of syndromes due to the underlying condition or to steroid therapy is often problematic especially in disorders like SLE which are known to cause many different psychiatric symptoms. The onset of steroid-induced mental changes does not seem to correlate with increase, decrease, or steady state of drug. Alterations in mental states may occur in patients who had previously tolerated, without difficulty, the same dose of drug in the past. Treatment usually consists of discontinuation of steroid medications. If steroids cannot be stopped, the best action is to treat symptoms with antipsychotic or antimanic agents (see Chapter 21).

Hypoadrenal states (Addison's disease) may also be associated with multiple psychiatric symptoms including depression, anxiety, irritability, paranoia, psychosis, and delirium (Smith et al., 1972). Apathy, fatigue, and negativism may appear as part of the primary constellation of symptoms of this disorder. Convulsions may occur. Hypoglycemia and other indirect effects of the illness may also contribute to the psychiatric syndrome.

Other endocrine disorders which may rarely present with depressive symptoms include hyperparathyroidism and hypoparathyroidism, although both of these are far more likely to give rise to delirious states (Smith et al., 1972). Klinefelter's syndrome may also be associated with affective illness (Nielson, 1969; Sachar, 1975; Sorensen and Nielsen, 1977; Caroff, 1978). Pituitary and hypothalamic disorders have also been occasionally misdiagnosed as depression.

Diabetes Mellitus.   Several authors have recently pointed out the association of diabetes mellitus and psychiatric disorders (Koranyi, 1977b, 1979, Hall et al., 1978). In our experience depression is often misdiagnosed when the diabetic patient begins to develop an organic brain syndrome characterized by apathy and anergy. Frequently, these patients are developing dementia secondary to cerebrovascular disease, although distant effects of failure of other organ systems (such as the kidney) may also play a part. Cognitive impairment may often be overlooked because the "depression" seems "understandable." As always, however, there is a strong likelihood that dementia and depressive illness may coexist in diabetic patients.

Drugs.   Alcohol and drug abuse—particularly sedative-hypnotic abuse—often give rise to syndromes indistinguishable from depression. Opiate abuse may also generate symptoms that appear to be depressive in origin. The physician should always be aware that *any* patient may abuse drugs or alcohol. Medical professionals such as nurses and doctors who have easy access to drugs may be particularly at risk.

Problems in correct diagnostic assessment may occur because drug and alcohol abusing patients usually conceal their substance usage. Once it is discovered, however, they may pressure the physician to treat their depression without acknowledging the significant contribution of substance abuse to their problems. Indeed, alcoholic patients in particular may require several months of abstinence before definitive psychiatric assessment can be made, since normalization of mood, sleep, energy, and appetite, may be a slow process after heavy drinking for long periods of time (see Chapters 15 and 16).

Minor tranquilizers like diazepam (Valium) and chlordiazepoxide (Librium) are widely prescribed, as are the barbiturates, meprobamate (Miltown), glutethimide (Doriden), ethchlorvynol (Placidyl) and others. All are CNS depressants and they may easily give rise to symptoms similar to those of true depressive illness. Elderly patients may frequently have depressive reactions with quite small doses, although paradoxic reactions, with excitement and agitation, are also very common in older patients taking these medications.

Other drugs such as the antihypertensive agents reserpine, methyldopa (Aldomet), and propanolol may give rise to depressive syndromes (Whitlock and Price, 1974; Bant, 1978). Diuretics often make patients weak and fatigued due to hypokalemia and these complaints may be mistaken for depression. As a general rule one should at least consider that medications used by the patient may be responsible for depressive or other psychiatric symptoms.

Infectious Diseases. Infectious diseases may be accompanied by symptoms that mimic depression. Primary and secondary syphilis may give rise to symptoms such as fatigue, irritability, and poor concentration (Mayer-Gross, 1969). Tertiary syphilis is more commonly associated with psychiatric syndromes characterized by

grandiosity, poor judgment, expansiveness, and euphoria. Mania may be diagnosed if the patient's neurologic and intellectual deficits are overlooked. Depressive syndromes, often with delusional overtones may occur. Syphilis must be considered in the differential diagnosis of all psychiatric syndromes. This is especially true since its relative rarity nowadays may lead to its diagnosis being missed. Simple laboratory tests, such as the VDRL or FTA-ABS, will easily exclude this possibility (Luxon et al., 1979).

Influenza and the common cold may be associated with depressed mood and neurovegetative changes. This is especially true in the prodromal and convalescent phases. Mayer-Gross (1969) notes that hepatitis has been complicated by depression and suicide. He also states that rabies, typhus, and typhoid have been associated with depressive symptoms although delirium is the most common manifestation. St. Louis encephalitis commonly gives rise to depression during recovery (Hall et al., 1979).

Systemic Diseases. Systemic diseases like Wilson's disease, SLE, and AIP have been associated with a wide variety of psychiatric symptoms. These disorders may *all* show mental changes masquerading as depression, although affective illness is not the most common psychiatric presentation for any of these symptoms (Cross, 1956; Feinglass et al., 1976; Cartwright, 1978). Screening tests for these diseases are easy and relatively inexpensive to perform. One should not hesitate to order these tests.

Anxiety

Anxiety is probably a ***ubiquitous*** symptom among all patients who come to a physician for any reason. Differential diagnosis may be complicated by the simultaneous presence of symptoms of anxiety and those of the underlying illness (Table 5–2). The evaluation, management and distinction between anxiety and anxiety disorders have already been discussed. Unlike depressive disorders, anxiety disorders are rarely life-threatening although they may cause significant disability and discomfort if they are severe and chronic (Woodruff et al., 1974; Noyes et al., 1978). The medical disorders that can masquerade as anxiety disorders are not so benign, however, and thus require vigilant attention.

As a general rule, anxiety disorders begin in the teens and twenties and rarely occur de novo after age 35 years (Woodruff et al., 1974). One study found that of all women between 15–30 years of age referred for neurologic consultation, 29% had hyperventilation syndrome as the sole cause of their presenting symptoms. In hyperventilation patients over age 30 years, however, almost half had an associated medical illness (Pincus and Tucker, 1978).

Endocrine Disorders. Hyperthyroidism is very commonly associated with symptoms similar to those of anxiety disorder. Thyrotoxic patients may be volatile, irritable, anxious, and jumpy. Anxious patients, however, are more likely to have a psychological precipitant for their illness, to experience depersonalization

---

TABLE 5–2
Medical illnesses presenting with anxiety

Hyperthyroidism
Pheochromocytoma
Carcinoid syndrome
Hypoglycemia/hyperinsulinism
Tachyarrythmias/paroxysmal tachycardia
Temporal lobe epilepsy (partial-complex
    seizures)
Alcohol, sedative-hypnotic withdrawal
Opiate withdrawal
Central nervous system stimulants
    (amphetamine, cocaine,
    sympathomimetics, caffeine)
Pulmonary disease (asthma, decompensated
    chronic lung disease)

---

and panic attacks, to have hysterical symptoms, and to have a younger age of onset. Thyrotoxic patients are more likely to have heat intolerance, to lose weight, and to show fatigue and shortness of breath on effort. Increased appetite and sweating are also common (Mayer-Gross, 1969). Thyrotoxic patients may show mixed syndromes with combinations of dysphoria, depression, anxiety, overactivity, agitation, and even paranoid thinking. Such a state may be mistaken for a major affective illness, such as mania or agitated depression. In general, however, adequate treatment of the underlying illness results in complete resolution of all psychiatric symptoms even those ascribed to "personality disorder" (Mayer-Gross, 1969; Smith, 1972; Sachar, 1975). Physical and laboratory symptoms are usually diagnostic.

Pheochromocytoma classically may cause symptoms easily confused with anxiety states (Mayer-Gross, 1969; Detre and Jarecki, 1971; Shulman, 1977). Symptomatic episodes correspond to periods of elevated arterial pressure, however, and should therefore be readily amenable to diagnosis. Carcinoid tumors may also produce symptoms which can be confused with anxiety disorder. Other endocrine disorders that may manifest symptoms similar to anxiety disorder include hypoglycemia or hyperinsulinism from any cause, hypoparathyroidism, and hyperparathyroidism.

Cardiac and Respiratory Conditions. Anxiety is prominent in cardiac conditions—especially those with disturbance of cardiac rhythm. In particular, paroxysmal tachycardias may be accompanied by symptoms often misdiagnosed as anxiety. A recent report describes a patient with mitral valve prolapse syndrome with tachyarrythmia who met stringent diagnostic criteria for anxiety disorder during episodes of arrhythmia (Pariser et al., 1978).

Asthmatics may show anxiety-like symptoms due to use of sympathomimetics and theophylline-containing drugs. Asthmatics and patients with respiratory failure may experience anxiety symptoms when they are dyspneic. It may be difficult to tell whether such patients are experiencing anxiety as a reaction to their illness or whether their complaints stem from respiratory compromise. Anxiety frequently coexists with pulmonary disease. Differential diagnosis may be aided if the anxiety symptoms seem out of proportion to the physical disability or if symptoms persist in the face of adequate treatment and return of pulmonary function to baseline. Tests of arterial blood gases and pulmonary function may be necessary to evaluate the situation.

Central Nervous System Disorders. Temporal lobe epilepsy may be accompanied by symptoms similar to those found in anxiety and panic disorders (Mayer-Gross, 1969; Detre and Jarecki, 1971). Depersonalization, feelings of ***deja vu***, disorders of perception, and paroxysms of fear, were found in epileptics and also in a group of severely anxious patients. Consciousness disturbances, self-injury, automatisms, disturbed speech, incontinence and, of course, abnormal electroencephalogram readings (EEG) tend to be more common among epileptics (Mayer-Gross, 1969). Dementia and Parkinsonism are other CNS syndromes which in their manifestations may have symptoms mimicking anxiety.

Drugs. Drug and alcohol abuse must always be suspected in the differential diagnosis of anxiety syndromes. Alcohol, barbiturate, and sedative-hypnotic withdrawal are entities with significant morbidity and mortality, which may initially present with tremulousness, restlessness, jumpiness, autonomic hyperactivity, apprehension, distractability, and easy startling. Abrupt discontinuation of high doses of benzodiazepines may result in a withdrawal syndrome similar to barbiturate withdrawal. There is evidence that sudden withdrawal of chronically used therapeutic doses of benzodiazepines may result in a mild withdrawal syndrome with manifestations similar to anxiety symptoms (Pevnick

et al., 1978). The initial manifestations of opiate withdrawal may also be confused with anxiety symptoms. This is not likely to have much relevance in treating the "street" addict who is usually quite obvious when it comes to the origin of his or her symptoms. There are cases, however, of chronically or terminally ill patients being treated with narcotics, when suddenly drugs are withdrawn for medical reasons. Although these patients often have multiple causes for the development of anxiety, reinstitution and then tapering of narcotics reduces their anxiety symptoms.

Central nervous system stimulants such as amphetamines, cocaine, sympathomimetics, and theophylline-related drugs, including caffeine, may all cause symptoms indistinguishable from anxiety. Users of amphetamines may appear with complaints of anxiety, irritability, and sleeplessness and request barbiturates or sedative-hypnotics, which they are liable to abuse as well. Intake of large amounts of caffeine-containing beverages or their sudden withdrawal may result in symptoms much like those of anxiety disorders (Greden, 1974). Hypertensive patients who abruptly stop the antihypertensive agent taking clonidine also appear anxious during withdrawal.

Confusion, Psychosis, and Disordered Thinking

The differential diagnosis of confusion, psychosis, and disordered thinking are discussed together since questions concerning them are often interrelated (Table 5–3). Current psychiatric thinking emphasizes that psychiatric symptoms or syndromes are best thought of as final common pathways with potentially diverse origins. Acute psychosis itself is seen as a relatively nonspecific state, representative of major disruption of the personality by any of a number of causes. Hallucinations, delusions, ideas of reference, and disordered thinking may be seen in acute schizophrenia, acute mania, and even acute depressions (see Pope and Lipinski, 1978).

In addition, such symptoms are almost invariably present in delirium from any cause (see Chapter 6 on differential diagnosis of confusion and organic brain syndrome).

TABLE 5–3
Medical illnesses presenting with confusion, psychosis, and disordered thinking
SYSTEMIC ILLNESSES

Infection (pneumonia, sepsis, etc.) ⎫
Pulmonary embolism ⎪ Particularly in
Congestive heart failure ⎬ the elderly
Myocardial infarction ⎭
Wilson's disease
Acute intermittent porphyria
Systemic lupus erythematosus
All causes of delirium (toxic, metabolic, endocrine, etc.)
Vitamin B_{12} deficiency

INFECTIOUS DISORDERS

Viral (especially herpes) encephalitis
Systemic infection

NEUROLOGIC DISORDERS

Temporal lobe epilepsy
Brain tumor
Subdural hematoma

DRUGS

Hallucinogens
Phencyclidine (PCP)
All drugs with CNS anticholinergic activity (phenothiazines, tricyclic antidepressants, OTC sleep preparations, narcotic analgesics etc.)
Amphetamine, cocaine
Alcohol withdrawal

Organic Brain Syndrome. A critical point about differential diagnostic concerns abnormalities of cognitive and intellectual functioning discovered during a mental status examination (see Chapter 2). Interference with orientation, memory, and cognition (thinking), is presumptive evidence of a medical etiology until proven otherwise. Rarely, patients with acute schizophrenic or manic psychoses are seen who have *apparent* disorientation and disturbance of higher cognitive functioning due to the patient's overwhelming anxiety or preoccupation with psychotic experiences. Patients with depressive disorders sometimes may show symptoms of cognitive impairment. Depressed patients may complain of a subjective sense of memory impairment. In general, many depressed patients with these complaints will be able to perform adequately on the mental status examination or on psychologic testing if they are able to make the effort. These patients may perform tasks very slowly because of psychomotor retardation and lack of energy; this in turn may lead to questions about organic deficits. Evaluation of depressed patients often requires CT scan, EEG tests, thyroid and metabolic screening, and even neuropsychological testing to exclude an organic etiology. Visual hallucinations and other nonauditory hallucinations are sometimes suggestive of a medical illness (Hall et al., 1978), while olfactory or gustatory hallucinations may reflect a seizure disorder (Pincus and Tucker, 1978).

In the elderly patient, differentiation between cognitive deficits due to brain disease and those caused by so-called depressive pseudodementia can be quite complicated. Many times the elderly patient with mild dementia is depressed as well, adding to the manifest signs of intellectual impairment. A depressed, pessimistic, melancholic mood in such patients may be helpful in diagnosis but often in the elderly only a sad face will be present (Shraberg, 1978). Changes in sleep, appetite, energy, or bowel movements, may be the key that depression is present when there is also reduction in cognitive abilities. Correction of abnormalities in metabolic, hematopoietic, and cardiorespiratory function, treatment of infection, removal of unnecessary medications or those with CNS effects, should be the first steps in trying to separate medical from psychiatric causes of cognitive dysfunction in elderly patients. Sometimes, only a successful trial of low-dose antidepressant medication or even ECT is the only way to make the diagnosis of a depression. Only after psychiatric consultation should ECT be undertaken, and antidepressant medication for the elderly should be administered or supervised only by someone experienced in the special complexities of using psychotropic medication in this special situation (Post, 1975).

Acute onset of confusion or acute deterioration of intellectual functioning is an important differential diagnostic feature and strongly hints at a medical illness rather than a psychiatric one. Sudden onset of symptoms of confusion or depression in an elderly patient may be the ***only presenting sign*** of an acute medical process such as pulmonary embolism, myocardial infarction, pneumonia, congestive heart failure, drug intoxication, and/or infection. Accurate history, including assessment of prior social and psychologic functioning (which must frequently be obtained from friends or relatives) is essential, as are appropriate physical and laboratory diagnostic measures. Elderly patients with treatable disorders who display acute confusional states may be regarded as "demented" or "organic." Appropriate testing is too often delayed and expectation for recovery of function unnecessarily pessimistic (Godber, 1975; Reichel, 1976). Acute organic brain syndromes can be caused by any number of infectious, toxic, endocrine, metabolic, and structural abnormalities (see Chapter 6).

Wilson's Disease. There are a few medical disorders that initiate psychotic symptoms with little or no obvious cognitive impairment, at least in the early phases. Some of these conditions may be accompanied by subtle cognitive deterioration which only in-depth psychological testing can elicit. Wilson's disease (a disorder of copper metabolism, which affects the liver and CNS), for example, may give rise to a variety of psychiatric syndromes including depression, mania, and schizophreniform psychosis. Often there are subtle neurologic symptoms such as tremor, dysarthria, dyskinesia, akinesia, rigidity, and excessive salivation. Treatment with phenothiazines actually worsens all of these neurologic symptoms, whose existence is then ascribed to the prescribed drugs, while their true importance is discounted (Malamud, 1975; Cartwright, 1978). If psychiatric symptoms of Wilson's disease are present, a Kayser-Fleischer ring will be detectable and biochemical evidence of altered copper metabolism should be present as determined by abnormally low ceruloplasmin and an elevated 24-hour copper excretion study result (Cartwright, 1978) Psychiatric symptoms of Wilson's disease frequently are completely reversible with penicillamine treatment, as are many other manifestations of the disease (Scheinberg, 1975; Cartwright, 1978). Some of the psychiatric symptoms seen with Wilson's disease may develop as a result of the patient's reaction to the situation of being ill and not only to effects of disturbed CNS function.

Acute Intermittent Porphyria. Acute intermittent porphyria (AIP) may also stimulate a variety of mental disturbances. A psychotic picture with delusions, hallucinations, catatonic symptoms, and bizarre gestures has been described as accompanying this disorder—they may progress to a delirium. Neurologic complications can lead to respiratory paralysis and death (Cross, 1956; Becker and Kramer, 1977; Reynolds, 1977). An association with hysterical personality traits has been proposed but there is no good epidemiologic evidence on this point (Roth et al., 1959; Reynolds, 1977). Persistent complaints of abdominal pain in patients with psychiatric disturbances of any kind should lead to consideration of the diagnosis of AIP. Sometimes pain complaints will seem bizarre because of the mental disturbance. Carter (1977) reports a case of a psychotic AIP sufferer who mutilated his abdomen with a razor because of severe pain which the patient ascribed to "demons," and "rotten bowels." The patient's pain complaints had been discounted until after self-mutilation, when medical evaluation was finally undertaken.

Systemic Lupus Erythematosus. Systemic lupus erythematosus (SLE) can present with a wide variety of psychiatric syndromes. Organic brain syndromes and schizophreniform psychoses are relatively common among SLE patients with neuropsychiatric complications (Feinglass et al., 1976; Hall et al., 1979). Feinglass and colleagues (1976) emphasize that subtle organic and neurologic symptoms, as well as an abnormal EEG reading are frequently associated with SLE-related mental changes. Although some researchers have postulated that treatment of SLE may cause CNS abnormalities, the presence of neurologic symptoms or other signs of active SLE suggest that mental changes are due to SLE itself and not from steroid therapy.

Infections. Certain infectious agents can produce psychotic disorders. Viral encephalitis, especially herpes encephalitis, may demonstrate psychiatric syndromes. Herpes encephalitis, like syphilis, is described as a "great imitator" (Wilson, 1976). In particular, herpetic encephalitis sufferers in the early stages might display a syndrome of psychotic disorganization most resembling schizophrenia. In a number of cases, severe emotional stress has been found preceding the episode of illness. The stress appears to be a "precipitant" of the psychosis. In early encephalitic cases, diagnosis may be extremely difficult until neurologic or other physical symptoms such as fever become apparent.

Wilson (1976) suggests a high index of suspicion and continual reevaluation of psychotic patients, especially when response to treatment

is atypical and soft neurologic signs and clouding of the sensorium are present. He cautions that once a "functional" diagnosis is made, organic symptoms tend to be dismissed or are subjected to psychological analysis which— although possibly apt—tends to ignore the contribution of the biological dimension. In general, even if one has established a psychiatric diagnosis, new data should always be considered to make sure that no underlying organic factor was missed.

Neurologic Disorders. Neurologic disorders frequently involve personality changes and symptoms of psychosis. Wilson's disease has already been discussed. Temporal lobe epilepsy may present with schizophrenialike psychoses (see Slater and Beard, 1963; Flor-Henry, 1969; Mayer-Gross, 1969; Malamud, 1975; Kristensen and Sindrup, 1978a and b). Psychotic features appear in a subgroup of patients with this disorder as their disease progresses, although usually only after a number of years. These patients may experience hallucinations, delusions, ideas of influence and reference, catatonic symptoms, thought disorder and hyperreligiosity (Slater and Beard, 1963; Mayer-Gross, 1969). Although these patients frequently progress to a more typical dementia, risk factors for development of psychosis associated with temporal lobe epilepsy include, left-handedness, history of brain injury, neurologic or radiographic evidence of frank brain damage, and seizures involving automatic behaviors. In addition, psychosis may be related to *frequency* of *temporal lobe seizures*, although unrelated to frequency of generalized seizures. It is probable that psychoses in these patients are a reflection of lesions in deep-seated temporal regions (Flor-Henry, 1969; Kristensen and Sindrup, 1978a, 1978b). Such patients may also show psychotic features during periods of frequent seizure activity, but this is due to cumulative effects of ictal events and is usually accompanied by disturbances of sensorium and cognitive function. Seizures themselves may be accompanied by visual, auditory, and olfactory hallucinations as well as perceptual distortion, feelings of unreality, and other strange sensations either as part of the aura or the seizure. Patients may fear to tell their physicians of these experiences out of concern that they will be labeled "crazy." Diagnosis of partial-complex seizures (temporal lobe epilepsy) may be extremely difficult. The EEG result often is normal, although sleep-deprived studies will increase the likelihood of detecting an abnormality. Instances of self-injury, automatisms, disturbed consciousness, amnesia, and incontinence increase the certainty of an epileptic diagnosis, but partial-complex seizures may occur in the absence of any of those. Frequently patients are diagnosed as having "hysterical" seizures because the EEG does not reveal obvious epileptic signs and the attacks are atypical. An additional complication is that in many epileptic patients "hysterical" and "nonhysterical" seizures coexist. In general, "hysterical" seizures tend to be overdiagnosed (see Chapter 13). It is important to remember, however, that to make a diagnosis of conversion symptoms one must demonstrate either the presence of a proximate psychologic stimulus for the development of conversion symptoms and/or that the symptom allows the patient to avoid otherwise anxiety-provoking activity (primary gain) and/or that the patient can gain support from the environment because of the symptom (secondary gain) (see *DSM-III*).

An important cause of partial-complex seizures is brain tumor. Deep temporal, limbic system, and hypothalamic tumors may cause mental symptoms which are most likely to simulate schizophrenia (Malamud, 1975). Diagnosing such tumors is difficult because localizing neurologic signs may be absent until quite late in the disease process and even CT scan may fail to visualize the lesion.

A possible misinterpretation involves failing to recognize that brain lesions may *cause* schizophrenia-like syndromes, either through epileptic activity or local tissue destruction. Treatment may be directed toward the "psychiatric" symptoms and a comprehensive workup is delayed. A number of factors may aid in diagnosis. In epileptic patients, as with schizophrenics, family history is more likely to be negative for mental disorder or schizophrenia. Findings of neurologic abnormalities on physical or mental status examinations increase the chances that psychosis is due to organic factors. Sudden change in personality or habits in a previously well-adapted person points to an organic etiology. Structural lesions must then be considered in the differential diagnosis.

Subdural hematoma must always be considered in the differential diagnosis of any mental or neurologic change. Subdural—either acute or chronic—hematoma is infamous for simulating almost any neurologic or psychiatric picture. Alcoholics, the elderly, and people with disorders of hemostasis are particularly at risk for developing subdural hematoma. A history of head trauma, no matter how trivial, should be sought and one should look carefully for evidence of injury.

Drugs. Drug use may simulate psychotic disorders. Amphetamines and cocaine can give rise to both an acute and chronic psychosis with notable paranoid features; this occurs without much alteration in cognitive function or in orientation. The psychosis caused by these drugs can simulate a manic attack with paranoia. A paranoid schizophrenic picture is more likely, however. Collateral history from friends and relatives may suggest correct diagnosis, but by the time the patient comes to medical attention, he or she may no longer attempt to conceal drug usage. Track marks may suggest intravenous amphetamine usage. Intranasal pathology may suggest cocaine abuse.

Use of psychedelics like LSD and mescaline may give rise to psychosis characterized by visual hallucinations and changes in perception. Prolonged usage of psychedelics is thought to be associated in a few patients with an acute schizophreniform psychosis or with an insidiously progressive chronic psychotic state characterized by withdrawal, hyperreligiosity, and apathy (Glass and Bowers, 1970; Bowers, 1972). Phencyclidine (PCP) is a common drug of abuse in recent years. It is associated with a number of severe mental alterations including hallucinatory, agitated, often violent, paranoid psychosis with confusional features. PCP intoxication can progress to convulsions, coma, and death. Physicians in emergency rooms must particularly be on the lookout for this form of intoxication.

Any drug with anticholinergic properties can cause an acute delirium. Drugs with anticholinergic effects include over-the-counter (OTC) sleep and cold remedies, antispasmodics, narcotic analgesics, tricyclic antidepressants, and phenothiazine tranquilizers. Children and the elderly may be particularly susceptible to the anticholinergic side effects of psychotropic medications. In these groups, treatment with these agents should be cautious with respect to initial dosage and rate of dosage increase.

CONCLUSION

Differential diagnostic determinations of patients with symptoms of emotional, cognitive, and behavioral dysfunction, must be made as skillfully, expeditiously, and inexpensively as possible. The state of the art, however, is such that the physician and patient have to bear considerable uncertainty in trying to understand the cause of a patient's complaints. Shulman (1977) states: "A doctor needs to concede that hidden knowledge, crucial for diagnosis, is often locked up in his patient, and that to gain access to this a special kind of . . . relationship has to be developed. To achieve this one has to tolerate ambiguity rather than risk premature and erroneous closure, to accept that answers are not always clear-cut and that symptoms do not fit into neat conceptual systems according to specialty." Shulman's quote of Francis Bacon is

quite apt: "If a man will begin with certainties he shall end in doubts; but if he will be content to begin with doubts, he shall end in certainties."

RECOMMENDED READINGS

Koranyi, E.K. 1979. Morbidity and rate of undiagnosed physical illnesses in a psychiatric clinic population. *Arch. Gen. Psychiatry* 36:414–19. A carefully researched paper representing the major statement so far of Koranyi's work, this addresses in a succinct way major issues concerning diagnosis of psychiatric and medical disorders.

Lipowski, Z.J. 1975. Psychiatry of somatic diseases: Epidemiology, pathogenisis, classification. *Compr. Psychiatry* 16:105–23. This is the best and most comprehensive review of the topics covered in this chapter. There is a complete review of the earlier literature in the field and this paper touches on most of the major clinical and theoretical areas relevent to psychosomatics, differential diagnosis, and psychophysiology.

Shulman, R. 1977. Psychogenic illness with physical manifestations and the other side of the coin: A practical approach. *Lancet* 1:524–26. The brief but complete, concise, well-written, and wise article addresses clinical management issues and strategies that can be undertaken by primary clinicians who must make differential diagnoses of medical and psychiatric illnesses.

REFERENCES

Akiskal, H.S., and McKinney, W.T. 1973. Psychiatry and pseudopsychiatry. *Arch. Gen. Psychiatry* 28:367–73.

American Psychiatric Association. 1980. Diagnostic and statistical manual of mental disorders. 3rd ed. Washington D.C., American Psychiatric Association.

Baldessarini, R.J. 1977. Schizophrenia. *N. Engl. J. Med.* 297:988–95.

Bant, W.P. 1978. Antihypertensive drugs and depression: A reappraisal. *Psychol. Medicine* 8:275–83.

Becker, D.M., and Kramer, S. 1977. The neurological manifestations of porphyria: A review. *Medicine* 56:411–23.

Blumer, D. 1975. Temporal lobe epilepsy and its

psychiatric significance. In Psychiatric aspects of neurologic disease, ed. D.F. Benson, and D. Blumer, pp. 171–98. New York: Grune & Stratton.

Bowers, M.D. 1972. Acute psychosis induced by psychotomimetic drug abuse 1. Clinical findings. *Arch. Gen. Psychiatry* 27:437–42.

Brenner, I. 1978. Apathetic hyperthyroidism. *J. Clin. Psychiatry* 39:479–80.

Capstick, A. 1960. Recognition of emotional disturbance and the prevention of suicide. *Br. Med. J.* 1:1179–82.

Caroff, S.N. 1978. Klinefelter's syndrome and bipolar affective illness: A case report. *Am. J. Psychiatry* 135(6):748–49.

Carroll, B.J. 1977. Psychiatric disorders and steroids. In *Neuroregulators and psychiatric disorders*, ed. E. Usdin, pp. 276–83. New York: Oxford University Press.

Carter, J.H. 1977. Updating acute intermittent porphyria: A case of self-mutilation. *J. Nat. Med. Assoc.* 69:51–52.

Cartwright, G.E. 1978. *Diagnosis of treatable Wilson's disease. N. Engl. J. Med.* 298:1347–50.

Cross, T.N. 1956. Porphyria—A deceptive syndrome. *Am. J. Psychiatry* 112:1010–14.

Davidoff, F., and Gill, J. 1977. Myxedema madness: Psychosis as an early manifestation of hypothyroidism. *Conn. Med.* 41:618–21.

Detre, T.P., and Jarecki, H.G. 1971. *Modern psychiatric treatment*. Philadelphia: J.B. Lippincott Co.

Eastwood, R.M. 1975. The relation between physical and mental illness. Toronto: University of Toronto Press.

Feinglass, E.J.; Arnett, F.C.; Dorsch, C.N., et al. 1976. Neuropsychiatric manifestations of systemic lupus erythematosus: Diagnosis, clinical spectrum and relationship to other features of the disease. *Medicine* 55:323–39.

Flor-Henry, P. 1969. Psychosis and temporal lobe epilepsy: A controlled investigation. *Epliepsia* 10:363–95.

Fras, I.; Litin, E.M.; and Pearson, J.S. 1967. Comparison of psychiatric symptoms in carcinoma of the pancreas with those in some other intra-abdominal neoplasms. *Am. J. Psychiatry* 123:1553–62.

Freedman, A.M.; Kaplan, H.I.; and Sadock, B.D. 1975. *Comprehensive textbook of psychiatry*. 2nd ed. Baltimore: Williams & Wilkins Co.

Freedman, R., and Schwab, P.J. 1978. Paranoid symptoms in patients on a general hospital psychiatric unit. *Arch. Gen. Psychiatry* 35:387–90.

Gelenberg, A.J. 1976. The catatonic syndrome. *Lancet* 1:1339–91.

Geschwind, N. 1975. The borderland of neurology and psychiatry: Some common misconceptions. In *Psychiatric aspects of neurologic disease*, ed. D.F. Benson, and D. Blumer, pp. 1–9. New York: Grune & Stratton.

Glass, R.M.; Allan, A.T.; Uhlenhuth, E.H., et al. 1978. Psychiatric screening in a medical clinic. *Arch. Gen. Psychiatry* 35:1189–95.

Glass, G.S., and Bowers, M.B. 1970. Chronic psychosis associated with long-term psychotomimetic drug abuse. *Arch. Gen. Psychiatry* 23:97–103.

Godber, C. 1975. The physician and the confused elderly patient. *J. R. Coll. Physicians Lond.* 10:101–12.

Greden, J.F. 1974. Anxiety or caffeinism: A diagnostic dilemma. *Am. J. Psychiatry* 131:1089–92.

Groves, J.E. 1978. Taking care of the hateful patient. *N. Engl. J. Med.* 298:883–87.

Hall, R.C.W.; Popkin, M.D.; Devaul, R.A., et al. 1978. Physical illness presenting as psychiatric disease. *Arch. Gen. Psychiatry* 35:1315–20.

Hall, R.W.; Gruzenski, W.P.; and Popkin, M.K. 1979. Differential diagnosis of somatopsychic disorders. *Psychosomatics* 20:381–89.

Kidd, K.K., and Mathysee, S. 1978. Research designs for the study of gene-environment interactions in psychiatric disorders. *Arch. Gen. Psychiatry* 35:925–32.

Kiev, A., ed. 1974. Somatic manifestations of depressive disorders. Amsterdam: Exerpta Medica.

Kline, N.S. 1976. Incidence, prevalence, and recognition of depressive illness. *Dis. Nerv. Syst.* 37:10–14.

Koranyi, E.K. 1972. Physical health and illness in a psychiatric outpatient department population. *Can. Psychiatr. Assoc. J.* (suppl) 17:109–16.

———. 1977a. Fatalities in 2070 psychiatric outpatients. *Arch. Gen. Psychiatry* 34:1137–42.

———. 1977b. Medical considerations at intake. Paper presented at a regional meeting, Pittsburgh, Oct. 28, 1977.

———. 1979. Morbidity and rate of undiagnosed physical illnesses in a psychiatric clinic population. *Arch. Gen. Psychiatry* 36:414–19.

Kristensen, O., and Sindrup, E.H. 1978a. Psychomotor epilepsy and psychosis I:Physical Aspects. *Acta Neurol. Scand.* 57:361–69.

———. 1978b. Psychomotor epilepsy and psychosis II: Electroencephalographic findings, *Acta Neurol, Scand.* 57:370–79.

Kubler-Ross, E. 1969. On death and dying. New York: Macmillan.

Lancet editorial. 1979. Psychiatric illness among medical patients. *Lancet* 1:478–79.

Lipowski, Z.J. 1975. Psychiatry of somatic diseases: Epidemiology, pathogenesis, classification. *Compr. Psychiatry* 16:105–23.

Lipton, M.A.; Killam, K.F.; and Dimascio, A., eds. 1977. Neuropsychopharmacology: A generation of progress. New York: Raven Press.

Luxon, L.; Lees, A.J.; and Greenwood, R.J. 1979. Neurosyphilis today. *Lancet* 1:90–93.

Malamud, N. 1975. Organic brain disease mistaken for psychiatric disorder: A clinicopathologic study. In *Psychiatric aspects of neurological disease*, ed. D.F. Benson, and D. Blumer, pp. 287–307. New York: Grune & Stratton.

Manschreck, T.C., and Petri, M. 1978. The paranoid syndrome. *Lancet* 2:251–53.

Mayer-Gross, W.; Slater, E.; and Roth, M. 1969. Clinical psychiatry. 3rd ed. Baltimore: Williams & Wilkins.

Moffic, H.S., and Paykel, E.S. 1975. Depression in medical inpatients. *Br. J. Psychiatry* 126:346–53.

Murphy, G.E. 1977. Suicide and attempted suicide. *Hosp. Pract.* Nov.: 73–81.

Nielsen, J. 1969. Klinefelter's syndrome. *Acta Psychiatr. Scand.* [Suppl] 209.

Noyes, R.; Clancy, J.; Crowe, R., et al. 1978. The familial prevalence of anxiety neurosis. *Arch. Gen. Psychiatry* 35:1057–59.

Paredes, A., and Jones, H. 1959. Psychopathology of acute intermittent porphyria: A case report. *J. Nerv. Ment. Dis.* 129:291–95.

Pariser, S.F.; Pinta, E.R.; and Jones, B.A. 1978. Mitral valve prolapse syndrome and anxiety neurosis/panic disorder. *Am. J. Psychiatry* 135:246–47.

Pevnick, J.S.; Jasinski, D.R.; and Haertzen, C.A. 1978. Abrupt withdrawal from therapeutically administered diazepam. *Arch. Gen. Psychiatry* 35:995–98.

Pincus, J.H., and Tucker, G.J. 1978. Behavioral neurology. 2nd ed. New York: Oxford University Press.

Pope, H.G., and Lipinski, J.F. 1978. Diagnosis in schizophrenia and manic depressive illness. *Arch. Gen. Psychiatry* 35:811–28.

Post, F. 1975. Dementia, depression, and pseudodementia. In *Psychiatric aspects of neurological disease*. ed. F.D. Benson, and D. Blumer, pp. 99–120. New York: Grune and Stratton.

Reichel, W. 1976. Organic brain syndromes in the aged. *Hosp. Pract.* May: 119–25.

Reynolds, N.C. 1977. Porphyrias: Neurologic aspects and the treatment of exacerbations. *Minn. Med.* 7:515–20.

Roth, N.; Friedman, I.; and Tomisch, R. 1959. Further remarks on porphyria and report of prolonged observation of a case. *J. Nerv. Ment. Dis.* 129:296–301.

Sachar, E.J. 1975. Psychiatric disturbances associated with endocrine disorders. In *American handbook of psychiatry*, 2nd ed., vol. 5, ed. S. Arieti, pp. 299–314. New York: Basic Books.

Scheinberg, I.H. 1975. Psychosis associated with hereditary disorders. In *American handbook of psychiatry*, 2nd ed., vol. 5, ed. S. Arieti, pp. 404–12. New York: Basic Books.

Shraberg, D. 1978. The myth of pseudodementia: Depression and the aging brain. *Am. J. Psychiatry* 135:601–3.

Shulman, R. 1977. Psychogenic illness with physical manifestations and the other side of the coin: A Practical Approach. *Lancet* 1:524–26.

Slater, E., and Beard, A.W. 1963. The schizophrenia-like psychoses of epilepsy. *Br. J. Psychiatry* 109:95–150.

Slater, E.T.O., and Glithero, E. 1965. A follow-up of patients diagnosed as suffering from 'hysteria.' *J. Psychosom. Res.* 9:9–13.

Smith, C.K.; Barish, J.; Correa, J., et al. 1972. Psychiatric disturbance in endocrinologic disease. *Psychosom. Med.* 34:69–86.

Sorensen, K., and Nielsen, J. 1977. Twenty psychotic males with Klinefelter's syndrome. *Acta Psychiatr. Scand.* 56:249–55.

Stewart, M.A.; Drake, F.; and Winoker, G. 1965. Depression among medically ill patients. *Dis. Nerv. Syst.* 26:479–85.

Swanson, D.W., and Stipes, A.H. 1969. Psychiatric aspects of Klinefelter's syndrome. *Am. J. Psychiatry* 126:814–22.

Taylor, J.W. 1975. Depression in thyrotoxicosis. *Am. J. Psychiatry* 132:552–53.

Weissman, M.M., and Myers, J.K. 1978. Affective disorders in a U.S. urban community. *Arch. Gen. Psychiatry* 35:1304–11.

Weller, D.J., and Miller, P.M. 1977a. Emotional reac-
tions of patient, family, and staff in acute-care period of spinal cord injury—Part I. *Soc. Work Health Care* 2:369–76.

———. 1977b. Emotional reactions of patient, family, and staff in acute-care period of spinal cord injury—Part II. *Soc. Work Health Care* 3:7–17.

Whitlock, F.A., and Price, J. 1974. Use of β-adrenergic receptor blocking drugs in psychiatry. *Drugs* 8:109–24.

Wilson, L.G. 1976. Viral encephalopathy mimicking functional psychosis. *Am. J. Psychiatry* 133:165–70.

Woodruff, R.A.; Goodwin, D.W.; and Guze, S.B. 1974. Psychiatric diagnosis. New York: Oxford University Press.

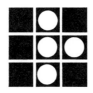

CHAPTER 6

Evaluation and Management of Confusion — Organic Brain Syndromes

Daniel C. Moore, M.D.

Organic brain syndromes exemplify the relationship between physical states (metabolic or structural damage to the brain) and mental/behavioral states (confusion, disorientation, cognitive deficits). Organic brain syndromes are some of the most commonly encountered psychiatric syndromes in general medical practice. Many are caused by an underlying physical disease or treatment regimens (for example, drugs) for such disease. In organic brain syndrome, unlike in some other psychiatric syndromes, the etiology is often definable; a search for etiology is crucial since many organic brain syndromes can be cured by removing the causative agent.

Organic brain syndromes are among the most common yet most misdiagnosed psychiatric disorders to be seen in a medical setting. Lipowski has estimated that approximately 30% of the 20–70-year-old population will experience an episode of delirium within their lifetimes (Lipowski, 1967a). In a study of an elderly community population, 17% were found to have chronic organic brain syndromes (Fisch, 1968). Often these disorders are missed because the prominent emotional or behavioral reactions are suggestive of other diagnoses and therefore obscure the underlying intellectual deficit. For this reason, "confusion" is the best single descriptive term for organic brain syndrome, since it suggests both the loss of intellectual functioning and the emotional reaction. The patients' confusion results from the failure of intellectual abilities that they once automatically relied upon to make their way in the world. These abilities include attention, memory, orientation, and logical thought.

In every case, the underlying cause of these disturbing changes in cognitive functions is a transient or permanent impairment of brain tissue function. In a definitive article on organicity, Engel and Romano (1959) have chosen to describe this impairment as a "syndrome of cerebral insufficiency." They specifically use this phrase to highlight the similarity of the central nervous system to other organ systems more familiar to the average physician. For example, with renal insufficiency, the compromise or damage of the renal tubular cells results in a failure of the primary function of the whole system, that is, filtering of the blood and excretion of bodily wastes. In the same manner, compromise of brain cells from whatever reason results in failure of normal brain function, which is the maintenance of orderly and coherent contact with the world. When this fails, the result is inattention, disorientation, and confusion. As with other organ systems, cerebral insufficiency can be the result of either temporary damage to the neurons or permanent loss of function through cell death. When the damage is temporary and reversible, it is due to altered metabolism of the neurons. Causes for this change may

---

CASE HISTORY 6–1

A 65-year-old married man was admitted to the hospital with chest pains; the electrocardiogram on admission revealed anterior wall myocardial infarction. He was placed in the coronary care unit and given morphine sulfate injections for pain, diazepam for anxiety, flurazepam for sleep, and lidocaine intravenously for cardiac arrhythmias. On the second day of admission, the patient began to accuse the nurses of being FBI agents who were spying on him and imprisoning him.

He wanted to call his attorney so that he could be released from the prison (referring to the room). He was, however, unable to remember the attorney's name or phone number, although he had recently made a will. When asked about the circumstances concerning his admission, he stated that he was arrested, put in a police van, and brought to this "prison." He was unable to remember how long he had been in the room, the current date, or day. He, however, wanted to leave immediately. (See the appendix at the end of this chapter for further discussion and PEG.)

include lack or excess of essential substances for neuronal function such as oxygen or glucose; presence of abnormal substances such as sedative-hypnotic drugs or toxins such as urea or ammonia; abnormal physical environments such as fever or electrolyte imbalance; or abnormal neuronal activity patterns such as sensory deprivation or seizure activity (Heller and Kornfeld, 1975). In the case of cell death, as from trauma, infection, or neoplasm, the insufficiency is permanent and leads to irreversible changes in intellectual function when sufficient numbers of cells have died.

SYMPTOMS OF ORGANIC BRAIN SYNDROME

In organic brain syndrome, primary symptoms result from compromise of intellectual, cognitive or perceptual abilities (Table 6–1). Many functions that previously occurred without effort now become laborious and difficult, if not impossible.

Orientation is often impaired so that the patient gives the wrong date, even when corrected several times, and may not be able to figure out his or her location, even though the

---

TABLE 6–1
Cognitive and perceptual deficits in organic brain syndromes

Poor attention
Decreased level of sensorium
Loss of orientation
Poor memory, especially recent
Lack of logical reasoning
Inability to abstract
Failure of comprehension
Inaccurate calculations
Deficient social judgment
Misperceptions
Illusions
Visual hallucinations

---

clinic sign was seen on the way in. With less severe cases, the patient may be able to name the place, but then be found wandering aimlessly after going to the lavatory because the sense of spatial orientation (location) is impaired. Only in the most severe cases does the patient lose orientation to self and forget his or her name.

Memory is a critical function that deteriorates in both acute and chronic organic brain syndromes. *Recent memory* for events occurring a few minutes to a few days before is most affected. As a result, patients are noted to forget where they put something and spend much time rummaging about for it in an aimless fashion. They may also ask the same question over and over again, unaware that they have just heard the answer a few moments before. By contrast, remote memory for events in the past often remains remarkably intact, so that the patient will remember the names of high-school classmates while forgetting repeatedly why he or she is in the hospital.

Calculations become inaccurate and the patient may slow down to the point of never finishing a problem or may race through several without arriving at a single right answer. Similarly, *comprehension* is drastically limited by the patient's inability to grasp more than one or two concrete concepts at a time. Understanding a series of ideas leading to a conclusion becomes impossible. The patient feels anchored in concrete concepts and feels more at home repeating simple, well-learned tasks or ideas. When a patient repeats a familiar action continually and compulsively, it is referred to as "occupational delirium." Thus, a truck driver may go through the motions of driving a truck, or a sailor may endlessly discuss the proper dimensions of catboats—length, breadth, sail size—because he knows these by rote. In comparison, grasp of abstractions or holistic concepts is shaky or nonexistent. The patient may insist on taking the old, familiar route to the hospital even though the map clearly shows a shorter route.

In more severe cases, the normally smooth organization of sensory *perceptions* into a coherent whole is spotty and unreliable. Patients consequently *misinterpret* what they see or hear. The pattern of venetian blinds on a wall are taken to be the bars of a jail cell. A nurse with a thermometer is thought to be an assailant. Frank hallucinations not based on misperceptions also occur; these are usually *visual* in nature. Auditory hallucinations are uncommon, but may occur.

Level of attention or *sensorium* is altered and fluctuates between normal and poor or may remain constantly depressed. This will show up in the patient's inability to concentrate on a topic for more than a few minutes. When sensorium fluctuates, it will often do so according to day and night cycles, a phenomenon called "sundowning." A patient may appear relatively coherent during the day, but in the evening or at night, may begin to become confused, wander about wondering where he is, searching for his motorboat. In the morning, he may speak seriously of having been transported to Mexico the previous evening.

Unfortunately, few organic brain syndrome patients or their relatives acknowledge these primary symptoms as their major complaint. The patient may complain, "I'm going crazy" or "I feel like I'm dying" or "What's happening to me?" Relatives may overlook the confused wandering or memory lapses, chalking it up to "that's just his way" or "his moods" because they are too close to the situation. This is especially true with a dementia which may develop slowly and insidiously over years, so that family members may come to expect that grandfather is "just getting odd." At other times, they may morally condemn confused behavior as willfully destructive. If the onset is more sudden, relatives may view organic brain syndrome as emotional illness. This interpretation is not surprising since most patients do have strong emotional reactions to their confused awareness of their intellectual deficits. These *secondary reactions* may be so marked as to temporarily obscure the primary cognitive changes from the family and friends (Table 6–2).

With a growing personal perception of their own confusion, patients may become anxious. Depending on the severity and degree of threat they feel, anxiety may progress to physical agitation or panic. They may try to escape or fight their way out of the situation. Other patients are seen as depressed—and some may be—though many only appear this way because they have withdrawn from active contact in an attempt to reduce the amount of confusing stimuli they have to deal with. Still others become highly suspicious and paranoid, believing that something has been done to them to cause this change. They may develop *delusions* to explain what has happened, though usually these are of an unsystematized, variable nature. *Mood* may be very *labile*, shifting from sadness to anger to contentment over a short period of time. This lability may partly be explained on the basis of a "release phenomenon," in which cortical cell damage removes higher cortical inhibition over emotional behaviors. This phenomenon may also result in *socially inappropriate* sexual or aggressive behaviors—as in the case of the distinguished older man who suddenly begins pinching nurses. In more advanced cases, the

---

TABLE 6–2
**Secondary emotional reactions
in organic brain syndromes**

Lability of mood
Anxiety, agitation, or panic
Depression
Anger
Paranoia
Delusions
Socially inappropriate sexual
    or aggressive acts
"Catastrophic reaction"
Personality change

impaired judgment may take the form of neglect of personal hygiene or even soiling.

Some organic brain syndrome patients appear to adapt well to even relatively severe intellectual deterioration but may have marked emotional reactions when faced with a problem which suddenly makes them aware of their deficit. The trigger may be a task requiring some degree of abstract thinking which the patient has been able to perform in the past. The patient tries, realizes he or she cannot succeed, and suddenly becomes irritable, angry, and at times even assaultive. More often they become highly agitated and try to run away, often in a wild and disordered fashion. This phenomenon is referred to as a *"catastrophic reaction"* (Goldstein, 1952).

Other patients may be described by relatives as having undergone a *personality change*. Their behavior may be different from usual, such as the patient who acts in a socially inappropriate manner, or there may simply be an accentuation of their normal personalities. A patient who was meticulous all his life may become unbearably compulsive, insisting on noting down minute, unimportant details no one else cares about. Accentuation of personality style can be seen as a characterologic response to an awareness of intellectual deficits. Whatever techniques worked best for dealing with the world before are heightened now in an attempt to stave off confusion. Unfortunately, these accentuations of personality do not help and often hinder cooperation or rapport with those around them.

The foregoing descriptions are of the more severe emotional reactions to the intellectual deficits caused by organic brain syndrome. The severe reactions of these patients call attention to themselves and the correct diagnosis is ultimately made. Other patients do not react in such dramatic ways and consequently their organic brain syndrome may be missed. These patients may respond to their confusion by trying to reduce the perceptual input with which they have to deal. They may withdraw and look depressed when in fact they are simply avoiding

stimulation. Others feign disinterest in new experiences and seem to be getting "stuck in their ways." Conversely, they may display a bland and happy response to everything but refuse to become engaged in ways that would challenge their reasoning powers. When faced with such tasks, they become evasive and vague and, if pushed to perform, may begin to show the more obvious emotional reactions of agitation, depression, or anger (Brosin, 1967). This *denial of defect* is often beneficial for patients in the short run, since it protects them from unpleasant experiences, but it also retards diagnosis and treatment. Although it has been estimated that 5%–10% of all patients in general hospital wards suffer from organic brain syndromes, few patients are diagnosed and even fewer receive psychiatric consultations (Lipowski, 1967b). For this reason, a high index of suspicion regarding organic brain syndromes is necessary. Any unusual behavior in a medical patient, whether wild emotions or quiet withdrawal, should be considered to be a possible symptom of organicity until it is ruled out by testing of intellectual capacities.

DIAGNOSIS

Up to now, the similarities in presentation of all organic brain syndromes have been emphasized. However, for purposes of diagnosis and treatment, they can be divided into acute or chronic syndromes based on the *rapidity of onset* and the *degree of reversibility*. The terms *delirium* and *acute organic brain syndrome* are used interchangeably to refer to cases with relatively rapid onset of confusion, usually within a few hours to a few days. Attention is significantly disturbed and the level of consciousness may fluctuate widely. The patient may have insomnia or may appear stuporous and sleep most of the time. Many delirious patients become restless and hyperactive. They may continually attempt to get out of bed, constantly pick at the bedclothes or pull at the intravenous line. Along with increased psychomotor activity, they may show signs of autonomic arousal with rapid pulse, increased blood pressure, dilated pupils, sweating, and flushed face. Alternatively, they may appear sluggish and have difficulty responding to even the simplest questions. Frequently there is an obvious medical cause for the delirium, but occasionally the delirium may be the presenting symptom. For example, it may be the first sign in a subdural hematoma—when the underlying medical disorder is corrected, the impaired but not permanently damaged brain cells can return to normal functioning. The usual course for a delirium is recovery within a brief period of time (a few days to weeks) or occasionally death from the medical illness.

By comparison, *dementia* and *chronic organic brain syndrome* usually refer to a more insidious onset of intellectual deficits over a period of months to years, usually caused by *irreversible loss of brain cells*. Agitation and strong emotional reactions are less common than a progressive inability to perform the usual tasks of daily life. This usually starts with failure at problems which require some abstracting ability, such as fixing a broken machine for the first time, and progress to difficulty with the simplest tasks. Personality change, depression, and loss of social inhibitions are more common presentations. Gradually the family finds the patient impossible to live with and considers institutionalization. At the end stage, patients are often incontinent and unable to perform any of the activities of daily living. They usually die from intercurrent infections such as pneumonia.

Not all disorders fit these categories easily. Pernicious anemia can have a slow onset of apparently irreversible dementia and other neurologic signs over a period of months before it is diagnosed and treated with vitamin B_{12}, at which point the mental deterioration is reversible. Similar recoveries can occur with slow, progressive illness such as normal pressure hydrocephalus and severe hypothyroidism. On the other hand, some irreversible dementias can have a rapid onset rather than insidious deterioration. Strokes or head trauma can leave a permanent dementia as a result of a single episode. To minimize terminological confusion, this chapter follows the conventions of the third edition of the *Diagnostic and Statistical Manual of Mental Disorders (DSM-III)*. According to *DSM-III*, mental deterioration of slow, insidious onset is called a dementia even though it may at some point be found to be reversible. Tables 6–3 and 6–4 contain the *DSM-III* criteria for delirium and dementia.

TABLE 6–3
Diagnostic criteria
for delirium (DSM III)*

A. Clouding of consciousness (reduced clarity of awareness of the environment), with reduced capacity to shift, focus, and sustain attention to environmental stimuli

B. At least two of the following:
   (1) perceptual disturbance: misinterpretations, illusions, or hallucinations
   (2) speech is at times incoherent
   (3) disturbance of sleep-wakefulness cycle, with insomnia or daytime drowsiness
   (4) increased or decreased psychomotor activity

C. Disorientation and memory impairment (if testable)

D. Clinical features that develop over a short period of time (usually hours to days) and tend to fluctuate over the course of a day

E. Evidence, from the history, physical examination, or laboratory tests, of a specific organic factor judged to be etiologically related to the disturbance.

*American Psyciatric Association. 1980. *Diagnostic and statistical manual of mental disorders:* 3rd ed. Washington, D.C: American Psychiatric Association. Reprinted with permission from the American Psychiatric Association.

Differential Diagnosis

Unfortunately, the correspondence between the degree of intellectual deficit and the extent of secondary emotional reactions can be highly variable. Patients with a slow onset of dementia may adapt to it relatively well in a familiar home or neighborhood setting and only show confusion when thrown into new situations. Some patients may suffer major memory difficulties and are easily confused, but still control their emotional reactions. With others, even mild intellectual impairments may be so distressing as to result in strong emotional outbursts. Various theories hold that those able to control their emotional responses have greater "ego strength" or that they are not as globally affected by cerebral deterioration, but there is no scientific basis for any of these ideas. Whatever the reason, this variability in presenting symptoms makes differential diagnosis of organic brain syndromes difficult since the prominence of intellectual deficits or of emotional reactions in one case or another can cause it to be confused with other psychiatric states. The disorders that can be confused with organic brain syndrome are discussed in the following sections.

Anxiety Disorders. Anxiety disorder (neurosis) is often the misdiagnosis made in the early stages of a slowly developing dementia. The

---

TABLE 6–4
Diagnostic criteria for dementia
(DSM-III) *

A. A loss of intellectual abilities of sufficient severity to interfere with social or occupational functioning.

B. Memory impairment.

C. At least one of the following:
   (1) impairment of abstract thinking, as manifested by concrete interpretation of proverbs, inability to find similarities and differences between related words, difficulty in defining words and concepts, and other similar tasks
   (2) impaired judgment
   (3) other disturbances of higher cortical function, such as aphasia (disorder of language due to brain dysfunction), apraxia (inability to carry out motor activities despite intact comprehension and motor function), agnosia (failure to recognize or identify objects despite intact sensory function), "constructional difficulty" (e.g., inability to copy three-dimensional figures, assemble blocks, or arrange sticks in specific designs)
   (4) personality change, i.e., alteration or accentuation of premorbid traits

D. State of consciousness not clouded (i.e., does not meet the criteria for delirium or intoxication, although these may be superimposed).

E. Either (1) or (2):
   (1) evidence from the history, physical examination, or laboratory tests, of a specific organic factor that is judged to be etiologically related to the disturbance
   (2) in the absence of such evidence, an organic factor necessary for the development of the syndrome can be presumed if conditions other than Organic Mental Disorders have been reasonably excluded and if the behavioral change represents cognitive impairment in a variety of areas.

---

* American Psychiatric Association. 1980. *Diagnostic and statistical manual of mental disorders*. 3rd ed. Washington, D.C.: American Psychiatric Association. Reprinted with permission from the American Psychiatric Association.

individual begins to perceive in a vague way that something is wrong with his or her performance. They forget things, make obvious errors, and are reprimanded by colleagues or family. They become anxious, work harder, but find that redoubled efforts result in further mistakes. Anxiety escalates and the individual begins to avoid friends or work. He or she may turn to alcohol to ease anxiety, but this worsens the condition. If such patients consult a physician for sudden "nervous state" or "performance anxiety," the disorder may be misdiagnosed as an anxiety reaction or anxiety neurosis and the patients receive a tranquilizer, which will sedate them and further impair performance. In delirium, the confusion is of more rapid onset and should be more obvious, but since this acute organic brain syndrome occurs most often in medically ill patients, the agitation may be taken as an upset over the medical condition.

Depression and Mania.   Differential diagnosis between *depression* and organic brain syndrome is the hardest one to make, particularly in elderly people. A comprehensive evaluation of the patient, using the PEG (Chapter 1), will help greatly in this type of differential. Like anxiety, depressive reactions often go hand-in-hand with a growing awareness of intellectual deficiency. The patient begins to withdraw, sees little future for him or herself, and may even develop vegeta-

tive signs of depression such as decreased appetite, weight loss, and sleep disruption (found in recent context of the PEG). Thus, the patient has a concurrent depression which may obscure the underlying organic brain syndrome. Often cognitive tests on the mental status examination help to separate purely depressed patients from those who also have a dementia, but particularly in severe depressions of the elderly it may be difficult to decide which disorder is primary (Cavenar et al., 1979). Depressed patients may be so self-preoccupied and so uninterested in the outside world that they fail to attend to the questions they are being asked and thus miss even when they are capable of answering. They are sometimes referred to as having a "pseudodementia" since the underlying cause is depression. More frequently, dementia is misdiagnosed because the patient appears depressed, a situation referred to as "pseudodepression." At times, even careful psychologic testing cannot establish which of the two states is primary. In these cases, a trial of antidepressants is often instituted. If the patient is primarily depressed, his spirits will improve and he will begin to be interested enough to perform better or repeat psychological tests. If the disorder is primarily organic, the patient will become more confused and disoriented on antidepressants. Naturally, if this occurs, the medication should be stopped immediately.

Another affective illness, *manic-depressive disorder* or bipolar illness, can also be confused with organicity. In this disorder, patients may have both depression and mania or, less frequently, mania only. The discussion here is limited to a description of mania since depressions have already been discussed. As with schizophrenia (discussed later), the first episode usually occurs before age 40 years, which helps distinguish it from the later-occurring organic brain syndromes. Mania consists of hyperactivity combined with elevated or irritable mood. The patient often feels expansive and grandiose and takes on immense projects, or starts spending

---

TABLE 6–5
Differential diagnosis of organic brain syndromes

Anxiety disorders (neurosis)
Depression and affective disorders
Drug-abuse and intoxication
Drug Withdrawal
Obsessive-compulsive disorder (neurosis)
Personality disorder
Schizophrenia

money that he or she cannot afford on trips, phone calls, cars, or entertainment. They are constantly on the move and talk in a rapid, pressured manner. They seem to be having a new idea every second and the listener is exhausted trying to keep up. Along with hyperactivity, they sleep less and eat less and sexual interest is increased. When thwarted in their grand designs, they become belligerent or even violent. If there are delusions, they are of a grandiose nature and involve some great plan on the patient's part. Less often, these delusions are accompanied by auditory hallucinations. Organic brain syndrome patients have been reported with symptoms similar to these, especially the hyperactivity and euphoric moods. They may become involved in feverish activity such as fixing a car or cleaning the house, but this "occupational delirium" is usually very confused, haphazard and unsuccessful. They have no elaborate, almost plausible plans like those of the manic-depressive. Once again, the failure of intellectual function distinguishes the patient with organic brain syndrome from the manic patient, whose cognitive abilities are intact.

There are certain etiologies of organic hyperactivity that are more likely to resemble a manic pattern. Diseases that specifically affect the brain, such as tumors, epilepsy, and encephalitis, are more likely to cause a manialike picture. In particular, tertiary syphilis can appear with sudden onset of euphoria and hyperactivity in an older patient, and so closely resembles mania that it was difficult to separate the syphilitics from the manic-depressives before serologic tests for syphilis were developed. Increased exogenous or endogenous cortisone also can cause manic or depressed picture accompanied by confusion.

Schizophrenia. Patients with organic brain syndromes, both acute and chronic, may do or say bizarre things when they are disoriented or confused. They may become psychotic, lose touch with reality, and have delusional ideas and

hallucinations. Their speech is often vague, rambling, or repetitive and seems to make no sense. These symptoms superficially resemble those seen in *schizophrenia* and as a result a psychotic organic brain syndrome may be misdiagnosed as acute schizophrenia. *Psychosis* only refers to a state; it is not a diagnosis (see Chapter 6). In psychosis, the patient no longer perceives reality clearly but rather sees it in distorted ways. He or she develops peculiar ideas, or delusions, to explain why the world has suddenly changed, why he is hearing or seeing things differently than others. Schizophrenia and organic brain syndrome can both be psychoses, but they differ in specific ways. Most commonly, the first episode of schizophrenia occurs in the teens, and almost always before age 40 years. It would be very rare for a man of 60 years to develop schizophrenia without a previous psychiatric history. On the other hand, delirium and especially dementia are most common in the over-55-years age group, and a *first episode of psychotic, bizarre behavior in this age group should be considered organic in origin until proven otherwise*, especially if it accompanies a medical illness (Fisch et al., 1968; Heller and Kornfeld, 1975). A delirium may occur at any age in association with serious illness, but vulnerability seems to increase with age.

Acute schizophrenia usually involves auditory hallucinations ("hearing voices") and the accompanying delusions often have a recurring theme—persecution for special powers, the FBI is wiretapping the patient, the patient thinks he is Jesus, or that there are x rays being beamed through his head. The patient maintains his preoccupation with a particular theme over a period of time. By contrast, the organic brain syndrome patient suffers primarily from *misperceptions* and *illusions*. When he or she does have hallucinations, they are usually *visual* or *tactile* in nature. Delusions are usually *unsystematized, less elaborate,* and *shifting*. They may have a vague belief that they are being attacked, whereas the schizophrenic usually has strong, fixed ideas about why and by whom he or she is being attacked. The schizophrenic will retain this fixed idea, while the organic patient may shift to some other vague belief, such as that he or she is being moved from room to room so parties can be held next door. Asked about it a while later, he or she may have still another idea. Schizophrenics may have a thought disorder in which they speak in a sing-song fashion, or switch subjects in midstream—so-called "looseness"—or block completely on a train of thought. The organic brain syndrome patient may appear more vague and rambling—moving from one topic to another with no specific purpose. They may also perseverate and repeat a phrase or idea over and over again.

The single most distinguishing difference between schizophrenia and organicity is in the area of *intellectual functions*. The schizophrenic should have intact orientation, memory, calculations, and comprehension, whereas the patient with a delirium or dementia will fail on these cognitive aspects of the mental status examination. If the schizophrenic is acutely agitated, he or she may have some initial difficulties correctly performing simple tasks because attention is so disrupted or because there are delusional fears of the examiner, but once calmed by seclusion or medication, schizophrenics should show intact intellectual abilities.

Obsessive-Compulsive Disorders. Chronic organic brain syndrome can be confused with *obsessive-compulsive disorders* (neuroses) because patients may react to their perception of decreased memory with obsessive preoccupation with detail. Fearing that they will forget something, they incessantly count to make sure they have hold of everything. They may develop rigid, compulsive behaviors, which they repeat again and again because they feel most comfortable with familiar actions and cannot learn new approaches. In the worst cases, the patient's intellectual deterioration is so advanced that he or she counts windows, doors, chairs, people,

anything to keep the world from dissolving into confusing, unrelated perceptions. By comparison, the patient with an obsessive-compulsive neurosis has an act or ritual which he or she feels compelled to repeat, even while knowing it is senseless. Beyond this one irrational act or thought, the obsessive-compulsive is intact intellectually and has no difficulty with attention, memory, or calculations.

Personality Disorders. Organic brain syndromes may at times resemble *personality disorders* (see Chapter 3) since organicity allows the accentuation of preexisting personality styles. This accentuation probably occurs because the deterioration of higher intellectual functions decreases the patient's ability to control and modulate emotional responses and he or she falls back on automatic, overlearned patterns of behavior. Patients with a dependent style may become unbearably demanding and clingy as they sense their ability to function alone slipping. The extremely neat, highly disciplined executive may begin to be overcontrolling with staff and require overdetailed, unrealistic information in the fear that failing memory will cause him or her to miss something. For example, a patient with a dementia secondary to an advancing brain tumor, who was initially quite affable, in later stages became suspicious of what the nurses were doing and began to wonder if his medicines were poison. This man had been a millionaire builder whose paranoid style had served him well in the construction business; only when it was accentuated by dementia could his personality disorder be called pathologic.

Drug and Alcohol Abuse. *Intoxications* due to drug abuse may be separated from other organic brain syndromes even though the mechanisms of causation are similar, because the treatment is very different. Intoxicating substances do cause a compromise of cerebral function (delirium), and for that reason intoxicated patients may have deficits of short-term memory, poor attention, and erroneous calculations. Differentiating the intoxicated substance abuse patient from other confused patients may be relatively easy in the case of alcohol abuse, but it can be more difficult in cases of sedative or tranquilizer abusers who do not volunteer information about their drug dependence. For this reason, it is important to ask every patient about drug and alcohol use.

Withdrawal from drugs or alcohol can result in disorientation and confusion, as well as, agitation or wild hallucinations and delusions. Cerebral cells are in an excitatory state during withdrawal from a CNS-depressant drug and in a depressed state during delirium from other causes. Engel and Romano (1959) have shown that during delirium from a variety of causes, the EEG reading is slowed compared to normal, while with alcohol or sedative withdrawal the EEG is faster than normal. Drug withdrawal states also differ from other organic brain syndromes in approach to treatment. Intoxication and withdrawal are treated by careful detoxification (Thompson et al., 1975), while delirium and dementia are treated symptomatically while a search is made for the basic cause. Treatment is discussed in detail later.

Measuring Intellectual Function

After intoxication or withdrawal have been ruled out by careful history-taking, the most useful tool in making the differential diagnosis is the cognitive part of the *mental status examination* (Table 6–6). (See Chapter 2 for broader discussion.) This section tests the intellectual functions which should be intact in all other diagnoses except organic brain syndrome. This important test can be administered in 5–10 minutes. All nonorganic patients should be able to give the date within a day or two as well as their location. In doubtful cases, the patient can be told the correct date or location and asked again later. For more subtle cases of organicity, the patient

can be asked to explain how to get from one well-known part of the city to another. *Memory* has three components to it: immediate, recent, and remote. Recent memory is most affected in organic brain syndrome, so that a patient asked to remember three objects such as a pencil, a boat, and a ball, will not be able to repeat them back when asked five minutes later. Another test is to ask patients what they had for breakfast. Remote memory can be tested by asking for the patient's birthdate and place of birth or a list of the last five presidents of the United States. Immediate memory is tested by having the patient repeat a set of random digits after the

---

TABLE 6–6
Mental status examination

INTELLECTUAL FUNCTION	TEST
Orientation	Date, location, name
Memory —remote	Place of birth and birthdate List last 5 presidents of the United States
—recent	Remember 3 objects after 5 minutes
—immediate	Repetition of digits forward and backward
Calculations	Serial subtraction of sevens from 100 Multiply 3 × 14 Add 17 + 15
Judgment	Reaction to hypothetical situation, for example, fire in a theater
Abstraction	Understanding proverbs or similarities

examiner. Start at three digits and keep increasing the number until the patient misses. Average response is seven digits forward and four backward; only four digits forward or two digits backward is a poor performance. *Calculations* are often dependent on native intelligence and educational level, but most patients should be able to subtract 7 from 100 and follow a command to keep subtracting by sevens. If they cannot do sevens, serial threes subtracted from 20 may be tried. This test also examines attention as well as calculation. Some patients make arithmetic mistakes but attend to the task. Others with attentional difficulties get lost and forget where they are or what they are doing. Multiplying 3×14 or adding 15 and 17 are other useful tests. *Judgment* is examined by asking the patient how he would react in a hypothetical situation. Organic brain syndrome patients usually have concrete emotional responses. For example, if they see fire in a theatre they may yell out instead of thinking out a rational plan such as informing the usher and helping open doors. Other psychiatric diagnoses may have unusual or bizarre reactions to social judgment questions, so this question cannot be used alone to distinguish the organic brain syndrome. Finally, the ability to *abstract* may be impaired in organicity. A classic concrete response to "People who live in glass houses shouldn't throw stones" is "They might break the glass." Concreteness is present in other diagnoses such as schizophrenia and manic-depressive illness, so it is not indicative of organicity alone. Very bizarre or personalized interpretations of a proverb are likely to be more characteristic of schizophrenia or mania.

Specific Diagnosis

Once the diagnosis of organic brain syndrome is made, it is useful to try to determine whether it is an acute delirium or a chronic dementia. As already mentioned, this is usually distinguished by the course of the illness. A delirium usually has a sudden onset with frequent fluctuation in level of attention and symptoms, whereas a dementia has a more insidious onset of slow intellectual deterioration and loss of previously learned abilities. It is also not unusual for an acute episode of delirium to be temporarily superimposed on a chronic, slowly progressing dementia. For instance, a man with Alzheimer's senile dementia may develop a pneumonia which makes him temporarily delirious. The acute-chronic distinction is important because *generally* a delirium indicates a reversible cause, and vigorous workup is indicated. However, it can often be difficult to make this distinction initially if the history is fuzzy, and in some cases it is only possible to make the diagnosis retrospectively.

In either case, even when the diagnosis of organic brain syndrome is made, the diagnostic work is not finished since this is only a syndromic diagnosis and not an *etiologic* one. There are hundreds of possible causes of organicity. Potentially, any illness can cause an organic brain syndrome, since any disease that either alters the metabolic environment or causes direct damage to brain cells is capable of causing temporary or permanent cerebral dysfunction. Many physicians assume that organic brain syndromes cannot be further diagnosed or treated and assign a nonspecific title like "idiopathic brain syndrome." Seltzer and Sherwin (1978) studied 80 patients with cases of suspected organic impairment who had a nonspecific primary neuropsychiatric diagnosis such as "organic psychosis" or "chronic brain syndrome." From examination of the charts for past history, laboratory tests, and special procedures, along with a neurologic examination, they were able to assign a specific diagnosis to 77 of the 80 subjects. Since even in chronic cases some specific causes are reversible, it is essential that all patients receive a workup of their organic mental state after the diagnosis is first made. A minimum evaluation (Table 6–7) should include a medical and psychiatric history especially sensitive to head trauma, drug and alcohol abuse, previous psychiatric hospitalizations, and family history. This should be followed by a careful medical and neurologic examination. A basic set of laboratory tests would be: chest roentgenogram, complete blood count, serology for syphilis, electrolyte levels, liver function tests, blood glucose, blood urea nitrogen (BUN) and creatinine levels, urinalysis, thyroid function tests (T_4), and vitamin B_{12} and folate levels. Other specific blood tests suggested by history or examination should be drawn. If a cerebral etiology is at all suspected, an EEG, computerized tomographic scan of the brain, or brain scan may help establish the diagnosis. The clinician is encouraged not to be too sparing with these tests since they can pick up diagnoses of reversible states, such as normal pressure hydrocephalus or chronic subdural hematoma, which might otherwise be missed. Both states

---

TABLE 6–7
Basic diagnostic evaluation procedure

A. Medical history (especially head trauma, family history)

B. Psychiatric history (especially previous hospitalizations, alcohol and drug abuse)

C. Phsyical and neurologic examination

D. Chest roentgenogram

E. Urinalysis

F. Blood tests
1. Complete blood count
2. Electrolytes, glucose, BUN, creatinine, liver function tests
3. Serology for syphilis
4. Thyroid function tests (T_4)
5. Vitamin B_{12} and folate levels

G. Optional tests:
1. Computerized tomographic scan of brain
2. EEG
3. Brain scan
4. Skull roentgenogram
5. Cerebrospinal fluid studies

---

have intellectual deterioration as their primary presenting symptom in the over-60-years age group.

Only when the underlying cause of the organic brain syndrome has been found can final decisions about reversibility or irreversibility be made. To aid the clinician in diagnostic thinking, refer to the tables listing common causes of acute, usually reversible, organic brain syndromes (Table 6–8) and chronic, usually irreversible, organic brain syndromes (Table 6–9). Some etiologies may appear on both lists since the extent or duration of exposure may determine whether permanent damage is done. These tables are by no means a full listing of all possible causes, since potentially that could include all diseases.

TREATMENT

The etiologic diagnosis and proper treatment of the underlying cause is the only specific treatment for the organic brain syndrome. In most of the acute cases of organicity, *medical or surgical intervention is the key to reversibility*. For example, a patient with severe hyponatremia may be confused, uncooperative, and hallucinating, even threatening suicide, but when the serum sodium level returns to normal, composure is restored. Another patient may have taken too many anticholinergic drugs and is wildiy hallucinatory and combative. Once he has received physostigmine (1–2 mg intramuscularly) a specific antidote, he will once again be oriented, calm, and cooperative (El-Yousef et al., 1973). A patient may suddenly begin to appear irritable and withdrawn and seem to have a depression until he is tested and found to be disoriented. The medical evaluation then reveals him to have tuberculous meningitis. With proper antimicrobial treatment, he recovers with intact mentation.

During the confusing initial stages of an organic brain syndrome, many patients are misdiagnosed and treated with a variety of sedatives

TABLE 6–8. Causes of acute (usually reversible) organic brain syndromes

METABOLIC	DRUGS	TOXINS	VASCULAR	DEFICIENCY
Sodium (especially hyponatremia) Potassium Magnesium (especially hypomagnesia) Calcium (especially hypercalcemia) Alkalosis or acidosis Glucose (especially hypoglycemia) Copper (Wilson's disease) Uremia	Overmedication with: anticholinergics sedatives analgesics tranquilizers Digitalis Quinidine Steroids many others Undermedication with: analgesics Idiosyncratic reactions: pentasocine propranolol many others	Heavy metals (lead, arsenic, etc) Organic phosphate compounds	Hypertensive encephalopathy Inflammatory diseases of blood vessels (for example, SLE, polyarteritis nodosa)	Pernicious anemia (B_{12}) Folate Thiamine Pyridoxine Pellagra (nicotinic acid)

ENDOCRINE	NEUROLOGIC	ENVIRONMENTAL	VENTILATION-PERFUSION	OTHER
Thyroid (hypo- or hyper-) Parathyroid (hypo- or hyper-) Addison's disease Cushing's disease Elevated corticosteroids from any cause	Concussion Acute subdural hematoma Epidural hematoma Tumor Epilepsy Abscess Meningitis (especially tuberculous, cryptococcal, viral) Encephalitis (especially herpes simplex) Normal pressure hydrocephalus	Room location Lack of stimulation Poor lighting	Hypoxic (anemia, chronic obstructive pulmonary disease) Congestive heart failure Hypovolemia (dehydration, hemorrhage, shock)	Fever Postcardiotomy Postanesthetic AIP Remote effects of malignancy (cancer of the pancreas or lung, pheochromocytoma)

and tranquilizers. It is not unusual to find a patient taking a benzodiazepine like diazepam and two different sleep medications prescribed by several different doctors. These sedating medications do not help and, in fact, often increase the agitation because they further depress the patient's sensorium. These medications should be tapered to avoid withdrawal and discontinued as soon as possible. Often this measure alone will result in an increase in the patient's attention and comprehension.

At times, especially with medical patients who are acutely ill, there is no one metabolic derangement which is significant enough to explain the acute delirium seen in that particular patient. In fact, there may be other patients with far more significant medical problems which would be expected to affect the brain, who are well oriented and clear. Two concepts help to explain these differences. In some patients, the cause of the delirium is not a single derangement but a combination of several minor changes which all together affect the brain cells enough to cause the organic brain syndrome. Thus, a diabetic in metabolic acidosis with a pneumonia and fever might not have organic brain syndrome from any of these causes alone, but the effect of all three results in cerebral dysfunction and confusion. The other concept which explains differential response of the brain to these metabolic changes is the differential vulnerability of the brain cells with increasing age. Younger patients have more reserves in the face of any illnesses in their bodily systems and the CNS is no exception. People over 60 years of age, especially, have higher rates of organic brain syndromes when admitted to hospitals (Lipowski, 1967b).

TABLE 6–9
Causes of chronic (usually irreversible) organic brain syndrome

DEGENERATIVE	SPECIFIC NEUROLOGICAL SYNDROMES	TOXIC

Presenile dementia
  Alzheimer's disease
  Pick's disease
Senile dementia
	Huntington's chorea
	Parkinson's disease
	Friedreich's ataxia
	Creutzfeldt-Jakob disease
	Wilson's disease
	Diffuse cerebral sclerosis
	  (Schilder's disease)
	Multiple sclerosis
		Alcoholic dementia
		Korsakoff's psychosis
		Heavy metal poisoning
		  (mercury, lead, magnesium)
		Carbon monoxide
		Postanoxic

INFECTIOUS	VASCULAR	STRUCTURAL

Abscess
Meningitis
Encephalitis
Tertiary syphilis (general
  paresis)
	Multi-infarct dementia
	  (replaces atherosclerosis)
	Cerebral thrombosis
	Cerebral hemorrhage
	Cerebral embolism
		Trauma (contusion)
		Chronic subdural hematoma
		Tumor
		Normal pressure
		  hydrocephalus
		Epilepsy

Even when a patient is discovered to have a dementia that is not reversible, specific medical procedures may be useful and important in preventing the progression of the organic brain syndrome. For example, a long-term Korsakoff's psychosis may show some irreversible short-term memory loss, but cessation of alcohol and a healthy diet with thiamine supplements will prevent the disease from getting worse and may even cause some improvement. Antibiotic treatment of tertiary syphilis will likewise prevent further progression in the dementia.

MANAGEMENT

Once the diagnosis of organicity is made and specific evaluation and treatments have been instituted, behavioral management of the syndrome can be considered. Management of delirium and dementia are similar, with the exception that management plans can be more short term for those patients who have reversible cases of organicity. *Explanation* to the family of the cause of the patient's behavior is essential, since relatives may have strange or erroneous ideas about the patient, particularly if his or her behavior has been socially inappropriate. Patients themselves need ongoing *reassurance* that the physician understands what is happening and is instituting treatment, but complicated explanations should be avoided since the patient will not remember them and may only be more confused. Whether in the hospital or at home, the patient will be helped by *orienting aids* such as a calendar, television or radio, as well as familiar objects such as pictures from home. Frequent family visits also help by lending the calming effect of familiarity in the strange atmosphere of a hospital.

If the patient has a dementia that is expected to be permanent, certain changes may be necessary at home, but these need to be carefully thought out. As a rule of thumb, it is better to keep things as familiar as possible, since marked or frequent changes will be more disorienting.

Thus, a family that passes the organic brain syndrome patient around several relatives' houses in a month may be increasing confusion despite their good intentions. Measures that simplify the patient's life and do not change it are the best. Often the Visiting Nurses Association can make evaluations of the home situation and the feasibility of the patient's continuing to live there.

With some patients, the deterioration may be so severe as to preclude the patient living at home. The patient may be wandering about outside at night or leaving gas burners on at the stove. Without someone to watch over them continually, they may become dangerous to themselves or others by accident. Families may have unrealistic hopes that they can care for the patient at home even when it is not feasible. In these situations, the physician needs to counsel the family about placement in safe settings, such as a nursing home. Such decisions sometimes arouse considerable guilt in families, which the physician can help reduce by indicating that institutionalization is not just socially but medically necessary for the patient as well as the family's well-being. Often the medical social worker can help to work through family discomfort about this step and also find appropriate placement for the patient.

Whether inpatient or out, the confused and uncooperative patient can be hard to handle. When patients' organic behavior becomes so severe as to hamper care and diagnostic evaluation, it becomes essential to try to calm them and induce cooperation with treatment. Restraints may be necessary to prevent them from pulling out intravenous lines, but this will not necessarily ease agitation and hallucinations. In these cases, a neuroleptic such as perphenazine, 2 mg three or four times a day, or haloperidol, 0.5–1.0 mg three or four times a day, provide the greatest calming effect with the least sedation. The doses can be given either orally or intramuscularly. Thioridazine, 10–25 mg orally three or four times a day, is also widely prescribed by psychiatrists for patients with dementias, but it must be used with care since it has considerable hypotensive and sedative effects compared to haloperidol and perphenazine. Haloperidol, in particular, has very mild sedative or hypotensive effects in the doses recommended. Although there has never been a formal scientific study, psychiatrists generally agree that these neuroleptics are more useful in delirium and dementia than minor tranquilizers like diazepam or sedatives like barbiturates.

CRITERIA FOR REFERRAL

Most cases of delirium or dementia can be handled by the primary care physician using the principles just outlined. Most of these patients benefit from a supportive, reassuring doctor-patient relationship and do not need special neuropsychiatric evaluation or psychotherapy. However, there are some situations in which referral to a psychiatrist is advised. At times it is impossible to distinguish depression and de-

mentia and more sophisticated evaluation is necessary. This might include neuropsychiatric testing, close observation on a psychiatric inpatient unit, and a diagnostic-therapeutic trial of antidepressants. Likewise, cases which do not seem to be following the usual patterns discussed here may be complicated combinations of depression and dementia, a personality disorder and dementia, or schizophrenia and delirium, which require the talents of a psychiatrist to separate out. Finally, when the family has difficulties accepting the changes in their relative, they may benefit from counseling from a social worker or a psychiatrist to understand and cooperate with the new needs of the patient.

CONCLUSION

In contrast to the common misconception, many cases of organicity are treatable and should not be ignored when recognized. If diagnosed and treated correctly, the devastating effects of an organic brain syndrome can be minimized for the patient and family.

APPENDIX: CASE HISTORY— THE CONFUSED PRISONER

A PEG constructed by the psychiatric consultant shows that the patient has evidence of acute organic brain syndrome (agitation, disorientation, poor recent memory, suspiciousness, labile affect, guardedness). In addition, there is question about possible dementing process (forgetfulness in last 2–3 years), perhaps due to heavy alcohol consumption. The acute organic brain syndrome may be caused by: (a) myocardial infarction and reduced perfusion of the brain, (b) CNS depressant drugs (morphine, diazepam, flurazepam), or (c) the coronary care unit environment with its sensory deprivation and stimulus overload.

Possible management plans that can take PEG data into account include the following:

1. **Biological dimension:** (a) Reduce CNS depressant tranquilizers (diazepam, flurazepam), and (b) give perphenazine 2 mg tid (for agitation and psychotic symptoms associated with the organic brain syndrome).
2. **Personal dimension:** (a) Orientation of the patient by the nursing staff at every opportunity. For example, "Hello, I am Susan, your nurse today. Today is May 25, 1982, Tuesday. You are in the coronary care unit of the Yale–New Haven Hospital. I will be taking your blood pressure and

PATIENT EVALUATION GRID

DIMENSIONS	CONTEXTS		
	CURRENT (Current States)	RECENT (Recent Events and Changes)	BACKGROUND (Culture, Traits, Constitution)
BIOLOGICAL	Acute myocardial infarction Morphine, diazepam, flurazepam, lidocaine	Mild angina—2 yr Essential hypertension —5 yr controlled with hydrochloro-thiazide	Heart disease in family
PERSONAL	Agitated Patient thinks chest pain is due to indigestion Feels nurses are FBI agents imprisoning him Mental status: disoriented to time and place; refused to do serial sevens or calculations; poor recent memory; suspicious; labile affect	Forgetful in last 2–3 yr Sleep: OK Increasing irritability—2 mo Increased drinking—6 mo	College education Hard-driving, active, coping style Tends to blame others when upset (information gained from wife)
ENVIRONMENTAL	Coronary Care Unit Restricted visiting hours Wife visits	Considering retiring from job—1 yr Has been working as the manager of a shoe retail store—increasing competition lately Lives with wife who seems supportive	Jewish, lower middle-class background One older brother died in accident 15 yr ago Married when at age 23 yr No children

Demographic data: 65-yr-old white married male; retailer.

pulse rate now," and (b) calm reassuring attitude by the staff when patient is delusional without arguing with the patient.

3. **Environmental dimension:** (a) Familiar objects (photographs) from home; (b) clock, calendar, and radio in the room; (c) night lights; (d) extend visiting hours for wife since she is supportive and has a calming influence on the patient; and (e) transfer to a regular medical floor as soon as possible.

With the above regimen, the patient's psychosis cleared within 3 days. After being transferred to a regular medical floor, the patient had only vague recollections of the events in the coronary care unit. Perphenazine was discontinued in 4 days without recurrence of agitation or delusion. The patient has no signs of dementia.

RECOMMENDED READINGS

El-Yousef, M.K.; Janowsky, D.S.; Davis, J.M., et al. 1973. Reversal of antiparkinsonian drug toxicity by physostigmine: A controlled study. *Am. J. Psychiatry* 130:141–45. This paper details treatment of atropinic delirium, one of the few organic brain syndromes with specific therapy.

Engel, G.L., and Romano, J. 1959. Delirium, a syndrome of cerebral insufficiency. *J. Chronic Dis.* 9:260–77. This classic paper discusses the physiologic bases and EEG findings in delirium.

Goldstein, K. 1952. The effect of brain damage on the personality. *Psychiatry* 15:245–60. Here is an elegant and definitive description of the intellectual defects and emotional reactions in dementia.

Heller, S.S., and Kornfeld, D.S. 1975. Delirium and related problems. In *American handbook of psychiatry, vol. 4*, ed. M.F. Reiser, pp. 43–65. New York: Basic Books. The authors provide an excellent review of the history, causes, diagnosis, and treatment of delirium.

Thompson, W.L.; Johnson, A.D.; and Maddrey, W.L. 1975. Diazepam and paraldehyde for treatment of severe delirium tremens. *Ann. Intern. Med.* 82:175–80. This excellent controlled study shows the superiority of diazepam for treating delirium tremens.

REFERENCES

American Psychiatric Association. 1980. *Diagnostic and statistical manual of mental disorders*. 3rd ed. Prepared by the Task Force on Nomenclature and Statistics. Washington, D.C.: American Psychiatric Association.

Brosin, H.W. 1967. Acute and chronic brain syndromes. In *Comprehensive textbook of psychiatry*, ed. A.M. Freedman and H.I. Kaplan, pp. 711–16. Baltimore: Williams & Wilkins Co.

Cavenar, J.O.; Maltbie, A.A.; and Austin, L. 1979. Depression simulating organic brain syndrome. *Am. J. Psychiatry* 136:521–23.

El-Yousef, M.K.; Janowsky, D.S.; Davis, J.M., et al. 1973. Reversal of antiparkinsonian drug toxicity by physostigmine: A controlled study. *Am. J. Psychiatry* 130:141–45.

Engel, G.L., and Romano, J. 1959. Delirium, a syndrome of cerebral insufficiency. *J. Chronic Dis.* 9(3):260–76.

Fisch, M.; Goldfarb, A.I.; Shahinian, S.P., et al. 1968. Chronic brain syndrome in the community aged. *Arch. Gen. Psychiatry* 18:739–45.

Goldstein, K. 1952. The effect of brain damage on the personality. *Psychiatry* 15:245–60.

Heller, S.S., and Kornfeld, D.S. 1975. Delirium and related problems. In *American handbook of psychiatry, vol. 4*, ed. M.F. Reiser, pp. 43–65. New York: Basic Books.

Lipowski, Z.J. 1967a. Delirium, clouding of consciousness and confusion. *J. Nerv. Ment. Dis.* 145:227–55.

———. 1967b. Review of consultation psychiatry and psychosomatic medicine, Part II. Clinical aspects. *Psychosom. Med.* 29(3):201–24.

Seltzer, B., and Sherwin, I. 1978. "Organic brain syndromes": An empirical study and critical review. *Am. J. Psychiatry* 135:13–21.

Thompson, W.L.; Johnson, A.D.; and Maddrey, W.L. 1975. Diazepam and paraldehyde for treatment of severe delirium tremens. *Ann. Intern. Med.* 82:175–80.

CHAPTER 7

Evaluation and Management of Psychosis

Malcolm B. Bowers, M.D.

Psychosis is the final common pathway of many possible contributing factors—physical disease, metabolic derangement, endogenous or exogenous toxins, as well as psychosocial stress and environmental factors. It is *essential* that any physician be able to recognize the presence of psychosis and manage acute psychosis intelligently. Psychosis is an important and extreme abnormality in the current context personal dimension of the patient. The presence of psychosis limits history taking and may call for emergency treatment approaches as outlined in this chapter.

This chapter is written by one of the foremost authorities in the biology and phenomenology of psychosis.

Psychosis is a generic term applied to pathologic states of mind characterized by a prolonged, distorted, and bizarre perception of self and external world, a state of mind that is not under conscious individual control. The foremost symptoms of psychosis, delusions and hallucinations, are unusual ideas and experiences based upon primary alterations in sensory experience in a context of extreme anxiety.

Psychosis is not an uncommon symptom in the primary care setting, particularly if this setting includes an emergency room or walk-in service. Psychotic symptoms are present in approximately one-third of the patients seen by psychiatrists working in general hospital emergency room settings. The first part of this chapter discusses the evaluation, diagnosis, management, and referral considerations that arise when psychotic patients are encountered in the primary care setting. The last part of the chapter discusses etiologic and management theories of schizophrenia.

CLINICAL EVALUATION OF PSYCHOTIC PATIENTS

The physician usually suspects the presence of psychosis prior to seeing the patient. Often reports that the patient is "talking strange" or "acting funny" are obtained from the family or referral sources. In such instances the examiner can prepare to modify the usual initial approach to the patient based upon knowledge of psychotic ideation. It is not unusual for the examiner to feel some anxiety when faced with the prospect of evaluating a psychotic patient. If the patient's mental status is unknown (due to muteness or catatonia, for example) or if there is violent behavior or threats, the examination should be performed in a setting where the examiner feels safe if the examination is to be effective. Precautions vary from the presence of one or two attendants to the use of restraints and a bedside interview.

CASE HISTORY 7–1

An 18-year-old man was brought to the emergency room of a general hospital because of "bizzarre" behavior. He was brought in by his roommate, who told the physician that the patient suddenly started conversing with people who were not there and was incoherent when the roommate tried to speak with him. The patient had a "stomach virus" for the last several days, for which he was taking Donnatal. On mental status examination, the patient was grossly disoriented, attention and concentration was poor with very poor recent memory. He was frightened of "little green men" who were trying to take him to a planet in another galaxy. The patient's blood pressure was 150/100 mm Hg, and the pulse rate was 120/minute. The patient is a journalism major in college and an avid fan of science fiction. (See the appendix at the end of this chapter for further discussion of this case and PEG.)

It is best if the psychotic patient is evaluated in a low stimulus setting; one that is quiet and relaxed. Since most primary care settings are relatively high stimulus environments, it is important to attempt to reduce ambient stimulation in the interview. Many psychotic patients have extreme sensitivity to stimuli from nearly all sensory modalities. In addition, they tend to interpret stimuli in a more personal way than nonpsychotic individuals. Thus adventitious environmental sounds which would usually not receive attention, reach awareness and are scrutinized for their personal meaning, which usually has a threatening cast for the psychotic. The pace of ideas and thinking is often accelerated in the mind of the psychotic individual, sometimes to the point that he or she is simply unable to think conclusively. Therefore, it is critical, if elementary, to recognize that most psychotic patients are very frightened. They are under the control of an aberrant mental state, in which there are usually strange and threatening intimations; it is a state of mind from which they cannot escape and which they cannot control. It is imperative that the examiner proceed in a manner which conveys concern, awareness of the altered mental state, and confidence that he or she, with the patient's help, can set in motion the process of recovery.

It is usually not possible to perform a complete psychiatric interview with an acutely psychotic patient. Whenever possible family members or other individuals who may accompany the patient also should be interviewed. Information should be sought about the following: onset period, premorbid level of adjustment, prior episodes, recent stressful events, known medical conditions, and the possibility of drug and alcohol use. The examiner should try to convey assurance that the patient is in a safe place, that he or she will be protected, and that others will be protected from the patient, if threatening behavior or loss of self-control has been an issue. It is important to establish some rapport with the psychotic patient, even if a toxic or organic etiology is suspected. An attitude of firm, benevolent control is usually reassuring to individuals suffering from acute psychosis. If at all possible, the interviewer should try to establish whether or not the patient is oriented to date (month, day, year) and place. If clear disorientation exists and the level of consciousness is thus decreased, the possibility of organic brain syndrome with psychosis should be seriously considered (see Chapter 6). This possibility is more likely in older individuals. It may be necessary in a primary care setting to administer medication before an interview can take place.

ETIOLOGY OF ACUTE PSYCHOSIS

Psychosis related to drug use

Pharmacologic agents may be involved in the production of acute psychosis. Three general classifications of drugs should be considered in this regard: general metabolic agents, anticholinergic compounds, and hallucinogens (see Chapter 16).

In the category of general metabolic or toxic compounds are included steroids, bromides, organic solvents, phencyclidine (PCP), antimalarial drugs, major analgesics, quinidine, and the class of sedative-hypnotic compounds. In general, these compounds produce a lowering in the level of consciousness, disorientation, and loss of recent memory. An exception to this general rule are the steroids which may produce psychosis with a clear sensorium. Psychosis associated with high-dose steroids use is usually associated with altered mood, either mania or depression. The sedative-hypnotic drugs, including ethyl alcohol, are true addicting drugs and produce a withdrawal syndrome (delirium tremens) upon discontinuation. This withdrawal syndrome is often associated with psychosis in addition to acute organic brain syndrome. Long-term ethyl alcohol abuse may be associated with chronic hallucinatory syndromes. Phencyclidine (PCP) is a substance that is used illicitly with increasing frequency. Acute intoxication with PCP is characterized by marked behavioral disinhibition (particularly of aggressive behavior), disorientation, mutism, nystagmus, and hypertension. In severe intoxication, coma may occur. Numerous prolonged psychotic reactions, resembling acute mania or schizoaffective psychosis, have been recently reported.

Many drugs used in general medicine and psychiatry have pronounced anticholinergic properties. These drugs include the antihistamines, antiparkinsonism drugs, antidepressants, and the major neuroleptics. Toxic amounts of these compounds produce the central anticholinergic syndrome (CAS) characterized by disorientation, flushed and dry skin, mydriasis, tachycardia, elevated temperature, visual hallucinations, and amnesia. When delirium is produced by excessive central anticholinergic activity, it can be reversed by physostigmine administration. Physostigmine (1 mg intramuscularly) must be administered every 2–3 hours to be effective since its therapeutic action in CAS is relatively short-lived. Phenothiazines are not indicated in anticholinergic psychosis since many of these compounds are strongly anticholinergic themselves.

Among the hallucinogenic compounds that may produce psychosis are amphetamines and related stimulants, cocaine, LSD, and cannabis derivatives (marihuana). In general these drugs produce psychotic syndromes in a clear sensorium so that in the primary care setting it may be initially impossible to differentiate hallucinogenic drug psychosis from psychosis unrelated to drug use. Amphetamines or related stimulants may be prescribed as appetite suppressants, in decongestant preparations, or as antidepressants. Tolerance may develop to the initial doses used so that patients may use increasingly higher doses to achieve a desired effect. At relatively high doses the amphetamine congeners may produce a paranoid psychotic syndrome in individuals who have no prior history of psychiatric disorder. If psychosis occurs

at lower doses, one suspects individual susceptibility to low-dose stimulant psychosis. These drugs, like all hallucinogens, can precipitate or exacerbate disorders in the schizophrenic-manic depressive spectrum. LSD and cannabis preparations can be associated with acute psychotic episodes. One may suspect LSD in the etiology of acute psychotic syndromes associated with florid visual illusions. Frequently there is a history of "bad trips," brief episodes of pronounced anxiety, associated with prior LSD or cannabis use. It should be emphasized that severe guilt and/or suicidal or self-mutilatory behavior may be associated with psychoses produced by hallucinogens. Other drugs that may produce psychosis in a clear sensorium are L-dopa, MAO inhibitors, and tricyclic antidepressants.

Psychosis Associated with General Metabolic Illness

Psychotic behavior (delusions, bizarre thinking, hallucinations) sometimes may form a major symptomatic component of generalized illness. These psychoses are usually characterized by acute brain syndrome (disorientation and memory loss). High fever is usually associated with altered mental states which may include delirium and psychosis. Psychotic behavior may occur in the long-term course of seizure disorders, particularly temporal lobe epilepsy, or may be associated with epileptic status. Catatonia is a syndrome sometimes seen in functional psychoses, but it may also be observed in a wide variety of CNS disorders, including encephalitis. Disorders of the endocrine system, including Cushing syndrome, hyperinsulinism, and thyroid disorders may be accompanied by psychotic syndromes. Abnormalities in electrolyte levels may lead to an altered sensorium and psychosis. In the primary care setting, therefore, the evaluation of the psychotic patient must include, insofar as possible, a medical history and a screening physical and neurologic examination, particularly if disorientation and memory loss (acute brain syndrome) are present.

Functional Psychoses

The term, *functional psychosis*, has a long tradition and is used here to include those major psychiatric disorders (schizophrenia, schizoaffective illness, manic-depressive illness, and delusional depression) that may be encountered in the primary care setting. It is evident from the discussion thus far that these diagnoses should be entertained if toxic or general illness factors seem unlikely and if there is a clear sensorium. Another clue to functional psychosis is a history of prior psychotic episodes. Such psychoses usually begin between age 15 and 35 years, and may have either an acute or indolent onset. Frequently there is a previous history of poor social and sexual development. Extreme motor disturbance may be seen, either restless agitation or stuporous immobility. If the clinical picture is one of premorbid poor social adjustment coupled with marked, bizarre disturbances in thought and speech, along with delusions and auditory hallucinations, the term *schizophrenia* is most appropriate. (Schizophrenia is discussed in Chapter 8.) If significant signs of depression, elevated mood, or irritability are present in addition, the term *schizoaffective psychosis* may be most fitting.

MANAGEMENT OF PSYCHOSIS

Evaluation and management of psychosis in the primary care setting are closely intertwined and ultimately depend upon a working diagnosis with respect to etiology. It was stressed earlier that evaluation of the patient's sensorium is the major clue to diagnosis. If consciousness is lowered and orientation and recent memory are impaired, a careful search in the history and general examination must be made for a toxic or general metabolic etiology. Medical and neurologic consultation should be utilized liberally. There is at least one diagnostic test which can be considered, namely, physostigmine reversal of central anticholinergic syndrome. In properly equipped settings, a urine toxicology screening may be obtained, although results are not usually available to assist immediate management.

With the acutely agitated or disruptive patient, it may be necessary to give medication in the course of evaluation. If CAS has been excluded, parenteral neuroleptic medication may be used. For the individual of average size who requires sedation, either chloropromazine (25 mg intramuscularly) or perphenazine (5 mg intramuscularly) may be given and repeated every 3–4 hours. If less sedation is desired, haloperidol (5 mg intramuscularly) may be used every 4–6 hours. It is usually advisable to administer parenteral anticholinergic drugs concurrently (for example, benztropine 1–2 mg intramuscularly) to avoid the acute dystonic reactions often associated with neuroleptic drugs. In the elderly or those suffering from generalized metabolic illness, acute neuroleptic doses are usually reduced to about one-third the usual dose. If the psychosis is part of a sedative withdrawal syndrome, benzodiazepines may be helpful in the overall management of the clinical picture. Usually chlordiazepoxide or diazepam, 10–20 mg is administered every 2–4 hours until control of the agitated syndrome has been obtained. Management approaches in relation to suspected etiology of psychosis are outlined in Table 7–1.

REFERRAL

If the diagnosis of functional psychosis is made, it is likely that the patient will require a period of psychiatric inpatient treatment. Acute neuroleptic drug administration should be limited to whatever is required to effect a rapid transfer of the patient to a psychiatric unit. If the patient is currently under the care of a psychiatrist or is being followed in an outpatient psychiatric setting, it is important to make every effort to contact the responsible clinician to obtain details of prior treatment and to plan for appropriate and timely reinstitution of continuing care.

If the acute psychotic episode seems clearly associated with recent drug use, there is a possibility that the picture will clear rapidly with or without neuroleptic drug treatment. The availability of a 24–48 hour clinical holding unit is very helpful in evaluating this possibility. However, one should err on the side of conservative management in such instances. The symptoms of acute psychosis may wax and wane so that a symptomfree period of 48 hours or so without neuroleptic drug treatment should be required before one concludes that the psychosis is strictly limited to the drug episode and will not involve a more prolonged psychosis. Such prolonged or drug-precipitated psychoses may run essentially the same course as func-

TABLE 7–1
Diagnosis and Management of Psychosis

ETIOLOGY	CLINICAL CHARACTERISTICS	PRIMARY CARE MANAGEMENT
Psychoses associated with acute brain syndrome	Disorientation, recent memory impairment, delusions, visual hallucinations; consider CAS or other general medical illness	Low-stimulus environment; search for drug or medical etiology; physostigmine as diagnostic test for CAS; low-dose antipsychotics or diazepam if CAS not likely
Psychoses related to sedative drug withdrawal (delirium tremens)	Disorientation, recent memory impairment, delusions, visual hallucinations, tremor, tachycardia, fever; history of ethanol or other sedative drug abuse and withdrawal	Low-stimulus environment, hydration, vitamin supplement; withdrawal schedule using benzodiazepines; low-dose antipsychotics for persistent psychotic symptoms
Psychoses related to phencyclidine (PCP) reaction	History of PCP use, nystagmus, hypertension, disorientation, mutism	Low-stimulus environment; gastric lavage, acidification of urine, conservative treatment of acute intoxication; prolonged psychosis requires psychiatric referral
Hallucinogen-related psychoses	Usually clear sensorium, delusions, visual illusions; history of hallucinogenic drug abuse (LSD, amphetamines, cannabis)	Low-stimulus environment; acute reaction may resolve in 24 hours with conservative management; prolonged psychosis requires psychiatric referral
Schizophrenia and related psychoses	Usually clear sensorium, delusions, auditory hallucinations, history of prior psychotic episodes; drug use not involved in onset	Low-stimulus environment; may require antipsychotic drug treatment in primary care before psychiatric referral can be effected

tional psychoses which have not been precipitated by drug use.

If psychotic behavior is found to be associated with other primary medical illness, the treatment locus should be one appropriate to the illness. Serious sedative drug withdrawal syndromes should be treated in an inpatient setting. The psychiatrist can function as a consultant in the management of psychosis in the appropriate setting for care of the primary illness or may refer the psychiatric management to a consultation-liaison team if such a group is available.

CHRONIC PSYCHOSIS

Some primary care settings may assist in the management of the chronic functional psychotic patient. In such a setting, with adequate linkages to mental health care clinics, patients with chronic psychosis may receive general medical care and appropriate neuroleptic medication. Chronic psychotic patients usually require a range of medical and social services, which are best delivered from a single locus of care. However, in some settings, such centralized, comprehensive care may not be possible. When primary care centers participate in the management of chronic psychotic patients it is particularly important that care be coordinated with the mental health care clinic or psychiatric consultant. Chronic psychotic patients often do have genuine unrelated medical problems—accordingly, any complaints of illness should not be automatically interpreted as part of their known psychiatric condition.

SUMMARY

Psychosis is a relatively common symptom in primary care settings, especially in emergency room and walk-in services. The psychotic patient should be examined in a low-stimulus environment with appropriate safeguards to assure the safety of both patient and examiner. Such patients are best approached confidently and with reassurance by an individual who has some appreciation for the profound alteration in experience that psychosis produces. Ancillary information should be obtained whenever possible from family, friends, or clinicians who have been previously involved in the patient's care. A screening medical and neurologic examination should be performed, particularly if drug use or general metabolic illness is suspected. The presence of a reduced level of consciousness, clouded sensorium, disorientation, and memory loss should raise the index of suspicion of a toxic or general medical etiology. Administration of medication may be required for management and/or evaluation of the patient. Toxic drug reactions may clear in a few hours, although long-lasting psychoses may be triggered by hallucinogenic drugs or PCP. If the patient who becomes psychotic after drug use is symptom-free without neuroleptic medication for 48 hours, it may be possible to discharge the patient to home care. However, it is best to be conservative in such instances and to admit the patient to a psychiatric unit for continued observation if there is reasonable concern. Psychoses associated with sedative drug withdrawal or general medical illness should be managed with psychiatric consultation in an appropriate inpatient setting. The primary care setting may function in the continuing care of the chronic functional psychotic patient if there is psychiatric consultation or close liaison with a primary mental health care clinic.

APPENDIX: CASE HISTORY—THE LITTLE GREEN MEN

The PEG of this 18-year-old patient reveals that he is currently suffering from acute psychosis characterized by visual hallucinations, paranoid delusion (the little green men want to kidnap him), agitation, and disorientation. The physical examination data reveal evidence of sympathetic hyperarousal (or anticholinergic drug intoxication). In the recent context, the patient has taken large doses of atropine (Donnatal) during the past several days for gastrointestinal disturbance. There is no history of any other drug ingestion. The psychotic symptoms occurred concurrently with large doses of atropine. Some environmental stressors were also present, including breakup with a girlfriend. The background history reveals no evidence of psychosis or drug abuse problems in this patient.

Diagnosis.   Psychosis caused by atropine intoxication.

Management.   An injection of physostigmine (1 mg) resulted in temporary clearing of the psychosis, confirming the diagnosis of atropine psychosis. Conservative management in the hospital resulted in complete and permanent clearing of the psychosis in 4 days.

PATIENT EVALUATION GRID*			
CONTEXTS			
DIMENSIONS	**CURRENT** (Current States)	**RECENT** (Recent Events and Changes)	**BACKGROUND** (Culture, Traits, Constitution)
BIOLOGICAL	BP 150/100 mm Hg Pulse rate 120/min Dry, warm skin Mydriasis	"Stomach virus"—3 days with diarrhea Donnatal—3 days; consumed whole bottle during last 24 hr No other drugs	Patient's uncle alcoholic Usual childhood illnesses No family history of other mental illness
PERSONAL	Seeing "little green men" who want to kidnap patient to another planet Agitated; disoriented to time and place; decreased attention, concentration, recent memory; frightened; feels doctors are "alien agents"	Increasing confusion last 24 hr Starting to see "little green men" in the last 12 hr Agitation, incoherence—6–8 hr Restless sleep—4–5 days Didn't eat much because of GI disturbance—3 days	"Shy and high-strung person" according to roommate No history of psychiatric illness
ENVIRONMENTAL	Brought in by roommate Lives in college dorm Parents live in another state	Did not attend classes—3 days Breakup with girlfriend 1 wk ago Came to college 6 months ago, leaving hometown	Middle-class Protestant background Older brother (24) a salesman Close to parents

*Demographic data: 18-year-old, single male; college student

RECOMMENDED READINGS

Allen, R.M., and Young, S.J. 1978. Phencyclidine-induced psychosis. *Am. J. Psychiatry* 135:1081–84. This is a clinical description of PCP-induced psychoses.

Bowers, M.B., Jr., 1974. *Retreat from sanity—the structure of emerging psychosis.* New York: Human Sciences Press. This is a discussion, using accounts written by patients, of the experience of psychosis.

Bowers, M.B. 1980. Biochemical processes in schizophrenia: an update. *Schizophrenia Bull.* 6: 393–403. Bowers gives an up-to-date review of various biochemical theories and findings in schizophrenia.

Bowers, M.B., Jr., and Freedman, D.X. 1975. Psychoses related to drug use. In *American handbook of psychiatry*, vol. 4, ed., M.F. Reiser, pp. 356–70. New York: Basic Books. This is a survey of various psychotic reactions that may be encountered in the context of drug use.

Cutting, J. 1978. A reappraisal of alcoholic psychoses. *Psychol. Med.* 8:285–95. This is a useful review and reassessment of alcohol-related psychoses.

Detre, T.P., and Jarecki, H.G. 1971. *Modern psychiatric treatment.* Philadelphia: Lippincott. This useful text has strong sections on psychotic reactions and organic brain syndromes.

Duvoisin, R., and Katz, R. 1968. Reversal of central anticholinergic syndrome in man by physostigmine. *J.A.M.A.* 206:1963–65. This article is an early report of the use of a cholinomimetic agent to reverse anticholinergic delirium.

Engel, G.L., and Romano, J. 1959. Delirium, a syndrome of cerebral insufficiency. *J. Chron. Dis.* 9:260–77. This classic paper describes the stages of delirium and EEG correlates.

Heller, S.S., and Kornfeld, D.S. 1975. Delirium and related problems. In *American handbook of psychiatry*, vol. 4, ed., M.F. Reiser, pp. 43–66. New York: Basic Books. The authors provide a survey of delirium and related syndromes.

Kaplan, H.I.; Freedman, A.M.; and Sadock, B.J., eds. 1980. *Comprehensive textbook of psychiatry*, 3 vols. Baltimore: Williams & Wilkins. This three-volume textbook is the standard authoritative textbook of psychiatry. Chapter 15, "Schizophrenic Disorders," by Robert Cancro has a comprehensive, timely discussion of schizophrenia, and is recommended for readers who wish to learn more about schizophrenia as well as any other psychiatric disorder. It uses *DSM-III* nomenclature.

Perry, D.C. 1976. PCP revisited. *Clin. Toxicol.* 9: 339–48. Perry gives a discussion of the clinical pharmacology of phencyclidine.

Showalter, C.V., and Thornton, W.E. 1977. Clinical pharmacology of phencyclidine toxicity. *Am. J. Psychiatry* 134:1234–38. This is a discussion of the clinical pharmacology of PCP.

Wynne, L.C.; Cromwell, R.L.; and Matthysse, S., eds. 1978. *The nature of schizophrenia: new approaches to research and treatment.* New York: Wylie. This multi-authored book has full discussions of the etiologic theories of schizophrenia and the course and the diagnosis.

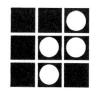

CHAPTER 8

Schizophrenia

Hoyle Leigh, M.D.

Schizophrenia, together with the affective disorders, is a major psychiatric disorder about which much has been written; much controversy exists as to its etiology and treatment. Schizophrenia is a chronic psychosis that affects the patient in several ways—the patient's perception, understanding, and adherence to medical regimen may be unusual, and the patient's capacity to work and socialize may be reduced. The patient may need to take medications indefinitely. His or her relationship with the physician may be strained. This chapter deals with the practical and most relevant aspects of schizophrenia for the nonpsychiatric physician.

Schizophrenia is a chronic psychotic disorder of unknown etiology. It is characterized by psychotic symptoms including thought disorder (looseness of association, tangentiality, delusions) and often hallucinations (especially auditory hallucinations) that occur relatively early in life (see appendix for case example).

Bleuler (1857–1939) coined the term "schizophrenia," and described the fundamental symptoms of schizophrenia known as the four A's—autism, association (disturbance of), affect (flat or inappropriate), and ambivalence. In addition to the four A's, he described many of the secondary symptoms such as hallucinations, delusions, bizarre behaviour, and so on. The diagnostic criteria for schizophrenia according to the *DSM-III* are presented in Table 8–1. The term, "schizoaffective disorder," is used when the patient has major features of both schizophrenia and affective disorder so that differential diagnosis between them is not possible.

The first psychotic break of schizophrenia usually occurs during adolescence or early adulthood and without treatment the course of the illness is usually downhill (thus the old term for schizophrenia, "Dementia Praecox"). Since the advent of antipsychotic medications, most patients' symptomatology can be greatly alleviated and with combined supportive psychotheraphy, family therapy, and medication, most patients can be expected to maintain some function in the community.

Approximately 1% of the population may be expected to become schizophrenic sometime in their lifetime.

ETIOLOGIC THEORIES

Since the etiology of schizophrenia is yet unknown, there are many theories. Etiologic theories may be broadly classified into biological and psychosocial theories.

Biological Theories

Genetics of Schizophrenia.   Schizophrenia clearly runs in families. The risk of developing schizophrenia for the general population is approximately 1%; for the parents of known schizophrenic patients, the risk is 12%; for full siblings of schizophrenic patients, the morbidity risk is 13%–14%. Children with one schizophrenic parent have a risk of 8%–18% of developing schizophrenia. If both parents are schizophrenic, the morbidity risk is as high as 50% for their children (Rosenthal, 1968). Studies of twins also indicate a high genetic influence. The concordance rate for schizophrenia in monozy-

---

CASE HISTORY 8–1

A 20-year-old single woman, a local college student, was brought to the physician by the police when she was observed talking to a refrigerator and started to undress in a department store. This patient was a rather shy but excellent student until approximately 1 year ago, when she started to withdraw socially, broke off with her only boyfriend, and started to develop psychotic symptoms, including delusions of being the Virgin Mary, auditory hallucinations in which two voices commented on her, and somatic hallucinations of feeling an "electrical sensation" in the spine. (See the appendix at the end of this chapter for further discussion and PEG.)

gotic twins is high, although the variability in the rate is also high depending upon the researcher (it varies from practically 0%–86%). Generally, the concordance rate in monozygotic twins is considered to be approximately 50%, while in dizygotic twins, the concordance rate is similar to that of a full sibling, approximately 10%–15%. Studies of adopted children also suggest that genetic factors play an important role in vulnerability to schizophrenia. It is interesting to note that many schizophrenic patients and their relatives have abnormalities in tracking an object visually (Holzman, 1974). Although few would deny a genetic component in the vulnerability to develop schizophrenia, the mode of transmission and the nature of the transmitted vulnerability is still unclear.

Biochemical Theories. In the past, various substances have been proposed as the abnormal biochemical substance present in schizophrenics. Such proposed substances included taraxeine (Heath, 1960) and 3,4-dimethoxyphenylethylamine (DMPE), and others. None of these abnormal substances are now generally believed to be present specifically in schizophrenic patients. Increased level of serum creatine phosphokinase (CPK) has also been reported in schizophrenia (Meltzer, 1976) but its significance is unclear.

TABLE 8–1
Schizophrenia: Definition and Diagnostic Criteria

DEFINITION

Schizophrenia is essentially a disorder characterized by certain psychotic features, especially related to thought processes, and delusions, and hallucinations, and deterioration from a previous level of functioning, that has a duration of at least 6 months and which has an onset before the age of 45 years.

DIAGNOSTIC CRITERIA (AFTER *DSM-III*)

A. At least one of the following during a phase of the illness:
1. Bizarre delusions, such as delusions of being controlled, thought broadcasting, thought insertion, or thought withdrawal
2. Somatic, grandiose, religious, nihilistic, or other delusions
3. Delusions with persecutory or jealous content if accompanied by hallucinations
4. Auditory hallucinations in which either a voice keeps up a running commentary on the individual's behavior or thoughts, or two or more voices converse with each other
5. Auditory hallucinations on several occasions with content of more than one or two words, having no apparent relation to depression or elation
6. Incoherence, marked loosening of associations, markedly illogical thinking, or marked poverty of content of speech if associated with at least one of the following:
    a. Blunted, flat, or inappropriate affect
    b. Delusions or hallucinations
    c. Catatonic or other grossly disorganized behavior

B. Deterioration from a previous level of functioning in work, social relations, or self-care

C. Duration: Continuous signs of the illness for at least 6 months

D. Onset before age 45

E. Absence of an identifiable medical disease or chemicals that might account for the symptoms

Reprinted with Permission. Copyright 1980, American Psychiatric Association, Washington, D.C.

Autoimmune and Infectious Agents.
Recently, there has been much interest in changes in the immunoglobulin levels in the serum of schizophrenic patients. Considerable numbers of schizophrenic patients have elevated serum immunoglobulin G and immunoglobulin M levels. The possibility exists that schizophrenia may be an autoimmune disease (Burch et al., 1968; Amkraut et al., 1973). Virus-like agents have been reportedly found in the cerebrospinal fluid of schizophrenic patients (Tyrrell et al., 1979; Crow et al., 1979). Although these findings are interesting, no specific pathogens or immune reactions unique to schizophrenia have been identified so far.

Central Neurotransmitters.   Currently much attention is paid to dopamine as a neurotransmitter which may be intimately involved in schizophrenia. Most antipsychotic medications are dopamine-receptor blockers (Snyder, 1978). Drugs that release dopamine or increase its level in the brain, such as amphetamine and L-dopa, may cause or worsen schizophrenic symptoms in some patients.

Psychosocial Theories

Socioeconomic Class.   Ferris and Dunham (1939) found an increased incidence of schizophrenia in the urban ghetto areas of Chicago. It appears that the prevalence of schizophrenia is in fact greater in low socioeconomic areas. Whether the environment of low socioeconomic areas contributes to the development of schizophrenia or whether schizophrenics drift down in social status to these areas is not known. The incidence of psychosis and schizophrenia seems to be increased in areas of rapid cultural change and stress.

Family Studies.   Some studies of the families of schizophrenics also indicate major abnormalities. There may be marital schism, or marital skew (Lidz and Fleck, 1965). In a skewed family,

one parent with idiosyncratic behavior dominates the whole family. Acceptance of bizarre behavior or major disturbance in communication may exist among family members of schizophrenics (Wynne et al., 1977; Singer et al., 1978). The so-called double-bind relationship has been described in the mother-child relationship, in which the child is put in a no-win situation; psychosis is the only escape (Bateson et al., 1956).

Psychological Studies.   Psychological studies of schizophrenic patients indicate that their major difficulties stem from disturbances of the so-called ego functions—disturbances in the ability to perceive and relate with reality, and an inability to control and keep in perspective their inner fantasy life. There is also difficulty with ego boundary—in maintaining the sense of self as a distinct entity discernible from the environment.

Conclusion

Various studies of schizophrenia seem to suggest that schizophrenia is a multifactorial illness in which the vulnerability may be inherited to varying degrees. This vulnerability may interact with developmental factors, such as family and social conditions, which determines whether or not the individual will actually develop the psychosis and if so, what form (delusions, hallucinations, and so on) the psychosis will take.

MANAGEMENT

Definitive management of an acute phase of schizophrenia usually requires referral to a psychiatrist. (A detailed discussion of treatment of schizophrenia is beyond the scope of this book, and the reader is referred to standard textbooks of psychiatry). The primary physician, however, should understand the principles of management, especially in chronic illness. Many schizophrenic patients have concomitant medical problems that require treatment and follow-up observation by the primary physician. A collaborative relationship between the primary physician and the psychiatrist is essential. The management of schizophrenia involves a three-dimensional approach, outlined in the following sections.

Biological Dimension

The advent of neuroleptic drugs (antipsychotic drugs) revolutionized the treatment of schizophrenia. Antipsychotic drugs commonly used in the treatment of schizophrenia are *phenothiazines* and *butyrophenones*. Representative among phenothiazines are chlorpromazine (Thorazine), perphenazine (Trilafon), thioridazine (Mellaril), trifluoperazine (Stelazine) and fluphenazine (Prolixin). Haloperidol (Haldol) is the representative butyrophenone. Thioxanthine and thiothixene are somewhat less commonly used neuroleptics. The choice of the antipsychotic drug depends to a large extent on their side effects. The common side effects that figure importantly in the choice of medication are sedation, cardiovascular effects (especially orthostatic hypotension), and extrapyramidal effects (pseudoparkinsonism, dystonia, akathisia). An often irreversible movement disorder, tardive dyskinesia, is also associated with the chronic use of any of the antipsychotic medications in a significant number of patients.

In commonly used therapeutic doses, the sedative and hypotensive effects are most often associated with chlorpromazine and thioridazine, less commonly with perphenazine and trifluoperazine, and least commonly with fluphenazine and haloperidol. On the other hand, the extrapyramidal side effects occur most commonly with haloperidol and fluphenazine, less commonly with trifluoperazine, perphenazine, and chloropromazine and least commonly with thioridazine. Thioridazine, however, has the most anticholinergic effect and may cause retinitis pigmentosa, thus it should not be given in doses higher than 800 mg per day. Fluphenazine

is available in depot injection form. Thus, patients with chronic schizophrenia may receive fluphenazine decanoate injections every 2 weeks or so.

When large doses of antipsychotic medications are used, the extrapyramidal effects may be prevented or reversed by concomitant use of an anticholinegic or antihistaminic agent, such as benztropine (Cogentin) or procyclidine (Kemadrin).

The dose of antipsychotic drug must be individualized depending upon the symptomology and the general health status of the patient and the side effects of the medication being considered. Usually, higher doses are required in the acute phase of the illness and, then, a smaller maintenance dose may be necessary for an indefinite period. The need for antipsychotic medication should be reassessed periodically in order to avoid chronic side effects, especially tardive dyskinesia.

There are a number of less common but potentially dangerous side effects associated with antipsychotic drugs such as agranulocytosis, jaundice, photosensitivity, electrocardiogram (ECG) changes, and so on. (For further discussion of the antipsychotic drugs and dosage, refer to Chapter 20.)

Personal Dimension

Psychotherapy is an important therapeutic tool in the management of schizophrenia. (See Chapter 20 for more discussion of psychotherapy.) Supportive psychotherapy in the form of regular contact and inquiry concerning the patient's symptomatology and interpersonal relationships may make the difference between compliance with an effective medication regimen or an acute exacerbation of psychotic symptoms. Although some schizophrenic patients benefit from insight-oriented intensive psychotherapy, the majority of patients receive optimal care through a combined supportive psychotherapy and antipsychotic medication regimen. An important consideration in the psychotherapy of the schizophrenic patient is that it should be geared to the continuing care of the patient on regular periodic intervals. In this sense, schizophrenia is somewhat like diabetes, a chronic condition for which the patient must be followed for a long period of time. The frequency of appointments should be individualized but, in general, at least once every 3 months is indicated.

Environmental Dimension

In the acute phase of schizophrenic psychosis, hospitalization is usually necessary. Hospitalization in a psychiatric service may provide the patient with protection and an environment conducive to a sense of mastery over the symptoms which perplex the patients. Even patients who have been managed well for long periods may develop acute psychosis under stress and require hospitalization. Negative emotions expressed by relatives who spend much time with the patient seem to contribute to relapse (Brown et al., 1962, 1972).

Many schizophrenic patients require some kind of sheltered environment even after the acute phase of the illness. This is especially so with those patients who have impaired function due to residual symptoms of schizophrenia. Such sheltered environment may be provided by halfway houses and other long-term facilities. For young, first-break schizophrenic patients, family therapy may be important in combination with medications and individual psychotherapy.

REFERRAL

Generally, a patient who is suspected of having schizophrenia should be referred to a psychiatrist for comprehensive evaluation and treatment. If the patient is known to have schizophrenia and has been in treatment with a psychiatrist, the primary physician should contact the psychiatrist for collaborative management of the medical condition. Since most schizophrenic patients are on maintenance medications, the primary physician should discuss with the psychiatrist the possible interactions of the antipsychotic drugs and medical management. Through this communication, the primary physician may also achieve a better understanding of the patient and, perhaps, some of the unique ways in which his or her patient may experience the world.

SUMMARY

Schizophrenia is a chronic psychotic disorder of unknown etiology. There is clear genetic predisposition, furthermore, abnormal family environment is often associated with the development of schizophrenia. Schizophrenic disorder is characterized by autism, disturbances of association and affect, and ambivalence. Most frequent symptoms include looseness of association, tangentiality, auditory hallucinations, and experiences of thought insertion, thought broadcast, and delusions. Management of schizophrenia involves antipsychotic medication, supportive psychotherapy, family therapy, and hospitalization when necessary. Most antipsychotic drugs used in treating schizophrenia are dopamine-receptor blockers. As a rule, patients with schizophrenic symptoms should be evaluated by a psychiatrist and managed jointly by the psychiatrist and the primary physician.

APPENDIX: CASE HISTORY—RELIGIOUS DELUSION AND SOMATIC HALLUCINATIONS

In considering this case, one should be cognizant that psychotic symptoms may be associated with organic brain syndromes due to metabolic disorders (see Chapter 6). In this case, the results of all laboratory tests including EEG were normal. (A syndrome that had to be ruled out was postviral infection encephalopathy in view of her recent bout of "flu"—the normal EEG and subsequent normal spinal tap militated against this possibility.)

On the basis of the quality of hallucinations, delusions, and mental status (loose associations in the absence of confusion as to time and place, and intact cognitive tests such as memory and calculations), and the duration of the symptoms (at least 6 months), the diagnosis of schizophrenia was made. The age of onset, and family history of mental disorder, and the family relationships ("schismatic"—see Lidz et al., 1965) all corroborate this diagnosis.

The treatment plans were as follows:

1. **Biological dimension:** Antipsychotic drug (perphenazine, 32 mg per day); anticholinergic drug to prevent extrapyramidal side effects of perphenazine (benztropine 2 mg per day).
2. **Personal dimension:** Supportive psychotherapy and evaluation of drug effect.
3. **Environmental dimension:** Psychiatric hospitalization; further family evaluation and family therapy.

The treatment plans follow this priority: first, psychiatric hospitalization; next, antipsychotic drug and psychotherapy; and finally, family evaluation and possible family therapy.

PATIENT EVALUATION GRID			
	CONTEXTS		
DIMENSIONS	CURRENT (Current States)	RECENT (Recent Events and Changes)	BACKGROUND (Culture, Traits, Constitution)
BIOLOGICAL	"Electrical sensation" in spine Physical exam within normal limits Routine lab tests—normal EEG—normal	"Electrical sensation" in spine (6 mo) "Flu"—3 mo ago No drug use	Mother's sister—mental disorder (in hospital) Menarche at age 13 yr
PERSONAL	"All electrical appliances send me messages that I am Virgin Mary" Auditory hallucination Two voices arguing about pt. loose association, orientation and cognitive tests intact	Started feeling "electricity"—approx 6 mo ago TV occasionally addressed patient directly Signed an exam "Virgin Mary" 4 mo ago sleep and appetite decreased	Shy, somewhat clumsy Excellent school records until recently One sexual experience at age 18 yr; not enjoyable
ENVIRONMENTAL	Lives with parents Father (47)—engineer Mother (44)—stays home Brother (25)—truck driver Parents constantly quarrel	Social withdrawal in last year Broke off with boyfriend—8 mo ago Stopped attending classes—6 mo ago	Irish Catholic background Parents fight constantly; mother tries to enlist pt. on her side against father. Brother not as smart as pt.
Demographic data: 20-year-old single female; college student.			

REFERENCES

Amkraut, A.P.; Solomon, G.F.; Allansmith, M., et al. 1973. Immuno-globulins and improvement in acute schizophrenic reactions. *Arch. Gen. Psychiatry* 28:673–77.

Bateson, G.; Jackson, D.D.; Haley, J., et al. 1956. Toward a theory of schizophrenia. *Behav. Sci.* 1:251–64.

Bleuler, E. 1950. *Dementia praecox and the group of schizophrenias*, trans. S. Zinkin. New York: International Universities Press.

Brown, G.W.; Birley, J.L.T.; and Wing, J.K. 1972. Influence of family life on the course of schizophrenic disorders: A replication. *Br. J. Psychiatry* 121:241–58.

Brown, G.W.; Monck, E.M.; Carstairs, G.M., et al. 1962. Influence of family life on the course of schizophrenic illness. *Br. J. Prev. Soc. Med.* 16:55–68.

Burch, P.R.J.; Rowell, N.R.; and Burwell, R.G. 1968. Schizophrenia: auto-immune or auto-aggressive? *Br. Med. J.* 2:50.

Crow, T.J.; Ferrier, I.N.; Johnstone, E.C., et al. 1979. Characteristics of patients with schizophrenia or neurological disorder and virus-like agent in cerebro-spinal fluid. *Lancet* April: 842–44.

Ferris, R.E.L., and Dunham, H.W. 1939. *Mental disorders in urban areas*. Chicago: University of Chicago Press.

Heath, R.G. 1960. A biochemical hypothesis on the etiology of schizophrenia. In *The etiology of schizophrenia*, ed. E.D. Jackson, p. 146. New York: Basic Books.

Holzman, P.S.; Proctor, L.R.; Levy, D.L., et al. 1974. Eye-tracking dysfunctions in schizophrenic patients and their relatives. *Arch. Gen. Psychiatry* 31:143–51.

Lidz, T.; Fleck, S.; and Cornelison, A.R. 1965. *Schizophrenia and the family*. New York: International Universities Press.

Meltzer, H.I. 1976. Neuromuscular dysfunction in schizophrenia. *Schizophrenia Bull.* 2(1):106–46.

Rosenthal, D., 1968. The heredity-environment issue in schizophrenia: Summary of the constant and present status of our knowledge. In *The transmission of schizophrenia*, eds., D. Rosenthal, and S.S. Kety, p. 413. London: Pergamon.

Singer, M.T.; Wynne, L.C.; and Toohey, M.L. 1978. Communication disorders and the families of schizophrenics. In *The nature of schizophrenia*, eds., L.C. Wynne; R.L. Cromwell; and S. Matthysse pp. 499–511. New York: Wiley.

Snyder, S.H. 1978. Dopamine and Schizophrenia. In *The nature of schizophrenia*, eds., L.C. Wynne; R.L. Cromwell; and S. Matthysse, pp. 87–94. New York: Wiley.

Tyrrell, D.A.J.; Parry, R.P.; Crow, T.J., et al. 1979. Possible virus in schizophrenia and some neurological disorders. *Lancet* April: 839–41.

Wynne, L.C.; Singer, M.T.; Barko, J., et al. 1977. Schizophrenics and their families: recent research on parental communication. In *Developments in psychiatric research*, ed., J.M. Tanner, pp. 254–86. London: Hodder & Stoughton, Ltd.

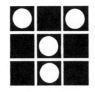

CHAPTER 9

Evaluation and Management of Depression and Affective Disorders

Hoyle Leigh, M.D.

Depression and mania are perhaps the most important psychiatric syndromes in medical practice. They are common among general medical patients and are often unrecognized until serious complications occur. Depression is a frequent contributing factor to a negative outcome of patient care—mortality, complications, and prolonged convalescence. The recognition of these syndromes and accurate differential diagnosis are crucial because effective treatment can be easily instituted by the primary physician.

The term "depression" may mean anything from mild dysphoric affect (feeling blue) to a serious pathological state in which the patient feels hopeless, apathetic, and suicidal. While mild depressive affect is commonly experienced by normal people in anticipation of or as a reaction to a loss or failure, a more severe form depression, the depressive syndrome, is always a pathological state that requires specific therapy (Leigh and Reiser, 1980). Mild depressive affect related to loss generally does not require antidepressant therapy—time and social support are usually all that are needed.

In psychiatry, "depression" usually denotes the depressive syndrome. Depressive syndrome may occur as a part of the psychiatric illness called *major affective disorder*. Major affective disorder may manifest itself in depressive episodes only (called unipolar depression), or there may be both depressive and manic episodes (called bipolar disorder). Depressive syndrome may also be secondary to a medical disease, an exogenous agent, or an environmental loss (such as prolonged grief reaction).

DEPRESSIVE SYNDROME

Depressive syndrome is characterized by a period of either depressive mood or a pervasive loss of interest or pleasure. Feelings of sadness, hopelessness, and helplessness are characteristic, although in severe cases, the patient may feel more apathetic than actively sad. There is loss of self-esteem and, frequently, guilt feelings and a sense of emptiness. Behaviorally, the patient usually withdraws from any social and family contact, and loses interest in hobbies and activities that used to bring pleasure. The neurovegetative symptoms of depressive syndrome include sleep disturbance (usually insomnia, especially early morning awakening, but in some cases, hypersomnia), decreased appetite and weight loss, psychomotor agitation or retardation, loss of sexual interest. There may be cognitive disturbances—indecisiveness, difficulty in concentration, slowed thinking, and so on. Small tasks often seem monumental to a depressed patient. The patient may become hypersensitive to vague discomfort and pains in his or her body, and may form delusions of a depressive nature (for example, my "brain is rotting"). Suicidal ideations are common, but the patient may not volunteer this information unless specifically asked.

Diurnal variation in mood is common in the depressive syndrome—the patient typically feels worst in the morning, but feels somewhat better as the day wears on.

CASE HISTORY 9–1

A 50-year-old married male attorney was referred by his family physician to a behavioral medicine clinic for evaluation and treatment of insomnia. The family physician, in his referral note, suggested possible relaxation training or biofeedback to help the patient's insomnia. The patient's insomnia was characterized by an inability to sleep through the night, usually waking up at 2 or 3AM and being unable to fall asleep again. In addition to the insomnia, the patient had moderate hypertension and was on chlorothiazide. Upon comprehensive evaluation, a depressive syndrome was diagnosed. (See the appendix at the end of this chapter for further discussion of this case and PEG.)

The *manic syndrome* is at the opposite pole of the depressive syndrome, characterized by extremely elevated, expansive, or irritable mood. There is often hyperactivity, indiscriminate enthusiasm for various projects and plans which are usually careless. Sometimes the manic patient shows irritability rather than euphoria. There is often pressured speech, which is loud and often incoherent (due to rapidity, associations based on sound rather than meaning— "clang association," inappropriate puns, flight of ideas, distractibility). Self-esteem is usually inflated; grandiosity and uncritical self-confidence are common. There is often increased sexual interest and sexual behavior (often inappropriate). Judgment is typically poor (indiscriminate spending of money, telephoning someone in the middle of the night for small talk). Characteristically, the manic patient sleeps very little and often professes no need for sleep.

ETIOLOGIC THEORIES

Psychological Theories

On the basis of the similarity between mourning and depression, Freud postulated that depression represented the symbolic loss of an ambivalently loved object, the loss of which was not consciously acknowledged and the aggressive impulse toward the object was redirected against the self (Freud, 1957). Later psychoanalysts such as Bibring (1965) postulated depression to occur when the person recognized inability to cope with an important task. Seligman and others postulated a "learned helplessness" model of depression based on the observation that some animals that had been exposed to inescapable shock showed impaired ability to avoid shock even when it was avoidable (Seligman and Maier, 1967). Depressed patients often exhibit the cognitive set of hopelessness and helplessness, even when it is obvious that they are not in fact so helpless. Beck (1967) postulated an altered cognitive style characteristic of depression—that of negative conception of the self, negative interpretations of one's experiences, and a negative view of the future.

Biological Theories

Biogenic amines seem to be involved in the depressive syndrome. Administration of reserpine depletes the storage of biogenic amines (especially norepinephrine and serotonin) in the brain. Patients treated with reserpine for hypertension sometimes develop a depressive syndrome. The monoamine oxidase (MAO) inhibitors are antidepressants that increase the available levels of catecholamines in the brain by reducing their intraneuronal degradation. Tricyclic antidepressants (for example, amitriptyline, imipramine) increase the available levels of norepinephrine (and/or serotonin) at the synaptic junction by blocking its reuptake into the presynaptic neuron and also increase the sensitivity of the post-synaptic receptors. The *catecholamine* theory postulates that the level of available norepinephrine in the synapses in the brain is increased in mania, and decreased in depression (Schildkraut and Kety, 1967). The *indoleamine* or *serotonin* theory of affective disorders postulates a decrease in the availability of serotonin in the brain in depression (serotonin levels in mania are inconsistent).

The *permissive theory* (Prange et al., 1974) of affective disorders postulates decreased serotonin levels in the brain in both mania and depression, with an increase in norepinephrine in mania, and a decrease in norepinephrine in depression.

The *two-disease* theory postulates two different kinds of depression: one associated with decreased functional levels of norepinephrine (and responding better to antidepressants selectively increasing norepinephrine levels in the brain, such as desipramine), and another associated with decreased functional levels of serotonin (and thus responding better to antidepressants increasing brain serotonin levels, such as amitriptyline). The norepinephrine metabolite,

3-hydroxy-4-methoxyphenylethylene glycol (MHPG), is low in the urine in some depressives, and these patients seem to respond better to tricyclic antidepressants that increase brain norepinephrine, such as desipramine and imipramine (Maas, 1978).

In addition to the biogenic amines, a number of other neurotransmitters and neuroregulators have been implicated in depression. For example, acetylcholine-mediated neurons may be hyperactive in depression and hypoactive in mania. Intracellular sodium may be increased in depression. Endorphins may also be involved in the modulation of affect.

Integrated Models

Depression may be seen as a "final common pathway" determined by various symbolic, environmental, genetic-chemical factors (Akiskal and McKinney, 1975; Leigh and Reiser, 1980). Psychosocial stresses such as bereavement or separation would be translated in the brain into neural impulses and neuroendocrine responses, which, in combination with genetic loading and preexisting vulnerability, may result in disregulation and thereby in the depressive syndrome. The cognitive functions of the neocortex may, in turn, be influenced by the disregulated neuroendocrine function.

Depressive syndrome, then, may be conceptualized as a disregulation of the normal affect of depression. The disorder may be caused when a threshold is reached in the final common pathway, contributed to by genetic factors, the state of the CNS, and the psychosocial and intrapsychic (or symbolic) stimulus.

EVALUATION

The first step in evaluating a patient who seems to be depressed is to determine whether the patient's depression qualifies as a depressive syndrome. This is necessary because treatment of depressive syndrome usually requires specific somatic therapies in addition to supportive psychotherapy. Supportive psychotherapy may suffice for less severe depressions. Table 9–1 shows criteria for diagnosis of depressive syndrome, which is called "major depressive episode" in the *DSM-III.*

Once the diagnosis of the depressive syndrome has been established, the probable underlying cause must be elucidated. Somewhat similiar to evaluation of hypertension, evaluation of depressive syndrome utilizes a process of elimination of known causes. Depressive syndrome due to known causes may be subclassified into arising from sources secondary to an external event (bereavement, loss, and so forth) or secondary to a known biological factor (disease, toxins, drugs, and so forth).

Grief reactions may be diagnosed by taking a careful history about recent losses and life changes supplemented by interviews with family and friends when indicated. Although uncomplicated grief reactions are best treated through family and interpersonal support, antidepressant therapy may be considered in severe and prolonged cases.

Depressive syndrome may be associated with a number of medical diseases and toxic states (Table 9–2). Any endocrinopathy (especially hyperparathyroidism), any occult carcinoma (especially carcinoma of the tail of the pancreas), any viral disease (especially hepatitis), and many medications (especially antihypertensive drugs) and toxic states are known to give rise to many or all features of the depressive syndrome. To rule in or out the various conditions listed in Table 9–2, careful *medical history, physical examination, and laboratory tests* should be performed on all patients exhibiting signs and symptoms of the depressive syndrome. In addition to routine laboratory tests, specific laboratory tests to rule out endocrinopathies, viral disease, and occult malignancies should be performed as indicated on the basis of the history, physical examination data, age and family history of the patient, and so on. Diagnosing or ruling

TABLE 9–1
Diagnostic criteria for depressive syndrome

A. Dysphoric mood or loss of interest or pleasure in all or almost all usual activities and pastimes. The dysphoric mood is characterized by words such as: depressed, sad, blue, hopeless, low, down in the dumps, or irritable. The mood disturbance must be prominent and relatively persistent, though not necessarily the most prominent symptom.

B. At least four of the following symptoms have each been present nearly every day for a period of at least 2 weeks:
   1. Poor appetite or significant weight loss (when not dieting) or increased appetite or significant weight gain
   2. Insomnia or hypersomnia
   3. Psychomotor agitation or retardation
   4. Loss of interest or pleasure in usual activities, or decrease in sexual drive not limited to a period when delusional or hallucinating
   5. Fatigue, loss of energy
   6. Feelings of worthlessness, self-reproach, or excessive or inappropriate guilt (may be delusional)
   7. Complaints or evidence of diminished ability to think or concentrate, such as slowed thinking, or indecisiveness not associated with marked losening of associations or incoherence
   8. Recurrent thoughts of death, suicidal ideation, wishes to be dead, or suicide attempt

After *DSM-III* diagnostic criteria for major depressive episode of major affective disorders (American Psychiatric Association, 1980. *Diagnostic and statistical manual of mental disorders.* 3rd ed. Washington, D.C.: American Psychiatric Association.)

To qualify as major affective disorder, the depressive syndrome must not be superimposed on schizophrenia or schizophreniform psychosis, and not due to a known organic cause such as endocrinopathies or drugs.

out the biological factors that may contribute to the depressive syndrome is essential because definitive treatment should be directed to the underlying biological factor (for example, removal of occult carcinoma) if one is found rather than to the depressive symptom alone. (See Case History 9–1, the appendix to this chapter, and chapter 5 for further discussion.)

If the depressive syndrome arises neither from an external event nor from a known

TABLE 9–2
Medical and toxic states associated with depression

ENDOCRINOPATHIES	Hyperparathyroidism (hypercalcemia) Cushing's syndrome Hypothyroidism Premenstrual tension syndrome
VIRAL DISEASE (OFTEN DURING INCUBATION AND CONVALESCENCE)	Influenza Infectious mononucleosis Infectious hepatitis Any other viral infection
MALIGNANCIES	Occult abdominal malignancies, especially cancer of the tail of pancreas Any other malignancy
DRUGS THAT MAY CAUSE OR AGGRAVATE DEPRESSION	Corticosteroids and ACTH Oral contraceptives Reserpine Alpha methyldopa (Aldomet) Propranolol (Inderal) Alcohol Benzodiazepines (such as diazepam or chlordiazepoxide)

internal biological derangement, then the diagnosis of "idiopathic depression" may be made, which is better known by the psychiatric diagnosis, *major depression of major affective disorders* (this is *DSM-III* nomenclature; in the past, this disorder was called by various names such as, manic depressive illness, depressed type, unipolar depression, melancholia, and so on).

When depressive syndrome not secondary to an external event or medical disease or toxins is associated with episodes of mania and/or hypomania as revealed by history or during the course of illness, then the depression may be a part of the psychiatric illness called *bipolar disorder of major affective disorder*. Sometimes, the physician sees patients who have mood swings; that is, cycles of depressed and rather hypomanic periods, but who do not quite meet the criteria for depressive syndrome or manic syndrome. These patients may have *cyclothymic disorder*, a milder form of bipolar disorder described earlier.

Both types of major affective disorders (major depression and bipolar disorder) have a strong genetic component, that is, they seem to run in *families*. About 15%–20% of first-degree relatives of people suffering from major affective disorders have histories of similar illnesses. It seems that major depressions and bipolar disorders are genetically separate, in other words, family history of bipolar disorder increases the probability of that particular patient's depression being a part of the bipolar disorder, while the family history of major depressions (unipolar disorder) increases the probability that the patient will not later have a manic episode. Thus family history is an invaluable tool in making the diagnosis of major affective disorders.

Recurrence is quite common in major affective disorders. About 95% of patients with an initial episode of major depression or mania are expected to have another episode in the next 10 years. Thus, past history of a depressive or manic episode is an important positive indicator for the

diagnosis of major depression or bipolar disorder.

There are some patients who are chronically depressed, who exhibit reduced interest or pleasure, but whose depression does not quite meet the criteria for the depressive syndrome. These patients may be said to have *dysthymic disorder* (or "depressive neurosis") according to the *DSM-III*. To diagnose dysthymic disorder, duration of the depression in an adult must have been more than 2 years without any period of normal mood lasting for more than a few months (in children, the duration of 1 year is sufficient for this diagnosis).

The category of *atypical affective disorders* is a residual category for those patients who have idiopathic depression or mania of varying degrees, but whose symptoms and duration of depression do not quite meet the diagnostic criteria of other affective disorders discussed in the foregoing paragraphs. A summary of the differential diagnostic categories for depressive syndrome is found in Table 9–3.

TABLE 9–3
Differential diagnostic categories for depressive syndrome

A. Secondary to
1. External event (grief reaction, situational adjustment reaction)
2. Demonstrable biological factor (medical disease, toxins, drugs)

B. Idiopathic
1. Major affective disorders
   a. Major depression
   b. Bipolar disorder
2. Cyclothymic disorder
3. Dysthymic disorder (depressive neurosis)
4. Atypical affective disorders

MANAGEMENT OF DEPRESSION

Depressive affect is a ubiquitous human experience that usually does not require specific treatment, unless it reaches the severity of the depressive syndrome.

Hospitalization Options

Once depressive syndrome has been diagnosed, regardless of under-lying cause, an important consideration is whether the patient should be hospitalized or treated as an outpatient. Generally, these are indications for psychiatric hospitalization for depression: suicidal potential, and inability to function in daily life. In addition, a medical disease requiring hospitalization for evaluation or treatment, or lack of home or work environment conducive to recovery from depression, are other indications for hospitalization in a medical or psychiatric service. If the patient is hospitalized in a medical service, psychiatric consultation should be obtained and collaborative management with a psychiatrist established.

The purpose of psychiatric hospitalization for depression is twofold, namely, for protection and therapy. The physical setting of a psychiatric inpatient service, trained personnel, and activity schedule for patients, all serve to protect the patient from potential suicide and severe social withdrawal. Opportunities to interact with the staff, regular medications administered by trained staff, and psychotherapy can be coordinated to render optimal therapy for the patient. When indicated, ECT can be given in an inpatient setting.

There are, however, some disadvantages in hospitalization for the patient. It may be seen by some patients as another defeat, and also a stigma. (Indeed, psychiatric hospitalization may, in reality, jeopardize some patients' careers or ambitions.) Hospitalization may actually allow some patients to withdraw further from social interactions. Also, hospitalization may strain the financial resources of some patients.

To hospitalize or not is in most instances a clinical decision that can only be made by the physician who has weighed the pros and cons for the particular patient. This decision is best made by a psychiatrist or by the primary physician in collaboration with a psychiatrist. In the presence of clear-cut suicidal plans or an attempt, however, hospitalization is mandatory, by commitment if necessary (see Chapter 10).

Once the decision has been made to treat the depressed person as an outpatient, management plans are made according to the nature of depression (secondary to other factors, idiopathic). Each time the patient is seen, the severity of the depression should be reevaluated, and hospitalization reconsidered (for example, if there is increasing suicidal thought).

Grief and Situational Adjustment Reaction with Depressive Features

Ordinary grief reactions and discouraged state in reaction to situational adjustment to life events commonly manifest some features of the depressive syndrome but fall short of the complete syndrome. Supportive interpersonal relationships, mobilization of family support, and time, usually suffice. The role of the physician is that of a sympathetic counselor, who can help mobilize the patient's social and family resources and give encouragement to the patient's efforts to cope with the loss. Mild tranquilizers such as diazepam, 2.5 mg three times a day, when necessary may be sufficient to reduce the anguish and acute pangs of psychologic pain in these patients. Flurazepam, 15 mg at bedtime, may help associated insomnia. (Because of the potential for dependence, caution is needed in prescribing benzodiazepines. They should be given only for acute distress in the initial phase of the grief syndrome.)

Many persons in a state of acute grief are preoccupied with the deceased, and may have illusions of seeing the deceased in a crowd, vivid images that are almost lifelike, or, occasionally, frank hallucinations of the deceased. Some become frightened by these experiences and seek the physician's advice. Reassurances that these vivid images and hallucinations are normal phenomena that will spontaneously subside can bring immense relief to the patient and family.

Although depression may be secondary to an external event, if a full-blown depressive syndrome develops (with suicidal thoughts, loss of self-esteem, anorexia, and so on), specific antidepressant therapy (discussed later) may be necessary.

Depression Secondary to Medical Disease, Toxins, or Drugs

Treatment of depression arising from medical conditions, or intoxication, must be directed to the cause, for example treatment of the medical disease (see Table 9–2), correction of the metabolic abnormality, or discontinuation of the depressogenic drug (such as reserpine). Antidepressant drugs are not indicated for depressive syndrome secondary to a medical disease, and their efficacy in these conditions is equivocal. When no definitive treatment for the underlying disease is feasible, however, a trial of antidepressant drugs might be considered.

Explaining to the patient and family that the depression being experienced is related to the medical condition and that it is expected to subside when the medical disease is treated, is an important aspect of management.

Depression in Major Affective Disorders

Management of depressive syndrome in major affective and bipolar disorders must be three-dimensional (see Chapter 1). In the *biological dimension*, specific somatic therapies (antidepressant drugs, ECT) are considered. Psychotherapy in the *personal dimension* is essential not only as a therapeutic modality but also as a prerequisite for compliance with the medication regimen, as is considered in a later section. Management in the *environmental dimension* include considerations concerning hospitalization, mobilization of interpersonal resources, and the like. It should be remembered that management of patients with major affective disorders is best accomplished in collaboration with a psychiatrist, and the possibility of referral to a psychiatrist should be always kept in mind before the primary physician embarks on this endeavor. Next, each of the therapeutic dimensions and modalities for the practicing non-psychiatric physician are treated briefly.

PSYCHOTHERAPY

Regardless of other treatment modalities used concurrently, psychotherapy is essential if the management plan for depressive syndrome is to be successful. Psychotherapy in this sense does not necessarily mean insight-oriented therapy, but, rather, the maintenance of a trusting doctor–patient relationship and an indication of concern and understanding conveyed to the patient by regular contact and listening to the patient. In this supportive psychotherapy, the physician should see the patient at least once a week (in the acute phase, daily if indicated, even if only for 15 minutes to assess any changes in mood or suicidality). During the sessions, which may last 30 minutes or an hour, the physician should specifically inquire about any changes in the patient's mood, sleep pattern, appetite, suicidal thoughts, and so on. The answers will give indications about the patient's responses to medications, and changes in the severity of depression. During each visit, the physician should reassess any indications for hospitalization.

A patient's family may be helpful in providing information for the physician about the patient's progress. It is of benefit for the physician to tell the patient that the depressive syndrome may color the patient's thinking process in such a way that everything may seem pessimistic and hopeless, but that with the resolution of the depressive syndrome, things may begin to look brighter. The physician should recognize, however, that suicidal potential of a depressed patient may increase just at the time that the depressive syndrome is beginning to abate as the patient may then gain enough energy to put suicidal plans into action. Sudden, apparent lifting of mood too early or unrelated to external events or treatment may be a sign that the patient decided on suicide as a solution.

As the patient's depressive syndrome abates with combined psychotherapy and somatic therapy to be discussed next, the frequency of psychotherapy sessions may be reduced to once every 2 weeks and then to once a month. At least 80%–90% of patients with depressive syndrome recover with a combination of judicious psychotherapy and antidepressant drugs.

ANTIDEPRESSANT DRUG THERAPY

There are two types of commonly used antidepressants—the tricyclics (imipramine, amitriptyline) and the MAO inhibitors (phenelzine, tranylcypromine). Because of their interaction with many foods and beverages as well as medications, MAO inhibitors are not usually used as the initial drug of choice (specific indications and interactions are discussed later).

Tricyclic Antidepressants

The most commonly used tricyclics are imipramine (Tofranil, among others) and amitriptyline (Elavil, and others). The nonpsychiatric physician treating patients with depression should be familiar with these two drugs and desipramine (Pertofrane, and others). Their mechanism of action is considered to involve sensitizing the receptors and increasing the functional levels of norepinephrine or serotonin at the synaptic junctions in the brain by blocking the reuptake of the biogenic amines by the presynaptic membrane. The choice of the tricyclic depends primarily on past history of efficacy (or family history, for that matter, since chemical efficacy of antidepressants seems to run in families), and the side effects of the drugs.

The most common *side effects* of the tricyclic antidepressants are: anti-cholinergic effects (dry mouth, blurred vision, tachycardia, precipitation of glaucoma attacks, and so on), sedation, orthostatic hypotension, cardiac arrhythmias, and heart blocks. In predisposed individuals, tricyclics may precipitate a psychosis. Tricyclics are contraindicated in serious heart disease, glaucoma, and in psychotic patients unless administered concomitantly with antipsychotic drugs. Patients who are given tricyclics should be warned about drowsiness that may interfere with attention while driving.

Among the tricyclics, amitriptyline has the most sedative action and most anticholinergic action. Desipramine is least sedative and least anticholinergic. Imipramine occupies an intermediate position. Amitriptyline is considered to have the highest serotonin-reuptake-blocking action at the synapse: desipramine is considered to block primarily noradrenergic reuptake; imipramine is again in an intermediate position. There is some evidence that patients who have low 24-hour urine levels of the norepinephrine metabolite MHPG, respond better to imipramine or desipramine, while those who have normal MHPG levels respond better to amitriptyline (Maas, 1978), but this urine test is not yet widely available.

Amitriptyline may be the first choice for a patient who has major insomnia, utilizing its sedative side effect. On the other hand, for a patient who has psychomotor retardation (sluggish and anergic), imipramine may be the drug of choice. For depressed patients with constipation, desipramine might be considered.

Dosage and Schedule. Although patients vary greatly in their absorption and blood levels of tricyclics after administration, the empirically effective dosage of imipramine and amitriptyline is 75–300 mg per day. For desipramine, it is 75–200 mg per day. As far as schedule is concerned, clinicians differ widely. Table 9–4 pre-

sents one of the many possible schedules for imipramine.

Administering all the tricyclic medication at night has the advantage of reducing the possibility of orthostatic hypotension and drowsiness during the daytime, and helping the patient's sleep. Patients should be cautioned, however, about possible dizziness when getting up, especially in the middle of the night. If patients have severe hangover, or other problems during the

---

TABLE 9–4
Sample schedule for imipramine dosage for depressive syndrome

Day 1.	Imipramine	25 mg p.o. h.s.*	In the absence of serious side effects, continue for next 6 days
2.		50 mg p.o. h.s.	
3.		75 mg p.o. h.s.	
4.		100 mg p.o. h.s.	
5.		125 mg p.o. h.s.	
6.		150 mg p.o. h.s.	
7.		150 mg p.o. h.s.	Reevaluate indications for hospitalization and side effects; reduce dose if necessary. If side effects are not serious, continue same dosage and schedule for another week
14.		150 mg p.o. h.s.	If good improvement, maintain dose If there is partial improvement, increase dose by 25 mg per day, up to 300 mg per day maximum
4 weeks.		300 mg p.o. h.s.	If no improvement at 300 mg at the end of 4 weeks, switch to amitriptyline (or to imipramine if on amitriptyline); if no response to other tricyclic; then refer to psychiatrist; at this point, the patient probably needs hospitalization, ECT, or MAO inhibitor; MAO inhibitors should not be given until 2 weeks have passed since tricyclic has been stopped

* p.o. h.s. = by mouth at bedtime.

night, the dose of imipramine may be divided (for example, 50 mg in the afternoon, 150 mg at bedtime, or other combinations, for example, 75 mg three times a day). If dry mouth is bothersome, patients may be instructed to chew gum or suck on sour candy. Severe tachycardias may be treated with propranolol, 10 mg three times a day or four times a day. If arrhythmia continues, the tricyclic should be discontinued.

Maintenance and Withdrawal.

Once the depressive syndrome has completely subsided, maintenance therapy should be instituted by reducing the drug very gradually (by 25 mg per week), until a dose of 50–75 mg imipramine or amitriptyline per day is reached. At any point during this reduction phase, the dose should be increased or reduction stopped if the patient shows any signs of increasing depression, sleep disturbance, or the return of any other signs. The patient should be maintained at the lowered dose for approximately 6–9 months. At the end of 6–9 months, withdrawal may be attempted by reducing the dose by 25 mg per week in the absence of recurrence of symptoms. Even after withdrawal, the physician should be cognizant of the probability of recurrence of the syndrome, and instruct the patient to contact the physician or the psychiatrist at the earliest sign of depressive syndrome. A successfully treated patient is likely to be aware of the early symptoms and to seek treatment before the depressive syndrome becomes severe.

Precautions.

In addition to considerations of the side effects just described, the physician should recognize that tricyclics are dangerous drugs if overdosed. Prescriptions should be given for one week at most until the maintenance phase is reached to avoid the possibility of a serious overdose in a suicidal attempt.

Tetracyclics and Trazodone

These antidepressants are essentially similar to tricyclics. Trazodone (Destrel) seems to have serotonergic function in the CNS and very little anticholinergic side effects.

Monoamine-Oxidase Inhibitors

Phenelzine (Nardil) and tranylcypromine (Parnate) are two commonly used MAO inhibitors. Their mechanism of action is considered to be that of increasing the functional levels of biogenic amines by blocking the enzyme, monoamine oxidase, which normally degrades norepinephrine and serotonin in the presynaptic neuron. MAO inhibitors interact with a variety of foods that contain the pressor amine, tyramine, such as aged meats, cheese, wine, pickled herring, and beer, and also with any sympathomimetic drug, including meperidine, cough medications, and so on. Interactions may cause serious hyperpyrexia, hypertension, cerebrovascular accidents, seizures, and other problems. MAO inhibitors are also potent rapid eye movement (REM) sleep suppressants. The use of MAO inhibitors are not usually recommended in primary care settings, unless in collaboration with a psychiatrist.

Lithium

Lithium is used most effectively to prevent recurrent manic episodes, and to a lesser extent, to prevent or reduce the severity of recurrent depressive episodes. It is recommended that the physician consult a psychiatrist before instituting lithium therapy for a patient with mania. In mania, antipsychotic drug therapy (for example, haloperidol) is usually indicated in addition to lithium in the acute phase, and inpatient psychiatric hospitalization is usually necessary because of the hyperactivity and poor judgment usually manifested by the manic patient. Recurrent depressive syndrome requiring lithium maintenance probably also requires psychiatric consultation. Lithium carbonate is the most commonly used lithium salt in major affective disorders. Lithium carbonate is usually given in 300 mg tablets in divided doses to maintain a plasma level of 0.6–1.2 mEq/L of lithium. This usually means a dosage of 900–1,200 mg per day. Plasma levels should be measured approximately 10 hours after the last dose, and at least once a week. Under no circumstances should the lithium level be allowed to reach or exceed 2 mEQ/L.

Lithium *toxicity* is manifested first by gastrointestinal symptoms (anorexia, gastric discomfort, diarrhea, nausea, vomiting, thirst), and by neuromuscular and CNS signs in severe toxicity (tremor, muscle twitching, fasciculation, ataxia, hyperreactive deep tendon reflexes, dysarthria, somnolence, confusion, seizures, coma, and death). Polyuria and nephrogenic diabetes insipidus may occur, and in some cases, hypothyroidism and goiter may occur with long-term lithium administration. Leukocytosis is not uncommon, and an increase in blood glucose level may accompany long-term lithium therapy.

Lithium is contraindicated in renal disease and serious cardiac disease. Extreme caution is necessary when lithium is given to a patient on low-salt diet, since inadequate excretion of lithium in the kidneys may elevate plasma lithium level to a toxic degree.

Electroconvulsive Therapy

ECT is the most effective therapy for the depressive syndrome (a higher proportion of depressive patients responds to ECT as compared to any other treatment), but it is usually reserved for drug-resistant depression. ECT is indicated as initial treatment modality for extremely suicidal hospitalized patients. ECT should be performed on hospitalized patients, with an anesthesiologist in attendance. Contrary to popular notions, ECT is not an inhumane or painful procedure, because patients are anesthetized with sodium pentobarbital, and muscles are relaxed with succinylcholine, when the electric shock is given. The only absolute contraindication to ECT is increased intracranial pressure (intracranial mass or recent cardiovascular accident). ECT may be the treatment of choice for patients who have serious cardiac problems precluding the use of antidepressant drugs. The usual number of electroconvulsive sessions required for de-

pressive syndrome is about eight. The most common complications of ECT are memory deficits, and confusion, both of which may persist in a mild form for months.

ENVIRONMENTAL THERAPY

While psychotherapy and pharmacotherapy is continuing, the physician should also begin therapeutic involvement of the patient with the environment. This includes encouraging socialization, continuing contact with family and friends, and above all, continuing contact with the physician. The physician may gently encourage the patients to participate in social activities, in activities that used to give them pleasure that they may have neglected of late (for example, hobbies), and the family may be counseled to encourage patients as well. The spouse and family of the depressed patient are often baffled and fearful—discussion of the treatable nature of the depressive syndrome may be a great antidepressant for them.

Referral to a psychiatrist may be another environmental change to be considered by the physician.

Referral

Specific indications for referral to a psychiatrist are (a) need for psychiatric hospitalization; (b) uncertainty concerning suicidal potential; (c) presence of symptoms suggesting another psychiatric disorder superimposed on depression, especially psychotic symptoms; (d) strong family history of suicide or schizophrenia; (e) patient expresses the wish to be treated by a psychiatrist; (f) lack of time (at least 1 hour once a week for a month) on the part of the primary physician; and (g) disinclination of the primary physician to treat this syndrome.

When the primary physician decides that a referral to a psychiatrist is indicated, he or she should discuss this with the patient in a tactful way. The physician should convey to the patient the information that depressive syndrome is a treatable condition and that the prognosis is good with specific therapy. Patients must also be told that the depressive feelings may make them feel more pessimistic and despondent about everything than reality warrants, and that these feelings will fade as the depressive syndrome abates. Since patients with depressive syndrome often do not have the energy to make contact with a new physician by themselves, the primary physician should obtain an appointment with the psychiatrist and relay the information to the patient and, preferably, also to a family member who will remind and accompany the patient to the psychiatrist.

SUMMARY

Although depressive affect is ubiquitous and a normal occurrence, depressive syndrome is a pathologic condition that requires careful evaluation and definitive treatment. In evaluating depressive syndrome, external precipitating factors of grief reactions, medical diseases, and drugs and toxins that frequently cause depression must be considered and ruled out before the diagnosis of a major affective disorder is made. Major affective disorder may be unipolar bipolar, and tends to be familial and recurrent.

Treatment of depressive syndrome should be etiologic if possible (as for example, treatment of an endocrinopathy). Management should be three-dimensional: in primary depressive syndrome, an antidepressant drug in combination with supportive psychotherapy and environmental support is usually indicated. Hospitalization should be reconsidered on each contact with the patient. Fortunately, depressive syndrome in major affective disorders is usually quite responsive to the therapy program outlined in this chapter.

APPENDIX: CASE HISTORY: THE HYPERTENSIVE INSOMNIAC

The PEG clearly shows that the initial complaint and the reason for referral may be only part of the true comprehensive picture of the patient. While the patient was initially referred for insomnia, the patient is shown to have moderate hypertension in the biological dimension, and in the personal dimension, he shows severe insomnia, depression, anxiety, occasional feelings of hopelessness, difficulty in concentration which progressed over a period of 3–8 months. The symptom complex described establishes the diagnosis of depressive syndrome, which requires definitive psychiatric treatment. The patient is intelligent, achievement-oriented and tends to be sometimes aloof and sometimes gregarious. This changeability of mood raises the question of a bipolar (manic-depressive) disorder. In the environmental dimension, increasing friction with his wife associated with the development of the depressive syndrome is noted. In establishing the diagnosis of depressive syndrome, it should also be noted that in the biological dimension background context, the patient's father died of complications of alcoholism and the patient's mother was hospitalized three times for depression. Alcoholism and depression in family tends to predispose an individual to the depressive syndrome.

On the basis of the PEG, the following treatment plans were developed.

PATIENT EVALUATION GRID			
	CONTEXTS		
DIMENSIONS	**CURRENT** (Current States)	**RECENT** (Recent Events and Changes)	**BACKGROUND** (Culture, Traits, Constitution)
BIOLOGICAL	Moderate hypertension Other physical exam and lab tests normal On chlorothiazide, a diuretic for hypertension	Mild hypertension discovered 6 mo ago—placed on diuretic	Father died of liver cirrhosis from alcoholism at age 50 when patient was 25 yr of age Mother was hospitalized for depression three times
PERSONAL	Insomnia (early morning awakening) Depressed, anxious Occasional feelings of hopelessness Difficulty in concentration No suicidal thoughts Does not smoke	Insomnia, esp. early morning awakening for 3 mo Increased drinking in past 6 mo Decreased sexual interest in past 8 mo Loss of appetite and weight loss of 10 lb in last 2 mo	Often aloof, intellectual, but at times a gregarious person Habitually uses rationalization and denial
ENVIRONMENTAL	Lives with wife (age 46 years, also attorney); no children Pressured work situation	Increasing friction with wife for 6 mo Mother died 3 yr ago of stroke at age 70 yr	Protestant, lower-middle-class background, 3rd among siblings; younger sister died of overdose (suicide) at age 27 yr, 10 yr ago
Demographic data: 50-year-old married male; attorney.			

1. **Biological dimension:** The hypertension should continue to be treated with diuretics and ongoing follow-up by the internist. Biological treatment for depressive syndrome should be instituted in the form of an antidepressant medication, imipramine.
2. **Personal dimension:** Treatment for depressive syndrome should be combined psychotherapy and antidepressant medication. The psychotherapy is to be provided by the psychiatrist who will also manage the medication and see the patient on an ongoing basis. Once the depressive syndrome has been treated, the associated symptoms of insomnia, loss of appetite, and loss of interest in sex should also subside. Then psychotherapy may be geared toward increased coping abilities.
3. **Environmental dimension:** In view of the conflict the patient developed with his wife, the psychiatrist should enlist the wife's support in treating the patient's depression. Eventually couples therapy may be considered. If the depressive syndrome continues despite the therapies, and the patient develops suicidal thoughts, hospitalization may be indicated, especially considering his sister's suicide.

The patient responded to combined psychotherapy and imipramine, as an outpatient, with the support of his wife who now understood that some of the frictions were caused by her husband's depressed mood and irritability. In 2 months' time, all depressive symptoms subsided but the patient continues in psychotherapy to increase his coping skills. Couples therapy was found to be unnecessary when the depressive syndrome subsided.

RECOMMENDED READINGS

Flach, F.F., and Draghi, S.C., eds. 1975. *The nature and treatment of depression*. New York: John Wiley & Sons. This multi-authored text is a comprehensive and eclectic discussion of various aspects of depression.

Leigh, H., and Reiser, M.F. 1980. *The patient: Biological, psychological, and social dimensions of medical practice*, Ch. 6. New York: Plenum Medical Book Co. Chapter 6 deals with the phenomenology, theories, and pathophysiology of depression, and is recommended for a basic, comprehensive survey of the topic.

Shader, R.I. 1975. *Manual of psychiatric therapeutics*, Ch. 3, 5. Boston: Little, Brown and Co. This is a very practical manual on psychopharmacologic treatment of psychiatric disorders. Chapter 3, "The classification and treatment of depressive disorders," by Schildkraut and Klein, and chapter 5, "The treatment of manic-depressive states" by Gershon are especially recommended in considering depression.

REFERENCES

Akiskal, H.S., and McKinney, W.T. 1975. Overview of recent research in depression. *Arch. Gen. Psychiatry* 32:285–87.

Beck, A. 1967. *Depression: Clinical, experimental, and theoretical aspects*. New York: Harper & Row.

Bibring, E. 1965. The mechanism of depression. In *Affective disorders*, ed., P. Greenacre. New York: International Universities Press.

Freud, S. 1957. Mourning and melancholia. In *Complete psychological works of Sigmund Freud*, vol. 14, ed., J. Strachey. London: Hogarth Press.

Leigh, H., and Reiser, M.F. 1980. *The patient: Biological, psychological, and social dimensions of medical practice*, New York: Plenum Medical Book Co.

Maas, J. 1978. Clinical and biochemical heterogeneity of depressive disorders. *Ann. Intern. Med.* 88:556–63.

Prange, A.; Wilson, I.; Lynn, C.W., et al. 1974. L-tryptophan in mania: Contribution to a permissive hypothesis of affective disorders. *Arch. Gen. Psychiatry*. 30:56–62.

Schildkraut, J., and Kety, S. 1967. Biogenic amines and emotion. *Science* 156:21–30.

Seligman, M., and Maier, S. 1967. Failure to escape traumatic shock. *J. Exp. Psychol.* 74:1–9.

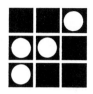

CHAPTER 10

Evaluation and Management of Suicidal Potential and Attempts

Andrew E. Slaby, M.D., Ph.D, M.P.H.

When a patient attempts suicide, the physician (family physician, internist, or psychiatrist) often feels a sense of failure, frustration, and anger. Was there something I could have done for the patient before this attempt had to be made? In fact, there are many behavioral indicators and risk factors in the road to suicide. This chapter discusses these important factors that any physician should know in dealing with potentially suicidal patients.

EPIDEMIOLOGY

Seventy people take their own lives every day in the United States (Schneidman and Mandelkom, 1967; Frederick and Lague, 1978). In 1976 there were 27,000 recorded suicides accounting for about 1% of all deaths in the United States that year. These figures, as shocking as they may seem, are felt to represent only a partial picture. They do not reveal what may be called hidden suicides in the form of such destructive events as single-car accidents and alcoholism; moreover, restrictions in insurance policies, societal taboos, and family shame obscure the complete picture. Experts estimate that a more accurate figure would be at least three times as great and that another 250,000 people attempt, but do not succeed, to take their lives (Slaby et al., 1981). Suicide is the nation's fifth leading killer. Only heart disease, cancer, stroke and accidents outrank it as health problems.

Compared to other countries, the United States is about average with yearly rates of 10–12.5 per 100,000 population (Yolles, 1968; Frederick, 1971; Slaby et al., 1981). Chile, Ireland, and New Zealand report significantly lower rates, while Austria, Denmark, Hungary, Japan, Sweden, and West Germany have high reported rates, in some instances greater than 20 per 100,000 (Slaby et al., 1981).

Two thirds to three fourths of people who eventually take their own lives *visit a physician* at least once in the last 4 months of their life. In many instances they are openly communicative about their situation, but the physician fails to pick up clues. They do not see the patients as having as serious an intent as they in fact do (Schneidman and Mandelkom, 1967; Frederick and Hendin, 1976). Physicians sometimes are surprised despite patients' long history of problems when they finally kill themselves. In one study (Neuringer and Lettieri, 1971) a *third of those who attempted suicide were found to have*

CASE HISTORY 10–1

A 51-year-old married woman with a chronic history of multiple somatic complaints and suicidal gestures was admitted to the hospital following a suicidal attempt with aspirin. The patient was well known to the hospital staff because she had been admitted to the hospital at least six times during the past 5 years—twice following a suicidal gesture with pills, for alcoholic pancreatitis, for evaluation of vague abdominal pains and aches (8 months ago), hysterectomy for dysfunctional bleeding (3 months ago). The patient's hospital chart consisted of four volumes; the patient had a reputation for being a somatizer and a manipulative person. No psychiatric consultation was obtained; psychiatric consultations had been obtained during previous admissions, amitriptyline had been prescribed, and the patient referred for outpatient therapy, which she did not follow through). On the fourth day she was discharged from the hospital with a prescription for 100 50 mg amitriptyline tablets and was told to take it twice a day. Three days after discharge, the patient was found dead after ingesting all 100 tablets of amitriptyline and a bottle of vodka. (See appendix at the end of this chapter for further discussion of this case and PEG.)

a serious physical complaint and *another third reported that someone in their family was sick or had been hospitalized just before the attempt.*

Suicide and Depression

It is a myth that an individual must be depressed or psychotic to want to kill himself or herself. Self-inflicted death is, indeed, 500 times more common among those with serious depressions (Frederick and Lague, 1978) but many people who kill themselves are simply angry, chronically ill, or lonely. Many individuals who deny any overt depression engage in very destructive behavior. For example, a patient with severe congestive heart failure may stop taking digoxin, or a diabetic may neglect proper diet and insulin. We all know of people who have driven a car when heavily intoxicated. A history of such behavior should make a clinician uncomfortable when evaluating a patient's suicide potential.

Self-inflicted death is counter to one of man's most essential drives, that of self-preservation. Lovers, friends, and family who survive the suicide relentlessly search out explanations. In some instances, the cause may be a readily preventable biological one, such as an instance in which a person on an antihypertensive medication, which has a side effect causing an alteration of mood, becomes depressed and kills himself. Diseases such as hypothyroidism, Huntington chorea, and Cushing disease may also be accompanied by depression. In other instances of suicide there is clear-cut evidence of psychopathology, as evidenced by a lifelong history of manic-depressive illness (as was the case with writer Virginia Woolf) or of schizophrenia (as in the instance of Michael Wechsler, whose parents poignantly describe their anguish over his illness and death in *In a Darkness* [1972]).

Sometimes, suicide is an existential choice. A patient dying of cancer or witnessing options constrict and health and ability to control one's own fate waning with advanced age, may consider taking one's own life as one of the few actions over which one has some control. The dual suicide of Henry P. Van Dusen, former president of Union Theological Seminary and his wife at age 77 and 80 years respectively appears to have been at least in part a statement that for the religious person, or any other human being, suicide may become an option to consider as the infirmities of old age set in.

Nonpsychiatric clinicians and lay people sometimes forget that the mood of depression, regardless of its origin, profoundly colors perception. The depressed person looks at the world through blue-tinted glasses: he or she minimizes personal achievements, withdraws from social supports and views all he or she has done, is doing, or may be able to do as worthless. To them, their situation seems hopeless and themselves helpless.

THEORIES ON SUICIDAL BEHAVIOR

A number of theories have been posited to explain why an individual would want to take his or her own life. As with many psychological theories, what appears to be valid in some instances does not necessarily always hold true. A lover scorned or someone who lost someone special through death may have quite different motivations for taking his or her life than a person who is dying of cancer, or has toxic side effects from an antihypertensive medication, or has just been given the diagnosis of Huntington chorea and has a history of family members dying demented and psychotic. In the example of the loss of a loved one, anger turned against the self may play a significant role. Biochemical alterations altering mood would be seen as responsible for depression and suicide ideation in cases of toxicity with antihypertensives. A reality-based rejection of another form of death more painful to a person than suicide may be a factor for individuals with cancer or who face the prospect of developing dementia.

Perhaps the best-known theory of suicide is that of the psychoanalysts. Freud and others (1950, 1955; Menninger, 1938) felt that in suicide one saw in the extreme the result of anger turned against the self. Suicide represented symbolically murder of another. A repressed unconscious desire to kill someone else was felt to be at the basis of suicide. Depression was a less extreme result of the same inverted rage. A person in the act of taking his or her own life may be acting out anger or revenge.

The relationship between suicide and homicide was of special interest to the analysts. Some felt that if anger was expressed one would expect to see lower suicide rates. In some countries it was found that when rates of suicide are low, rates of homicide are high. In other countries, however, this relationship does not hold true and rates for both are high or low. It is interesting to note that during the wars in the nineteenth-century Europe, and the two world wars, and Korean War during this century, suicide rates declined in both the United States and Europe (Slaby et al., 1981).

A somewhat different perspective to suicide is that of Durkheim (1897), the French sociologist who used statistical data from France and Switzerland to develop a nosology of self-destructive behavior. Suicides were found to be more common in cities (as opposed to rural areas), among the divorced and single (as opposed to the married), among Protestants (as opposed to Catholics and Jews), among the wealthy (as opposed to the poor), and among men (as opposed to women). From these observations, Durkheim conceptualized suicidal behavior as having four major forms: *egoistic*, *altruistic*, and *anomic*, which reflected respectively lack of social integration, extreme social integration, and loss of cultural guideposts. Although his explanations lack a psychodynamic dimension and consideration of biological bases of depression, they do draw attention to the strong role social factors play in suicidal behavior. In *egoistic suicide*, for instance, the

individual is not integrated into any social group be it family, community, or religion. Thus, one would expect to see greater rates among the single, divorced, and widowed than among the married and the lowest rates among the married with children. Protestantism is a less cohesive religion than Judaism or Catholicism, and urban communities tend to have less cohesion than rural communities. Hence, lower suicide rates among Jews and Catholics than among Protestants and rates higher in cities than rural areas. *Altruistic suicide* represents extreme integration into a group, as occurs in some societies with rigid social classes. An example was the Japanese military group, in which an individual may sacrifice life for "honor." *Anomic suicide* occurs when an individual is left without customary norms of behavior, as happens in economic depressions in which the wealthy are suddenly impoverished, or instances in which individuals move from a marital state to the divorced state.

Hendin (1964) looked to child-rearing practices to explain the differences in Scandinavian suicide rates. He contends that just as children learn different languages in different countries, they learn different ways of coping with stress. Danish passivity and Swedish competitiveness were felt to relate to higher rates in Denmark and Sweden.

Another theory of suicide is based on learning theory (Frederick & Resnik, 1971; Frederick, 1978). According to learning theorists, depression is an inability to behave in such a way as to evoke stimulating or pleasurable responses from others. The depressive state, as well as suicide, is seen as a lack of social skills needed to maintain stimulation through social interaction. Karen Horney's (1950) ideas represent a variation of the classic psychoanalytic explanations of Abraham, Fenichel, Freud, and others, which to some degree can be reconceptualized in learning theory terms. Horney emphasized the presence of defiance, self-hate, vindictiveness, and despair in depression and suggested that therapists attend to less dramatic signs in an attempt to diffuse anxiety before it mounts to unbearable heights. This, she felt, could help avert suicidal behavior.

EVALUATION OF SUICIDE POTENTIAL

There is an old adage taught to surgeons: "Man proposes; God disposes." By this is meant that the individual physician may perform an operation, remove an offending lesion, and suture the wound, but it will heal only by the "grace of God." So, too, in the evaluation of suicide, great clinical and technical skill and interpersonal sensitivity may be exerted in dealing with suicide potential, but in some instances, especially with patients having borderline personalities, suicide may still result. There are, however, a number of epidemiologic and sociological characteristics of those who have successfully taken their own lives which can assist clinicians in evaluating the suicidal potential in a clinical situation. The correlates of successful suicide are discussed in the following sections.

Age

Suicide rates *increase steadily with age.* In the United States in 1976, the annual rate in the 15–24-year-old range was 11.7 per 100,000 and in the 25–34-year-old range was 16.5 per 100,000. By age 55–64 years, the rate was 20.0 per 100,000. Suicide is the fourth leading cause of death among both sexes in the age group 15–44 years. For young males in the age range 15–24 years old, there has been a 250% increase fom 6.8 per 100,000 to 17.4 per 100,000 over the last two decades.

After adolescence there is a decline in suicide rates until age 40 at which time rates begin a gradual rise. The rate of the 20–24-year-old range is not equaled again until age 55 years. Thereafter, rates rise continuously to a peak at 75–79 years, which has a range of 42.5 per 100,000 per year (Frederick, 1978), the highest in any age group. Although suicide is always a concern, after age 75 years the number of suicides yearly are considerably less than that found in the younger age ranges. The small increase in recent years in this older age range has actually resulted in a decrease in suicide rate, considering the increase in population in this age group. One reason given for the decline is that more attention in recent years has been given to the issues of aging and need for continuing social supports.

Adolescent suicide has been the cause of considerable concern. There are an estimated 60,000 suicide attempts in the 15–19-year-old age group each year (Teicher and Jacobs, 1966a). As early as 1960, suicide attempt was given as the reason for admission for 10% of child and adolescent patients to New York's Bellevue Hospital. In addition, the suicide rates of young blacks and other nonwhites, which have characteristically been lower than whites, have increased in recent years to rates equal to or greater than corresponding white rates. For instance, the rate for nonwhites in the age group 20–24 years was 4.9 per 100,000 per year. In 1973, it was 14.1 per 100,000, nearly that of whites (race and ethnic group suicide risks are discussed in another section).

A number of factors play roles in adolescent suicide. These include family problems, lack of acceptance into school peer groups, breakdown of the nuclear family, unemployment, failure to make good grades, and a desire to be united with someone who has died. Children may imitate the behavior of older children or a loved one, such as a parent, sibling, aunt, or uncle, who has committed suicide. To a child's or young adolescent's mind death may be romanticized as a reunion. In other instances, an adolescent may be seeking revenge in suicide ("they'll be sorry when I'm gone"). Alcoholism and drug use may be a correlate of suicidal behavior or symptomatic of the self-destructive behavior of an underlying depression.

In a Los Angeles study of suicidal youths (Neuringer and Lettier, 1971), a history of mental illness in the family in the previous 5 years was commonly found. The children were often of unwed mothers or their mothers were pregnant at the time of the marriage. Suicidal girls were often pregnant and rejected by their parents and boyfriends when they needed acceptance most. Of the youths, 72% had had one or both of their natural parents away from home because of death, divorce, or separation in early childhood. This sometimes resulted in institutionalization of the child or placement in a foster home, or leaving the child with relatives. Many had to change schools and residence frequently. One third were out of school at the time of the attempt because of illness, pregnancy, or earlier suicide attempt. One fourth were out of school because of acting out in school (for example, involved in fights) or because of emotional instability. Of 46% who reported their suicide attempt, less than half told their own parents despite the fact that 88% of the attempts occurred at home usually with the parents in the other room. Two thirds reported it to someone other than their parents, such as a peer they "trusted."

It is unclear whether a young child understands sufficiently the finality of death to actually posit suicide as a permanent act. It is felt by some (NAMH Reporter, 1972/73), however, that children before age 8 years can commit suicide even though the Division of Vital Statistics does not list suicide in this age group. Children who have killed themselves by drowning, overdose with aspirins or jumping out of windows, in some instances, have been found to have left notes implying revenge for what they perceived as rejection by parents.

Sex

Women attempt suicide more frequently, but men succeed more often. In one study (Frederick and Lague, 1972) the percentage of successful suicides for men was 70%; for women 30%. Ratios of male to female suicide range from 2:1 to 7:1. The gap appears to be closing in recent years. Nearly 90% of all adolescent suicide attempts are made by females. Men, however, on the whole kill themselves three times as frequently as women.

Men tend to use more lethal means: hanging, jumping, and firearms. Women tend to use drug overdose. Many suicide attempts by women may be seen as a cry for help, while male suicides are often silent attempts to end an intolerable condition. With increasing opportunity for women to participate in the competitive professional and business world, we are seeing a rise in the pathologic conditions traditionally associated with men: coronary heart disease, suicide, and alcoholism. Women are beginning to suffer more from such stresses as failure to get tenure or being passed up for a promotion. In addition, the aggression that is sometimes needed to succeed in highly competitive systems, if turned against the self, can be quite destructive—even resulting in suicide.

Marital Status

The suicide rate for singles is twice that of marrieds (Slaby et al., 1975) and the rate for the widowed, divorced, and separated is four to five times that of the married. Rates are lowest among the married with children. The only major exception to this rule is that the married female adolescent is at greater risk than the single teenage girl (NAMH Reporter, 1972/73).

At first, it was believed that the reason suicide rates were greater among the divorced, separated, and single than among the married was that less stable people either were unable to maintain a marriage, or to even contract one in the first place. This seems unlikely as a full explanation, however, since the widowed have as high suicide rates as the divorced or separated and, in fact, greater than the single. A more complete explanation perhaps is that of *lack of social support*. The married more than any other group are part of a social matrix in terms of children, spouse, extended family, or community. This is, to various degrees, less true for other marital statuses.

Race and Ethnic Group

Until relatively recently, suicide rates were re-markably *higher among whites than among nonwhites*. Now, however, just as the gap is narrowing with increasing job and other oppor-tunities for women in society with a concomitant rise in suicide, so too for minorities. *Young urban blacks in the age range 20–35 years now have rates of suicide greater than white males of the same age.* In Schneidman's and Farberow's earlier work, 95% of successful suicides were white. The rate among blacks was usually said to have been one-third that of whites. In a study in New Orleans, (Breed, 1966) the rates were 10 per 100,000 for whites and 2 per 100,000 for blacks. The segregation blacks experienced, it was felt, forced them to limit their ambitions and, there-fore, reduced the strain of the competition. In a more recent study (Pederson et al., 1973) rates of suicide attempts by nonwhites were found to be 160 per 100,000 per year compared to 53 per 100,000 for whites, with the women to men ratio 6:1 for whites and 3:1 for nonwhites. The authors reviewing this data felt that whites and nonwhites attempting suicide may comprise two psychologically different populations and, there-fore, require two different types of intervention. The nonwhite group was younger and from lower socioeconomic classes, with the women more frequently separated from spouses. Over one half of the nonwhite males were single. The nonwhites were less frequently in psychiatric care before or after the attempt and less fre-quently diagnosed as having a psychiatric dis-order. A high risk group for suicide was most obvious among the white group. Suicide oc-curred at a young age and there was a relatively short time interval between the attempt and a successful suicide. For the white group, the successful suicide rate among those who pre-viously attempted suicide was 64 times greater than for whites in the general population. For nonwhites, suicide attempts appeared to be not as predictive of future suicide as for the whites.

Suicide is a special problem among *Native Americans*. There was a 36% increase in Indian suicide rates between the years 1970 and 1975 compared to a 6% increase during the same period for all whites and a 17% increase for blacks. The 1975 overall Indian suicide rate was 21.6 per 100,000 per year—64% higher than that of whites and 254% higher than that of blacks for the same year (Frederick, 1978). Not all tribes have suffered the same increase (Frederick and Lague, 1972). Some American Indian tribes have rates five times the national average while others are considerably lower.

Most suicides appear to occur among young Native Americans from adolescence through early adulthood. Adolescent Indians are looking for an identity in a rapidly changing pluralistic society marred by bigotries and economic con-straints. There is a dissolution of traditional family ways. Housing is poor and unemployment and poverty rampant. Young Indians experience conflict over remaining on reservations or attempting life in mainstream society where they will probably be working at menial jobs. Frus-trated and angry, with feelings of worthlessness and hopelessness, they often turn to drink to quell the strains of poverty, unempolyment, and discrimination. Excessive drinking is a form of self-destruction which may, like single-driver automobile accidents, be seen as a suicidal equivalent. The rate of death for cirrhosis of the liver for Native Americans exceeds that of all races for all age groups. In the age range 15–34 years, the figures exceed those of all other races by an average of 12:1 (Frederick, 1978).

One final point in ethnic or social considera-tions in evaluation of suicide risk concerns migration. Immigrants on the whole have rates consistent with those of their country of origin. The picture, however, is complicated by the fact that immigration brings with it displacement and dissolution of social matrixes. The new immi-grant is isolated in a new country and, especially if nonwhite in the United States, often discrimi-nated against in job opportunities and education.

Thus, one sees that rates of suicide are higher for first-generation immigrants than for the second-generation ones and those for the second generation are greater than those for the third. As an ethnic group becomes assimilated and new social bonds form, suicide rates fall.

Occupation

Suicide rates differ remarkably among professions, with physicians, other professionals, and business executives ranking quite high. Rates are lowest among artisans and farm workers.

Several studies have shown rates to be *highest among health professionals* (Frederick, 1978). Rates of male health professionals exceeded those of others by a ratio of 2.3:1. Female health professionals showed an excess of 1.7:1. Physicians over age 65 years showed the highest rates, but half of deaths from suicide occur during the most productive years of a physician's career: the two decades between ages 35 and 54 years. High risk factors for physicians are divorced marital status and increasing age. The ratio increases to 12:1 after retirement compared to 3:1 for the general population. While divorced men in the general population have rates three times those of married men, divorced physicians are 13 times as likely to kill themselves as their married colleagues. Personality disorders and manic-depressive illness are other variables increasing risk for health professionals. Physicians and residents in training tend not to reach out for help, while others burden them with their problems. There are no readily available outlets for physicians to ventilate their own anguish over being confidants and making daily decisions that bear on the life and death of others. They cannot deny the unhappiness that life has in terms of illness and human frailty and psychiatric disturbances. In other instances, some physicians may have turned to medicine as a career that allows altruism as a mechanism of defense—taking care of others as they wish they themselves were taken care of. The increased sensitivity to their own and other's problems makes them more susceptible to depression and feelings of hopelessness when confronted with their own human limitation to help others and themselves. Of the specialties, psychiatrists, ophthalmologists, and otolaryngologists have the highest rates; pediatricians and pathologists, the lowest. The rate for psychiatrists is 61 per 100,000 per year and that for pediatricians 10 per 100,000 per year (Slaby et al., 1981).

Other professional groups with equally high rates reported per 100,000 population annually are chemists with 120 (California); pharmacists, 104 (California); nonmedical technicians, 88 (California); dentists, 83 (California) and 78 (Oregon); lawyers, 54 (California and Oregon); and engineers 45 (California) and 43 (Oregon) (Frederick, 1978).

Family History

A family history of suicide increases risk, particularly if the event occurred before pubescence and the relationship with the victim was close (Frederick, 1973). In Farberow's and Schneidman's (1965) series 25% of those who attempted suicide had a history of suicide in the immediate family. A particularly high risk time for a same sex child of a suicide is when he or she reaches the age and/or anniversary of the parent's suicide.

Location

Rates of suicide for *urban* areas are nearly always greater than rural and suburban areas even when overall rates are low. More suicides are committed in the eastern and western states than in other parts of the country. The state of Nevada has the highest rates. Wyoming, California, Maine, and Vermont are other states with high rates. The northcentral states and midwest have characteristically had the lowest rates. Interestingly, New Jersey and New York have low rates (Frederick, 1978).

Method

The more potentially *lethal* the mode employed or planned to be used in a suicide attempt, the greater the risk. Women tend to use poisonous substances, analgesics, or psychoactive and soporific drugs. In 1965, only 7% of males used these means while 37% of women employed these methods. In 1975, 60% of deaths from substances were by women while 82% of deaths from firearms and 62% of deaths by jumping were male (Frederick, 1978). People tend to use a *method available to them*. Although only 3% of all suicides in the nation are a result of jumping from high places, in New York City where there are many tall buildings 33% of suicides are the result of jumping from high places (Frederick and Lague, 1972). Jumping from the Golden Gate Bridge has a long-time reputation as a place of self-inflicted death in San Francisco.

Beck and associates (1975) found that suicidal intent correlates highly with medical lethality *when* the attempter has sufficient knowledge to properly assess the outcome of an attempt. If a patient naively felt that death could result from an overdose of diazepam, risk is considerably greater than if he or she knew that such was a relatively nonlethal mode of exodus. Wrist cuttings and minor ingestion are usually relatively nonlethal. The *more violent and painful an attempt was*, the *greater the risk of future suicide and need for protection*. The acquiring of firearms, knives, rope, poisons, or other items that can be used in a successful suicide attempt should make family members, friends, and therapists wary. Over the decades the percentage of deaths from firearms and explosives has increased.

Education

College students are at high risk for suicide although the overall mortality rate is lower for their nonacademic peers (NAMH Reporter, 1972/73). The rates are especially high at so-called high prestige schools. For instance, Lyman (1961) reported that the annual rates per 100,000 per year for students at Oxford and Cambridge Universities respectively was 26.4 and 21.3. For the University of London it was 16.3

and for seven unnamed British universities it was 5.9. The overall rate at the time of the study for this group in the United Kingdom was 4.1 per 100,000 per year. In the United States when the rates were 7–10 per 100,000 per year for this age group, the rates at Harvard (Tembly, 1961) and Yale (Parrish, 1957) were respectively 15 and 14. One explanation posited for the high rates is that such schools tend to be highly competitive with overt and covert stresses to achieve. Others (Frederick and Lague, 1972) have pointed out that in studies of male student suicides, the fathers of the victims were often found to be absent through death or divorce before the suicide victim was 16 years old or when alive and still married to the mother was heavily involved in business away from home. Instead of feeling a part of the family, the victim had often been sent off to boarding school.

Psychiatric Illness

There are certain psychiatric illnesses in which suicide is high. These include affective disorders (depression, mania), schizophrenia, and borderline personality. Obviously, when a person is depressed with feelings of worthlessness, helplessness, and hopelessness, regardless of the etiology, risk of self-destruction is great. A thought disorder combined with depressed mood is especially ominous. If voices suddenly tell an individual to enter the "other world," to kill himself or join someone in a grave, it is hard to argue with them. If the voice commanding someone to kill himself is felt to be that of God, the risk is especially great. Suicide risk is greatest in affective disorders, including manic-depressive disease, when they are accompanied by sleep disturbance, anhedonia, decreased sex drive, somatic complaints, guilt, and motor or verbal retardation.

Religion

Suicide rates are highest among Protestants and lowest among Jews and Catholics. This observation was first made by Durkheim (1951) and has been found to hold true in subsequent studies. *Active* membership in a religious organization afforded by the traditional extended Jewish factor (Breed, 1966). As discussed earlier in this chapter, Durkheim and many others have felt that the social support afforded by the traditional extended Jewish family and the parish community of the Catholic church as opposed to the individualistic Protestant ethic was felt to mollify the vicissitudes of human existence.

Socioeconomic Factors

In the United States in recent years, one sees high rates of suicide at *both ends of the economic continuum*. At one time, rates appeared higher among lower socioeconomic individuals, with agricultural workers and unskilled laborers having quite high rates but this is changing (Slaby et al., 1981).

The peak time for suicide in this country was during the Great Depression (17.4 per 100,000 per year) when both suicide and homicide rates were great (Frederick, 1978).

Suicide rates for whites seem more sensitive to business fluctuations than for nonwhites, and rates for upper socioeconomic strata are greater than those less financially able. Henry and Short (1954) found in a study of Chicago during the 1930s that economic shifts influenced male suicide rates more than women. An exception, however, were blacks. The rates for black women increased disproportionately to those of black men during the Depression. In addition, the rates for those in the age group 15–65 years were more sensitive to the economic shift than those over 65 years. Interestingly, the suicide rate for whites living in high-rent districts in Chicago fell sharply over the years from 1930 to 1941 while the rates for whites in the low-rent districts remained relatively constant. People who stood to suffer the greatest loss from unemployment (white men in the age range 15–65 years and black women) and from the crash of the stock market (whites living in the high-rent

districts) showed the greatest increase in suicide rates.

Season and Day of Week

During the 1950s and 1960s, April and May were the months of greatest suicide. Since then, however, there has been a bimodal change with high rates in both spring and fall. December has very low rates save for the Christmas holidays when both depression and suicidal attempts increase. In spring, the theme is one of hope and rebirth. For depressed people, the air of renewal and hope for the future in spring and the happiness and songs of joy during the Christmas season make them feel all the more alone, and all the more hopeless and depressed. In addition, for college students spring signals the end of the school year and for seniors, the transition to jobs and choosing life's goals.

Of the days of the week, Friday and Monday have the highest suicide rates, partially corroborating the old notion of "blue" Monday. Sunday is the third likeliest day (Frederick and Lague, 1972).

Pregnancy, Abortion, Surgery, and Physical Illness

Recent studies show both *childbirth* and *surgery* are associated with increased rates of suicide (Slaby et al., 1975). Self-inflicted death because of pregnancy itself is felt to be unusual. (Resnik and Wittlin, 1971) When a pregnant woman attempts suicide, it is often precipitated by arguments with spouse, parents, or lovers. Suicide rates do increase, however, *following delivery*. Refusal to grant an abortion at a time when medical permission was required does not appear to influence suicide rates remarkably (Resnik and Wittlin, 1971).

The question of whether individuals should be allowed to take their own lives in the face of severe or debilitating illness (such as terminal cancer or quadriplegia) is both a philosophic and religious question for which an answer can only be found within the individual. There have been several attempts to develop guidelines to help physicians to provide answers for their patients (Slaby and Tancredi, 1975), but such decisions are never without pain and conflict for all concerned: patient, family, and physician.

Previous Attempts

Some 50%–80% of individuals who ultimately commit suicide have histories of *previous attempts* (Slaby et al., 1975). The ratio of attempted suicide to completed suicide has been given as between 5.5:1 to 7.2:1 (Pederson et al., 1973). Given the relationship between suicidal gestures and ultimate suicide, one would expect to see a rise in the death rate from suicide over the next several years. Although it has been shown that untreated suicide attempters are at higher risk for a future successful suicide, most attempters referred for outpatient treatment never actually begin therapy (Kirstein et al., 1975). This has led some physicians in Great Britain to adopt a policy to routinely hospitalize all suicide attempters.

Psychological Correlates

A number of psychological characteristics of those who attempt and ultimately succeed at taking their own lives have been identified. The first and most obvious is *depression*, although many who atttempt suicide are not depressed. Depression is especially ominous when accompanied by neurovegetative changes such as difficulty falling asleep, sleep interruption, early morning awakening, hypersomnia, variations in mood, reduced appetite, weight loss, and decreased libido. The presence of a thought disorder, as already mentioned, coupled with depression is particularly disturbing. If after an evaluation a patient continues to feel worthless, hopeless, and helpless, a clinician should be particularly concerned. *Suicidal patients usually conceptualize death as the only possible solution to a situation they see as desperate and hopeless* (Beck et al., 1975). In fact, some researchers feel that the cognitive element of **negative expecta-**

tions is a stronger indicant of suicidal intent than is depression, and therefore aim at alleviating hopelessness with the goal of successfully preventing suicide (Minkoff et al., 1973). *Treatment with antidepressants may bring energy back before the thoughts of guilt, worthlessness, and hopelessness have faded and, therefore, increase suicide risk during the first few weeks of treatment.*

The histories of many people who attempt suicide are filled with evidence of *emotional instability* and *difficulty in maintaining close and intimate relationships*. Parental deprivation (Paffenbarger et al., 1969), disorganization in the family (Resnik and Dizmang, 1971), and a history of violence in the home may have been present. Prior to an attempt, relatives may report an individual, especially a child, to be more morose and withdrawn. Decreased job efficiency and poor work attendence is also in evidence. Loss of a parent or parents through death, divorce, or separation is common. Interestingly, despite the earlier formulation that suicide represents anger turned inward, many suicidal people have been found to be more overtly *hostile*, both by history and during psychiatric interview (Weissman et al., 1973). If anger is turned inward, it appears that it is also directed outward—destroying interpersonal relationships with friends, family, employers, and lovers. This observation has led some researchers to question the role of loss in suicide. What appears in some instances to be a loss that precipitated a suicide in fact may have been a loss that was the result of the same angry depressive posture that caused the person to attempt to take his or her life. The anger that preceded the attempt may have brought about a loss of job or lover and caused family members and friends to withdraw.

Other Correlates of Suicidal Behavior

The following other correlates of suicide attempts and successful suicide have been identified.

Accident Proneness. Suicidal individuals may have a history of increasing accidents at home, work, and on the road. As insurance assessors well know, accidents are not randomly distributed. A small number of people are responsible for a disproportionate number of accidents. Single-car accidents and cutting or burning of oneself "by accident" may suggest underlying depression.

Suicide Equivalents. Alcoholism, experimentation with dangerous drugs, and risk-taking adventures may be in some instances suicidal equivalents. A person may "drink himself to death," "fry his brain in drugs," or simply "kill himself one of these days" by racing motorcycles or by engaging in other high-risk ventures. Alcoholism may be considered a form of subtle suicide. Hepatic, cardiac, and brain disease are but a few of its complications. An intoxicated person may drive an airplane or car or motorcycle to his or her death, or swim away from shore, tire, and drown. Alcoholism and drugs may act in a synergistic manner. The usual amount of sleep medication when taken with alcohol may lead to respiratory depression. In other instances, a person intoxicated from drugs or alcohol may awaken in dreamlike states repeatedly and take additional amounts of drugs to the extent of fatal doses.

Ignoring medical advice is another possible instance of suicidal equivalent. Patients with chronic medical illness, such as diabetes mellitus and epilepsy, may neglect their medication and go into coma or end up in car accidents. They may not overtly address their anger and frustration over being physically infirm but rather act it out by not following medical advice.

Sometimes, what appears to have been a death by hanging may have in fact been an accidental death in the form of sex play, eroticized repetitive hanging (Resnik, 1972). Such deaths, known since medieval times, usually involve adolescent or young adult men who hang themselves while masturbating to heighten the pleasure. If, however, no one else is present or they are unable to release the noose in time, they may die. The practice is clearly in the genre of behavior classified as suicide equivalents. There were 20 such fatal cases in the Los Angeles area between 1958 and 1968 and it is felt at least two such cases with resultant death occur in Massachusetts each year. The intent of the act is usually apparent from the partial nudity and evidence of autoerotic activity.

Severe Insomnia. Sleep is a very sensitive indicator of a person's emotional life and even in the absence of overt depression severe insomnia increases suicide risk.

Hypochondria. Excessive somatic concerns may be a sign of depression and therefore reason for concern. Suicide attempts may be seen by the individuals concerned as an escape from fantasized physical limitations without ever addressing the issue of an underlying depression.

Command Hallucinations. Mandatory or imperative hallucinations are always ominous and usually just reason for hospitalization. It is difficult to argue with the voice of God or a dead parent calling one to the grave.

Crisis Event. Losses and gains alike can stress people to the point that they take their own lives. Loss of a loved one, job, money, or self-esteem may all lead to depression and self-destructive behavior. Comparably, what may be seen as a gain, such as birth of a child or occupational advance, may in fact be felt as a loss or crisis. A child may frustrate the dependent needs of a parent and force him or her to give more than received. Job advance may leave a person without peers or superiors to turn to for advice. In addition, successful people may become the object of jealousy and anger because they do not fulfill everyone's individual expectations.

Lack of Secondary Gain or Discovery.
When someone attempts suicide and there is no apparent gain or change in environment or circumstances that may result from the act, the prognosis is worse than when the attempt may be seen as a manipulation or cry for help. Lack of "message value" in an attempt suggests a greater sense of despair and unhappiness. In the same way, if a suicide attempt takes place in a visible setting, such as a home where parents are present, it usually is less serious than if it takes place in the middle of a forest. What is the possibility of discovery? Did the person tell anyone he or she was going to attempt suicide? Most individuals have told someone they were going to attempt suicide before they act. It is a myth that people who talk about it don't do it. Most people who ultimately kill themselves have told someone that they planned to end their lives. All threats should be taken seriously.

Other Signs. Other signs of concern in evaluation of suicide include *giving away of prized possessions* or *getting things "in order"* and *making out a will.* The giving away of cherished pets or other belongings in essence is a way of symbolically making out a will and executing it.

The fact that someone is living alone is always a dangerous sign if the person is morose and talking of suicide. If no one is present to assuage the depression, help the individual to seek aid or, in the extreme, find him or her if suicide is attempted, risk is heightened. Finally, if a person has been physically active and is left severely limited by illness or accident, risk is increased.

MANAGEMENT

The first step in the management of a suicidal patient is *ascertaining whether the individual can be treated outside of a hospital setting.* While most individuals who talk of suicide do not need to be in a hospital if appropriate supports are available in the community, there is a core group of individuals who are mentally ill and may in fact, in the extreme, need to be forcibly detained in a manner consistent with extinct state laws to prevent them from taking their own lives.

The decision of whether or not a patient must be hospitalized is based on good clinical judgment after all information about past history, the patient's current living situation, degree of depression (if present), available social supports, the effect of evaluation, and initiation of treatment has been taken into account. A moderately suicidal individual is easier to manage outside of the hospital in the presence of supportive family members and friends than a midly suicidal person who is a loner. All suicidal threats and gestures must be taken seriously and evaluated in the total context of the individual and his or her situation. In no case should a suicidal person be challenged, argued with, or given facile interpretations, no matter how true, in an acute situation of threatened suicide. Advanced age; divorced, widowed, or single marital status; male sex; alcoholism; previous attempts; and predominant homosexual orientation are all variables that increase risk, while being married, young, female, and without physical or mental illness conversely decrease it. If hospitalized or treated at home, access to any objects or drugs that could be used in a suicide attempt should be guarded.

When hospitalization is required at a *general hospital* in the community, a first-floor room with *unbreakable windows* and without easy ways for patients to hang or otherwise harm themselves should be used. One-to-one nursing observation may be required in the acute setting, especially if mandatory hallucinations are present. Orders for staff should be clearly written, and a schedule is determined by the severity of the suicidal ideation for observational checks. Less suicidal patients may be placed with another patient for observation. Physician notes should contain statements regarding any worsening or bettering of the condition accompanied by appropriate nursing orders.

If the depression is one that responds to antidepressant medication, it should be remembered that *suicidal risk may increase during the first weeks of treatment*. Psychomotor retardation, appetite and weight disturbance and associated changes in sleep usually respond to adequate doses of antidepressants in 7–10 days. Depressive ideation, patterns, however, with attendant feelings of hopelessness, helplessness, and guilt usually take 3–6 weeks to respond. Thus, energy returns while feelings of despair remain. Individuals who have been immobilized by depression may find renewal of energy to carry out suicide plans that they were unable to accomplish during states of marked psychomotor retardation. If the depression is profound and suicidal potential great, a clinician may feel it is unwise to wait for the effect of medication and may decide to employ ECT. Suicidal patients often respond rapidly to ECT. However, effects of ECT on depression are unfortunately usually short-lived and maintenance antidepressant medication is necessary to keep depression in check.

If the suicidal ideation and depression are *secondary to an organic process* that is treatable, appropriate therapy should be initiated. In the case of depression as a toxic effect of drugs such as steroids or antihypertensives, the medication may be discontinued or reduced or substituted for a similar drug with less likelihood to cause depression. Hydralazine, for instance, is said to be less likely to cause depression than reserpine or methyldopa (all three are antihypertensives). Depression and suicidal ideation associated with electrolyte imbalance or vitamin deficiency may be corrected by restoration of fluid and electrolyte balance and correction of the vitamin deficiency. In instances of chronic illness, such as degenerative diseases of the brain or neoplasia, all that may be able to be offered are *social support*, a *protective environment*, and a *therapeutic trial* with antidepressants. In all instances of prescribing medication, especially drugs such as the tricyclic antidepressants and MAO inhibitors, care must be given so that a suicidal patient does not have access to lethal amounts of medication during the acute phase of depression. As little as one week's supply of antidepressants can kill a patient if taken all at once because of their cardiovascular toxicity. Single-dose preparations taken at night are especially dangerous in the acute phase because a patient may underestimate their potency. In addition, if certain foods, such as chianti wines or aged cheeses, are taken with MAO inhibitors, a hypertensive reaction may result. Alcohol may react with some drugs to produce CNS depression. Whenever suicidal potential remains, despite initiation of an active treatment program, a primary care clinician should seek consultation from a psychiatrist.

When depression is less profound and a suicidal attempt unlikely because of rallied social support or initiated treatment, there are a number of therapeutic maneuvers to reduce even further the likelihood of suicide. Patients and their family or friends should be given the *primary care physician's telephone number* as well as that of a *backup clinician* or *emergency room* where someone would be immediately available for reevaluation and disposition if the need should arise in the absence of the primary physician. Remarkable reduction of patient's and family's concern is possible if the physician calls to see how both the patient and family are doing during the stress of the acute phase. Such a call serves to keep the primary care physician abreast of the situation as well as perhaps reducing the suicide risk. A return visit should be scheduled, even the next day if there is serious concern that the decision not to hospitalize might need to be reconsidered. Family and friends should be alerted to ominous signs such as withdrawal, moroseness, and silence. Careful records should be kept in all instances documenting why a patient was or was not hospitalized.

The thrust of the crisis work in suicide prevention is establishment of *social supports,* opening lines of *communication*, and initiating *therapeutic interventions.* Patients and their families should feel something definitive has been done after an evaluation. A sufficient number of options should be elucidated so that any problems that may accompany home care are minimized and every effort made to treat patients with as little interference with daily routine as possible. Reevaluation of the patient's self-destructive potential during the acute phase should be done as frequently as clinical judgment dictates. The frequency of visits, if the individual is treated as an outpatient, depends to a great degree on the degree that the primary care physician feels able to depend on others in the community (family, friends, and clergy) to provide rapport, social support, opportunity for ventilation, and option exploring, and to call the physician should the condition worsen.

SUMMARY

All suicidal threats and gestures should be taken seriously and evaluated in the context of the patient in his or her total environment. A decision to or not to hospitalize and need for the primary care clinician to consult a psychiatrist should be based on: (a) depth of depression; (b) level of social supports in the patient's environment; (c) past history; (d) the presence or absence of physical or mental illness; (e) sociodemographic characteristics; (f) the presence of a plan and its lethality; and (g) the effect of evaluation and initiation of treatment on the patient's level of suicidal tension. It should always be remembered that family members or spouse may be ambivalent and covertly encourage self-destructive behavior. Following evaluation, the primary care clinician should act definitively and assertively in formulating and implementing a treatment plan. Social supports in terms of family, friends, lovers, and clergy should be rallied. Opportunities for suicide should be minimized. Access to windows, firearms, poison or drugs, sharp objects, and other potential modes for self-harm should be guarded. When there is an endogenous basis to the depression, psychopharmacotherapy and/or electroshock treatment, as appropriate, should be initiated. If the depression has an organic basis, the medical condition should be treated. The direction of crisis work with suicidal patients is evaluation, diagnosis, establishment of social supports, opening lines of communication, and initiation of active treatment.

APPENDIX: CASE HISTORY—SUICIDAL COMPLAINER

In this unfortunate case, had the physician constructed a PEG at the time of the patient's admission to the hospital following the aspirin overdose, attention might have been drawn to the following items: (a) strong family history of depression and suicidality, (b) the patient's clear history of depression and suicidal attempts, and (c) major recent changes which increase the risk of suicide (living alone, separation and rejection from significant others, alcohol intake, presence of pain). Prescribing large doses of an antidepressant drug, without close followup and psychotherapy, provided the patient with an effective means of suicide.

Management in this case should have been:

1. Transfer to a psychiatric service following a psychiatric consultation
2. Antidepressant therapy in an inpatient setting with combined psychotherapy
3. Outpatient therapy with antidepressant drugs when the patient's suicidality has abated.

PATIENT EVALUATION GRID*			
	CONTEXTS		
DIMENSIONS	CURRENT (Current States)	RECENT (Recent Events and Changes)	BACKGROUND (Culture, Traits, Constitution)
BIOLOGICAL	Aspirin ingestion—50 tablets Vague abdominal pains	Vague abdominal pains—18 mo Hysterectomy for dysfunctional Bleeding—8 mo Menopause—approx. 5 yr ago	Patient's mother had recurrent depression Father alcoholic Patient had alcoholic pancreatis—8 yr ago Patient had multiple psychiatric admissions since age 32 yr for depression and suicidal attempts; also, multiple somatic complaints and hospitalizations—no organic pathology found
PERSONAL	Suicidal attempt with aspirin Feels hopeless, helpless Feels she has cancer of colon Frightened of being left alone Feels rejected by family	Depressed mood, chronic increase in depression—3 mo Decrease in appetite—3 mo Insomnia—difficulty falling asleep and early morning awakening—4 mo Increased drinking—2 yr Two overdoses with aspirin and amitriptyline—16 mo ago and 3 yr ago	Chronically complaining, depressed and "manipulative" person Patient is high school graduate
ENVIRONMENTAL	Currently lives alone Separated from husband Two children (ages 19 and 35 yr) in another state	Husband left her for another woman—6 mo ago 19-year-old son went to college out of state—1 yr ago Patient's maternal cousin died of colon ca—2 yr ago Six hospitalizations in 5 yr Frequent visit with MD for vague pains in abdomen—2 yrs	Lower middle-class, Catholic background Mother died age 49 yr of overdose Father died age 60 yr of liver failure One older brother—alcoholic Patient married at age 20 yr to a salesman; two children

*Demographic data: 51-year-old married woman, mother of two children, housewife.

RECOMMENDED READINGS

Farberow, N.L., and Schneidman, E.S., (eds). 1965. *The cry for help*. New York: McGraw-Hill. This book is edited by two pioneers in the study of self-destructive behavior and reviews a number of topics germane to suicide including assessment of suicide potential in both emergency and nonemergency situations, the development of suicide prevention centers, and statistical comparisons between those who attempted and those who sucessfully committed suicide. In addition, it summarizes speculations on the etiology of suicide.

Frederick, C.J. 1972. Ecological aspects of self-destruction: Some legal, legislative and behavioral implications. In *Health and human values*, ed. A. Jefcoat, New York: John Wiley & Sons. This chapter provides an overview of the legal aspects of suicide evaluation and treatment with an outline for emergency mental health procedures.

Frederick, C.J., and Lague, L. 1978. *Dealing with the crisis of suicide* 8th rev. ed. New York Public Affairs pamphlet no 406A. New York: Public Affairs Committee Inc. Dr Calvin J. Frederick, of the National Institute of Mental Health, and Louise Lague have written a very readable introduction for the lay person to suicide, its extent, circumstances, and victims. Their goal is to help concerned individuals who are not psychiatric professionals to understand personality groups in which suicide is most likely to occur, motivations, and techniques for helping individuals going through suicidal crises.)

Slaby, A.E.; Lieb, J.; and Tancredi, L.R. 1981. *Handbook of psychiatric emergencies: A guide for emergencies in psychiatry*. Flushing, New York: Medical Examination Publishing Co. This handbook is written in outline form for on-the-lines clinicians dealing with psychiatric emergencies in which suicide may be prominent. It provides techniques for treating suicidal patients as well as evaluating crises and illnesses which may feature self-destructive behavior.

Slaby, A.E., and Tancredi, L.R. 1975. Suicide and the right to die. *Collusion for conformity*. New York: Jason Aronson. In the chapter on suicide and the right to die in this book, the ethical and legal aspects of taking one's own life are discussed.

Present attitudes and legal sanctions are placed in historic and sociologic context.

REFERENCES

Alcohol, Drug Abuse and Mental Health Administration. 1976. Dr. Frederick notes suicide increase during spring. *ADAMHA News*, p. 1 (April 30, 1976).

Beck, A.T.; Beck, R.; and Kovacs, M. 1975. Classification of suicidal behaviors: I. Quantifying intent and medical lethality. *Am. J. Psychiatry* 132:285–87.

Blachly, P.; Disher, D.; and Roduner, G. 1968. *Suicide by physicians. Bull. Suicidology*, pp. 1–19. Washington, D.C.: U.S. Government Printing Office.

Breed, W. 1966. Suicide, migration and race: A study of cases in New Orleans. *J. Soc. Issues* 22:30–43.

Davidson, M. and; Hutt, C. 1964. A study of 500 Oxford student psychiatric patients. *Br. J. Soc. Clin. Psychol.* 3:175–85.

Dorpat, T.; Anderson, W.F.; and Ripley, H.S. 1968. The relationship of physical illness to suicide. In *Suicidal behaviors*, ed. H.L.P. Resnick. Boston: Little, Brown.

Dublin, L. 1967. Suicide: A public health problem. In *Essays in self-destruction*, ed., E.S. Schneidman. New York; Science House.

Durkheim, E. 1951. *Suicide*. New York: Free Press.

Farberow, N.D., and Schneidman, E.S., eds. 1965. *The cry for help*. New York: McGraw-Hill.

Frederick, C.J. 1970. The school guidance counselor as a preventive agent to self-destructive behavior. New York: State Personnel and Guidance Journal, vol 5:1–5.

———1971. The present suicide taboo in the United States. *Ment. Hygiene* 55:178–83.

———1972. Ecological aspects of self-destruction: Some legal, legislative and behavioral implications. In *Health and human values*, ed., A. Jefcoat. New York: John Wiley & Sons.

———1973. The role of the nurse in crisis intervention and suicide prevention *J. Psychiatry. Nurs.* 2:27–31.

———1977. Current trends in suicidal behavior in the United States. Paper presented in abridged form at thirteenth national scientific meeting of the Association for the Advancement of Psychotherapy, Toronto, Canada, May 1, 1977.

————1978. Current trends in suicide in the United States. *Am. J. Psychiatry* 32:172–200.

Frederick, C.J. and Farberow, N.L. 1970. Group psychotherapy with suicidal persons: A comparison with standard group methods (*Int. J. Soc. Psychiatry* 16:103–11.)

Frederick, C.J. and Lague, L. 1978. Dealing with the crisis of suicide. 8th rev. ed. New York Public Affairs pamphlet no 406A. New York: Public Affairs Committee Inc.

Frederick, C.J.; and Resnik, H.L.P. 1970. Interventions with suicidal patients. *J. Contemp. Psychother.* 2:103–9.

————1971. How suicidal behaviors are learned. *Am. J. Psychother.* 25:37–55.

Freud, S. 1950. *Beyond the pleasure principle.* London: Hogarth.

————1955. *Mourning and melancholia.* Vol. 18. Translated by James Strachey. London: Hogarth.

Hendin, H. 1964. *Suicide and Scandinavia.* New York: Grune & Stratton.

Henry, A.F.; and Short, J.F. 1954. *Suicide and homicide: Some economic, sociological and psychological aspects of aggression.* New York: Free Press.

Henslin, J.M. 1971. Problems and prospects in studying significant others of suicides. *Bull. Suicidology*, pp. 81–84. Washington, D.C.: U.S. Government Printing Office.

Horney, K. 1950. *Neurosis and human growth.* New York: Norton.

Kirstein, L.; Prusoff, B.; Weissman, M. et al., 1975. Utilization review of treatment for suicide attempters. *Am. J. Psychiatry* 132:22–27.

Kelly, W.A. 1973. Suicide and psychiatric education. *Am J. Psychiatry* 130:463–68.

Lieb, J.; Lipsitch, I.I.; and Slaby, A.E. 1973. *The crisis team: A handbook for the mental health professional.* New York: Harper & Row.

Lyman, J.L. 1961. Student suicide at Oxford University. *Student Medicine* 10:218–34.

MacMahon, B.; Johnson, S.; and Pugh, R.F 1963. Relation of suicide rates to social conditions. *Public Health Rep.* 78:285–93.

Menninger, K.A. 1938. *Man against himself.* New York: Harcourt, Brace.

Minkoff, K.; Bergman, E.; and Beck, A.T., et al. 1973. Hopelessness, depression, and attempted suicide. *Am. J. Psychiatry* 130:455–59.

Mintz, R.S. 1964. A pilot study of the prevalence of persons in the City of Los Angeles who have attempted suicide. Paper presented at the 120th annual meeting of the American Psychiatric Association, Los Angeles, May 4, 1964.

Murphy, G.E.; Armstrong, J.W.; Hermele, S.L., et al. 1979. Suicide and alcoholism: Interpersonal loss confirmed as a predictor. *Arch. Gen. Psychiatry* 36:65–69.

National Association of Mental Health. 1972/73. Females lead suicide attempts. *NAMH Reporter* (Winter 1972/73).

Neuringer, C.; and Lettieri, D.J. 1971. Cognition attitude and affect in suicidal individuals. *Life-Threatening Behav.* 1:106–24.

Ogden, M.; Spector, M.I.; Hill, C.A. 1970. Suicides and homicides among Indians. *Public Health Rep.* 85:75–80.

Paffenbarger, R.S.; King, S.H.; Wing, A.C. et al. 1969. Chronic disease in former college students: IX characteristics in youth that predispose to suicide and accidental death in later life. *American Journal of Public Health* 59:900–8.

Parrish, H. 1956. Cause of death among college students: A study of 209 deaths at Yale University, 1920–1955. *Public Health Rep.* 71:1081–85.

Parrish, H.M. 1957. Epidemiology of suicide among college students. *Yale J. Biol. Med.* 29:585–95.

Peck, M.; and Schrut, A. 1971. Suicidal behavior among college students. *Health Services and Mental Health Administration Health Reports* 86:149–56.

Pederson, A.M.; Aruad, G.A.; and Kindler, A.R. 1973. Epidemiological differences between white and nonwhite suicide attempters. *Ment. Health Digest* 5:27–29.

Reasons Sought for Adolescent Suicide Increase. 1976. *The Washington Post* (June 4, 1976).

Resnik, H.L.P. 1968. *Suicidal behaviors: Diagnosis and management.* Boston: Little, Brown.

————1972. Erotized repetitive hangings: A form of self-destructive behavior. *Am. J. Psychother.* 26:4–21.

Resnik, H.L.P.; Dizmang, L.H. 1971. Observations on suicidal behavior among American Indians. *Am. J. Psychiatry* 127:882–87.

Resnik, H.L.P.; Wittlin, B.J. 1971. Abortion and suicidal behaviors: Observations on the concept of "endangering the mental health of the mother." *Mental Hygiene* 55:10–20.

Rosen, D.H. 1975. Suicide survivors—a follow-up study of persons who survived jumping from the Golden Gate and San Francisco-Oakland Bay bridges. *West. J. Med.* 122:289–94.

Sainsburg, P. 1955. *Suicide in London.* London: Chapman and Hall.

Schneidman, E.; Farberow, N.; and Litman, R 1970. *The psychology of suicide.* New York: Science House.

Schneidman, E.S., and Mandelkom, P. 1967. How to prevent suicide. New York Public Affairs pamphlet no. 407.

Seiden, R. 1969. *Suicide among youth.* Washington, D.C.: U.S. Government Printing Office.

Slaby, A.E.; Lieb, J.; and Tancredi, L.R. 1981. Handbook of psychiatric emergencies: A guide for emergencies in psychiatry. Flushing, New York: Medical Examination Publishing Co.

Slaby, A.E., and Tancredi, L.R. 1975. *Collusion for conformity.* New York: Jason Aronson.

Suicide: How to keep patients from killing themselves (Interviews with C.J. Frederick and H. Hendin). 1976. *Med. World* News (July 1976) pp. 86–95.

Suicide rate for young rises sharply. 1975. *The Washington Post* (April 28, 1975).

Susser, M. 1968. *Community psychiatry: Epidemiologic and social themes.* New York: Random House.

Teicher, J.D., and Jacobs, J. 1966a. Adolescents who attempt suicide: Preliminary findings. *Am. J. Psychiatry* 122:1248–57.

Teicher, J.D., and Jacobs, J. 1966b. The physician and the adolescent suicide attempter *J. School Health* 36:406–15.

Tembly, W.O. 1961. Suicide. In *Emotional problems of the student,* ed. G.B. Blane and C.C. McArthur. New York: Appleton-Century-Crofts.

Wechsler, J.A. 1972. *In a darkness.* New York: W.W. Norton.

Weissman, M.M. 1974. The epidemiology of suicide attempts, 1960 to 1971. *Arch. Gen. Psychiatry* 30:737–46.

Weissman, M.; Fox, K.; and Klerman, G.L. 1973. Hostility and depression associated with suicide attempts. *Am. J. Psychiatry* 130:450–55.

Yolles, S.F. 1968. Suicide: A public health problem. In *Suicidal behaviors,* ed, H.L.P. Resnik. Boston: Little, Brown.

Young suicides. 1976. *Harper's Bazaar* (June 1976).

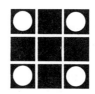

CHAPTER 11

Evaluation and Management of Anxiety

Hoyle Leigh, M.D.

Although anxiety is a ubiquitous human experience, and an adaptive one in the face of danger, it also can be paralyzing. Its physiologic correlates may endanger a medically ill patient. Some individuals respond to relatively mild stresses with overwhelming anxiety. In others, the anxiety symptoms may be secondary to drugs or physical illness. In this chapter, the signs and symptoms of anxiety, the classification and phenomenology of anxiety disorders, and practical management strategies are discussed.

Anxiety is a feeling of dread and apprehension, often accompanied by a sense of impending doom and signs of autonomic activation, for example, palpitations, sweating, muscle tension, dyspnea, urinary frequency, and diarrhea. (Refer to case study below.) When anxiety is associated with a specific, identifiable object or situation, the term "fear" is often used. When anxiety is severe and overwhelming, the term "panic" is appropriate. The function of anxiety is protective—it signifies the presence of a potential danger situation either externally or within the personality system (Leigh and Reiser, 1980). In this sense, anxiety, like pain, warns the individual so that action may be taken to avoid or master the danger situation. How, then, can we explain the fact that anxiety occurs at times when no identifiable danger can be recognized?

Two psychological theories concerning such nonfunctional anxiety are widely accepted. *Learning theory* or Pavlovian theory postulates that anxiety is a conditioned fear reflex (Pavlov, 1927). According to the classic conditioning paradigm, the pairing of a neutral stimulus (for example, entering an elevator) with a frightening experience (for example, being mugged) may result in the neutral stimulus acquiring frightening qualities. The frightening experience then produces anxiety symptoms in normally nonanxiety-provoking situations.

Psychoanalytic theory, on the other hand, proposes that anxiety (as opposed to fear) is a reaction of the personality system (ego) to a conflict between unconscious wishes for pleasure gratification (id impulses) and the person's moral standards and inhibiting influences (superego) (Freud, 1953; Brenner, 1955). This theory further postulates that *psychological defense mechanisms*, such as repression, denial, and rationalization, among others, are mobilized to attenuate the anxiety. It is only when the defense mechanisms fail that one experiences severe clinical anxiety.

To sum up, anxiety may be experienced in the presence of a life-threatening situation, as a conditioned reflex to an early frightening experience, or as a sign of an intrapsychic conflict with which the personality system is unable to deal effectively through the use of psychological defense mechanisms. Anxiety may also occur secondary to a malfunction of the biological system normally involved in anxiety mechanisms—that is, any disease of the CNS, autonomic nervous system (ANS), and the neuroendocrine system (Leigh and Reiser, 1980).

CASE HISTORY 11–1

A 35-year-old divorced male junior executive in an electronics company came to his physician complaining of palpitations and choking sensations. Recently, he had been promoted to a position that required him to give presentations in public to customers and executives of the company. The patient was concerned that he might have a heart attack during these presentations and wanted to have a thorough workup to make sure that his heart was healthy. The patient stated, "You know, doctor, I've always been a Type A personality." (See appendix at the end of this chapter for further discussion and PEG.)

EVALUATION OF ANXIETY

The presence of anxiety is manifested by subjective symptoms, objective signs, and/or signs of autonomic arousal. Subjective symptoms include fear (often irrational and recognized as such by the patient), dread, apprehension, or a sense of impending doom. Objective signs include tense muscles, anxious facial expression, shakiness, jumpiness, hypervigilance, distractibility, insomnia, restlessness, or signs of autonomic arousal. Some signs of autonomic arousal are dyspnea, hyperventilation, heart pounding or racing, cold clammy hands, dry mouth, dizziness, paresthesias, hot or cold spells, urinary frequency, diarrhea, gastrointestinal discomfort, "butterflies in the stomach," lump in throat, tachycardia, tachypnea, or hypertension.

Once it is determined that the patient is anxious, the physician must decide whether the anxiety requires further evaluation and possible treatment. The construction of a PEG, as described in Chapter 1, is helpful in this process.

Consideration of the biological dimension should include the symptoms and signs of anxiety, the organ systems most affected by it, and the presence or absence of drugs that might modify anxiety. Many medical diseases and drugs (or drug withdrawal) may cause anxiety symptoms (discussed later in the section on differential diagnosis). Personal dimension factors include the patient's interpretation of the anxiety symptoms (for example, "I am afraid I will drop dead because my heart is pounding so"), the status of psychological defense mechanisms, personality style, and coping mechanisms. Environmental dimension factors include any actual external danger situations, recent life stresses, and cultural expectations concerning expression of anxiety. For example, is expression of fear culturally unacceptable for this patient? This may explain why the patient has all the objective signs of anxiety without subjective admission of feelings of apprehension.

The current context factors to be considered are: What are the patient's principal signs and symptoms of anxiety? Are they primarily subjective or autonomic? What are the immediate circumstances under which the anxiety is experienced? Is the patient receiving any antianxiety medications? Is she or he attempting self-medication with alcohol? The recent context factors important in evaluation include any identifiable danger situations (or life stresses), recent awareness of these, or their aftereffects. Have there been any physical illnesses that might contribute to anxiety? Recent drug abuse (such as amphetamines), or withdrawal from drugs (such as barbiturates, narcotics, antianxiety drugs, alcohol) may cause anxiety symptoms. The background context is important in determining whether the anxiety being experienced is a personality trait or a new phenomenon. Also relevant are the habitual defense mechanisms the patient uses. How is anxiety usually handled in the patient's family and social culture?

If anxiety symptoms are persistent, and not related to identifiable life stress situations, or to a progressive or disabling disease, the diagnosis of an *anxiety disorder* (as opposed to normal adaptive anxiety) may be considered. When anxiety is manifest primarily through symptoms of the ANS, psychophysiologic symptoms may occur (see Chapter 12).

DIFFERENTIAL DIAGNOSIS

When severe anxiety is related to an identifiable life stress, the diagnosis of an *adjustment disorder with anxious mood* is indicated (see Chapter 14 for further discussion).

Anxiety syndrome *secondary to an identifiable medical disorder* should be ruled out by appropriate tests and procedures. Any disease of the CNS, especially of the limbic system and hypothalamus, or any disease of the ANS and the neuroendocrine system, can cause various aspects of anxiety syndrome. Some medical diseases commonly associated with anxiety symptoms are: hyperthyroidism, pheochromocytoma, partial complex (temporal lobe) seizures, hypoglycemia, and carcinoid syndrome.

Drug *intoxication* and drug *withdrawal* often are accompanied by anxiety symptoms. Any CNS stimulant drugs or psychotomimetics (such as amphetamines, LSD, phencyclidine) may cause anxiety. Withdrawal from CNS-depressant drugs, such as barbiturates, benzodiazepines, narcotics, and alcohol, is one of the most common causes of the anxiety syndrome.

Major psychiatric syndromes such as **schizophrenia** and **major affective disorders** may be associated with anxiety symptoms (see Chapters 8 and 9). The clinician should determine their presence or absence in a patient who has anxiety symptoms because definitive treatment may need to be directed toward the underlying major psychiatric disorder.

Anxiety may be a prominent symptom in **organic brain syndromes**, especially if there is agitation. When a patient with organic brain syndrome is suddenly confronted with cognitive deficits (perhaps during mental status examination), panic may ensue, in what is termed "catastrophic reaction" (Goldstein, 1975). (For further discussion of organic brain syndrome, see Chapter 6.)

Classification of Anxiety Disorders

After ruling out secondary anxiety syndromes due to problems of everyday living, medical diseases, drug intoxication or withdrawal, and major psychiatric disorders (schizophrenia and major affective disorders), the clinician is in a position to make a more specific diagnosis of an anxiety disorder.

According to the third edition of *Diagnostic and Statistical Manual of Mental Disorders*, (*DSM-III*), anxiety disorders are divided into four broad categories. They are: anxiety states

(anxiety neuroses); phobic disorders (phobic neuroses); posttraumatic stress disorder; and atypical anxiety disorder. These entities are discussed in the following sections to familiarize the primary physician with the basic concepts underlying the classification of anxiety disorders.

Anxiety States.   Included in the category of anxiety disorders characterized by spontaneous manifestations of anxiety are: panic disorder, generalized anxiety disorder, and obsessive-compulsive disorder.

In panic disorder, recurrent attacks of extreme fear or agitation occur either unpredictably or in association with particular activities, such as driving a car. At least three panic attacks in a 3-week period must take place to meet the criteria for this diagnosis. In addition, there must be at least four autonomic or motor signs of anxiety, as described earlier in the section on evaluation. In situations of extreme physical exertion or actual life-threatening events, the diagnosis of panic disorder does not apply.

Generalized anxiety disorder is diagnosed when there is pervasive, persistent anxiety of at least one month's duration in the absence of panic attacks or other specific symptoms justifying another designation such as phobia or obsessive-compulsive behavior.

Obsessive-compulsive disorder or neurosis is characterized by anxiety that must be reduced by performing ego-dystonic (that is, not congruent with the wishes of the individual) rituals, or by anxiety-provoking ego-dystonic recurrent thoughts or ideas, called obsessions. When the ego-dystonic ritual, or compulsion, is resisted consciously or by external force, anxiety may increase to an intolerable degree. Some common obsessions involve thoughts of violence, fears of contamination (such as being infected by shaking hands), and doubt. Hand-washing, counting, and checking and rechecking are common compulsions. Patients with obsessive-compulsive disorder may have either obsessions (recurrent involuntary thoughts, or ideas) or compulsions (usually repetitive and unnecessary acts that have to be performed to alleviate mounting anxiety), or both. This disorder should be differentiated from the compulsive personality disorder (see Chapter 4), which is a personality trait rather than an anxiety disorder.

Obsessions and compulsions may be seen as symptoms in schizophrenia, major affective disorders, and Tourette disease (see Chapter 22). The mechanism of obsessive-compulsive disorder is not completely known, but the obsessions and compulsions are usually considered to be attempts to reduce the anxiety generated by an unconscious intrapsychic conflict.

Phobic Disorders. Included in the category of anxiety disorders characterized by irrational fears are phobic disorders or neuroses. Agoraphobia, social phobia, and simple phobia are three main types of phobias. Phobias in general are characterized by a persistent and irrational fear of an object or situation, called the phobic stimulus. This results in a compelling desire to avoid the object or situation. When avoidance is not possible, panic ensues. The fear is recognized by the individual as being irrational or excessive.

Agoraphobia is characterized by an irrational fear of being alone, or being in public places from which escape may be difficult or help unavailable in case of sudden incapacitation. Common agoraphobic situations arise when the person must deal with crowds, public transportation, tunnels, or bridges. Patients with this disorder may progressively restrict their activity to the point of complete disability. Agoraphobia is the most common phobia for which people seek help, although the prevalence of simple phobias (discussed later) is probably greater. Agoraphobia may also occur as a symptom in many major psychiatric disorders and personality disorders, such as schizophrenia or paranoid personality disorder.

Social phobia is characterized by a persistent and irrational fear of situations in which the person may be exposed to scrutiny by others. The affected individual thus avoids any social situation. Fear of public speaking, eating in public, or using public lavatories are examples of social phobia. The patient may express the fear that he or she may act in a humiliating or embarrassing fashion in social situations.

A *simple phobia* is a long-standing irrational fear of an object or a situation not subsumed under agoraphobia or social phobia. The individual has a compelling desire to avoid exposure to this feared object or situation. Common specific objects of simple phobia include animals (dogs, cats, snakes, insects, or mice) and closed space (claustrophobia) or high places.

The mechanism of phobias is not known. In some agoraphobias with panic attacks, there may be an instability of biogenic amine systems in the brain. Simple phobias may be related to early experiences (classical conditioning), or to fear of objects that symbolize certain conflictual wishes.

Posttraumatic Stress Disorders. The category of anxiety arising as an effect of stress includes the acute and chronic or delayed development of characteristic symptoms following a severe psychological trauma, which is generally outside the range of usual human experience. The characteristic symptoms include: numbed responsiveness to the external world ("psychic numbing"); recurrent nightmares; anxiety symptoms with hyperalertness; and insomnia. "Survivor guilt" may exist. Recurrent and intrusive recollections of the traumatic event are common, and environmental cues may precipitate a feeling that the traumatic event is reoccuring.

Traumatic stressors may include assault, rape, natural catastrophes (earthquakes, floods, volcanoes), accidents (automobile or airplane crash, fire), or man-made disasters (bombing, torture, incarceration in concentration camps). The designation of chronic posttraumatic anxiety after trauma is made when the duration of the symptoms is at least 6 months. If the onset of symptoms occurs at least 6 months after the trauma, it is called "delayed" posttraumatic anxiety.

MANAGEMENT OF ANXIETY

Anxiety in response to a *life-threatening situation* usually does not require specific treatment. Social support and discussion of possible ways of coping with the situation may suffice. If anxiety is incapacitating, antianxiety drugs may be useful on a temporary basis as well as behavioral techniques such as learning the relaxation response (Benson, 1975) or self-hypnosis (Spiegel and Spiegel, 1978).

Anxiety is common among hospitalized medical and surgical patients. Misunderstandings about nature of illness and proposed treatments are very common causes of excessive anxiety. When a patient seems to manifest severe anxiety in the hospital, it is useful to ask specific questions of the patient concerning what his or her own ideas and imaginations are about the hospitalization, nature of illness, and possible treatment procedures. Then the clinician can offer specific information or reassurance. For example, a patient awaiting nephrectomy showed severe signs of anxiety. The psychiatric consultant found that the source of anxiety was the patient's mistaken notion that the loss of a kidney would cause impotence. When this was clarified, the anxiety symptoms subsided.

Anxiety syndromes secondary to medical diseases, drug intoxication and/or withdrawal should be handled by treating the underlying disorder. Anxiety associated with organic brain syndrome may be managed by first, treating the underlying cause of the organic brain syndrome, if possible; next providing a supportive social and physical environment; and finally, by prescribing small doses of neuroleptics such as perphenazine (2 mg three times a day when

necessary) for severe anxiety and agitation (see Chapter 6).

In treating anxiety disorder per se, a three-dimensional perspective is necessary, although intervention in one particular dimension may be especially important depending on the subtype of disorder.

Biological Dimension

Many different types of drugs have been used to treat anxiety, including barbiturates, propanediols, antihistamines, beta-blocking agents, neuroleptics, antidepressants, and benzodiazepines. Currently, the most commonly used antianxiety drugs are the benzodiazepines, antidepressants, beta-adrenergic-blocking agents, and neuroleptics.

Benzodiazepines. Chlordiazepoxide and diazepam are most commonly prescribed benzodiazepines. Benzodiazepines are rapidly absorbed in the gastrointestinal tract and reach peak blood levels within 2–4 hours. Oral administration is preferred to the intramuscular route, because the latter is often slow and incomplete. When rapid sedation is necessary, intravenous injection may be used cautiously. Disadvantages of benzodiazepines are their relatively long half-life (20–50 hours for diazepam), the fact that they potentiate other CNS depressants (such as alcohol), and that they are habit-forming. When taken in combination with other CNS depressants, respiratory depression may occur. The most common side effects of benzodiazepines are drowsiness and ataxia. Some elderly patients may develop a paradoxical reaction to benzodiazepines and experience a disinhibition phenomenon, such as irascibility, rage attacks, or impulsive behavior. Benzodiazepines should be used *temporarily* and *sparingly* to control severe anxiety. Physicians should caution patients about driving an automobile and engaging in activities requiring fine-motor coordination when taking benzodiazepines.

When prescribing benzodiazepines, the physician should be aware of their addictive and abuse potential, and also that the drug can never be a substitute for a comprehensive evaluation of the anxiety-causing situation, and a supportive physician-patient relationship.

A typical dosage schedule for diazepam is 5 mg three times a day as needed and for chlordiazepoxide, 10 mg three times a day as needed.

In attempting to stop benzodiazepines, the physician should first determine the *actual* amount the patient is taking, which is sometimes much higher than the prescribed dose. If the patient was taking at least the equivalent of 100 mg of chlordiazepoxide every day for a few months or more, the drug should be tapered gradually to avoid withdrawal symptoms (see Chapter 16).

Oxazepam, flurazepam, clorazepate, and prazepam are also commerically available benzodiazepines. In organic brain syndrome, benzodiazepines should be used with caution because they may increase confusion owing to the CNS depressant action.

Antidepressants. Tricyclic antidepressants such as imipramine and amitriptyline, and MAO inhibitors (such as phenelzine) have been used successfully to prevent the panic attacks in ***panic disorder*** and ***agoraphobia with panic attacks***. Dosage must be individualized, but as little as 10 mg of imipramine at bedtime might be effective (See Chapter 9 for further discussion on antidepressants). Antidepressants are also useful in anxiety associated with depression.

Beta-blocking Agents. Beta-blocking agents are particularly useful when autonomic manifestations of anxiety predominate the symptomatology. The contraindications are bronchial asthma, obstructive lung disease, and congestive heart failure. Propranolol, a beta-blocking agent, may be used to block autonomic manifestations of anxiety such as dyspnea, palpitations, and tremor. The usual dose is 10–20 mg of propranolol three or four times a day.

Neuroleptics. Neuroleptics such as phenothiazines or haloperidol may be used in small doses to reduce anxiety symptoms, particularly agitation, in certain patients for whom benzodiazepines are problematic (for example, patients with organic brain syndrome or elderly patients).

The physician should be aware of possible side effects such as orthostatic hypotension, lowering of seizure threshold, dystonias, parkinsonian tremor, and tardive dyskinesia with prolonged use of neuroleptics. A typical regimen is haloperidol, 0.5 mg twice a day orally or perphenazine, 2 mg three times a day orally.

Personal Dimension

Psychotherapies. *Supportive psychotherapy* is essential for all anxious patients. This involves listening to the patient, understanding the patient's sufferings, and conveying to the patient the physician's hopeful attitude concerning alleviating the suffering. Reassurance, to be effective, must be specific and not all-encompassing. For example, say, "I understand that you feel that your heart might be damaged or break down when it beats so fast. Fortunately, the EKG shows that your heart is strong enough to endure that. I think it is useful to talk about when you have these palpitations though, because we may be able to identify what is contributing to your anxiety response..."

Intensive psychotherapy or insight-oriented psychotherapy may be indicated if the anxiety seems to be associated with conflicts within the patient's personality system. This is often the case in patients who have generalized anxiety disorder or obsessive-compulsive disorder. Some patients with agoraphobia, social phobia, or simple phobia may also benefit from intensive psychotherapy, often in conjunction with drugs and behavioral therapy.

Intensive psychotherapy aims at identifying the intrapsychic conflicts that may manifest themselves in the form of anxiety or obsessive-compulsive or phobic symptoms, and helps resolve them by retracing the developmental roots of the conflicts. This is a specialized technique requiring special training (see Chapter 20).

Behavioral Therapy is often the treatment of choice for persons suffering from phobias. Behavioral therapy utilizes the learning theory concepts of extinction and reciprocal inhibition, that is, by thinking about relaxing and pleasant things while being exposed repeatedly to the phobic stimulus in a controlled fashion, the phobic quality of the stimulus is extinguished. Progressive relaxation, relaxation response, biofeedback, and self-hypnosis are all techniques of achieving relaxation to counteract anxiety experience. Special training is necessary to use these techniques effectively in treating patients.

Environmental Dimension

Environmental manipulation may be effective in reducing stress factors causing chronic anxiety. Alteration of environmental stress may include change of residence, change of occupation, planned vacations, and the like. Family or marital therapy may be necessary if the family or couple's relationship is identified as being contributory to the anxiety response. Hospitalization may be considered in severe, crippling anxiety states and for disabling obsessive-compulsive behavior.

REFERRAL

A persistent and disabling anxiety syndrome in the absence of associated medical disease or drug withdrawal or intoxication usually requires referral to a psychiatrist. Referral to a psychiatrist may be useful even if a threatening life situation can be identified, when the anxiety symptoms are profound and disabling. Referral is indicated especially if the anxiety syndrome does not subside after a course of counseling and therapy (whether drug or relaxation therapy) by the primary physician.

When referring a patient to a psychiatrist, it is a good idea for the primary physician to call the psychiatrist to discuss the patient. The referral note should include all pertinent medical history and laboratory findings so that unnecessary duplications of evaluation can be avoided.

The primary physician should be aware that not all psychiatrists or therapists use the same techniques to treat anxiety syndromes. Some may use only intensive psychotherapy while others may have expertise primarily in drug therapies. For initial consultation, it is a good idea to select a general psychiatrist who will determine the optimal therapeutic approach (see Chapter 20 for further discussion of psychotherapies).

SUMMARY

Anxiety is an adaptive response to a perceived threatening situation which may be external or within the personality system (intrapsychic). Anxiety syndrome ensues when the normal regulatory mechanisms of anxiety, such as psychologic defense mechanisms and coping strategies, are ineffective. Moreover, physical diseases, drug intoxication, and drug withdrawal states may also cause anxiety syndromes. Prolonged anxiety states may also generate physiologic disregulation resulting in psychophysiologic syndromes. (See Chapters 5 & 12 for further discussion.)

Persistent and disabling anxiety should be evaluated in the biological, personal, and environmental dimensions since factors in each may be playing an important role in the anxiety syndrome.

Anxiety disorder is diagnosed after anxiety syndromes secondary to problems of everyday living, medical diseases, and drug-related states, and major psychiatric disorders (schizophrenia and major affective disorders) have been ruled out. There are two large categories of anxiety disorders: anxiety characterized by *spontaneous* manifestations of anxiety (panic disorder, generalized anxiety disorder, and obsessive-compulsive disorder), and anxiety characterized by *irrational fears* (phobias).

Anxiety syndrome may be managed by administering drugs, psychotherapies (including behavior therapy, relaxation response, and so on), and initiating environmental change. Anxiety disorder may be managed by the primary physician on a temporary basis, but if the symptoms persist, or if the patient requires prolonged use of antianxiety drugs, referral to a psychiatrist is indicated. Referral is usually indicated if diagnoses of generalized anxiety disorder, panic disorder, obsessive-compulsive disorder, or agoraphobia arc made.

APPENDIX: CASE HISTORY—THE CHOKING TYPE A

The PEG reveals that the patient had always been a rather "nervous" person with high achievement orientation. The symptoms of palpitations and choking sensation increased since his promotion and were especially severe just before public speaking engagements. The biological dimension reveals tachycardia, tense musculature, and mild systolic hypertension. The ECG was normal as well as laboratory tests for thyrotoxicosis, pheochromocytoma, hypoglycemia, and so on. The diagnosis of generalized anxiety disorder was made. Contributing factors include his work demands, relative lack of supportive relationships, and his Type A personality trait. The treatment plans were as follows:

1. **Biological Dimension:** Propranolol was felt to be indicated for this patient in view of the sinus tachycardia, mild systolic hypertension, and tense muscles, which were his primary symptoms and signs of anxiety. In addition, since the patient has an anxious personality trait, potential habituation to a benzodiazepine drug with long-term use was considered a hazard. Thus, a regimen of propranolol, 10 mg, every 4 hours orally for anxiety symptoms was instituted.
2. **Personal dimension:** The patient was first reassured that his heart was healthy. He then received supportive psychotherapy to increase his coping skills and increase interpersonal skills. In the course of this supportive contact with the primary physician to discuss his situation and evaluate drug response, the patient also decided to take a course to build his public-speaking skills.
3. **Environmental dimension:** The physician encouraged the patient to develop supportive relationships outside of work, renewing old friendships and communicating with his supportive parents. Vacations (which he had not taken for some time) were also encouraged.

With this regimen, the patient's anxiety diminished considerably, and the severe symptoms prior to public speaking were successfully suppressed with propranolol. Eventually, as the patient's self-confidence increased, his need for propranolol decreased to none or, at most, 10 mg once a day.

PATIENT EVALUATION GRID			
	CONTEXTS		
DIMENSIONS	CURRENT (Current States)	RECENT (Recent Events and Changes)	BACKGROUND (Culture, Traits, Constitution)
BIOLOGICAL	Sinus <u>tachycardia</u> Blood pressure: 145/90 Heart rate: 110 beats per min <u>Tense musculature</u> Physical exam and laboratory results normal, including normal ECG	Valium (from friend) taken occasionally in last 2 mo	<u>Parents anxious</u> Paternal grandfather was <u>alcoholic</u> Mother's sister has diabetes
PERSONAL	<u>Palpitations</u> <u>Choking</u> sensation <u>Anxiety (continuous)</u> <u>Fear of heart attack</u> Fear of failure at work Mental status: normal except for anxiety	<u>Anxiety</u> (6 mo) <u>Problems with sleep</u> (esp. difficulty falling asleep) <u>Decreased appetite</u> (lost 5 lb in 6 mo) <u>Increased alcohol consumption</u> (to relax) Does not smoke	"Always nervous" <u>Competitive</u> but fearful, <u>Type A</u> College education, high achiever
ENVIRONMENTAL	Lives alone Work <u>demanding, esp. interpersonally</u> Several casual girlfriends Parents living and well, in another state	<u>Promoted</u> to a position with <u>increased responsibility</u> for presentations to public, 6 mo ago	Protestant, middle-class background Only child Father—stock broker Mother—operates clothing store Patient married at 22 yr, divorced at 25 yr, no children

*Demographic data: 35-year-old divorced male, junior executive.

RECOMMENDED READINGS

Fann, W.E.; Ismet, K.; Pokorny, A.D., et al. 1979. *Phenomenology and treatment of anxiety.* New York: Spectrum Publications. This comprehensive, multi-authored book dealing with various aspects of anxiety includes its assessment by questionnaires and scales, anxiety in children and in the elderly, biochemistry of anxiety, psychoanalytic theories, psychopharmacology, and so on.

Leigh, H., and Reiser, M.F. 1980. *The patient: Biological, psychological, and social dimensions of medical practice.* New York: Plenum Medical Books Co. Chs. 4 and 5. A comprehensive discussion of the basic mechanisms of anxiety, including the brain mechanisms, psychologic theories, and environmental aspects is found in Chapter 4, "Anxiety," and Chapter 5, "Psychological defense mechanisms." Defense mechanisms against anxiety are described with illustrative case vignettes.

REFERENCES

American Psychiatric Association. 1980. *Diagnostic and statistical manual of mental disorders*, 3rd ed. Washington, D.C.: American Psychiatric Association.

Benson, H. 1975. *The relaxation response.* New York: William Morrow & Co.

Brenner, C. 1955. *An elementary textbook of psychoanalysis.* New York: International Universities Press.

Freud, S. 1953. Inhibition, symptoms, and anxiety. *The Standard Edition of the Complete Psychological Works of Sigmund Freud*, vol. 20, ed., J. Strachey, London: Hogarth Press.

Goldstein, K. 1975. Functional disturbances in brain damage. In *American handbook of psychiatry*, 2nd ed., vol. 4, ed., M.F. Reiser, pp. 182–207. New York: Basic Books.

Leigh, H., and Reiser, M.F. 1980. *The patient: Biological, psychological, and social dimensions of medical practice.* New York: Plenum Medical Book Co. Ch. 4.

Pavlov, I.P. 1927. *Conditioned reflexes.* London: Oxford University Press.

Spiegel, H., and Spiegel, D. 1978. *Trance and treatment: Clinical use of hypnosis.* New York: Basic Books.

CHAPTER 12

Psychophysiologic Symptoms—Headache

David R. Rubinow, M.D.

This chapter and Chapter 13 are concerned with physical symptoms in which psychological factors, especially anxiety, may play an important role. We begin with a brief discussion of the evolution of the concept of "psychosomatic relationships." Then, the principles of evaluating suspected psychophysiologic symptoms are presented, followed by a discussion of headache, a common psychophysiologic symptom. The evaluation of headache is presented as a paradigm or illustration since it is beyond the scope of this book to discuss all common psychophysiologic symptoms in detail.

Chapter 5, which gives an overview of the relationships between physical and mental disorders, is helpful in understanding the material presented in Chapters 12 and 13.

PSYCHOSOMATIC RELATIONSHIPS

Despite the suggestion of the existence of a relationship between emotion and physical symptoms, the meaning of the term "psychophysiologic symptom" is not totally clear. The notion that the emotions can affect the body and the idea that *psyche* and *soma* are interrelated are Aristotelian concepts—yet after 2,000 years, these essential notions have not gained widespread acceptance. A number of historic forces have served to prevent the development of holistic medical paradigms. The Renaissance fascination with natural science and the material world and Cartesian dualism with its emphasized schism between mind and spirit and body and matter served to expel the study of the mind from the house of science. The mind came to be viewed as the province of theologians and philosophers; influence of the psyche on the body was immeasurable, hence deemed unscientific, and therefore disregarded. Mental processes were relegated by some of the more ardent nineteenth-century somaticists to the realm of somatic epiphenomena (Friedman, 1975). Freud attempted to reunite *psyche* and *soma* by demonstrating the role of emotion in physical and mental illness and by emphasizing, through the introduction of the concept of therapeutic alliance, the necessity of treating the patient and not just his or her symptoms.

In the early twentieth century, a number of joint medical and psychological investigations were performed which convincingly demonstrated the importance of the role played by psychologic factors in the precipitation and course of a variety of medical illnesses. However, it was with Franz Alexander and his specificity theory that the so-called psychosomatic disorder became identified. Alexander attempted to define the *etiology* and pathogenesis of the seven psychosomatic diseases (duodenal ulcer, bronchial asthma, rheumatoid arthritis, ulcerative colitis, essential hypertension, neurodermatitis, thyrotoxicosis) in terms of specific unresolved core conflicts, with associated emotions and physiologic responses. The specificity theory as an etiologic model was incomplete and reductionistic and gave way to the somato-psychosomatic disease model—one that is multifactorial and views coincident somatic and psychic phenomena as "separate and parallel reflections of a common underlying constitutional factor(s) usually postulated to be related to genetic and early experiential factors" (Reiser, 1975). While the somato-psychosomatic model as described by Reiser has certain specific applications, its underlying assumption may be generalized to apply to practically the entire class of medical disorders: to best understand an illness or symptom, one must understand the *person* who is afflicted. The predisposition toward development of illness as well as the

---

CASE HISTORY 12–1

A 45-year-old married accountant came to his family physician complaining of persistent headaches. The pain was described as being a dull, aching, nagging pain in the back of the head. The patient was concerned that he might have brain tumor. It turns out his cousin died of brain tumor approximately six months ago. (See the appendix at the end of this chapter for further discussion and PEG.)

precipitation and course of illness are functions of physiologic and psychosocial factors and the relationships that exist between them. The significance of these relationships and particularly their bidirectional nature cannot be overstated. Certainly the profound interconnection between the cerebral cortex and limbic system on one hand, and the hypothalamus on the other, suggests a means whereby thoughts and feelings could produce widespread physiologic effects through the mediation of the hypothalamo-pituitary-adrenal axis and the ANS. The extent to which this process actually takes place has been appreciated only relatively recently in the work of Mason (1974, 1975, 1978) and others.

Stress, Defense Mechanisms, and the Endocrine System

Mason demonstrated that emotions, social environment, and defense mechanisms were powerful forces in determining not only basal hormonal levels, but even more dramatically, the *direction* (as well as degree) of endocrine response to stress (Mason, 1974, 1975, 1978). Thus, people whose defense mechanisms (for example, denial) were very ineffective and who were acutely stressed in the context of chronic stress, experienced an extreme increase in their already elevated baseline cortisol levels, while people with highly effective defense mechanisms under similar circumstances demonstrated a stress-induced *decrease* in their already low baseline cortisol levels. Further studies have suggested that, in contrast to Selye's (1950) conceptualization of absolute nonspecificity of the pituitary-adrenocortical response to "stressors," multiple hormonal response patterns to various stimuli appear highly distinctive with the earlier noted nonspecificity a probable function of uncontrolled psychological factors. "New knowledge that the psyche is superimposed upon the humoral machinery for endocrine regulation drastically complicates our whole

view of physiologic homeostasis, says Mason, who as a physiologist, was greatly impressed "by the extent to which such psychological factors as anticipatory responses, neurotic process, reactions to subtle social conditions, and the operation of psychological defenses are sensitively reflected in hormonal balance," in chronic and acute cases (Mason, 1974). Thus, one's physiologic reaction to stress appears to be individualized as a product of the interaction and integration of psychological and physiologic variables.

Personality and Sick Role

Imagine a 35-year-old married man with two children, employed as a fireman, who is febrile with a chief complaint of chest pain. Following a bout of respiratory illness, which resulted in the patient's absence from work, he develops a steady constrictive chest pain that radiates into his left arm and that is exacerbated by inspiration. A diagnosis of viral pericarditis is made, and the patient is reassured and treated with bed rest. At this point, a number of factors related to the process of interpretation of the symptoms *by the patient* may alter the course of the illness.

Assumption of the sick role with its forced dependence, helplessness, powerlessness, inactivity, and lack of control can be an extremely difficult task, particularly in the case of individuals for whom the issues of control and autonomy play a major role in their personality organization. Such people may, while inpatients, complain about or refuse to cooperate even with seemingly trivial aspects of their management, or they may, as outpatients, simply fail to comply with their prescribed regimens (Kahana and Bibring, 1964). The sick role, as will be discussed later, can also be incorporated into one's adaptational system, thereby producing another set of problems. Alteration of body-image and/or self-image as a result of illness may exert a profound effect upon the patient's life. The patient in the example might experience an exaggerated sense of vulnerability and develop an increased awareness of his heart's activity. His concern about his heart may decrease his stress tolerance while increasing the anxiety associated with autonomic arousal. He may feel that a new set of limitations (actual and/or fantasized) have been imposed upon him, and his sense of effectiveness and self-worth may suffer further consequences because of the disruption of his customary social and familial roles. The significance of the particular organ system involved cannot be ignored. Perhaps this patient had a friend or relative who suffered a fatal myocardial infarction after a bout of chest pain or who became severely depressed and unable to resume normal life activities after a mild cardiovascular insult.

Reactions to current stressors are often colored by past experiences and identification with others. In short, the assumption of the sick role, alteration of self-confidence and body-image, disruption of sociofamilial roles and relational patterns, and investment of the symptomatic organ with predetermined meaning, all affect the course of the illness through the following five pathways:

1. Generation of anxiety and elicitation of a neuroendocrine-mediated stress response involving cardiovascular, adrenal, and generalized autonomic hyperactivity

2. Psychosocially-induced disturbance of immunologic competence (Schiavi and Stein, 1975)

3. Stimulation of behavior which may, in the case of lack of compliance, decrease the effectiveness of the therapeutic regimen or which, in the case of deviant illness behavior, may produce additional stress and increase the severity of the adaptive challenge of the illness

4. Anxiety-related alteration of pain perception and tolerance

5. Stress-mediated compromise of adaptive function with increased susceptibility in certain cases to development of affective and cognitive dysregulatory states.

Although what is provided here is an example of the dynamic interplay of psychological and physiologic factors in the *course* of an illness, a similar set of interactions can be postulated for the *predisposition* to and *precipitation or exacerbation* of illness. According to this model then, psychophysiologic responses are the norm rather than the exception. The remainder of this chapter offers a framework for evaluation of symptoms in psychophysiologic terms and describes the application of this framework to a representative disorder—headache.

EVALUATION

Physical diagnosis is often complicated by an uncertainty regarding the presence or absence of psychological symptoms which are mimicking, accompanying, or masking "physical disease." This uncertainty can best be mitigated by collecting a complete data base—one that includes biological, psychological, and environmental data viewed in the context of the present, recent past, and distant past. (For a complete discussion of data recording in the biopsychosocial model, see Chapter 1 and Leigh and Reiser, 1980.) While the acquisition of a thorough history is time-consuming, it is critical for effective clinical diagnosis and treatment and often results in savings of time, money, and energy otherwise spent on unnecessary laboratory tests, procedures, and therapeutic regimens which are ineffective as a result of misdiagnosis or failure of compliance. The following sections outline a series of questions that should probably be asked of all patients but which deserve particular attention for patients who pose diagnostic problems.

Current Emotional State

It is important to remember first that the depressive syndrome includes many physiologic symptoms—disorders of sleep, appetite, energy, libido, bowel function, as well as any of as many as

27 peripheral manifestations of anxiety (Shader, 1975); and secondly, in our culture, people can and do complain of physical distress without suffering the stigma (real or imagined) that they would receive were they to complain of emotional distress. Thus, as a result of a patient's wish to present "legitimate" physical symptoms to a physician and the physician's failure to consider psychiatric disorders in the differential diagnosis of physical complaints, many cases of depression are missed with both the physician and patient thereupon experiencing the frustration that comes from unsuitable, ineffective treatment plans. Numerous studies (Lipowski, 1967; Goldberg and Blackwell, 1970; Glass et al., 1978) describe a prevalence of psychiatric illness of between 25% and 80% in various medical patient populations. The illness is usually undetected. Moffic and Paykel (1975) note that of 43 medical inpatients rated as depressed, only 6 even had mention of depression in their hospital charts. The observation that 82% of suicides have visited a physician within 6 months prior to their attempt (Murphy, 1975) further emphasizes the fact that physicians need to be aware of their patients' psychological state and, of equal or greater importance, need to actively evaluate it.

The evaluation of so-called state-related phenomena requires knowledge of those more enduring "trait" characteristics (for purposes of differentiation) as well as any history suggesting that current symptoms may be recurrent rather than *de novo*. In spite of their shortcomings, the various psychiatric screening questionnaires (Hamilton, 1959, 1960; Zung, 1965, 1971) provide a simple means for rapidly establishing a symptomatic baseline against which future ostensible state alterations can be measured. The administration of such questionnaires as part of a patient's intake evaluation can therefore provide data, the importance of which may only become apparent at a later date.

Complaints of change of function in the following three areas should alert the physician to the possible existence of a depressive syndrome:

1. Vegetative functions—sleep disturbance (difficulty falling asleep, early morning awakening, decreased or increased total sleep); appetite disturbance (decrease or increase); weight change (loss or gain); change in libido (decrease)

2. Activity—physical (fatigue, lethargy, anergy, constipation, and decreased speed, amount, and effectiveness of activity); cognitive (decreased concentration, memory disturbance, rumination, somatic preoccupation, inability to make decisions, decreased speed of ideational flow and speech)

3. Psychological functions—mood (apathy, anhedonia, sadness, anxiety, irritability); investment (decreased interest in specific life activities or global decrease).

In patients who complain of physical symptoms without obvious explanation, inquiries as to the patient's functioning in the just-noted areas (Shulman, 1977) may suggest the presence of a masked depression despite a patient's failure to acknowledge "feeling depressed" or an assertion that his or her mood alteration is solely the product of physical symptoms. (For further discussion of masked depression, see Lesse, 1974.)

Why seek help now?

Some patients develop new symptoms or first seek help with chronic symptoms as a direct outgrowth of difficulties in other life areas. Disturbance of relationships with family, friends, or job can serve to decrease one's threshold for concern or complaint. Thus, it is often necessary to ask the additional question, What has changed in this person's life and social environment? to determine if symptom emergence is related to a situational adjustment reaction or depressive syndrome or to the issues of secondary gain (for example, a patient whose symptom elicits the concern and attention of previously emotionally unavailable family members or patients whose symptoms prevent them from attending a job that has become unpleasant).

How Do Symptoms Affect Ability to Function?

Another way of finding out how a patient's symptoms influence everyday life is to ask, "What is the patient's current disability, and is the degree of disability reported disproportionate to what one would predict on the basis of the actual physical complaint?" An example is a young mother with a complaint of headaches that have "prevented" her from venturing forth from her home and have "forced" her to abandon all household and child-care activities. Again, on the basis of this information the physician may be alerted to the possible existence of a depressive disorder or to the operation of a secondary gain.

Object of Complaint

Does the patient wish to obtain symptomatic relief, or does he or she wish to demonstrate the presence of a disease? Patients who suffer from the somatoform disorder previously know as hypochondriacal neurosis are preoccupied with the idea of having a disease, for they can thereby provide an explanation for the inadequacy and failure that figures so prominently in their lives. Such individuals focus attention away from their poor self-image and deficient adaptive mechanisms and tend to view themselves as victims of a depriving world and an infirm constitution. The "somatic displacement" (McCranie, 1979) of their problems permits them to seek help without experiencing an increased sense of inadequacy. Treatment for these people therefore consists not in labeling them as "crocks" and rejecting them, thereby aggravating the condition which led to the development of the somatization, but in recognizing that *their symptoms represent their attempt to deal with their suffering* (McCranie, 1979). As the core problem is usually long-standing, a psychiatric referral is often indicated to help the patient learn that failure and frustration result from maladaptive pattern of relating to the world and not from a defect in the self.

Personal Meaning of Symptoms

Fears and fantasies can serve as powerful modifiers of symptoms. Simple reassurance and an opportunity to discuss one's fears can have a startlingly salutary effect on even chronic syndromes (Shulman, 1977). Unless the physician inquires, patients' fears will often remain undisclosed to the physician, who is therefore not able to provide reassurance effectively.

Does the Patient Know of Someone Else with the Same Symptoms?

Identification with significant others is a process by which symptoms can be inbued with *personal meaning*. Development of a symptom identical or related to that experienced by a close friend or family member may suggest to the patient that he or she has the identical illness (for instance, multiple sclerosis or cancer) or that he or she will suffer the same untoward course. If, for example, a patient's father after developing angina suffered a cerebrovascular accident and became totally incapacitated, the patient, upon developing angina, may react to what he or she fears to be inevitable progression to incapacitation by undertaking excessively arduous tasks in an attempt to give self-assurance that he or she is not an invalid. In the case of an unresolved *grief reaction,* sharing the mourned one's symptoms may serve as expiation for feelings of anger toward the lost significant other. Knowledge of the date and age of the patient's parents at the time of their death may help to identify symptoms which appear as part of an anniversary reaction. Again, through recognition of the patient's identification process, the physician can more effectively reassure the patient and can, where appropriate, reduce the significance of the symptom by helping the patient to articulate grief.

Nature of the Stress Response

The concept of "response specificity" implies that people have individualized patterns of physiologic response to various stressors (Malmo and Shagass, 1949; Sainsbury and Gibson, 1954; Lacey, 1967). Depending upon the individual and the conditions, the elicited stress response might take the form of a headache, an altered cardiac rhythm, an alteration in gastrointestinal motility, and so on. If a physician can help make the patient aware of how he or she typically reacts to stressful situations, that is, which physiologic subsystem appears more reactive to stress—then both physician and patient will be better able to more confidently label symptoms as representing a stress diathesis, or, in the case of atypical or new symptoms, as deserving special diagnostic attention. It goes without saying that all symptoms deserve a differential diagnosis, since the stressor that might be activating a patient's patterned constellation of symptoms may be a demonstrable organic one.

It is, as has been mentioned before, important to determine current stresses acting in the patient's life. Schless and Mendels (1978) and Hudgens and colleagues (1970) have demonstrated that an interview with a patient's significant other can contribute 29% additional information about a patient's life stressors as compared with that provided by the patient alone. Particularly in the case of puzzling and/or chronic symptoms, the conduction of a separate or conjoint interview with the patient's significant other may yield critical psychosocial data.

Physician's Emotional Response

Finally, the physician should ask, "What are my reactions to this patient?" By so doing, the physician may gain insight into the nature and quality of the patient's interpersonal relationships as well as identify affects and adaptational strategies of the patient that directly influence response to treatment. For example, if the physician notices that he or she is struggling with a rambling patient to control the course of the interview, he or she might infer that the patient is anxious and deals with his anxiety and fears of being out of control by attempting to direct the interview. In such a case, the physician should determine, if possible, the source of the anxiety and devise a treatment regimen that allows the patient to feel in control, as, for example, with the use of self-monitoring and self-recording of pain. Similarly, a physician who feels irritated or nervous with a particular patient may be sensing the patient's hidden feelings—the anger of a passive-aggressive patient or the anxiety of someone with a depressive or anxiety disorder, organic brain syndrome, situational adjustment reaction, or impending psychosis. The good physician uses himself or herself as a clinical instrument when evaluating and treating patients.

HEADACHE

Pain

Any discussion of the evaluation and treatment of the common psychophysiologic symptom of headache or of any of the pain syndromes must avoid employing a reductionistic conceptualization of the complex phenomenon that we call pain. Pain is not the impingement of a critical number of nociceptive afferent stimuli upon the CNS. Rather, it is a complicated subjective experience with many determinants in *addition* to the nociceptive stimuli. One has only to recall Beecher's (1946) oft-cited observation that many severely wounded World War II soldiers experienced little or no pain, to realize that factors such as setting and significance of the injury—relief and evacuation in Beecher's case—can powerfully influence pain perception.

The neuroendocrine and neuroanatomical basis of this multidetermined phenomenon remains speculative at present. Melzack and Wall's gate theory of pain (1962) proposes that the "gate" that controls the admission of nociceptive stimuli to the CNS is opened or closed as a function of both the ratio of small nerve afferent stimuli to large nerve afferent stimuli, and the modulating influence of descending spinal pathways. The descending cortical influence is mediated at least in part through the reticular activating system (Frazier, 1975) and, probably as well, through the endogenous opiate system (Calner, 1978). This latter system involves opiate-like polypeptides (endorphins) and pentapeptides (enkephalins) which are widely and differentially distributed throughout the brain (including the thalamus, limbic system, and locus ceruleus). It thus provides a comprehensive model for pain perception which could account for the variability of central interpretation of pain as well as, more specifically, the profound relationship that exists between pain and affect. Goldstein suggests that endorphins/enkephalins not only mediate the placebo response (Levine et al., 1978) and accupuncture analgesia, but also "control the mood in response to stress" (Goldstein, 1978). Endorphins may further function as neurotransmitters in the descending spinal pathways which inhibit the excitatory activity of Substance P—a putative nociceptive neurotransmitter or neuromodulator in the substantia gelatinosa. It appears that recent neuropharmacologic discoveries support the clinical observation that cognitive and emotional factors and noxious stimuli interact in a complex manner to produce the pain experience.

Sternbach (1968) defined pain as consisting of: (a) a noxious stimulus; (b) a perception of "affective-cognitive response" (Maltbie et al., 1978); and (c) a coping response. The stimulus is a signal of actual or potential tissue damage. It is "perceived" in the context of the person's level of attentional arousal, current emotional state, and past experience including the cultural, personal, and interpersonal meaning assigned to the communication to others of one's complaint of pain. If immediate efforts to relieve or eliminate the pain are unsuccessful, there is an "affective escalation" (Maltbie et al., 1978) with emergence and intensification of fear and anticipatory anxiety (Chapman, 1977). A personalized coping reaction based largely on the individual's personality style and defensive structure is then elicited, and it is with this coping response that the physician often deals in the process of evaluating and treating pain syndromes. In the face of chronic pain, a patient may become depressed—preoccupied with the pain experience and incapable of successful adaptation; regressed—with assumption of the sick role and loss or impairment of independent activity; invested in maintaining the pain in order to gratify (in fact or fantasy) unconscious needs; or inured to the pain and capable of continued effective functioning in the various life areas. Engel (1959) suggests that the existence of certain patient characteristics increases the likelihood that pain will serve the patient's psychological needs, therefore producing a coping response "designed" to perpetuate the pain. Among the six characteristics identified by Engel, the prominence of guilt and the inability to express anger are frequently described factors in the headache syndrome, discussed in detail later.

In sum, the perception of and reaction to pain are profoundly affected by emotional factors. As such, assessment of pain syndromes requires a careful attempt to identify a physical source of noxious stimuli as part of a more comprehensive evaluation which includes attention to the patient's mental status, personal and family history, past medical history, and situational stressors.

HEADACHE CLASSIFICATION

In headache, the source of the noxious afferent sensation is the stimulation (pressure, compression, destruction, traction, tension, displacement, distension, distortion, or inflammation) of intracranial and extracranial "pain-sensitive structures," including the skin of the scalp and its blood supply, the head and neck muscles, venous sinuses and their tributaries, dural and intracerebral arteries, at least the fifth, ninth, and tenth cranial nerves, and the cervical nerves. (The cranium, most of the dura mater and pia mater, the brain parenchyma, the ependymal lining of the ventricles, and the choroid plexuses are not sensitive to pain.) According to Ray and Wolff (1940), the fifth cranial nerve serves as the pain pathway for stimuli arising from intracerebral structures lying on or above the tentorium cerebelli with the pain referred from these structures to the anterior two thirds of the head. Stimuli from the extracranial tissues are also transmitted by various branches of the fifth cranial nerve. Pain from structures below the tentorium cerebelli is referred to the occipital region of the head and is carried by the glossopharyngeal and vagus nerves and the upper three cervical spinal roots. As the headache syndrome may result from any number of diverse origins, a thorough medical, neurologic, and psychologic evaluation is warranted in all cases.

The American Medical Association (AMA) (1962) described 15 types of headache in their classificatory scheme of which the first five (vascular migraine, muscle contraction, combined, vasomotor, conversion or delusional) are both more common and more likely to be strongly related to life events than are the remaining types. What follows is a description of these five types of headache, with special attention paid to significant psychological factors and treatment. (The complete AMA classification is reviewed by Dalessio, 1969.)

Vascular Migraine

The cause of migraine is unknown. However, the sequence of arterial (particularly extracranial and scalp) constriction (the prodromal phase) followed by dilatation with sterile inflammation of the arterial wall (the pain phase) is generally regarded as the best available pathophysiologic model for vascular headache. The source of the cerebrovascular instability as well as the specific roles of various vasoactive substances implicated in the prodromal and pain phases remain topics for speculation. The epidemiology of migraine is more well defined. Migraine is reported as occurring in 10% of the national population,

with a family history of headache existing in approximately two thirds of cases. There are a number of commonly recognized subvarieties of the vascular headache. These include: classic migraine; common migraine; hemiplegic and ophthalmoplegic migraine; basilar artery migraine; cluster headache; and migraine equivalents.

In *classic migraine*, the head pain is part of a symptom complex which may include photophobia, nausea, vomiting, constipation or diarrhea, cyclic edema, bouts of fever, tachycardia, scotomata or visual field defects, paresthesias, benign postural vertigo, elevation of blood pressure, and pain in thorax, pelvis, or extremities (Dalessio, 1969). Many of these symptoms may appear without headache in a paroxysmal, recurrent fashion as migraine equivalents— a phenomenon which has been estimated as occuring in 20% of migraine subjects (Catino, 1965).

Classic migraine typically has a sharply defined, pain-free prodromal phase during which various neurologic symptoms, most often scotomata, but occasionally paraesthesias or motor deficits, occur. The head pain is characterized as intense, unilateral, throbbing or pulsating, and with nausea, anorexia, or vomiting as associated symptoms. Mood disturbance may accompany either or both of the two phases.

The most frequent type of migraine, *common migraine*, does not have a sharply defined prodrome. Mood, gastrointestinal, and fluid balance disturbances may precede the headache by hours or days. The pain is throbbing or steady and is variable in duration, lasting (like classic migraine) from hours to days. While a variety of factors, including certain foods, birth control pills, alcohol, bright light, hormonal changes, and so on, can precipitate attacks of either common or classic migraine, the common migraine headache is more frequently clearly related to environmental stressors. The fact that the headache often follows a stressful period is reflected in the descriptive terms, "weekend headache" or "vacation headache." The "premenstrual headache" also is included in the common migraine group.

Hemiplegic migraine is a strongly familial disorder in which the classic migraine attack is preceded, accompanied or rarely, followed by, unilateral extremity and facial weakness with numbness, paresthesias, and, depending upon the side involved, dysphasia.

Ophthalmoplegic migraine most often begins in childhood and is characterized by the occurrence of third cranial nerve paresis 3–5 days following the onset of headache. The deficit may persist for as long as 2–3 months and may become permanent if attacks are frequent (Friedman, 1978).

In *basilar artery migraine*, the prodrome may consist of vertigo, ataxia, dysarthria, and tinnitus, as well as visual disturbances. Syncope occurs in approximately 30% of the cases (Kudrow, 1978b; Bickerstaff, 1961).

Finally, the *cluster headache* is an intense, almost exclusively unilateral headache which, in contrast to migraine, occurs far more frequently in men, is of short duration (minutes to several hours) and recurs from one to as many as ten times in a 24-hour period (Lance, 1975). This pattern of frequent attacks may continue for weeks or months and then suddenly disappear, only to return after a remission period of months or years. Some 20% of people with cluster headache have the chronic variety, with pain recurring regularly without the pattern of episodic bouts and remissions. The pain in cluster headache is extraordinarily severe and is described as "boring, burning, piercing, tearing, and screwing" (Lance, 1975). It is felt behind one eye in about 60% of cases with radiation to the ipsilateral forehead, temple, cheek, or gum. Most patients experience unilateral lacrimation and rhinorrhea or nasal congestion associated at times with a partial Horner's syndrome consisting of conjunctival suffusion, lid lag, and miosis (Kudrow, 1978a). Again, as with migraine, both central and peripheral factors have been implicated in the pathogenesis of cluster headache.

Many studies have investigated the role of *personality traits* and *situational factors* in migraine (see Boag, 1969). The results of these studies suggest that while there is no "personality profile" shared by all migraine patients, certain personality traits do occur with striking frequency. These key traits appear to be rigid perfectionism, compulsivity, and inability to express anger. Other characteristics are: ambitious; efficient; resentful of authority; competitive; and inability to delegate responsibility, face new situations, or limit acceptance of burdens and responsibility. Thus, many patients with vascular headache appear to have an obsessional, controlling personality style that precludes the direct or verbal expression of anger. When placed in a situation where their ability to tolerate suppressed anger, frustration, and fatigue is surpassed, a headache develops. Although it is true that a variety of personality manifestations and emotional factors other than compulsivity and repressed anger may be involved for patients with vascular headaches, treatment nonetheless depends upon the recognition of maladaptive coping strategies that emerge from the patient's personality development and which predispose the patient to a life of tense control and stressful existence.

Treatment. If one views the vascular headache as the end product of the interaction of constitutional, personality, and situational factors, then the methods of therapeutic intervention become clear. *Pharmacotherapy* is basically symptomatic or prophylactic. Ergotamine tartrate remains the drug of choice for treatment of the acute migraine attack, although it cannot be used daily without the potential development of physical dependence, rebound headaches (Rose and Wilkinson, 1976), and possible toxic vascular change (Dige-Peterson et al., 1977). Ergotamine is frequently used in combination with caffeine (a synergist) and/or an antiemetic. Patients with frequent headaches or severe headaches occurring more often than twice a month deserve a trial of daily prophylactic therapy. Propranolol and methysergide are the two most successful prophylactic medications available, although treatment with the latter agent may be complicated by rather significant short-term and long-term adverse side effects. A host of other prophylactic agents including cyproheptadine, lithium carbonate, MAO inhibitors, and clonidine may be effective in certain cases, but widespread efficacy has not been demonstrated.

Biofeedback training has been successfully used in the treatment of vascular headaches, although it is not clear to what extent the relaxation associated with biofeedback may have been responsible for the clinical improvement noted (Diamond and Medina, 1978).

Assessment of headache patients requires knowledge of work and play habits, social and family life, long-range goals, personality traits, life stressors, and method of coping with stress, in addition to the more symptom-specific information related to the onset, location, duration, and modifying factors of the headache. In other words, the physician should create a model of the patient that will serve to organize the constitutional, psychological, and environmental data that the physician collects from the patient. By so doing, the physician can help the patient *learn to recognize which situational factors are stressful*, and can, where possible, suggest ways of avoiding or changing the stressful situation. Prescription of adequate *relaxation*, rest, exercise, and a well-rounded diet as well as proscription or reduction of provoking factors such as fasting, fatigue, exposure to light glare, irregular sleep, excessive responsibility, and offending allergens, foods, or drugs, can prove very beneficial. Additionally, however, the provision by the physician of a warm, *supportive environment* in which the patient is encouraged to express his or her feelings and feels comfortable doing so can often provide the patient with considerable

relief as a result of emotional decompression and subsequent enhancement of coping capacity.

Psychotherapy should be considered for patients who are resistant to pharmacologic management and for whom headache is severe and disabling, as well as for patients who are well motivated and who wish to examine their perceptions and patterns of behavior to learn to function in a less rigid, more adaptive manner.

Muscle Contraction Headache

"Tension," "psychogenic," and "nervous" headache are other names for the most common headache syndrome which involves sustained contraction of scalp, neck, face, and shoulder muscles. The headache is variously described as dull, aching, pressing, constricting, and bandlike and is most often bilateral and suboccipital, although frontal, temporal, and facial regions may be similarly affected. The pain may be transitory and intermittent or may persist for days, weeks, months, and even years. There is no prodrome, and nausea and vomiting occur rarely. Family history is usually unremarkable. Examination of the muscles of the neck, scalp, and face will often reveal areas which are taut and/or tender, and limitation of motion of the neck is occasionally present.

The muscle contraction is usually a component of the patient's *reaction to life stressor* and is frequently associated with *anxiety* and *depression*. There is no specific personality type for those with muscle contraction headache; however, an underlying dynamic frequently observed is that of inhibited expression of emotional arousal which becomes translated into somatic terms with a resultant increase in muscle tension (Shulman, 1979). While *situational factors* often serve as the precipitants of the emotional arousal, the existence of certain personality traits appears to increase the likelihood of the somatic translation. Plutchik (1954), in an excellent review of muscle tension and personality, presented evidence suggesting that patterns of movement, posture, facial expression, and general level of tension are highly individualized and "consistent aspects of personality." He further cited numerous studies which support the view that *frustration*—interference with actual or desired activity—and indecision are associated with increased muscle tension and a decreased threshold for pain, while removal of frustration and *successful problem-solving* produce changes in the opposite directions. These findings lend credence to the group of personality traits described as being frequently seen in people with muscle contraction headache: apprehensive, afraid or unable to express anger, scrupulous, overconscientious, avoidant of confrontation, unassertive and indecisive in situations requiring direct action (Boag, 1969; Shulman, 1979).

Treatment.   As with the vascular headache, the treatment of the muscle contraction headache should employ biopsychosocial strategies. *Antianxiety agents* (benzodiazepines), *muscle relaxants*, *heat*, *massage* and *manipulation* all can provide symptomatic relief on a short-term basis, but should not be substituted for careful evaluation and problem definition. While muscle contraction headache can develop secondarily to migraine, sustained muscle contraction can itself produce a relative muscle ischemia with intermittent compensatory throbbing which may be misdiagnosed as migraine but will not respond to ergot alkaloids. "Depressive syndromes" are generally reported as occurring with muscle contraction headaches more frequently than with migraine, although, in both cases, treatment of the depression with anti-depressants may afford considerable relief.

Hypnosis, meditation, biofeedback, and various other *relaxation therapies* are in many cases successful pain relief modalities and further provide patients with an enhanced sense of control, thereby decreasing their fear of loss of control. *Psychotherapy* may serve to clarify the relationship of attitudes and patterns of behavior to the muscle contraction headache and thus create a setting for potential behavioral change. This change may be accomplished through the development of new and more adaptive problem-solving methods and strategies for coping with anger and stress, including identification of stressful situations with subsequent avoidance or removal of stressors; acceptance of assertive and hostile feelings; and formulation of realistic goals and self-expectations.

Combined Headache.   Combined headaches contain both vascular and muscle contraction components occurring concurrently or sequentially. Sustained muscle contraction may result from a wide variety of headache-generating stimuli (such as, inflammation of the neck and scalp; migraine; hypertension; intracranial tumor; eye, ear, nose, sinus, and tooth pathology, and so on), or as previously mentioned, prolonged muscle contraction headache may develop a vascular component. Evaluation and treatment require utilization of the same strategies described for muscle contraction and vascular headaches.

Vasomotor Reaction Headache.   In vasomotor reaction headaches, nasal pain and discomfort accompany anterior head pain in the presence of engorged paranasal sinuses and in the absence of precise paranasal disease. Anxiety, resentment, menstruation, and sexual excitement have been implicated as the stimuli leading to vascular engorgement and a resulting headache, commonly referred to as "vasomotor rhinitis" (Dalessio, 1969). Causative factors (such as allergy, infection, and structural defects) must be ruled out before treatment, at the least consisting of identification and management of stress, is initiated.

Delusional, Conversion, or Hypochondriacal Headache.   Headaches that occur in delusional, hypochondriacal, or conversion states are characterized by their pronounced *symbolic importance* as well as by the minimal presence or absence of local tissue changes. In our culture at least, the head has acquired great symbolic significance as the residence of cognition and self and as the agency of control and adaptation, ideas that are revealed in sayings such as "Don't lose your head," or "That's using your head." It is not surprising that concerns related to intellect, cognition, emotional capacity, and self-worth are frequently expressed in terms of head-referred complaints. Additionally, in these headaches which represent somatic delusion, conversion symptoms or hypochondriacal over-elaboration, "the distribution and transformations of the pain do not follow patterns of vascular and muscular change" (Boag, 1969). Successful treatment of the headache therefore can only follow identification and treatment of the primary psychologic disorder. Monosymptomatic or somatic delusions may occur in major affective disorders (bipolar or unipolar) as well as in schizophrenia. Conversion headaches should more properly be classified as *psychalgia* rather than as conversion disorder unless another conversion symptom not involving pain is also present (*DSM-III*, 1980). Nonetheless, the headache may, in a way similar to more classic conversion symptoms, represent the operation of the mechanisms of primary gain—keeping an internal conflict unconscious—and secondary gain—avoidance of noxious stimuli or elicitation of compensation and support. While psychalgia is frequently (although not exclusively) seen in people with histrionic and dependent personalities, typical histrionic features (such as, dependency, seductiveness, or "la belle indifférence") are seldom present. A history of "doctor-shopping" or analgesic abuse supports the diagnosis of psychalgia.

Complaint of pain in the head may accompany complaints of any of a variety of other aches and pains in the patient with atypical somatization disorder (hypochondriasis) for whom a normal sensation appears to be transformed to a painful stimulus by means of the mediating effects of enhanced attention and autosuggestion. As previously noted, preoccupation with illness enables patients with this disorder to express resentment and concern while it provides them with an acceptable explanation for personal failure and inadequacy.

Headache that appears in the context of a history of recurrent, multisystem somatic complaints, frequent physician visits, and an onset of symptoms prior to age 25 years suggests the presence of *somatization disorder*, also known as Briquet's syndrome (see Chapter 13). Anxiety and depressive features are commonly observed in Briquet syndrome as is the occurrence of histrionic personality disorder and, less frequently, antisocial personality disorder. Baseline depressive symptoms or those secondary to a superimposed episodic affective disorder may sometimes be of sufficient severity to induce the patient to seek psychiatric treatment.

Notwithstanding the paucity or absence of demonstrable organic findings in this general class of conversion headache disorders, the pain complained of should be regarded as *real*, with the primary task of the physician then becoming that of *decoding the meaning of the symptom.* Psychiatric consultation or treatment may be of great potential benefit in this deciphering process.

One final headache disorder generally included in this category is the *posttraumatic headache.* Merritt (1979) reports that 35%–40% of people who sustain head injury develop a "posttraumatic syndrome," in which, in addition to headache, they may complain of anxiety, depressed mood, personality change, irritability, difficulty in concentration, dizziness or vertigo, hyperhidrosis, and insomnia with difficulty falling asleep, restless sleep, and terrifying dreams (also see posttraumatic stress disorder in *DSM-III*, 1980). In most cases, improvement can be anticipated with decrease in the headache's frequency and severity progressing to complete disappearance of the headache within 6 months to a year. The severity of the injury does not appear correlated with either the development of the syndrome or its duration. The headache is characterized as dull, aching, throbbing, pressing, or bursting, and exhibits both muscular contraction and vascular elements. Lance (1975) posits that "any blow to or laceration of the scalp arteries renders them more liable to the painful dilation that gives rise to the post-traumatic migraine." Further, there is evidence that suggests that premorbid psychopathology, domestic or financial problems, or a desire to obtain financial compensation, escape from a stressful occupation, or elicitation of environmental support may facilitate production and/or persistence of posttraumatic headache symptoms. It thus appears that this headache syndrome reflects the operation of both physiologic and psychological factors, namely, subtle organic changes secondary to trauma, and psychological reaction to the injury and setting of the injury, as well as to the protracted litigation so often an associated feature of this syndrome.

As previously noted, the head is of great symbolic importance, and head injury may thus evoke many frightening fantasies and concerns. Accordingly, education and reassurance are key elements in treatment and possibly prevention of the posttraumatic syndrome. Fairly rapid engagement by the patient in mild to moderate activites can often serve to prevent escalation of somatic concern, and expeditious resolution, if possible, of insurance or liability claims can similarly help avoid prolongation of symptoms (Merritt, 1979).

CONCLUSION

Graham (1967) has proposed that a mind-body dualism does exist but that it is only a linguistic dualism; that is, the terms "physical" and "psychological" are different languages for describing the same event. "Physical" and "psychological" then, are not rival etiologic hypotheses but rather are two different ways of describing some aspect of a person. The implications of this proposition can be seen in the nature of the processes of referral and collaboration as well as evaluation.

A psychiatrist can often be of help in the evaluation and, in some cases, the treatment of patients with any of a variety of complaints. It is important, however, for the primary care physician to remember that patients are extraordinarily emotionally invested in their relationship with their physicians and will, therefore, react strongly and negatively if they sense that they are being "dumped" on the psychiatrist or "accused of having psychiatric problems." The nature of the referral can dramatically influence its efficacy. If the patient can view referral to a psychiatrist as a manifestation of the physician's sensitivity to and interest in him or her, rather than as an act of frustration, rejection, or hostility, the patient is more likely to comply with and benefit from the referral. Patients who are willing to look at their emotional distress, to examine and alter their maladaptive behavioral patterns, or to learn, when necessary, to adjust to and "live with" their dysfunction, may profit from psychiatric treatment.

A group of medical students who participated in a clinical exercise were asked to take a "conventional medical history." For several, "conventional" meant that they should actively eschew any emotionally charged topics, as evidenced by one student's decision to interrupt a patient's tearful description of her husband's illness in order to determine the precise extent of her orthopnea. If the medical history is no more than a sterile information-collecting process, then the physician's perceptual field will be constricted with consequent impairment of his or her ability to use data the patient provides. To the extent that physicians are able to entertain a number of different paradigms for human distress, so will they be able to listen to patients more effectively, evaluate more efficiently, and treat them more successfully.

The physician who is able to listen to the patient and to attend to the details of that patient's environment and personality style can potentially enhance the effectiveness of any and all therapeutic interventions. For such a physician, the term "psychophysiologic" may have meaning as a description of a positive approach to patients—an approach that maximizes the opportunity for therapeutic success and personal gratification.

APPENDIX: CASE HISTORY—THE PERSISTENT HEADACHES

The PEG shows that the patient had occasional headaches for a long time, but that they increased in frequency and severity in the past 4 months. The location and description of the headaches are consistent with muscle tension headache, and laboratory tests including CT scan of the head did not reveal other causes such as brain tumor, of which the patient is afraid. It is also noted that the patient is a controlling, orderly person who tends to "hold in emotions," which may tend to predispose the individual to muscle tension. His father's frequent headaches also might have contributed to the patient's illness through both biological vulnerability and illness behavior. In addition, the recent stressors (death of cousin due to brain tumor, wife starting work again, increased work pressure) probably contributed to his anxiety symptoms (sleep problems, decreased appetite and sexual desire) and possible depression. It was concluded, however, on the basis of the degree of symptomatology that he did not have a complete depressive syndrome. The three dimensional diagnoses were:

1. **Biological dimension:** Muscle tension headache
2. **Personal dimension:** Adjustment disorder with anxiety and mild depressive features; obsessive-compulsive personality trait
3. **Environmental dimension:** Environmental stressors—moderate

On the basis of the assessment, the following three-dimensional management plans were made

1. **Biological dimension:** Diazepam 5 mg three times a day was initially prescribed with aspirin as needed for anxiety and pain.
2. **Personal dimension:** Supportive psychotherapy with electromyographic biofeedback for relaxation was given concurrently with above. This was arranged through the psychiatrist with whom the family physician has a collaborative relationship. In discussion with the psychiatrist, the patient was able to understand that his preoccupation with brain tumor was related to his grief over the cousin's death, who was quite close to him (and the same age). As he gained control over the occipital muscles through biofeedback relaxation, the diazepam was tapered off.
3. **Environmental dimension:** No specific treatment was given immediately other than dealing with the stressors in psychotherapy. Although couples' therapy was considered, it turned out to be unnecessary as the patient's symptoms improved in a matter of several months.

	CONTEXTS		
	Patient Evaluation Grid		
DIMENSIONS	**CURRENT** (Current States)	**RECENT** (Recent Events and Changes)	**BACKGROUND** (Culture, Traits, Constitution)
BIOLOGICAL	Persistent headache —bilateral, occipital Blood pressure 138/86 mm Hg Pulse rate 86/min Physical exam normal except for pain on pressure in the musculature on the occipital and dorsal cervical regions Lab tests & CT scan normal	Headaches began approximately 4 mo ago (December) Aspirin helped, but duration and severity of headache have been increasing	Father had frequent headaches and died of stroke (age 63 yr) Patient had occasional headaches since childhood
PERSONAL	Patient thinks he may have brain tumor Anxious, with tense facies Mental status otherwise normal	Feeling anxious and preoccupied about brain tumor—5 mo Difficulty falling asleep—3 mo Decreased sexual desire—3 mo Appetite decreased— 4 mo Does not drink or smoke	Controlling, orderly person "Never shows anger" Holds in emotions
ENVIRONMENTAL	Wife (age 42 yr) supportive Work is "pressured" Two married children	Cousin (age 45 yr) died of brain tumor—6 mo ago (the cousin had headaches as first symptom) Wife started working again—8 mo Increase in workload and "pressure" in patient's work— 1 yr (especially severe now because of income tax time)	Lower middle-class, Catholic background Average in school Married (age 23 yr) when in college. Worked for a bank for many years before becoming a CPA (night school) Patient's mother died in an accident when patient was 18 yr of age

Demographic data: 45-year-old married male, accountant.

RECOMMENDED READINGS

Graham, D.T.: 1967. Health, disease, and the mind-body problem: Linguistic parallelism. *Psychosom. Med.* 34:52–71. Here is an interesting summary of mind-body dualism in medicine.

Kahana, R.J., and Bibring, G.L. 1964. Personality types in medical management. In *Psychiatry and medical practice in a general hospital*, ed., N.E. Zinberg, pp. 108–23. New York: International Universities Press. This chapter is a must for anyone who works with patients.

Shulman, R. 1977. Psychogenic illness with physical manifestations and the other side of the coin. *Lancet* 1:524–26. Shulman gives an excellent presentation of a practical approach to diagnostic problems.

Vinken, P.J., and Bruyn, G.W., eds. 1969. *Handbook of clinical neurology*, vol. 5. New York: American Elsevier, pp. 15–24; 247–257. These two chapters, "Psychogenic headache," and "Headache mechanisms," are well-written, comprehensive, and extremely informative.

REFERENCES

Ad Hoc Committee on Classification of Headache. 1962. Special report. *J.A.M.A.* 179:717–18.

American Psychiatric Association. 1980. *Diagnostic and statistical manual of mental disorders (DSM-III)*, 3rd ed. Washington, D.C.: American Psychiatric Association.

Beecher, H.K. 1946. Pain in men wounded in battle. *Ann. Surg.* 123:96–105.

Bickerstaff, E.R. 1961. Basilar artery migraine. *Lancet* 1:15–17.

Boag, T.J. 1969. Psychogenic headache. In *Handbook of clinical neurology*, vol. 5, eds., P.J. Vinken, and G.W. Bruyn, pp. 247–57. New York: American Elsevier.

Calne, D.B. 1978. Pain and analgesic mechanisms. In *Psychopharmacology: A generation of progress*, eds. M.A. Lipton; A. Dimascio; and K.F. Killam, pp. 777–81. New York: Raven Press.

Catino, D. 1965. Ten migraine equivalents. *Headache* 5:1–11.

Chapman, C.R. 1977. Psychological aspects of pain in patient treatment. *Arch. Surg.* 112:767–72.

Dalessio, D.J. 1969. Headache mechanisms. In *Handbook of clinical neurology*, vol. 5, eds., P.J.

Vinken, and G.W. Bruyn, pp. 15–24. New York: American Elsevier.

Diamond, S. and Medina, J.L. 1978. The value of biofeedback in the treatment of chronic headache. Paper presented at twentieth annual meeting, American Association for the Study of Headache in St. Louis, June 1978.

Dige-Paterson, H.; Lassen N.A.; Noer, I., et al. 1977. Subclinical ergotism. *Lancet* 2:65–66.

Engel, G.L. 1959. Psychogenic pain and the pain-prone patient. *Am. J. Med* 26:899–918.

Frazier, S.H. 1975. Complex problems of pain as seen in headache, painful phantom, and other states. *American handbook of psychiatry*, ed., M.F. Reiser, pp. 838–53. New York: Basic Books.

Friedman, A.P. 1975. Headaches. In *Comprehensive Textbook of Psychiatry II*, 2nd ed., Vol. 2. eds., A.M. Freedman, H.I. Kaplan, and B.J. Sadock, pp. 1624–31. Baltimore: William & Wilkins Co.

Friedman, A.P.; Harter, D.H.; and Merritt, H.H. 1978 Ophthalmoplegic migraine. *Arch. Neurol.* 7:82–87

Glass, R.; Allan, A.T.; and Uhlenhuth, E.H. 1978. Psychiatric screening in a medical clinic. *Arch. Gen. Psych.* 35:1189–95.

Goldberg, D., and Blackwell, B. 1970. Psychiatric illness in general practice: A detailed study using a new method of case identification. *Br. Med. J.* 2:439–43.

Goldstein, A. 1978. Opiate receptors and opioid peptides: A ten-year overview. In *Psychopharmacology: A generation of progress* eds., M.A. Lipton; A Dimascio; and K.F. Killam, pp. 1557–63. New York: Raven Press.

Graham, D.T. 1967. Health, disease, and the mind-body problem: Linguistic parallelism. *Psychosom. Med.* 34:52–71.

Hamilton, M. 1960a. A rating scale for depression. *J. Neurol. Neurosurg. Psychiatry* 23:56–62.

———1959. The assessment of anxiety states by rating. *Br. J. Med Psychol.* 32:50–55.

Hudgens, R.W.; Robins, E; and Delong, W.B. 1970. The reporting of recent stress in the lives of psychiatric patients. *Br. J. Psychiatry* 117:635–43.

Kahana, R.J., and Bibring, G.L. 1964. Personality types in medical management. In *Psychiatry and medical practice in a general hospital*, ed. N.E. Zinberg, pp. 108–23. New York: International Universities Press.

Kaplan, H.I. 1975. History of psychophysiological medicine. In *Comprehensive textbook of psychia-*

try II, 2nd ed., vol. 2., eds., A.M. Freedman; H.I. Kaplan; and B.J. Sadock, pp. 1624–31. Baltimore: Williams & Wilkins Co.

Kudrow, L. 1978a. Managing migraine headache. *Psychosomatics* 19:685–93.

———1978b. Current aspects of migraine headache. *Psychosomatics* 19:48–57.

Lacey, J.I. 1967. Somatic response patterning and stress: Some revision of activation theory. In *Psychological stress*, eds., M.H. Appley and R. Trumbull, pp. 14–37. New York: Appleton-Century-Crofts.

Lance, J.W. 1975. *Headache: Understanding, alleviation*. New York: Charles Scribner's Sons. pp. 87–100; 188–96.

Leigh, H., and Reiser, M.F. 1980. *The patient: Biological, psychological and social dimension of medical practice*. New York: Plenum Publishing Co.

Lesse, S. 1974. Hypochondriasis and psychosomatic disorders masking depression. In *Masked depression*. New York: Jason Aronson. Ch. 4

Levine, J.D.; Gordon, N.C.; and Fields, H.L. 1978. The mechanism of placebo analgesia. *Lancet* 2:654–57.

Lipowski, Z.J. 1967. Review of consultation psychiatry and psychosomatic medicine: II. Clinical aspects. *Psychosom. Med.* 24:201–24.

Malmo, R.B., and Shagass, C. 1949. Physiologic study of symptom mechanism in psychiatric patients under stress. *Psychosom. Med.* 11:25–29.

Maltbie, A.A.; Cavenar, J.O., Jr.; and Hammett, E.B. 1978. A diagnostic approach to pain. *Psychosomatics* 19:359–66.

Mason, J.W. 1974. The integrative approach in medicine. Implications of neuroendocrine mechanisms. *Perspect. Biol. Med.* (Spring 1974) pp. 333–48.

Mason, J.W. 1945. Clinical psychophysiology: psychoendocrine mechanisms. In *American handbook of psychiatry*, vol 4, ed., M.F. Reiser. New York: Basic Books, Inc.

Mason, J.W. 1978. Psychoendocrinology: A future perspective, Yale-New Haven Hospital, New Haven, Conn. *Psychosom. Grand Rounds* (Sept. 1978).

McCranie, E.J. 1979. Hypochondriacal neurosis. *Psychosomatics* 20:11–15.

Melzack, R., and Wall, P.D. 1962. Pain mechanisms: A new theory. *Science* 150:969–79.

Merritt, H.H. 1979. *A textbook of neurology.* Philadelphia: Lea & Febiger, pp. 352–55.

Moffic, H., and Paykel, E.S. 1975. Depression in medical inpatients. *Br. J. Psychiatry* 126:346–53.

Murphy, G.E. 1975. The physician's responsibility for suicide. II. Errors of omission. *Ann. Intern. Med.* 82:305–9.

Plutchik, R. 1954. The role of muscular tension in maladjustment. *J. Gen. Psychiatry* 50:45–62.

Ray, B.S., and Wolff, H.G. 1940. Experimental studies on headache: Pain-sensitive structures of the head and their significance in headache. *Arch. Surg.* 41:813–56.

Reiser, M.F. 1966. Toward an integrated psychoanalytic-physiological theory of psychosomatic disorders. In *Psychoanalyisis—a general psychology*, ed., R.M. Loewenstein, pp. 477–500. New York: International Universities Press.

———1975. Changing theoretical concepts in psychosomatic medicine. In *American handbook of psychiatry*, vol. 4. ed., M.F. Reiser, pp. 477–500. New York: Basic Books.

Rose, F.C., and Wilkinson, M. 1976. Ergotamine tartrate overdose. *Br. Med. J.* 1:525.

Sainsbury, B., and Gibson, J.G. 1954. Symptoms of anxiety and tension and the accompanying physiological changes in the muscular system. *J. Neurol. Neurosurg. Psychiatry* 17:216–24.

Schiavi, R.C., and Stein, M. 1975. Disorders of immune mechanisms. In *American handbook of psychiatry*, vol, 4, ed., M.F. Reiser, pp. 709–25. New York: Basic Books.

Seyle, H. 1950. *The physiology and pathology of exposure to stress; a treatise based on the concepts of general-adaptation-syndrome and the diseases of adaptation.* Montreal: Acta.

Shader, R. 1975. *Manual of psychiatric therapeutics.* Boston: Little Brown & Co. pp. 27–38.

Schless, A.P., and Mendels, J. 1978. The value of interviewing family and friends in assessing life stressors. *Arch. Gen. Psychiatry* 35:565–67.

Shulman, B.H. 1979. The psychotherapist and the headache patient. *Psychosomatics* 20:175–81.

Shulman, R. 1977. Psychogenic illness with physical manifestations and the other side of the coin. *Lancet* 1:524–26.

Sternbach, R.H. 1968. *Pain: A psychophysiological analysis.* New York: Academic Press.

Zung, W.K. 1965. A self-rating depression scale. *Arch. Gen. Psychiatry* 12:63–70.

——— 1971. A rating instrument for anxiety disorders. *Psychosomatics* 12:371–79.

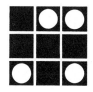

CHAPTER 13

Hysteria and Hypochondriasis

Craig Van Dyke, M.D.

Hysteria is one of the most misused terms in medicine. Patients who are suspected of having hysteria or hypochondriasis are often branded "crocks," and adequate medical workup is rarely performed. This chapter discusses the general concepts concerning these often perplexing syndromes and suggests ways of recognizing and managing them. The syndromes grouped under "somatoform disorders" in *DSM-III*, the material discussed here, differ from the psychophysiologic symptoms discussed in Chapter 12. The somatosensory nervous system and special sensory organs are primarily affected in somatoform disorders, while in psychophysiologic symptoms the autonomic nervous system is primarily affected.

Since antiquity physicians have had to deal with patients who complain of signs or symptoms for which no apparent medical explanation can be offered. Nothing is more frustrating for the physician than to be unable to determine the cause of a patient's complaints. Obviously, as we learn more about human physiology and disease processes, there are fewer instances of confusion about the etiology or treatment of a patient's condition. Nevertheless, there remain many patients who seek medical attention, for whom the physician cannot find a cause or successful treatment for their problems. Sooner or later these patients are labeled as "hysterical."

HISTORICAL NOTE

The diagnostic label "hysteria" originated with the Greeks and Romans, who thought the fundamental cause was a disorder of the uterus. Their differential diagnosis included such problems as "wandering," "suffocation," or "furor" of this organ. In the Middle Ages, hysteria was thought to be a result of the patient being in league with the devil and an expression of a sinful sexuality. Pinel, in early 1800s, noted that hysteria could be contagious. In the latter half of the nineteenth century, Charcot began to focus medical attention on patients suffering from hysteria. Charcot had already achieved fame in his work describing multiple sclerosis, amyotrophic lateral sclerosis, and lesions of the spinal cord. He subsequently turned his attention to patients with hysteria, recognizing that there were three different forms of the illness: (a) sensory disturbances; (b) disturbances of vision and hearing; and (c) motor disturbances. Although he recognized a psychological component to this condition, he steadfastly maintained that the major problem was a neurologic disorder. Charcot based this idea on the fact that he was able to hypnotize patients with hysteria and his certainty that only neurologically impaired individuals could be hypnotized. His views were strongly challenged and eventually overcome by Bernheim, who pointed out that normal individuals could be hypnotized and that hypnosis merely represented a state of increased suggestibility. In this sense hysteria was not a disease but rather an exaggerated or distorted reaction to emotional trauma. Somewhat later, Janet pointed out that a key element in hysteria was a dissociation of consciousness. A dissociated idea was not available to conscious awareness but was active and operated autonomously, much as a post-hypnotic suggestion may be carried out by an individual who is unaware of why he or she is performing a certain behavior (Veith, 1965).

CASE HISTORY 13–1

A 19-year-old single, female, college student was brought to the University Health Service by her classmate when her voice became strained, and in a matter of hours, she was totally unable to speak. The patient was able to make mouth movements, had no difficulty in breathing, but no sound would come out her mouth. She was, however, able to write without any difficulty. Complete physical examination, laboratory tests, and ENT examination were normal except for the aphonia. (See the appendix of the end of this chapter for further discussion and PEG.)

In their *Studies on Hysteria* (1895), Freud and Breuer revolutionized understanding of hysteria and introduced the psychoanalytic movement. They noted that some symptoms without medical basis could be cured by hypnotizing their patients and having them relive traumatic aspects of their lives. Their work especially focused on sexual traumas early in life, and they felt that patients with hysterical symptoms were suffering from "reminiscences." Because of the unacceptable nature of the emotions, the patient was not able to express or discharge these emotions at the time of the traumatic event. (Later, Freud realized that many of these sexual traumas did not really occur but rather were part of the patient's childhood fantasies.) They felt that the emotions associated with these sexual traumas, whether real or imagined, were converted into a physical symptom that symbolically expressed the underlying conflict. Their hypothesis was that by converting the psychologic conflict into a physical symptom the patient could remain unaware of the conflict and yet achieve relief from anxiety. They emphasized that the symptoms were defensive in nature by preventing the discomfort associated with feeling anxious. In fact, these patients classically expressed "la belle indifference" (that is, not feeling anxious about their physical symptoms). Freud also cautioned against the pejorative use of the term "hysteria." He believed that these patients were not weak-willed or suffering from a neurologic disorder, since they exhibited normal behavior once their symptoms had been cured by hypnosis and abreaction (reexperiencing their traumatic life event).

At the turn of the century and even into the early 1900s the attention of psychiatry was focused on curing symptoms. It was not until the 1920s and 30s that much thought was devoted to personality styles or disorders. Wittels (1930) and Reich in his famous *Character Analysis* (1933) finally drew the attention of psychiatrists to the patient's life style. These authors felt that the goal of psychoanalysis was not to relieve symptoms but rather to restructure the patient's character. One of the styles they characterized was the "hysterical personality." As Reich defined it, this style included: obvious sexualized behavior with apprehension about sexual relationships, body agility, excitability, suggestibility, infantile behavior, vivid imagination, and lying. Implied in this concept were certain psychodynamics that were thought to form the basis for this behavior (Marmor, 1953). Because individuals with hysterical personalities were unusually dramatic and suggestible, it was thought that they were highly susceptible to developing conversion symptoms. This concept was even carried to the point that only patients with hysterical personality were deemed able to develop conversion reactions.

With this history it is not surprising that the term "hysteria" has accrued so many different meanings as to be practically useless. It may be used to describe conversion symptoms, a personality style, or as a euphemistic term for malingering. When psychiatrists use the term, they often are referring to a cognitive style characterized by global and impressionistic thinking (Shapiro, 1965). In the final analysis, this term always seems to denote the frustration of the physician and a desire on the physician's part to be rid of the patient or to have the patient transferred to the care of a psychiatrist.

This chapter describes the current understanding and classification of the multiple syndromes often classed together under the rubric "hysteria." Where possible the term "hysteria" will be avoided and replaced by more specific terms. Although it seems somewhat silly to us today, the notion still persists that hysteria is primarily a disorder of women, and it is not uncommon for hysterectomies to be performed in an attempt to cure it. To help counteract this stereotype, references in this chapter can apply to male patients. Also included are the diagnostic criteria for each category as set forth in the *DSM-III* (1980). Although this new method provides a reliable method for diagnosing the different syndromes previously grouped together under the "hysteria" label, it remains to be determined whether the classifications actually represent clinically valid criteria. The syndromes formerly assigned to the label "hysteria" are:

1. Conversion disorder

2. Psychogenic pain disorder (psychalgia)

3. Histrionic personality

4. Somatization disorder (Briquet syndrome)

5. Hypochondriasis

6. Factitious illness (malingering or compensation neurosis)

RECOGNITION AND DIAGNOSIS

Conversion Disorder

Traditional Model. Since the early 1900s, several revisions have been made in the concept of conversion disorder as initially outlined by Freud and Breuer. To begin with, sexual repression is not the paramount issue today that it was in Vienna in the 1890s. It is now apparent that many emotions (other than anxiety related to sexual conflicts) can be converted into physical symptoms. For instance, guilt, anger, or depression can serve as a basis for conversion symptoms. Usually, the symptom develops in close temporal relationship with an emotionally charged event in the patient's life. For instance, a husband may develop paralysis of his arm following an argument with his wife. In this situation, anger is converted into the physical symptom of paralysis. Symbolically, the symptom expresses the forbidden impulse to hit his wife, yet at the same time prevents the husband from doing this. Traditionally it has been taught that conversion disorders involve the sensory or voluntary components of the nervous system. Typical examples include paralysis, decreased sensation, pain, deafness, blindness, and aphonia. However, vomiting also has been considered a classic conversion disorder and this phenomena clearly involves the ANS. Lending further complexity are recent studies with biofeedback techniques, demonstrating that the ANS may be under partial voluntary control (Miller, 1975). At the present time, it seems that conversion disorders usually involve the voluntary or perceptual components of the nervous system; however, occasional symptoms may also involve the "autonomic" component.

For many years it was also presumed that conversion disorders occurred only in individuals with hysterical personality and that only women had hysterical personalities—a rather simplistic and unjustified view. This notion was finally abandoned during World War II when it became evident that men could develop conversion disorders under the stress of combat. It is also apparent now that conversion disorders can occur in all categories of personality styles and in a variety of psychiatric conditions (Chodoff and Lyons, 1958).

Patients with conversion disorders traditionally were said to manifest "la belle indifference," meaning that they appear unconcerned about the impact or import of their symptoms. Unfortunately this has not held up as a basis for differentiating conversion disorders from other causes of physical symptoms. For instance, it is not uncommon for patients with multiple sclerosis or other neurologic conditions to deny or minimize the serious implications of their physical symptoms. Indeed, their denial is indistinguishable from "la belle indifference."

Social-Communication Model. The traditional concepts of conversion disorder have emphasized primary gain. By this is meant that physical symptoms relieve the anxiety associated with the underlying psychological conflict. More recently, emphasis has been placed on secondary gain as an important factor to consider in conversion disorders (Ziegler and Imboden, 1962). These authors have envisioned the physical symptom as metaphorically expressing psychological distress. The symptom is viewed as a language that negotiates interpersonal transactions, especially used by a powerless or dependent person who cannot cope with other individuals or a stressful situation. It is an enactment of a social role whereby the patient expresses psychological discomfort of unacceptable feelings through a more socially accepted organic symptom. It is obviously much easier to avoid a stressful situation as the result of a physical symptom than to admit openly that one is unable to cope with this difficult problem. Clearly, this model stresses observable social behavior rather than inferred notions about the patient's underlying psychological conflict.

The social-communication theory can be quite useful clinically since a patient's behavior may be apparent almost immediately, while determining the underlying psychological conflict may require a lengthy psychotherapeutic relationship. What must be carefully sorted out, however, is that *all illnesses have secondary gain and this fact is not synonymous with etiology.* An example may make this clear. A patient who undergoes amputation of his leg may feel that he is unable to work, that the government owes him a living, and that his wife must care for him. All of these factors represent secondary gain. Yet it is also evident that this is not the etiology of his amputation. The secondary gain may serve as a strong conflict of interest to his psychosocial rehabilitation and may have to be resolved in psychotherapy; however, it certainly does not imply that his amputation is not real.

Although Freud speculated on the underlying mechanisms that may be responsible for conversion disorders, there has been little progress since then in deepening our understanding of this phenomenon. It has been suggested by Moldofsky and England (1975) that the brain stem may be responsible for altering sensory input from the periphery (for example, decreasing input for anesthesia and increasing it for hyperthesia). Others (Galin et al., 1977; Bishop

et al., 1978) have suggested that conversion disorders may be an expression of the right cerebral hemisphere, which in most individuals does not contain language skills. This theory presumes that conflicts that arise in the right hemisphere cannot be expressed through language but rather through nonverbal somatic communication. Despite these sophisticated theories, it may be that conversion disorders are nothing more than physical symptoms that occur when the affect has been dissociated from our awareness—much as a scowl might occur in somebody who is obviously angry to others yet is unaware of this anger himself.

Certainly, the most important factor in the differential diagnosis is whether the patient has a conversion disorder or a physical illness. Sometimes the diagnosis of conversion disorder can be made on the basis of the patient's symptoms not being compatible with human anatomy or physiology. The classic example is so-called glove anesthesia (anesthesia of the hand that ends at the wrist). Most of the time, however, conversion disorders are *diagnosed* after extensive and repeated medical evaluations have failed to provide an explanation for a patient's symptoms. Unfortunately, psychological testing has not proved useful in separating patients with conversion disorders from those with physical illnesses (Lair and Trapp, 1962). Even more complex are patients with a *combined* physical problem and a conversion disorder. For instance, it is not unheard of for patients with a real seizure disorder to also have "hysterical seizures." Sorting out the various causes of the patient's seizures and treating them represents a real challenge to the clinician.

What is more worrisome are hints in the literature that a certain number of patients who are given the diagnosis of conversion disorder are in fact suffering from the early (and presumably undiagnosable) stages of a physical illness. Slater and Glithero (1965) completed a 7–11-year follow-up study of 85 patients given the diagnosis of conversion disorder or hysterical (histrionic) personality. Some 60% of these patients went on to develop neurologic illnesses. In the final analysis only 7 patients had a conversion disorder and 14 had histrionic personalities. In another study, Watson and Buranen (1979) found that after a decade, 10 of 36 patients diagnosed as having conversion disorders had gone on to develop physical problems. This represented a 28% false-positive rate for the diagnosis of conversion disorder. The most common physical illnesses to be misinterpreted as conversion disorders were degenerative diseases and structural failures affecting the spinal and peripheral nerves, bones, muscles, and connective tissues. Table 13–1 gives the *DSM-III* criteria for diagnosing a conversion disorder.

Psychogenic Pain Disorder

In many ways the category for psychogenic pain disorder or psychalgia represents a variant of the issues involved in conversion disorders. Here, pain without adequate physical explanation is the cardinal feature. The major problem for physicians is that they have no means for reliably verifying the patient's report of pain (Szasz, 1957). Usually, psychological features are inferred to be important because of the close temporal relationship between the onset of pain and the occurrence of an emotionally laden event in the patient's life.

It must be remembered that pain has a number of psychosocial meanings, in addition to signaling tissue damage. For instance, it may be associated with being either comforted or punished by a loved one. In certain individuals pain may act as a substitute for the suffering associated with loss. Many of these issues are well illustrated in Engel's (1959) description of the "pain-prone patient." Typically these patients had parents who were abusive and made the patient feel humiliated and defeated. Clearly, being treated in this way as a child can lead to anger and resentment of one's parents. If subsequently one of the parents develops an illness,

the patient may feel guilty and responsible because of his hostile feelings toward that parent. The patient may go on to develop a chronic pain syndrome that serves to assuage guilt by punishing him for his hostile feelings. The location of the pain is usually determined by a

---

TABLE 13–1
Diagnostic criteria for conversion disorder

A.   The predominant disturbance is a loss of or alteration in physical functioning suggesting a physical disorder

B.   Psychological factors are judged to be etiologically involved in the symptom, as evidenced by one of the following:
  1.   There is a temporal relationship between an environmental stimulus that is apparently related to a psychological conflict or need and the initiation or exacerbation of symptom
  2.   The symptom enables the individual to avoid some activity that is noxious to him or her
  3.   The symptom enables the individual to get support from the environment that otherwise might not be forthcoming

C.   It has been determined that the symptom is *not* under voluntary control

D.   The symptom cannot, after appropriate investigation, be explained by a known physical disorder or pathophysiological mechanism

E.   The symptom is not limited to pain or to a disturbance in sexual functioning

F.   Not due to somatization disorder or schizophrenia

From American Psychiatric Association. 1980. *Diagnostic and statistical manual of mental disorders*, 3rd ed., p 247. Washington, D.C.: American Psychiatric Association. Reprinted with permission from the American Psychiatric Association.

previous painful lesion suffered by the patient or by the location of the parent's disease. In the latter instance the pain may only be imagined or wished for by the patient. For example, if a patient's abusive father dies of abdominal cancer, it would not be unheard of for the son to develop abdominal pain. Under Engel's hypothesis this would be viewed as a means for the son to resolve his ambivalent feelings over the loss of his father. The pain represents both an indentification with his father and punishment for any of the negative feelings he may have harbored towards him.

Alternatively, a psychogenic pain disorder can occur when secondary gain plays a prominent role. A common scenario is for a patient to develop a painful physical disorder or injury. As with all illnesses, secondary gain ensues and serves to perpetuate the pain syndrome long after the physical disorder has resolved.

In interviewing patients with chronic pain syndrome it is important to explore their life histories, the events at the time the pain began, and the meaning the pain has for each patient. Usually, the more complex the patient's description and explanation for the pain, the greater the psychological component to his pain syndrome. Important questions to ask the patient are: What do you think is causing the pain? Have you had this pain before? Have you known anyone else with this pain? and even, Do you deserve to have this pain?

Dramatic presentations of pain may represent the patient's style (see the next section on histrionic personality) and should not automatically be used as evidence that the patient is suffering from a psychogenic pain disorder. *Placebos* must be used cautiously, if at all, in patients with chronic pain and *cannot* be used to differentiate "real pain" from psychogenic pain. For instance, it is not uncommon for individuals with painful peripheral lesions to respond to placebos, while those with a major psychogenic component to their pain to be unresponsive to placebos. The other critical issue to be aware of is the relationship between chronic pain and depression. It is not hard to understand that chronic pain easily can lead to irritability, discouragement, and depression. However, it is less appreciated that primary depression may have as one of its central features the somatic complaint of pain. Regardless of what comes first, a vicious cycle of ever-increasing pain and depression can quickly develop. Table 13–2 gives the *DSM-III* criteria for diagnosing psychalgia.

Histrionic Personality

Because of its historical development it is not surprising that the histrionic personality style (formerly called hysterical personality) represents an exaggeration of the traditional stereotype of women. It is now apparent, however, that this personality style can occur in either men or women and that such individuals are not uniquely predisposed to developing conversion disorders. In 1958, Chodoff and Lyons reformulated the hysterical personality to include such characteristics as egoism, vanity, exhibitionism, dramatization, labile affects, emotional shallowness, sexualization of nonsexual relationships, and sexual unresponsiveness. They emphasized *observable* behavior rather than tying such behavior to underlying psychodynamics.

Individuals with this disorder are overly dramatic and exhibitionistic. They draw attention to themselves by excessive expressions of emotion. Initially they are usually perceived as warm and charming with the ability to form friendships easily. Where they run into trouble is in sustaining relationships. Their initial charm quickly dissolves into vain and demanding behavior. They are seen as egocentric and inconsiderate of the feelings or wishes of others. In addition, they may be "helpless" or extremely dependent on their friends. It is not uncommon for histrionic patients to experience dysphoric moods in response to the many difficulties in their interpersonal relationships.

Recent work (Celani, 1976) has emphasized that this personality style may function as a way to communicate and negotiate in social and interpersonal situations. For instance, it may be a way for a weak and helpless individual to maintain another person's interest and limit that person's aggressiveness toward the weaker individual. Table 13–3 shows diagnostic criteria for histrionic personality disorder.

Somatization Disorder

Somatization disorder, or Briquet's syndrome, may actually represent a subcategory of the histrionic personality style just described. The

---

TABLE 13–2
Diagnostic criteria for psychogenic pain disorder

A. Severe and prolonged pain is the predominant disturbance

B. The pain presented as a symptom is inconsistent with the anatomic distribution of the nervous system; after extensive evaluation, no organic pathology or pathophysiological mechanism can be found to account for the pain; or, when there is some related organic pathology, the complaint of pain is grossly in excess of what would be expected from the physical findings

C. Psychological factors are judged to be etiologically involved in the pain, as evidenced by at least one of the following:
1. A temporal relationship between an environmental stimulus that is apparently related to a psychological conflict or need and the initiation or exacerbation of the pain
2. The pain enables the individual to avoid some activity that is noxious to him or her
3. The pain enables the individual to get support from the environment that otherwise might not be forthcoming

D. Not due to another mental disorder

From American Psychiatric Association. 1980. *Diagnostic and statistical manual of mental disorders*, 3rd ed., p. 249. Washington, D.C.: American Psychiatric Association. Reprinted with permission from the American Psychiatric Association.

TABLE 13–3
Diagnostic criteria for histrionic personality disorder

The following are characteristic of the individual's current and long-term functioning, are not limited to episodes of illness, and cause either significant impairment in social or occupational functioning or subjective distress.

A. Behavior that is overly dramatic, reactive, and intensely expressed, as indicated by at least three of the following:
1. Self-dramatization, for example, exaggerated expression of emotions
2. Incessant drawing of attention to oneself
3. Craving for activity and excitement
4. Overreaction to minor events
5. Irrational, angry outbursts, or tantrums

B. Characteristic disturbances in interpersonal relationships as indicated by at least two of the following:
1. Perceived by others as shallow and lacking genuineness, even if superficially warm and charming
2. Egocentric, self-indulgent, and inconsiderate of others
3. Vain and demanding
4. Dependent, helpless, constantly seeking reassurance
5. Prone to manipulative suicidal threats, gestures, or attempts

From American Psychiatric Association. 1980. *Diagnostic and statistical manual of mental disorders*, 3rd ed., p. 315. Washington, D.C.: American Psychiatric Association. Reprinted with permission from the American Psychiatric Association.

term is used to describe polysymptomatic individuals who seek medical attention (Purtell et al., 1951; Woodruff et al., 1971). Usually the syndrome has its onset before age 35 years and often before age 20 years. Frequent complaints include fatigue, headaches, nausea and vomiting, fainting, palpitations, allergies, or menstrual difficulties. For the diagnosis to be made the symptoms must have sufficient intensity for the patient to alter his life style, seek medical attention, or take medication other than aspirin. Often such patients reveal complicated medical histories or give vague statements such as "I have been sick all my life," or "I am feeling sore all over." They usually have a long-standing pattern of seeking help from physicians, and it is not uncommon for these patients to have a number of hospitalizations or even surgical procedures (especially hysterectomies) in an effort to diagnose and treat their symptoms. They may also have become dependent on antianxiety agents, sedatives, or analgesics that they have received on their many trips to the doctor. See Table 13–4 for diagnostic criteria.

TABLE 13–4
Diagnostic criteria for
somatization disorder

A. A history of physical symptoms of several years' duration beginning before the age of 30.

B. Complaints of at least 14 symptoms for women and 12 for men, from the 37 symptoms listed below. To count a symptom as present the individual must report that the symptom caused him or her to take medicine (other than aspirin), alter his or her life pattern, or see a physician. The symptoms, in the judgment of the clinician, are not adequately explained by physical disorder or physical injury, and are not side effects of medication, drugs, or alcohol. The clinician need not be convinced that the symptom was actually present, for example, that the individual actually vomited throughout her entire pregnancy; report of the symptom by the individual is sufficient.
1. Sickly: Believes that he or she has been sickly for a good part of his or her life
2. Conversion or pseudoneurologic symptoms: Difficulty swallowing, loss of voice, deafness, double vision, blurred vision, blindness, fainting or loss of consciousness, memory loss, seizures or convulsions, trouble walking, paralysis or muscle weakness, urinary retention or difficulty urinating
3. Gastrointestinal symptoms: Abdominal pain, nausea, vomiting spells (other than during pregnancy), bloating (gassy), intolerance (for example, gets sick) of a variety of foods, diarrhea
4. Female reproductive symptoms: Judged by the individual as occurring more frequently or severely than in most women: painful menstruation, menstrual irregularity, excessive bleeding, severe vomiting throughout pregnancy or causing hospitalization during pregnancy
5. Psychosexual symptoms: For the major part of the individual's life after opportunities for sexual activity: sexual indifference, lack of pleasure during intercourse, pain during intercourse
6. Pain: Pain in back, joints, extremities, genital area (other than during intercourse); pain during urination; other pain (other than headaches)
7. Cardiopulmonary symptoms: Shortness of breath, palpitations, chest pain, dizziness

From American Psychiatric Association. 1980. *Diagnostic and statistical manual of mental disorders*, 3rd ed., pp. 243–244. Washington, D.C.: American Psychiatric Association. Reprinted with permission from the American Psychiatric Association.

Hypochondriasis

Hypochondriasis as a diagnostic category can probably best be thought of as a variant of somatization disorder discussed previously. In this category are patients who have only a few somatic complaints (that is, not in enough *DSM-III* diagnostic categories to qualify for the diagnosis of somatization disorder) or the symptoms are not of sufficient intensity for them to alter their life style or take medication. Another example of hypochondriasis is a patient who is worried that he might have ulcerative colitis and seeks diagnostic evaluation with every gastrointestinal symptom he develops. This situation must be distinguished from the delusional patient, who is *convinced* he has ulcerative colitis and thinks his physician is incompetent when he fails to make the diagnosis.

Mechanic (1972) feels that hypochondriasis represents a process whereby individuals with low self-esteem and feelings of vulnerability wrongly attribute somatic sensations as representing physical illness. As with the social-communication model of conversion disorders, multiple somatic complaints are viewed as a means of expressing psychological distress. Seeking medical attention for these somatic sensations may be related to the patient's culture, family tradition, degree of psychological stress, and social supports. For example, a lonely individual who is under stress may visit a medical facility with vague somatic complaints, especially if the individual comes from a culture and family that lacks a vocabulary or behavior for directly expressing psychologic discomfort. See Table 13–5 for the criteria for diagnosing hypochondriasis.

It is not hard to see that there are a number of common elements in the diagnostic categories of histrionic personality, somatization disorder, and hypochondriasis. All three categories emphasize behavior rather than psychodynamics or psychological conflicts. Although histrionic personality emphasizes dramatic behavior and somatization disorder and hypochondriasis emphasize complaining about somatic symptoms, diagnostic confusion might result if a patient presents with dramatic complaints of somatic symptoms.

Despite the potential for diagnostic confusion, all three types of patients present the same problems for physicians. First, they present their symptoms in such a fashion that it is difficult for the physician to find them credible. This can lead to a vicious cycle in which the physician doubts that the symptoms result from "real" medical problems, resulting in the patient escalating his complaints and dramatic behavior, which in turn makes the physician even more certain that the symptoms are not the result of

---

TABLE 13–5
Diagnostic criteria for hypochondriasis

A. The predominant disturbance is an unrealistic interpretation of physical signs or sensations as abnormal, leading to preoccupation with the fear or belief of having a serious disease

B. Thorough physical evaluation does not support the diagnosis of any physical disorder that can account for the physical signs or sensations or for the individual's unrealistic interpretation of them

C. The unrealistic fear or belief of having a disease persists despite medical reassurance and causes impairment in social or occupational functioning

D. Not due to any other mental disorder such as schizophrenia, affective disorder, or somatization disorder

From American Psychiatric Association. 1980. *Diagnostic and statistical manual of mental disorders*, 3rd ed., p. 251. Washington, D.C.: American Psychiatric Association. Reprinted with permission by the American Psychiatric Association.

organic illness. In addition, these patients use physical symptoms as a means of establishing a supportive relationship with a physician. For the patient, continuation of the relationship requires that the complaints of physical problems must continue. This can be quite frustrating to the physician, who is attempting to diagnose and cure these symptoms. Not uncommonly, these opposing desires result in friction between the patient and physician, with the physician getting angry and rejecting the patient or referring the patient to a psychiatrist.

Factitious Illness

The critical issue that distinguishes factitious illness from the previously discussed diagnostic categories is that here the patient's behavior is under voluntary control. Typical examples include factitious infections or fever (Aduan et al., 1979). The most dramatic form of this illness is chronic factitious illness, more popularly known as Munchausen's syndrome.

Baron Hieronymus Karl Friedrich von Munchausen was a real person who wandered from city to city in Europe in the 1700s telling grand tales of adventure. Rudolph Erich Raspe popularized this character by publishing a volume purporting to describe Baron von Munchausen's fairy-tale life. The label has been appropriated for a group of patients who wander from hospital to hospital, telling fantastic stories about their medical problems. Variants of this syndrome have been called "laparotomaphilia migrans, hemorrhagica histrionica, neurologica diabolica, dermatitis autogenica, and hyperpyrexia figmentatica" (Asher, 1951; Spiro, 1968).

As the colorful nomenclature suggests, these patients have a dramatic flare. At times they cooperate in their evaluation and treatment, often submitting to invasive procedures for the sake of maintaining their role as a patient. However, at the same time they usually exhibit aggressive, hostile, or evasive behavior. Since they are quite familiar with hospital routines, it is easy for them to be demanding of the staff or noncompliant with hospital schedules and regulations. If evaluation of one set of symptoms proves to have negative results, they may develop a whole new set of problems. Seeking analgesics or antianxiety agents is another ploy. If not suspected of fabrication early in their hospitalization, their continued disruptive behavior usually arouses the suspicion of the medical staff. When confronted about their multiple hospitalizations and factitious medical history they usually become indignant and end the episode by signing out of the hospital against medical advice.

Munchausen's syndrome can occur in both men and women. Because it is extremely difficult to engage these individuals in any sort of an ongoing relationship the natural history of the disorder is poorly understood. There are reports documenting that the syndrome may last for years and the assumption of the patient role is so consuming as to disrupt family ties and make them unable to hold a job. The etiology or underlying psychodynamics of these patients are not clearly delineated. Certain authors emphasize the dramatic nature of this syndrome and believe that a desire to be the center of attention is the basis for this behavior. Others believe that a sadomasochistic relationship with physicians is the primary cause, and view this as a reenactment of the patient's relationships with parents. Common elements in many of these patients are a history of maternal deprivation and hospitalization early in life for a real medical illness. For instance, it is not hard to imagine that spending a year in the hospital for rheumatic fever can involve a great deal of anxiety for an 8-year-old child. Just a few of the issues that this young patient must cope with are separation from parents, anxiety over health, and fear of hospital procedures. The impostership of the patient role as an adult is viewed as an attempt to relive and master this early traumatic event (Spiro, 1968; Cramer et al., 1971). See Table 13–6 for diagnostic criteria for chronic factitious disorder with physical symptoms.

Malingering

When psychiatrists are asked to see a patient with "hysteria," it often means that the referring physician feels the patient is consciously and actively simulating medical illness for the purpose of achieving some goal. An example is an individual who actively simulates illness to gain access to a hospital because it provides food and shelter. Malingering is a type of factitious illness in that the patient voluntarily simulates or induces physical signs or symptoms and seeks medical attention for them. By definition malingering means simulating a physical symptom with the purpose of achieving a specific and immediately apparent goal. To most people, malingering usually has a negative connotation; that is, patients should not seek medical attention or be hospitalized for the treatment of these signs or symptoms, since it is a waste of socioeconomic resources and staff time. However, there are times when malingering may be adaptive. For instance, in times of war malingering in the face of harsh circumstances may allow the individual to survive a situation that he would otherwise not survive. Another example in which value judgment is very difficult concerns patients who use the hospital as a haven from difficult psychosocial situations. For instance, a single parent who is caring for a chronically ill child may on occasion complain of physical symptoms that require hospitalization for assessment and treatment. In some patients this may represent a conscious simulation of medical illness with the purpose of gaining some temporary relief from a difficult and taxing home situation. The situation may not become clear until there is a recurring pattern of hospitalization and negative diagnostic evaluations.

In summary, malingering has a social value judgment associated with it in that either the physician or the psychiatrist must make a judgment as to whether this simulation of physical signs or symptoms is adaptive or maladaptive (Szasz, 1961). The distinction between malingering and Munchausen's syndrome rests in the nature of the patient's goals. In malingering the goals are specific and usually time-limited, while in Munchausen's syndrome the goal is the lifelong pursuit of the patient role.

Compensation Neurosis

One issue that may closely resemble malingering is the hope for financial compensation for physical disability. This factor has been best studied in the industrial sector where on-the-job accidents may lead to prolonged disability even in the absence of physical findings. Nonet (1969) has described how the workman's compensation system evolved from its initial humanitarian intent (that is, protecting the worker from loss of income as the result of an industrial accident) into a complex administrative-legal system. Quite often the process is adversary in nature with the degree of disability and amount of compensation being contended. Clearly, many compensation or disability claims are justified

---

TABLE 13–6
Diagnostic criteria for chronic factitious disorder with physical symptoms

A. Plausible presentation of physical symptoms that are apparently under the individual's voluntary control to such a degree that there are multiple hospitalizations

B. The individual's goal is apparently to assume the "patient" role and is not otherwise understandable in light of the individual's environmental circumstances (as is the case in malingering)

From American Psychiatric Association. 1980. *Diagnostic and statistical manual of mental disorders*, 3rd ed., p. 290. Washington, D.C.: American Psychiatric Association. Reprinted with permission from the American Psychiatric Association.

on the basis of the individual's injury, personal suffering, and impaired ability to work. However, psychosocial issues may also play a role in these cases.

Brodsky (1978) summarizes some common issues involved in compensation cases. Premorbidly these patients are usually uneducated and unskilled laborers, who are finding it more difficult to compete in the labor market because of advancing age. They may be depressed, angry, or litigious, and often they feel exploited by their employer. Following an industrial accident, recovery is delayed if the injury is the result of an obvious safety hazard or a willful act. If the accident occurred at a time when the worker was in conflict with boss, fellow workers, or family, then a prolonged recovery is more likely. Similarly, if the patient's fellow workers or family are unsympathetic then the patient is more likely to extend the convalescent period to justify the extent of the injury.

Critical points for the patient in the recovery phase are contacts with physicians and the insurance company. Delays in being treated give the patient the ready-made and difficult to counter argument that, "If I had been treated earlier I wouldn't be disabled." Crisis may occur when the physician accuses the patient of abusing narcotic analgesics or tranquilizers or declares the person fit to return to work. In this regard, the medical opinion of company physicians are trusted less by the patient than the opinion of his own physician. In addition, the patient and the insurance company usually distrust one another. As a result the patient contacts a lawyer and the subsequent litigation greatly extends the period of disability.

Psychiatric referral often occurs at the end of this complex process. In evaluating these patients it is important to assess their adaptation to their disabled status. Some may lead quietly desperate lives while others may pursue hobbies or volunteer activities, and still others may use it as a period of transition in terms of developing new skills or changing their occupation. Some use the period of psychotherapy to prolong recovery and further their disability claims.

MANAGEMENT AND REFERRAL

Two basic errors are possible in managing patients with "hysteria" (Lewis, 1974). One is failure to *identify* symptoms, signs, or behavior as representing one of the syndromes described previously. Overly zealous diagnostic and therapeutic endeavors may result in considerable risk and expense to the patient and also prevent or delay more appropriate therapies. The second mistake is *labeling* patients as "hysterical" when in fact they are suffering from another illness. The problems arising from this mistake are legion. Multiple sclerosis, SLE, seizure disorders, and degenerative diseases of the CNS may be especially puzzling to diagnose because the somatic symptoms, along with the associated emotional symptoms, may be attributed to an underlying psychiatric condition. In these situations, primary treatment should be directed towards the medical condition. Occasionally, it may also be necessary to treat the psychiatric symptoms as well. Patients with schizophrenia may also present with perplexing somatic complaints that are confusing until the proper diagnosis is made.

Although it may sound absurd, making a proper diagnosis of one of the disorders just discussed does not convey immunity to other diseases or death. Patients with conversion disorders, histrionic personalities, malingering, and so on do sometimes develop very serious medical illnesses. Clearly, these patients require a vigilant primary physician, as well as close collaboration with a psychiatrist.

In view of the many different meanings of the diagnosis "hysteria," it is not surprising that there is very little reliable information about how to treat these multiple conditions. Discussed here are the current thoughts about how to treat conversion disorders, psychogenic pain, histrionic personality, somatization disorder, and hypochondriasis. It must be remembered that this information is not based on rigorous research but rather on clinical impression. Perhaps the new and more reliable diagnostic criteria of the *DSM-III* will allow therapeutic outcome studies to be done in the near future. For the conditions of factitious illness, malingering, and compensation neurosis, it is unclear whether any psychiatric treatment is effective. The major role of psychiatric consultation in these cases is to assist in evaluation and diagnosis.

Patients with a conversion disorder should be referred to a psychiatrist. Traditionally these patients are treated with psychoanalytically oriented psychotherapy, which is probably helpful whether the problem requires a resolution of a psychologic conflict or modification of the secondary gain associated with the physical symptom. On some occasions hypnosis or amobarbital (Amytal) interviews (that is, narcoanalysis) are helpful (Naples and Hackett, 1978; Spiegel and Spiegel, 1978). Hypnotherapy actually seems more helpful in controlling the pain from peripheral lesions than it does in curing patients with "psychogenic pain." The latter group seems to respond better to more traditional psychotherapy.

Individuals with somatic complaints as a result of having a histrionic personality, somatization disorder, or hypochondriasis require the same form of treatment. The major desire of these patients is to establish a supportive relationship with a physician. They usually will not comply with a referral to a psychiatrist, since they view this as the end of their relationship with the primary physician, as well as a de facto redefinition of their problems as psychological (the very idea they are defending against). The appropriate treatment of these patients is for the primary physician to form a supportive rela-

tionship with them. This can be managed by giving them regular but brief appointments. Trying to provide them with insight or trying to convince them to give up their symptoms is counterproductive, while sympathetically listening to their symptoms and conveying a sense that their suffering is being understood is critical. Not being forced or provoked into making a final diagnosis or into diagnostic procedures or therapeutic trials is equally important for such patients.

If by chance the patient does accept a referral to a psychiatrist, the therapeutic strategy is similar. The goal of psychotherapy is to form a supportive relationship with the patient. The unspoken message from the psychiatrist to the patient is, "I will see you regularly and be interested in you as a person, whether or not you have physical symptoms." The psychiatrist talks about whatever the patient has on his or her mind, whether it is physical symptoms or personal problems. In this context, patients begin to see that it is not necessary to talk about their physical problems in order to keep the psychiatrist's interest. Once this happens, they start discussing more pertinent problems with concomitant improvement in their personal lives.

SUMMARY

Hysteria has a long and complex history in medicine. It has developed so many different meanings that the word is now useless as a diagnostic entity. The *DSM-III* has developed more specific clinical entities to categorize the many different types of patients who have physical symptoms that defy medical diagnosis or treatment. It offers the first real chance for pursuing systematic research into the cause, natural history, and treatment of these fascinating patients.

APPENDIX: CASE HISTORY—THE APHONIC STUDENT

The PEG constructed at the time of initial interview essentially reveals no observable organic pathology or evidence of any major psychosocial stressors except for the move to start college. The psychiatric consultant tested the patient for the ability to be hypnotized and found her to be highly hypnotizable. During hypnosis, in deep relaxation, the patient was able to talk; initially her voice was hoarse, but it became progressively normal with further suggestions of relaxation. During this time, the patient gave the following additional history.

The patient developed a serious love relationship with a classmate shortly after arrival in college, but he broke up with the patient approximately a month ago because he feared the intensity of their relationship. She was very saddened by this event and found that she had difficulty in concentrating on school work. The night before the onset of the aphonia, while speaking with her mother on the telephone, she learned that her brother had just become engaged to a classmate. She narrated this additional history with a considerable amount of sadness, envy, and anger. During hypnosis the patient was told that she would remember as much as she wanted to of the hypnotic session and she would be able to speak as much as she was ready to do so. Following termination of hypnosis, she remembered everything that happened and was able to speak without difficulty. The patient agreed to see the psychiatrist for outpatient therapy. A diagnosis of conversion disorder was made.

PATIENT EVALUATION GRID			
	CONTEXTS		
DIMENSIONS	**CURRENT** (Current States)	**RECENT** (Recent Events and Changes)	**BACKGROUND** (Culture, Traits, Constitution)
BIOLOGICAL	Physical examination, ENT examination, routine laboratory tests all <u>normal</u> <u>except for aphonia</u>	<u>Stopped birth control</u> <u>pills</u>—1 wk ago <u>No medications or</u> <u>drugs</u>	<u>Frequent sore throats</u> <u>as a child</u>
PERSONAL	<u>Total aphonia</u>—6 hr Patient <u>can write well</u> Mental status exam: (through written communication) all within <u>normal</u> limits; patient somewhat anxious	<u>Sleeping more than</u> <u>usual</u>—2–3 wk <u>somewhat increased</u> <u>appetite</u>—2–3 wk <u>Denied any change in</u> <u>mood</u>	<u>Bright, outgoing,</u> "organized" person who tends to <u>suppress feelings</u>
ENVIRONMENTAL	Parents in another state Lives in <u>college dorm</u> <u>Close, supportive</u> <u>friends</u> One brother in graduate school in another state	<u>Started college</u>—4 mo ago Move to come to college from a distant state	Middle-class, Protestant background One brother, 4 yr older
Demographic data: 19-year-old single, female, college student.			

RECOMMENDED READINGS

Bean, W.B. 1959. The Munchausen syndrome, *Perspect. Biol. Med.* 347–53. This is a wonderful poem describing Munchausen syndrome.

Breuer, J., and Freud, S. 1955. *Studies on hysteria* (1895). Complete Psychological Works of Freud. London: Hogarth Press. This presents the classic description of patients with hysteria and their treatment by Freud.

Hyler, S.E., and Spitzer, R.L. 1978 Hysteria split asunder. *Am. J. Psychiatry* 135:1500–04. This article presents a summary of the new diagnostic criteria of the traditional hysterical disorders.

Veith, I. 1965. *Hysteria: The history of a disease.* Chicago: University of Chicago Press. This scholarly book presents a history of the multiple concepts of hysteria.

REFERENCES

Aduan, R.P.; Fauci, A.S; Dale, D.C., et al. 1979 Factitious fever and self-induced infection. *Ann Int. Med.* 90:230–42.

American Psychiatric Association. 1980. *Diagnostic and statistical manual of mental disorders*, 3rd ed. Washington, D.C.: American Psychiatric Association.

Asher, R. 1951. Munchausen's syndrome. *Lancet* 1:339–41.

Bishop, E.R.; Mobley, M.C.; and Farr, W.F. 1978. Lateralization of conversion symptoms. *Compr. Psychiatry* 19:393–96.

Breuer, J., and Freud, S. 1955. Studies on hysteria. *Complete psychological works of Freud*. London: Hogarth Press.

Brodsky, C.M. 1978. The genesis of a problem population. In *Communication and social interaction*, ed., P.F. Ostwald. New York: Grune & Stratton.

Celani, D. 1976. An interpersonal approach to hysteria. *Am. J. Psychiatry* 133:1414–18.

Chodoff, P., and Lyons, H. 1958. Hysteria, the hysterical personality and "hysterical" conversion. *Am. J. Psychiatry* 114:734–40.

Cramer, B.; Gershberg, M.R.; and Stern, M. 1971. Munchausen syndrome—its relationship to malingering, hysteria, and the physician-patient relationship. *Arch. Gen. Psychiatry* 24:573–78.

Engel, G.L. 1959. "Psychogenic" pain and the pain-prone patient. *Am. J. Med.* 899–918.

Galin, D.; Diamond, R.; and Braff, D. 1977. Lateralization of conversion symptoms: More frequent on the left. *Am. J. Psychiatry* 134:578–80.

Lair, C.V., and Trapp, P. 1962. The differential diagnostic value of the MMPI with somatically disturbed patients. *J. Clin. Psychol.* 18:146–47.

Lewis, W.C. 1974. Hysteria: The consultant's dilemma. *Arch. Gen. Psychiatry* 30:145–51.

Marmor, J. 1953. Orality in the hysterical personality. *J. Am. Psychoanal. Assoc.* 1:656–671.

Mechanic, D. 1972. Social psychologic factors affecting the presentation of bodily complaints. *N. Engl. J. Med.* 286:1132–39.

Miller, N.E. 1975. Applications of learning and biofeedback to psychiatry and medicine. In *Comprehensive textbook of psychiatry*, eds., A.M. Freedman; H.I. Kaplan; B.J. Sadock. Baltimore: Williams & Wilkins.

Moldofsky, A., and England, R.S. 1975. Facilitation of somatosensory average-evoked potentials in hysterical anesthesia and pain. *Arch. Gen. Psychiatry* 32:193–97.

Naples, M., and Hackett, T.P. 1978. The amytal interview: History and current uses. *Psychosomatics* 19:98–105.

Nonet, P. 1969. *Administrative justice*. New York: Russell Sage Foundation.

Purtell, J.J.; Robins, E.; and Cohen, M.E. 1951. Observations on clinical aspects of hysteria. J.A.M.A. 146:902–9.

Reich, W. 1972. *Character analysis*, 3rd ed., pp. 204–09. New York: Farrar, Strauss and Giroux.

Shapiro, D. 1965. *Neurotic styles*. New York: Basic Books.

Slater, J.E., and Glithero, E. 1965. A follow-up of patients diagnosed as suffering from hysteria. *J. Psychosom. Res.* 9:13.

Spiegel, H., and Spiegel, D. 1978. *Trance and treatment*. New York: Basic Books.

Spiro, H.R. 1968. Chronic factitious illness—Munchausen's syndrome. *Arch. Gen. Psychiatry* 18:569–79.

Szasz, T. 1957. *Pain and pleasure*. New York: Basic Books.

Szasz, T.S. 1961. *The myth of mental illness*. New York: Paul B. Hoeber.

Veith, I. 1965. *Hysteria: The history of a disease.* Chicago: University of Chicago Press.

Watson, C.G., and Buranen, C. 1979. The frequency and identification of false-positive conversion reactions. *J. Nerv. Ment. Dis.* 167:243–47.

Wittels, F. 1930. The hysterical character. *Medical Review* 36:186–90.

Woodruff, R.A.; Clayton, P.J.; and Guze, S.B. 1971. Hysteria: Studies of diagnosis, outcome and prevalence. *J.A.M.A.* 215:425–28.

Ziegler, F.J., and Imboden, J.B. 1962. Contemporary conversion reactions. *Arch. Gen. Psychiatry* 6:37–45.

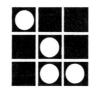

CHAPTER 14

Problems of Everyday Living

Vincenta Leigh, R.N., M.S.N.
Jane S. Sturges, M.S.W.

We discussed, in earlier chapters, the concepts of anxiety and depression, and how they may be associated with physical symptoms, signs, and diseases in interaction with constitutional vulnerabilities. Problems of everyday living, important factors in the recent context environmental dimension of the patient, are common stressors that may predispose an individual to illness. This chapter focuses on the recognition of stress and stress-related disorders in the medical setting. Chapters 1, 3, 9, 11, and 12 complement this chapter and should be referred to for detailed discussion of specific approaches and syndromes mentioned here.

The phrase, "problems of everyday living," refers to the emotional difficulties and problems experienced as a result of some stressful event. Usually the event is quite ordinary. The difficulty is sometimes called "situational disturbance" or "adjustment reaction" (*DSM-III*, 1980).

DIAGNOSIS

The three essential features of the situational disturbance syndrome according to the *DSM-III* are:

1. An identifiable stressor or life event

2. The reaction to which it occurs within 3 months, is maladaptive, and results in:
   a. A noticeable decrease in ability to function as usual at home, at work, with friends; or
   b. A reaction in excess of the normal, expected reaction to the stressor

3. The disturbance is brief and transient—when the stressor ceases, the disturbance is expected to clear.

RECOGNITION

Primary care physicians often come into contact with individuals experiencing "problems of everyday living." Case History 14–2 illustrates an example.

CASE HISTORY 14–1

A 40-year-old housewife came to her family physician complaining of lower back pain. She had a herniated lumbar disk some 20 years ago, it had been treated successfully without surgery, and she has been pain free for the last 18 years. Physical examination and laboratory tests were normal, including x-ray films of the spine. On further questioning, the patient admits experiencing anxiety and depression for the last 2 months, along with difficulty in falling asleep and occasional crying spells. She attributed these feelings to the recurrence of back pain after 18 years. (See the appendix at the end of this chapter for further discussion and PEG.)

CASE HISTORY 14–2

Mrs. B., a 46-year-old married female complains of dull headaches of 4 weeks' duration. The headaches, each lasting 5–6 hours, have been severe enough to require bed rest and are only slightly relieved by aspirin. Physical examination results were normal except for slightly elevated diastolic blood pressure. Subsequent laboratory tests did not indicate the presence of a serious medical disease. Closer examination revealed that the onset of the headaches coincided with the marriage of the last of her three sons.

A last child leaving home is only one of the many stressors that might cause an emotional upset of this kind. Some other stressors are retirement, getting married, starting school, or becoming a parent. Such stressors obviously may be related to a developmental phase in the patient's or the family's life, as in the case of Mrs. B., whose children are growing up and leaving home just as the parents are dealing with their own feelings about becoming middle-aged. The stressor may be a crisis, such as bereavement, loss of employment, unwanted pregnancy, trouble with the law, severe marital disputes or divorce, and a variety of other family and occupational upheavals. The stressor may be recurrent, as with seasonal business crises. It may be limited to the patient, as with the victim of a crime such as rape, or mugging, or perhaps, after the diagnosis of a serious physical illness has been made. Stress may occur in a family setting, as with discordant intrafamilial relationships. A group or community, in the case of persecution based on religious, racial, social, or other group characteristics, may be the setting for stress.

The emotional disturbance that occurs as a reaction to the stressor is marked by a noticeable change above and beyond the expected "normal" reaction to the stressor (*DSM-III*, 1980). This alteration may be evidenced by decreased productivity at work, or doing less "extras" or "goodies" for friends or family (as in the case of a woman who no longer bakes cookies for the family and does only the essential housework) and by decreased interest in other activities that used to provide pleasure. Coworkers, friends, or relatives may comment or express concern about this change or might even suggest seeing a doctor.

The presenting symptoms of this disorder are varied (*DSM-III*, 1980). They include:

- depressive or anxious feelings

- combination of mixed emotional features

- interpersonal and social withdrawal

- physical symptoms (as with the case of Mrs. B.)

- disturbances of conduct, such as assaultiveness, reckless driving, excessive drinking, or other defaulting of legal responsibilities

- disturbances of conduct mixed with disturbances of emotions

The onset and remission of symptoms may be immediate or delayed, and either sudden or gradual. They must, however, have a chronologic relationship with some stressor. Thus, the condition is expected to remit, and the behavior and functioning to resume normal levels, when the stressor ceases.

The primary causative factor of the emotional disturbance or "distress" then, is the stressor (life event) or stressors. Holmes and Rahe (1967) attempted to quantify the stressfulness of frequently encountered life events. They gave death of spouse the highest score of 100 and marriage 50 on the basis of studies on large populations (see Table 14–1). The severity of the disturbance, however, is only in part a function of the severity of the stressor, the number of stressors, and their nature and duration. On the opposite pole, the factors that tend to reduce the strain caused by the stress include a person's available resources (Warheit, 1979). Such mitigating factors are:

1. Personal characteristics—constitution, genetic predispositions, and the individual's personality style, the way the person tends to react, especially in the face of problems

2. Social environment—private wealth, socioeconomic resources, social support, family support, both nuclear and extended, interpersonal networks (a friend whom he or she can call on), and secondary organizations (professional agency, clinic, and so on)

3. Culture—belief systems, values, group norms, and symbolic meanings and definitions attached to events

TABLE 14–1
Life change events

DIMENSION	EVENT	LCU VALUES
Family:	Death of spouse	100
	Divorce	73
	Marital separation	65
	Death of close family member	63
	Marriage	50
	Marital reconciliation	45
	Major change in health of family	44
	Pregnancy	40
	Addition of new family member	39
	Major change in arguments with wife	35
	Son or daughter leaving home	29
	In-law troubles	29
	Wife starting or ending work	26
	Major change in family get-togethers	15
Personal:	Detention in jail	63
	Major personal injury or illness	53
	Sexual difficulties	39
	Death of a close friend	37
	Outstanding personal achievement	28
	Start or end of formal schooling	26
	Major change in living conditions	25
	Major revision of personal habits	24
	Changing to a new school	20
	Change in residence	20
	Major change in recreation	19
	Major change in church activities	19
	Major change in social activities	18
	Major change in sleeping habits	16
	Major change in eating habits	15
	Vacation	13
	Christmas	12
	Minor violations of the law	11
Work:	Being fired from work	47
	Retirement from work	45
	Major business adjustment	39
	Changing to different line of work	36
	Major change in work responsibilities	29
	Trouble with boss	23
	Major change in working conditions	20
Financial:	Major change in financial state	38
	Mortgage or loan over $10,000	31
	Mortgage foreclosure	30
	Mortgage or loan less than $10,000	17

*The life change units are weighted according to the disruption each causes. (From Gunderson, E.K., and Rahe, R.H. eds., *Life stress and Illness*, Springfield, Ill: Charles C Thomas, Chapter 4. pp. 60–61.) Reprinted with permission.

Thus, the degree of emotional disturbance in the face of stress is a complex function of numerous interacting factors.

When confronted with a stressful life event, the individual tends to rely on existing resources in his or her psychological, physical, and genetic makeup. If this proves insufficient, the person usually seeks to extend resources of support, calling for assistance from spouse, children, parents, or other family members. If they are unavailable or inadequate, the individual often turns to interpersonal networks, that is, to friends whom he or she can trust and go to for help. When even friends fail to provide enough support, the next step customarily involves seeking assistance from professional persons (physicians), agencies (clinics), or turning to culturally provided assistance—beliefs, values, and symbols (Warheit, 1979).

It is not unusual, then, that large numbers of patients with problems of everyday living come to the medical care system, a source of professional assistance, in an attempt to meet the demands of a life event and restore their usual sense of well-being (McWhinney, 1972; Mechanic, 1978). The patient may initiate contact with a physician for the relief of physical symptoms which may be minor, of long duration, or vague and unexplained. In addition to illness behavior and utilization of medical services, recent life events also appear to be associated with medical illness, coronary disease, psychiatric distress, and possible death, (Gunderson and Rahe, 1974; Mechanic, 1978; Rahe and Arthur, 1978).

Practical Suggestions for Identifying Patients

Although life events and stressful situations are common to most people, individuals differ in how they respond to those stressors and events. Data about stress-producing life events will aid the physician, not only in identifying patients who have a direct dysfunction as the result of some life event or have problems of everyday living, but also, in shaping future treatment plans based on a patient's anticipated response to major events, like surgery. In addition, the presence of certain life events may alert the physician to possible increased risk of morbidity, or susceptibility to illness. Therefore, it is helpful to routinely gather relevant information on all patients. The following questions might be asked during the course of the history-taking to ascertain recent life events and major changes: How have things been going? What has happened since the last time I saw you? How's the family? How is your job going? How do you spend your free time? Have you been busy lately? Or, one might simply ask, if appropriate: Why are you so nervous? You seem depressed, blue—are you? You don't seem your usual self; how come? Has anything been going on that might have contributed, caused, triggered this apparent change in your mood?

The nurse is in an ideal position to gather invaluable diagnostic data concerning a patient's major changes or recent life events. At times, patients confide information or minor problems to a nurse that they would be reluctant to tell a doctor. Nurses usually have developed a rapport with the patients and their families, and their proximity to the waiting room helps too. Once this information is communicated, the primary physician can then explore, in depth, the effects of this event.

After identifying the stressor(s), the physician can evaluate the reaction to the stressor, and the usual everyday functioning of the patient. He or she may consider questions such as, because of the distress, is there a change in functioning? Is it maladaptive—has the usual functioning been disrupted? Is the person less productive than usual? In establishing the chronology of life events and their reactions, one should consider whether the change in functioning and symptoms occur after or soon after the life event.

After ascertaining that there is a problem and that it is related to a life event, the physician should determine the severity. This will give clues for treatment. The physician decides at this point which resources can be mobilized to assist the individual to adjust and meet the demands of the stress-producing life event. He or she must also decide whether the patient's day-to-day functioning is severely impaired. If the patient is so disturbed as to raise the question of psychosis or a depressive syndrome (see Chapters 8 and 9), referral to a psychiatrist is indicated. If the disturbance is noticeable but not of such severity to warrant the diagnosis of psychosis or depressive syndrome then the diagnosis of *situational disturbance* (or problems of everyday living) may be made.

MANAGEMENT

The primary physician may decide to help the patient with the emotional disturbance related to the problems of everyday living or may refer the patient to a mental health professional. This decision to manage the patient depends on many interrelated factors, including time available, physician's training and experience, current and past relationship with the patient and the family, severity of the problem and symptoms of the patient, patient's and family's preference and motivation, and availability of mental health professionals in the community.

The goals of management of the patient by the physician are to prevent the patient's symptoms from becoming worse and to assist the patient to return to a prestress level of functioning as quickly as possible. This would include:

- Elimination of the stressor when possible. For example, if the problem is loss of employment, this means helping the patient with feelings about this and with ways of handling the situation, including free time, handling of money, consideration of career opportunities.

- Elimination of the physical and emotional symptoms, that is, the maladaptive reaction to the stressor when it is not possible to eliminate the stressor itself. For example, this means if the

problem is retirement, helping the patient with feelings about this and with ways of handling the adjustment, including consideration of substitute activities, such as a volunteer job, or hobbies, management of an adjusted income, and changes in family relationships related to retirement.

Ideally, a third goal in the management of the patient is the prevention of future maladaptive reactions to stress through learning new ways to handle problems of everyday living.

Techniques for achieving the goals vary according to the personalities and styles of the physician and the patient, the relationship between the physician and patient, and the nature of the problem and patient's reaction to it. Following are some techniques (Hansell, 1976; Schless and Mendels, 1978) that may be useful in helping the patient:

1. Empathic, nonjudgmental, thorough questioning about details of the patient's life

2. Education of the patient about symptoms as related to problems of living in a nonthreatening manner

3. Supportive comments such as letting the patient know that it is common for people to react to problems of everyday living with physical and emotional symptoms

4. Helping the patient to express his or her feelings and thoughts in order for patient and physician to understand what is going on

5. "Partialization" of the problem by determining with the patient which part of his or her life is proceeding smoothly and which part has the problem that is causing the stress

6. Encouraging the patient to look at the situation more objectively, to view it from different perspectives, and to consider various ways of handling it

7. Selecting with the patient concrete tasks that are capable of giving a sense of mastery

8. Time-limited psychotherapy, with specific, reasonable goals, and with a definite plan for follow-up appointments to assess progress.

9. Involving other family members for history-taking, assessment of the problem and the reaction, and participation in the solution

10. Hopeful, positive attitude on the part of the physician that the situation can improve with time and effort

REFERRAL

The physician may decide to refer the patient to a psychiatrist or a mental health professional such as a clinical psychologist, clinical (psychiatric) social worker, or psychiatric nurse-clinician. This decision depends on time available to the physician, amount of interest in managing the patient and the problem, degree of training and experience, symptoms that are too severe to be handled by the primary physician, or symptoms that persist in spite of management by the primary physician. When problems in living are causing symptoms in other family members, it indicates the need for a broader focus of treatment. The willingness and/or preference of the patient to see a psychiatrist or a mental health professional is another strong reason for referral.

The immediate goal of the primary physician in making a referral is to encourage and assist the patient in seeking psychological help, to assist the mental health professional to whom the patient is referred, and to continue to follow through on the outcome. The patient and/or family may feel very threatened by the referral, wondering if this means the patient is having a "nervous breakdown" and fearful of the outcome. This means a referral may itself require much time and energy on the part of the physician. Useful techniques to accomplish a smooth referral might include the nonthreatening explanation that physical and emotional symptoms are often related to everyday problems of living rather than to mysterious forces beyond the patient's control. The physician can encourage the patient that it is possible to help himself or herself with the aid of a physician or a mental health professional. Finally, there should be consideration with the patient of alternatives available, for example, psychiatrists, psychologists, clinical (psychiatric) social workers, psychiatric nurse-clinicans, or psychiatric clinics based on type of services needed and fees charged. Then the physician may provide names of qualified professionals.

If a referral is made, it is important to collaborate with the professional by offering medical backup for psychologist, clinical (psychiatric) social worker, or nurse-clinician through prescribing tranquilizers or antidepressant medication for a patient. The primary physician also assists psychiatrists or mental health professionals through providing information about patient's medical history, including medication history as is needed for treatment plan. In addition there should be a follow-up session with the patient and mental health professional to assess progress.

Whether the referral should be made to a psychiatrist, psychologist, clinical (psychiatric) social worker, or psychiatric nurse-clinician depends on the nature and severity of the problem, the physician's contacts with and knowledge of the work of mental health professionals in the community, as well as the preference of the patient (see Chapter 20).

Members of the mental health team specifically trained to deal with psychiatric problems are psychiatrists, clinical psychologists, clinical social workers, and nurse-clinicians. Others who may assist in the treatment include clergymen, school counselors, family agencies, the police, and friends. Referrals to trained individuals should be made according to the specialized help each is best equipped to render. As there is sometimes an overlap of services provided. physicians should, ideally, have familiarity with mental health professionals in the community so that they can make referrals with confidence. Psychiatrists are experts in serious psychiatric disorders and in evaluation and comprehensive management of behavioral problems. Some nonpsychiatrist mental health professionals, such as clinical social workers and nurse-clinicans, may be more interested and experienced than the psychiatrist in dealing with problems of everyday living and situational difficulties arising from it. Social workers may be the most skilled in dealing with couples and families. If this is not feasible, referral to a psychiatrist who can assume the coordinating responsibility is indicated. The primary physician can assume total responsibility for treating and managing the patient or, for coordinating the management efforts of all involved, using appropriate referrals and community resources to effectively maximize the treatment potential. Some examples of various referral decisions follow.

In the following pages, examples of referral decisions are presented in case histories. The referrals are to a psychiatrist (Case History 14–3), a primary care physician (Case History 14–4), and a clinical social worker (Case History 14–5).

CASE HISTORY 14–3

Mrs. C., a 51-year-old married woman, presents with complaints of loss of appetite, early morning awakening, loss of interest in sex, and decreased interest in social activities. Physical examination was normal. Questioning revealed that her favorite sister was being treated with chemotherapy for inoperable carcinoma. Mrs. C.'s previous medical history included two psychiatric hospitalizations for acute depression both following deaths in the family. After discussion with Mrs. C. it was decided to refer her to a psychiatrist who had treated her in the past. The treatment plan was to help her deal with her sister's illness in the hope of preventing an acute depressive episode.

CASE HISTORY 14–4

Mr. R., a 41-year-old man recently separated from his wife, visits the physician with symptoms of extreme fatigue, difficulty in falling asleep, and irritability. After noting that the physical examination results were normal, the physician spent some time with Mr. R. discussing his life situation. Mr. R. said he felt better after expressing some of his sadness and anger over the breakup of his marriage. Since the physician had treated the family for a number of years, he decided to work with Mr. R. to help resolve his problem of everyday living. Four follow-up appointments were set up with the hope of helping Mr. R. through this crisis in his life.

SUMMARY

"Problems of everyday living" refers to the emotional distress and behavioral disruption resulting from a stress-producing life event. The troubling event is usually a quite ordinary event. The essential features of this disorder are that the stressor or life event can be identified, and the reaction to it results in a maladaptive change in functioning. The change may be evidenced by impairment in work performance, role functioning, or the fact that symptoms or reaction are in excess of the usual reaction to that particular stressor. Moreover there is a causal and temporal relationship between the life event and the disturbance, and the disturbance is brief and transient. It can be expected to subside once the stress is relieved.

The presenting symptoms vary and include:

- Emotional features (depressed, anxious, irritable, and so on)

- Physical symptoms

- Disturbance of behavior or conduct (withdrawal, assaultiveness, reckless driving, excessive drinking)

- Any combination of the above

The severity of the disturbance produced by the life event is a complex function of:

- The severity of the stressor(s)

- The number of stressors

- The nature of the stressor(s)

- The duration of the stressor(s)

CASE HISTORY 14–5

Mrs. P., a 33-year-old married female, complained of insomnia, lethargy, occasional nausea, a 10-pound weight loss, and vague aches and pains of 6 weeks' duration. Physical workup was negative. From knowledge of the family, the physician was aware that Mrs. P.'s oldest son had drowned in a freak accident in a lake 8 months previously. Sensitive questioning about this led to Mrs. P.'s stating that she would "never forgive" herself for his death and that she was annoyed that her husband and daughter were gradually resuming their normal lives "as though nothing had happened." An interview with Mr. P., along with his wife, indicated that he seemed to be handling his grief appropriately but that his wife appeared to be suffering from a prolonged, intense grief reaction. The physician recommended counseling for Mrs. P. to help her deal with her son's death. Mrs. P. knew of a clinical social worker in her community who had been recommended to her by a friend. The physician prescribed antidepressant medication to relieve her depressive symptoms and scheduled a follow-up appointment to review her response to the medication. Following her second visit to the clinical social worker, with Mrs. P.'s permission the physician contacted the social worker to discuss Mrs. P.'s situation. An agreement was made with the social worker to collaborate in the interest of Mrs. P.'s medical and psychosocial treatment.

Resources available to the patient may mitigate the reaction to stressful circumstances. Such resources include the individual's personal characteristics—genetic predisposition, biological constitution, and personality style; his or her social environment—social support, family friends, professional organizations, socioeconomic status, or wealth; and the cultural background—beliefs, values and so on.

Often, patients experiencing problems of everyday living seek assistance from primary physicians, as this is a professional resource that is known and available to them. The primary physician can, depending on interest, time, experience, severity of the disturbance, and past relationship with the patient, assume responsibility for managing the patient alone or for coordinating management efforts using appropriate referrals and resources available.

The goals of management include:

- Eliminating the stressor when possible
- Alleviating physical and emotional symptoms
- Preventing worsening of symptoms and behavior
- Assisting the patient to return to the prestress level of functioning
- Educating the patient in more satisfactory and effective ways to handle problems to prevent future maladaptive reactions

Techniques for achieving the goals vary according to the particular physician, the patient, their relationship, and the nature of the problem.

Referral to individuals specifically trained to deal with psychiatric problems, including psychiatrists, psychologists, social workers, nurse-clinicians, or others should be made according to the specialized help each is best equipped to render. The coordinating role of the primary physician includes not only the appropriate use of referrals and community resources, but also helping the patient understand the referral decision, initiating and maintaining treatment and management, and prescribing of indicated medical treatments.

APPENDIX: CASE HISTORY—ANXIETY, DEPRESSION, AND LOWER BACK PAIN

No organic pathology was demonstrable that might explain the lower back pain. The patient's anxiety may have contributed to her pain through increased muscle tension; her depression, although mild, also may have contributed to her tendency to feel increased pain. The PEG also indicates that there was a major stressor—the impending move to another city following her husband's promotion and transfer. For the patient this would mean being away from her close friends, children, and parents. In addition, the recent irregularity of her menses and possible menopause would be another stressor. The three dimensional diagnoses and management are as follows:

1. *Biological dimension:* Diazepam 2.5 mg three times a day, was prescribed for both anxiety and muscle relaxation; she was also advised to take aspirin when needed

2. *Personal dimension:* The family physician talked with the patient at some length, pointing out in a sympathetic manner that it must be upsetting for her to contemplate leaving the city she lived in for so long, although the move is because of her husband's promotion. He pointed out that this natural anxiety might contribute to back pain through muscle tension. Also, the physician recommended that she see a social worker, who might look into resources in the new city. The patient then saw a social worker, who in collaboration with the physician, provided not only counseling but also arranged for the patient to look into hospital volunteer jobs and other organizations that she might join in the new city. Through this planning, with the help of the physician and the social worker, her back pain, anxiety, and depression subsided. Medications were no longer necessary in a few weeks.

3. *Environmental dimension:* The impending move was treated successfully by intervention in the biological and personal dimensions just described, which included plans geared toward the environmental dimension.

PATIENT EVALUATION GRID

DIMENSIONS	CONTEXTS		
	CURRENT (Current States)	RECENT (Recent Events and Changes)	BACKGROUND (Culture, Traits, Constitution)
BIOLOGICAL	Lower back pain Physical examination and laboratory tests including x-ray films are normal	Lower back pain—1 mo Aspirin—helps some but not much Irregular menses—4 mo	Herniated disk 20 yr ago conservatively treated No pain for 18 yrs No family history of depression or anxiety
PERSONAL	Feels anxious and mildly depressed Mental status examination was normal except for anxiety	Anxious and depressed mood—2 mo Difficulty falling asleep—1 mo Occasional crying spells—1 mo Some increase in wine drinking Increase in smoking (two packs/day)	"Shy person", but likes people No past history of depression or anxiety
ENVIRONMENTAL	Lives with husband Two grown children live in same city Patient works as volunteer in local hospital Close friends with several other volunteers Parents live in same city	Husband's promotion and transfer to another city announced— 3 mo	Middle-class, Catholic background Married at age 20 yr

Demographic data: 40-year-old housewife.

RECOMMENDED READINGS

Caplan, G. 1964. *Principles of preventive psychiatry.* New York: Basic Books. Caplan deals in depth with crisis intervention strategies and management.

Gunderson, E.K., and Rahe, R.H., ed. 1974. *Life stress and illness,* Springfield Ill. Charles C Thomas. This book contains several of the early but significant papers relating life events to psychosocial stress and medical illness, coronary disease, and death.

Hansell, N. 1976. *The person-in-distress.* New York: Human Services Press. This book is helpful for specific strategies in patient management.

Janis, I.L. 1958. *Psychological stress.* New York: John Wiley & Sons. This book deals with the differences in patients' response to a stressful life event, namely, surgery. Using a psychodynamic approach, preoperative emotional reactions are linked with postoperative adjustment. Chapter 25, "Psychological preparation," is a must reading.

Lazarus, R.S. (ed.) 1966. *Psychological stress and the coping process.* New York: McGraw Hill. This compilation of papers by Mason, Selye, Mechanic, Rahe, and others deals with the processes by which stressors act as precursors to physical and/or mental disorders.

REFERENCES

American Psychiatric Association. 1980. *Diagnostic and statistical manual of Mental Disorders,* (*DSM-III*), 3rd ed. Washington, D.C.: American Psychiatric Association.

Hansell, N. 1976. *The person-in-distress.* New York: Human Services Press.

Holmes, T.H., and Rahe, R.M. 1967. The social readjustment rating scale. *J. Psychosom. Res.* 11:213–18.

McWhinney, I.R. 1972. Beyond diagnosis: An approach to the integration of behavioral science and clinical medicine. *N. Engl. J. Med.* 287:384–87.

Mechanic, D. 1978. Effects of psychological distress on perceptions of physical health and use of medical and psychiatric facilities. *J. Hum. Stress* 4:26–32.

Rahe, R.H. 1974. Life change and subsequent illness reports. In *Life stress and illness,* eds., E.K. Gunderson and R.H. Rahe, pp. 58–78. Ch. 4. Springfield. Ill. Charles C Thomas.

Rahe, R.H., and Arthur, R.J. 1978. Life change and illness studies. *J. Hum. Stress* 4:3–15.

Schless, A.P., and Mendels, J. 1978. The value of interviewing family and friends in assessing life stressors. *Arch. Gen. Psychiatry* 35:565–67.

Warheit, G.J. 1979. Life events, coping, stress, and depressive symptomatology. *Am. J. Psychiatry* 136:502–07.

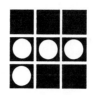

CHAPTER 15

Evaluation and Management of Alcoholism

Mary E. Swigar, M.D.

The moment I got sober, I became so horrified at my behavior that I got drunk again.

Diana Barrymore, actress dead at age 38 years* Alcoholism is perhaps the most common and most serious drug abuse problem in terms of morbidity and mortality. Diseases associated with alcoholism range from hepatic coma and acute pancreatitis to peripheral neuropathy and dementia. Its acute withdrawal state, delirium tremens, is often mistakenly diagnosed as "functional psychosis," and is associated with significant mortality if not properly treated. Chronic alcoholism is often not diagnosed until serious and irreversible complications occur. The recognition and treatment of alcoholism, discussed in depth in this chapter, is an essential skill for all physicians.

*Barrymore, D., and Frank, G. 1961. *Too much, too soon*. New York: Holt.

Evaluating the multifaceted phenomenon of alcohol use and abuse and its consequences is a supreme test of assessment capability. Much of evaluation and management of any illness ideally includes taking multiple factors into account; alcoholism especially demands this complex process. Pharmacologic, medical, comprehensive neuropsychological, familial, and social factors in acute and chronic management are all part of assessment of alcoholism. Furthermore, largely unspoken but widely prevalent negative attitudes on the part of health care personnel toward the alcoholic compounds the problem. They range from helplessness in the face of deterioration to a moralistic and punitive attitude toward the person who sets about bringing such a calamity upon himself or herself and seemingly refuses to stop the self-destructive behavior.

This chapter surveys facets of alcohol use and abuse. It discusses definitions, various widely used classifications, epidemiology, and considers predisposition and special groups at risk. It covers problems of evaluation and management in the acute stage of alcoholism—associated medical problems, problems particularly referable to the central nervous systems (CNS), manifestation and management of alcohol abstinence syndromes, and circumstances mandating certification and continued psychiatric hospitalization. Problems related to the subacute stage include assessment of coexisting psychopathologic states, and continuing dysfunction, defensive postures, assessment of emotional state and motivation for further therapy. Discussion of chronic stage problems addresses assessment of persisting central and peripheral nervous system dysfunction, and the impact of this on the nature of craving and loss of control, participation in treatment, and treatment outcome. Treatment options include inpatient or outpatient approaches, continuing pharmacologic, therapies, Alcoholics Anonymous (AA), group, and aversive-behavioral therapies. Concurrent family problems are important, and the role of the alcoholic's spouse, effects, of parental drinking and its effects on children, and adolescent alcohol abuse are also included.

CASE HISTORY 15–1

A 53-year-old executive of a large corporation was admitted to the hospital for emergency surgery because of a strangulated hernia. Although he tolerated the procedure well, the patient became progressively agitated postoperatively; on the third post-operative day, he appeared to be grossly psychotic. In a fearful voice, he complained that huge bugs and monsters were after him. He was unable to stay still and fought against the bed restraints. He seemed not to recognize his family who were visiting him. He was soaked in sweat and his extremities were quite shaky; the heart rate was 120 beats per minute. A psychiatric consultation was requested. (See the appendix at the end of this chapter for further discussion and PEG.)

DEFINITION AND CLASSIFICATION

Given that alcohol use and abuse is a multifaceted phenomenon, simple definitions are difficult. In general, an alcohol drinking problem may be defined as: *repeated drinking to the extent that an individual compromises any combination of health, work, or interpersonal relationships.* In view of these medical, behavioral, and sociologic components, the condition takes a considerable toll in decreased productivity, physical and psychological illness, accidents, and crimes. And, it disrupts many a close relationship or life situation.

Attempts at developing classification systems reflect not only the complex nature of alcohol abuse, but recognize it as a process that may also resurge and regress. Several classification schemes are in use, however, none have been systematically tested in multiple samples or populations to determine which cluster of symptoms, especially in early stages, provides reliable and more effective diagnosis.

The etiology or etiologies of alcoholism remain obscure. Thus, classification is geared to aid in assigning stages and patterns and treating concomitant conditions.

National Council on Alcoholism Classification

The most ambitious classification was published simultaneously in 1972 in *The Annals of Internal Medicine and The American Journal of Psychiatry* of criteria listed by an expert panel for the National Council on Alcoholism (NCA, 1972). It consists of two comprehensive tracks of criteria: Track I, physiologic and clinical, and Track II, behavioral, psychological, and attitudinal. In addition, there are major and minor criteria for each track. At least one major and several minor criteria are sufficient for diagnosis of alcoholism. Physical and laboratory findings are included,

and the NCA system also requires a separate psychiatric diagnosis when the patient is "dry." The criteria are shown in Table 15–1 and 15–2. This classification is primarily used to establish the degree of certainty in the diagnosis of alcoholism.

International Statistical Classification of Diseases

Classifications that focus more on neurobehavioral aspects of abuse and diagnoses of CNS dysfunction are found in the World Health Organizations *Manual of International Statistical Classification of Diseases, Injuries, and Causes of Death (ICD-9)* (WHO, 1977). Section 303 of the *ICD-9* manual includes the *alcohol dependence syndrome,* in which compulsion to ingest alcohol and discomfort with its absence are prominent, with or without tolerance. Alcoholic psychosis (Section 291) includes diagnostic criteria for delirium tremens, Korsakov psychosis, other alcoholic dementia and hallucinosis, pathological drunkenness, alcoholic psychosis, and nondelirium tremens alcohol withdrawal syndrome. The alcohol dependence syndrome may coexist with alcoholic psychosis (Table 15–3).

Diagnostic and Statistical Classification of Mental Disorders

The Diagnostic and Statistical Manual of the American Psychiatric Association (*DSM-III*) classification numerically coincides with *ICD-9* and subsumes alcohol use under Substance Use Disorders. It places emphasis on length of time of use and course of use, as well as behavioral and pharmacologic criteria. Briefly, the Substance Abuse category implies use for at least 1 month with social complications and psychological dependence. Substance Dependence is diagnosed when criteria for abuse are present and tolerance or withdrawal occur as well. Course of use has three categories: continuous (use over

TABLE 15–1
*Major criteria for the diagnosis of alcoholism** *

CRITERION	DIAGNOSTIC LEVEL[†]	CRITERION	DIAGNOSTIC LEVEL[†]
Track I. Physiologic and Clinical		Fatty degeneration in absence of other known cause	2
		Alcoholic hepatitis	1
A. Physiologic dependency		Laennec's cirrhosis	2
1. Physiologic dependence as manifested by evidence of a withdrawal syndrome when the intake of alcohol is interrupted or decreased without substitution of other sedation		Pancreatitis in the absence of cholelithiasis	2
		Chronic gastritis	3
		Hematologic disorders:	
Gross tremor (differentiated from other causes of tremor)	1	Anemia: hypochromic, normocytic, macrocytic, hemolytic with stomatocytosis, low folic acid	3
Hallucinosis (differentiated from schizophrenic hallucinations or other psychoses)	1	Clotting disorders: prothrombin elevation, thrombocytopenia	3
Withdrawal seizures (differentiated from epilepsy and other seizure disorders)	1	Wernicke-Korsakoff's syndrome	2
		Alcoholic cerebellar degeneration	1
Delirium tremens; minimally includes tremors, disorientation, and hallucinations		Cerebral degeneration in absence of Alzheimer's disease or arteriosclerosis	2
		Central pontine myelinolysis diagnosis only possible postmortem	
2. Evidence of tolerance to the effects of alcohol. (There may be a decrease in previously high levels of tolerance late in the course.)		Marchiafava-Bignami's disease	2
		Peripheral neuropathy (see also beriberi)	2
		Toxic amblyopia	3
A blood alcohol level of more than 150 mg without gross evidence of intoxication	1	Alcohol myopathy	2
		Alcoholic cardiomyopathy	2
The consumption of one fifth of whiskey or one quart of wine or beer daily, for more than one day, by a 180-lb individual	1	Beriberi	3
		Pellagra	3
		Track II. Behavioral, Psychologic and Attitudinal	
3. Alcohol "blackout" periods. (Differential diagnosis from purely psychological fugue states and psychomotor seizures.)	2	All chronic conditions of psychologic dependence occur in dynamic equilibrium with intrapsychic and interpersonal consequences. Alcoholism produces vocational, social, and physical impairments. The following behavior patterns show psychologic dependence on alcohol in alcoholism:	
B. Clinical: major alcohol-associated illnesses		1. Drinking despite strong medical contraindication known to patient	1
Alcoholism can be assumed to exist if major alcohol-associated illnesses develop in a person who drinks regularly. In such individuals, evidence of physiologic and psychological dependence should be searched for.		2. Drinking despite strong, identified, social contraindication (job loss for intoxication, marriage disruption because of drinking, arrest for intoxication, driving while intoxicated)	1
		3. Patient's subjective complaint of loss of control of alcohol consumption	2

* From *National Council on Alcoholism* (Criteria Committee), 1972.
† 1 = definite
  2 = probable, strong suspicion
  3 = possible, arouse suspicion

TABLE 15–2
Minor criteria for the diagnosis of alcoholism*

CRITERION	DIAGNOSTIC LEVEL[†]	CRITERION	DIAGNOSTIC LEVEL[†]
Track I. Physiologic and Clinical		mOsm/L reflects 50 mg/100 mL alcohol	2
A. Direct effects (ascertained by examination)		Minor — indirect	
		Results of alcohol ingestion:	
1. Early:		Hypoglycemia	3
Odor of alcohol on breath at time of medical appointment	2	Hypochloremic alkalosis	3
		Low magnesium level	2
2. Middle:		Lactic acid elevation	3
Alcoholic facies	2	Transient uric acid elevation	3
Vascular engorgement of face	2	Potassium depletion	3
Toxic amblyopia	3	Indications of liver abnormality:	
Increased incidence of infections	3	SGPT elevation	2
Cardiac arrhythmias	3	SGOT elevation	3
Peripheral neuropathy (see also Major Criteria, Track I, B)	2	Bromsulphthalein elevation	2
		Bilirubin elevation	2
3. Late (see Major Criteria, Track I, B)		Urinary urobilinogen elevation	2
		Serum A/G ratio reversal	2
B. Indirect effects		Blood and blood clotting:	
1. Early:		Anemia: hypochromic, normocytic, macrocytic, hemolytic with stoma-tocytosis, low folic acid	
Tachycardia	3		
Flushed face	3		
Nocturnal diaphoresis	3		
2. Middle:		Clotting disorders: prothrombin elevation, thrombocytopenia	
Ecchymoses on lower extremities, arms, or chest	3		
Cigarette or other burns on hands or chest	3	ECG abnormalities: Cardiac arrhythmias: tachycardia; T waves dimpled, cloven, or spinous; atrial fibrillation; ventricular premature contractions; abnormal P waves	
Hyperreflexia, or if drinking heavily, hyporeflexia (permanent hyporeflexia may be a residuum of alcoholic polyneuritis)	3		
			2
3. Late:		EEG abnormalities:	
Decreased tolerance	3	Decreased or increased REM sleep, depending on phase	3
C. Laboratory tests		Loss of delta sleep	3
1. Major — direct		Other reported findings	3
Blood alcohol level at any time of more than 300 mg/100 mL	1	Decreased immune response	3
Level of more than 100 mg/100 mL in routine examination	1	Chromosomal damage from alcoholism	3
2. Major — indirect			
Serum osmolality (reflects blood alcohol levels): every 22.4 increase over 200			

* From *National Council on Alcoholism* (Criteria Committee), 1972.
† 1 = definite
  2 = probable, strong suspicion
  3 = possible, arouse suspicion

TABLE 15–3
International statistical classification of diseases criteria*

303. Alcohol dependence syndrome

Continuous or periodic use of alcohol
a. For psychic effect
b. To avoid physical or psychic discomfort of absence of alcohol,
c. With compulsion to drink
d. Not yet necessarily tolerant to alcohol

291. Alcoholic psychoses

Etiology is either excessive alcohol use or withdrawal effect producing psychotic organic state. Nutritional deficit thought to be important.

291.0 Delirium tremens
Organic psychotic states in alcoholics with the following signs and symptoms:
a. Clouded consciousness with disorientation
b. Illusions, delusions, and hallucinations (esp. visual and tactile)
c. Fear
d. Restlessness, tremor
e. Fever

291.1 Korsakoff's psychosis, alcoholic Prominent and persistent loss of memory, occurring as a sequel to acute alcoholic psychosis and/or with chronic alcoholism
a. Temporal disorientation

b. Loss of recent memory is striking with confabulation
c. Usually accompanied by peripheral neuropathy
d. Associated with Wernicke's encephalopathy

291.2 Other alcoholic dementia
Designated for alcoholic dementias where there is no delirium tremens, Korsakoff's or hallucinosis

291.3 Other alcoholic hallucinosis
a. Prominence of auditory hallucinations—threats or insults are characteristic
b. No or slight clouding of consciousness
c. Duration usually less than 6 months

291.4 Pathologic drunkenness
a. Acute psychotic state induced by relatively little alcohol intake
b. Few neurologic signs of intoxication

291.5 Alcoholic jealousy
a. Presence of delusional jealousy
b. Chronic paranoid state associated with alcohol abuse

291.8 Other—alcohol withdrawal without delirium tremens

291.9 Unspecified

* From World Health Organization. 1977 International classification of diseases, 9th ed., Geneva.

---

5 years), episodic (one or more episodes in the past), and in remission. Age at onset, description of impairment, complications, and familial patterns are also classified. Psychotic states related to alcohol are somewhat changed from those in *ICD-9*. These will be discussed further in the section on Alcohol Abstinence Syndrome.

Jellinek's Phases of Alcoholism

Jellinek's symptoms of phases of alcoholism are largely sociobehavioral with elements of behavior descriptively elaborated. He compartmentalizes these criteria into four (Alpha through Delta) groups (Jellinek, 1960). Alphas drink to deal with discomfort and have not yet lost control but may have experienced unpleasant social consequences on occasion. There are no withdrawal symptoms noted. Beta alcoholics begin to experience physical problems such as gastritis, mild hepatic problems, but withdrawal symptoms as such are uncommon.

Gamma alcoholism progresses to loss of control, tissue tolerance, withdrawal states, and marked behavioral change. Delta alcoholism is the most severe phase in which the person is unable to avoid drinking for even a day. Jellinek's Prodromal, Crucial, and Chronic Phases of Alcoholism are summarized in Table 15–4.

TABLE 15–4
Criteria for phases of alcoholism— prodromal, crucial, and chronic phases

PRODROME-TO-ADDICTION PHASE	CRUCIAL PHASE	CHRONIC PHASE
Is preoccupied with alcohol	Alcohol-centered behavior increases	Thinking is impaired
Has guilt feelings about it	Loses control of drinking	Is indefinably fearful
Avoids referring to alcohol	Rationalizes drinking	Drinking is obsessive
Gulps drinks	Periodically abstains, attempts control	Rationalizations fail
Drinks secretly	Self-pity and resentment begin	Ethical deterioration is noted
Blackouts begin	Is remorseful after drinking	Has vague religious desires
	Alcoholic jealousy begins	Goes on benders, loses tolerance for alcohol
	Libido decreases	Tremors are noted
	Loses outside interests	Psychomotor inhibition is present
	Neglects nutrition	Drinks mouthwash, shaving lotion, and so on, when no access to ethanol
	Has aggressive or grandiose behavior	Drinks in more degraded circumstances
	Has regular morning drinking	Suffers alcoholic psychoses
	Protects alcohol supply	Hospitalizations become multiple
	Changes drinking pattern, further attempt at control	
	Social pressures begin	
	Drops friends, reinterprets interpersonal relations	
	Changes habits in relation to family	
	Quits or is fired from jobs	
	Contemplates or attempts "escape" with geographic relocation	
	Has first hospitalization	

*From Jellinek, E.M. 1960. *The disease concept of alcoholism.* New Brunswick, N.J.: Rutgers Center of Studies on Alcohol.

The major focus of all of these classifications is on later phases of alcoholism. It is to be hoped that this focus will change when earlier identification of the problem drinker is more widely practiced. Early detection and screening are always possible if the evaluator asks about alcohol use. Development of a similar system internationally would also aid cross-cultural studies. Even at present it is important that health care personnel become familiar with the standardized approach to diagnosis, no matter which classification is chosen.

EPIDEMIOLOGIC AND SOCIAL PROBLEMS AND ALCOHOLISM

In the United States 9 million people, or 4% of the population, are estimated to be alcoholic (Chafetz, 1975). One adult in 25 has an alcohol problem (Bates, 1965) and the figure may be higher since much of the problem is hidden. The ordinariness of most alcoholics contributes to the problem of early identification—they are usually "respectable citizens living quietly in our communities, their problems unknown to us." The corollary is that detection requires "considerable ingenuity as well as a high level of suspicion" (Selzer, 1961).

Of the entire population of the United States, two groups stand out as being significantly at risk: the American Indian whose alcoholism rate is twice that of the national average (Chafetz, 1975), and urban ghetto males under age 25 years (Mulford, 1964; Cahalan et al., 1969). "Skid row" alcoholics represent only 3–5% of the entire alcoholic group, which knows no socioeconomic or class boundaries.

Alcoholism costs our economy an estimated $15 billion per year, and $10 billion in lost work time. Alcoholics are thought to comprise 5% of the work force and another 5% suffers significant abuse (Chafetz, 1975).

In the United States, as in other countries, per capita consumption of alcohol remains fairly stable, while regional trends may vary. Thus, when per capita consumption increases, it is because of an increase in prevalence of a single subgroup, that is, heavy users of alcohol. Control of alcoholism from a public health standpoint is strongly related to identification and treatment of heavy abusers (Chafetz, 1975). This group is also most at risk for developing "core" alcoholism, defined as loss of control, development of tolerance, and relapsing drinking.

Heavy and repeated alcohol consumption can certainly lead to alcoholism. However, no single social or biological variable has been found that determines this completely. Furthermore, there is evidence to suggest that even heavy drinking patterns can spontaneously shift. From a representative survey of over 2700 persons in the United States, 32% were totally abstinent. Two thirds of Americans used alcohol at least occasionally and 12% were characterized as heavy drinkers. Follow-up studies 3 years later revealed that 15% shifted in or out of the heavy drinking group (Cahalan et al., 1969; Cahalan, 1970). Understanding the nature of these spontaneous shifts in usage of alcohol could facilitate apportioning of therapeutic energies.

Alcohol abuse does not exist in isolation from other substance abuse. Polydrug abuse, both opiate and nonopiate, is strongly associated with alcohol abuse. It is unclear whether this represents a shift in patterns of abuse or recognition of the nature of drug abuse problems. Alcohol abuse and coincident increase in tobacco (Dreher and Fraser, 1967; Griffiths et al., 1976), barbiturates and sedatives (Devenyi and Wilson, 1971; Freed, 1973), marijuana (Fisher and Brickman, 1973; Tec, 1973), and heroin—with or without methadone maintenance (Schut et al., 1973; Bourne, 1975; Raynes et al., 1975) have been identified.

Approaches to the evaluation and management of alcoholism at present are constrained by inadequate information concerning its etiology and the shifts in usage patterns. Current diagnostic approach consists of: (a) pursuing the goal of *early identification* by inquiring into this perhaps concealed area of patients' lives; (b) using *standardized assessment* techniques; (c) awareness that abuse of alcohol may also involve *abuse or other substances*; and (d) not contributing to substance abuse by *prescribing* more drugs.

The hardcore substance abuser or "skid row" type may continue to exist, since this has been true through man's history. However, countless emotional, physical, and social resources could be retrieved earlier. Crimes, accidents, destruction to persons and property could be prevented, and shattered interpersonal relationships and psychiatric illness treated.

PREDISPOSITION TO ALCOHOLISM

Genetics

Is alcoholism genetically determined? Goodwin, (1979) in his excellent review summarizes the evidence. At least 25% of alcoholics' male relatives are alcoholic (3%-5% of males in populations surveyed), 5%-10% of alcoholics' female relatives are alcoholic (compared to 0.1%–1% of females being alcoholic in total population surveys). That alcoholism is familial to a great extent is not new information, but the genetic factor remains unclear. Results of four twin studies as reviewed by Goodwin vary somewhat. Higher concordance for more extensive alcohol consumption among monozygotic than dizygotic twins was found in all four studies, but only one study demonstrated concordance for actual alcoholism (that is, pathologic consequences of drinking). Thus, the extent of drinking seems to have a genetic component but it is not necessarily central to alcoholism itself, namely, the loss of control, development of tolerance, and relapsing drinking.

Adoption studies approach to the genetics of alcoholism suggest that sons of alcoholics compared to those of nondrinking controls, are highly likely to become alcoholic whether reared by adopted or natural parents (Schukit et al., 1972; Goodwin, 1979). Thus, for males, the biological effect of having an alcoholic parent appears to outstrip environment in importance for producing alcoholism. Adoption studies on alcoholics' daughters need to be studied further. Inconclusive and confusing data came from Goodwin's Danish study (1977) that showed that daughters of alcoholics and daughters of the control group had a higher incidence of alcoholism (at least double) than that of the Danish general population of women. One finding that did emerge, however, was that daughters of alcoholics reared with the alcoholic parent were more likely to suffer depression than were control daughters. This was not true of alcoholic sons. Female adoptees, whether born to alcoholic parent or not, did not develop alcoholism or depression. Generally, men in alcoholic families are more likely to develop antisocial problems in contrast to women who tend to become depressed. Clearly, in future genetic studies, male/female differences and the distinction between heavy drinking and core alcoholism will be important.

Goodwin discusses an interesting hypothesis about *what* gets inherited in alcoholic families. Alcoholics might inherit a different way of metabolizing alcohol that predisposes them to difficulty. The large portion of the population who do *not* become alcoholic may (a) lack a particularly euphoriant response to alcohol, or (b) in fact, with relatively small amounts, may suffer a negative reenforcing effect and stop. Conversely, the person predisposed to becoming alcoholic may (a) experience a singularly pleasant euphoria, and (b) obtain a positive reenforcing effect over time. These patterns of experience may lead to two separate sets of learned responses —a positive or a negative feedback loop may form about alcohol consumption. The majority of the population appears to experience the negative reenforcing effect and does not continue on the path leading to alcoholism and avoid engaging in repeated and excessive drinking. This is an interesting hypothesis that warrants further testing.

Genetic marker studies have attempted to link some biological or phenotypic traits and alcoholism. Replication studies, in particular, are needed to resolve contradictions and to enlarge the scope of the findings. As with genetic studies, making the distinction between heavy drinking and true core alcoholism using standard criteria is very important. Findings showing promise in aiding in early identification are: first, having blood groups A, SS, Lewis a − b+ and a − b−, Duffy a + − a −; and in the second place, having genetically determined HL-A antigens HL-A-7, W10, and W16 and absence of autoimmune antibodies and HL-A-13. Dermatoglyphic characteristics and tendency to blue-yellow color blindness associations with core alcoholism may also be significant. Controversy exists about the reversibility of the color blindness, perhaps due to toxic effects of alcohol, with cessation of drinking (Kojić et al., 1977).

Gender and Alcoholism

Gender differences in relation to alcoholism exist and the examiner needs to know about these to better evaluate men and women for alcoholism. Sex differences, in addition to those discussed in the genetics section, are similar across studies and are not particularly controversial. Both alcoholic men and women are likely to have family histories of alcoholism. *Women* are highly likely also to have a history of parental loss by death, divorce, or desertion, and also to have suffered childhood deprivation (Lisansky, 1957; Delint, 1964; Curlee, 1970; Rathod and Thomson, 1971). While hormonal influences may play a part, shifts in sex roles and attitudes toward femininity are important (Schukit and Morrissey, 1976). At present, women have different drinking patterns than men. However, both have similar first drinking experiences in that they begin to drink in early teens, though women usually drink initially with their families.

In contrast, males are more likely to drink first with friends (Waller and Jorch, 1977). Women begin to drink more heavily at a later age (Winokur and Clayton, 1968; Curlee, 1970; Rathod and Thomson, 1971; Efron et al., 1974) and have a more rapid progression to late stage symptoms if they develop (Delint, 1964; Efron, et al. 1974). *Contextual drinking* is different for men and women. Men drink in a variety of contexts. Women are inclined to drink with their spouses and family on weekends (Irgens-Jenson, 1978) or to drink at home and alone (Wanberg and Horn, 1970; Horn and Wanberg, 1973).

The effect of alcohol on performance in moderate to heavily drinking men and women with comparable blood levels of alcohol is similar (Burns and Moskowitz, 1978). However, fantasy themes with drinking are dissimilar. Men report increase of physical sex and aggressive power fantasies with drinking. Women relate concerns about impact on others and concern for self-control. Boyatzis (1977) has reviewed this area and has attempted to establish a potential relationship between alcohol-induced arousal and increases in epinephrine, norepinephrine, and other hormonal substrates.

In future studies of alcoholics, controlling for gender differences will be important. Currently, the examiner must be aware that different motivations for drinking and different age-related patterns exist for men and women.

Personality Factors and Alcoholism

Alcoholics are most persistently described as immature, narcissistic, dependent, hostile, and socially isolated. As Mello and Mendelson (1975) have noted, reviewing studies in this area at present is an ungratifying exercise. Myths and untested belief systems are pervasive in problems of alcoholism, and personality is probably the area where this is most true. As with many studies of other facets of problem drinking, several problems arise.

1. Retrospective studies abound. Abuse of alcohol over months to years alters the person's self-assessment, social interactions, and coping, and, therefore, others' assessment of him or her, CNS function, and nutritional and metabolic status. This constellation of ongoing secondary problems makes it difficult to pinpoint personality traits that are "causative" or even associated with alcoholism.

2. Too many studies assess personality in the context of acute or subacute alcohol abuse when CNS function is altered and metabolic-nutritional state is in flux.

3. The distinction between heavy drinking versus core alcoholism is not sufficiently stringent, since, as noted earlier, 15% of heavy drinkers move in and out of that category.

4. Early identification of persons at risk for alcoholism and prospective assessment of personality traits is currently not possible. Since alcoholism is a chronic relapsing illness that often goes on in secret, becomes a central and consuming focus, and alters the person's ability to manage in situations, the previously mentioned personality "traits" may well be the result of alcohol abuse. These traits could be described as being shared with other chronic relapsing conditions, notably with other substance abuse.

EVALUATION AND MANAGEMENT

Acute Stages of Alcoholism

Any good medical textbook can serve as a source book for evaluation and treatment of medical conditions associated with acute alcoholism. Important ones are briefly summarized in Table 15–5.

Central Nervous System. There are a variety of acute neuropsychiatric problems in acute alcoholism. The most important, by virtue of being life-threatening, is delirium tremens. *Anyone likely to have a significant withdrawal reaction should be hospitalized.* Three conditions are necessary for withdrawal: (a) dose dependence; (b) tolerance; and (c) abrupt cessation or a large decline in intake (Victor and Adams, 1953). As Isbell and colleagues (1955) discovered, this spectrum could be produced in ten healthy, well-nourished volunteers kept intoxicated for 6–12 weeks, then abruptly withdrawn. Malnutrition and other complications are not necessary for the production of seizures, psychosis, or even of delirium tremens. *Any* beverage form of alcohol consumed steadily and in sufficient quantity (defined as 1 pint whiskey, $\frac{4}{5}$ quart of wine and 1 quart of beer per day) over enough time will result in development of alcohol dependence (Mello, 1975).

Alcoholism knows no bounds of social class or socioeconomic status. Accidental alcohol withdrawal can occur with any patient admitted to the hospital for any reason, and an appropriate degree of suspicion must be maintained with *all* patients. Concurrent sedative intake by the patient increases chances for withdrawal when both cellular and metabolic tolerance (due to induction of hepatic microsomal enzymes) have developed both to alcohol and sedatives.

Alcoholic Blackout. A blackout is a delimited memory disorder, a period of dense amnesia which occurs during drinking. It usually lasts from one to several hours, though rarely, it may persist for several days. The amount drunk and the level of intoxication do not necessarily predict when a blackout will occur, but they happen much more frequently in conjunction with drinking hard liquor, rather than wine or beer. Other associated factors are neglect of meals, gulping drinks, and a history of head trauma (Goodwin et al., 1969). The blackout is felt to be prodromal to core alcoholism (Jellinek, 1960). Sometimes the person can remember entering a blackout. Typically, the onset is abrupt, and complex behavior occurs during the blackout. If it is triggered by an unacceptable, threatening event, a blackout is clinically indistinguishable from deliberate denial. However, most blackouts are not induced by such occurrences and are frightening to the person.

Occasionally, events that happen during a blackout will be remembered only during another blackout. Not all alcoholics experience blackouts—the reasons for this are unknown. Controlled experiments using psychometric testing appear to show that blackouts are related to the effect of alcohol upon the rate at which immediate events are perceived and stored, not by the negative effect of alcohol on short-term memory (Goodwin, 1973; Parker et al., 1974; Moskowitz and Murray, 1976b).

Alcohol Abstinence Syndromes

The mildest form of alcohol abstinence syndrome is known as a hangover, the result of a

---

TABLE 15–5
Derangement associated with acute alcoholism

CONDITION	ASSESSMENT*
Infection	
Pneumonia	Exam, CXR, WBC & diff, sputum
Tuberculosis	Above plus acid-fast exams
Meningitis	Exam, LP
Trauma, especially CNS	Exam, skull x-ray films, CT scan, LP
Gastrointestinal.	
Bleeding—esophageal varices gastritis, peptic ulcer	Stools, appropriate GI x-ray films
Hypoglycemia	Blood glucose level
Malabsorption and diarrhea—gastritis, duodenitis jejunitis, hepatic and pancreatic insufficiency (Lindenbaum, 1977)	Mucosal structural change
Pancreatitis—in those with high protein and high fat diets (Sarles, 1977)	Amylase, lipase level
hepatitis-cirrhosis (Lieber, 1977) and portal hypertension	LFTs, biopsy, plasma ammonia
Hematopoietic (Lindenbaum, 1977)	Marrow examination
Megaloblastic anemia (not in folate-containing beer)	CBC, indices, folate and B_{12} levels
Thrombocytopenia (secondary to shortened platelet lifespan)	Platelet count
Sideroblastic anemia (with malnutrition)	Marrow, pyridoxine replacement Vacuolization of WBC/RBC precursors
Dehydration and electrolyte deficiency	Electrolytes and magnesium levels, then hydration, replacement
Cardiomyopathy and arrhythmias	Auscultation, ECG, potassium and magnesium levels

*Vital signs are important to monitor for a variety of reasons but are nonspecific and may be confounded by effects of withdrawal.

single heavy dose of alcohol. A hangover is mild rebound *neuronal hyperexcitability*, complicated perhaps by a spell of gastritis, sleep deprivation, water and electrolyte disturbance. With more prolonged and heavier drinking, this hyperexcitability manifests itself with graded intensity and severity, which is variable to some extent among individuals (Gross et al., 1974). As the blood alcohol level falls, early warning signs of withdrawal appear. *Photomyoclonus* is the first sign (Wolfe and Victor, 1971). *Tremor*, enhanced by heightened emotion or activity follows within a few hours, and is found in 100% of patients in early stages of withdrawal. Anorexia, nausea, vomiting, and diarrhea, as well as tachycardia and diaphoresis, occur as manifestations of *increased central autonomic tone*. The skin is cold and clammy, rebounding from the cutaneous vasodilatation of intoxication. The patient is *anxious*, *irritable*, and *startles readily*. He may suffer illusions and disorders of perception that precede hallucinosis. Insomnia occurs but its relationship to stages of sleep is as yet undefined. Alcohol-induced suppression of rapid eye movement (REM) sleep gives way to *REM rebound* during withdrawal in some, but not all, patients. At one time, REM suppression and rebound and the development of hallucinosis in alcoholics were thought to be associated, but this is no longer clear (Gross and Hastey, 1976). Hallucinations may occur in 39% of cases of this mild type of early (6–36 hour) withdrawal (Wolfe and Victor, 1971). Tremor, which may be treated by propranolol (Zilm et al., 1975) and hallucinations subside in most after 1–4 days, but the chronic alcoholic may suffer the other symptoms for several weeks.

Seizures and Alcohol Withdrawal.

If withdrawal progresses, *seizures* or "rum fits" may occur. About two-thirds of alcoholics have multiple episodes up to 3 days after withdrawal begins (Sereny and Kalant, 1965). Only 3% develop *status epilepticus*, and in these cases, other substance withdrawal or CNS infection or trauma must be suspected. In 25% of cases the seizure heralds onset of *delirium tremens*, though in 40% a deceptive lucid period follows (0.5–5 days) only to progress to delirium tremens after all. Temporally, seizures will have occurred within 3 days, hallucinosis within 4 days, and delirium tremens in 7 days in 100% of alcoholics in withdrawal. Some 90% of patients have onset of delirium tremens within 4 days. Thus, the risk of severe alcohol abstinence symptoms is over in a week.

Delirium Tremens.

Delirium tremens still carries at least a 15% risk of *mortality*, usually in those with medical complications, especially psychomotor agitation, underhydration, hyperthermia, cardiovascular collapse, meningitis, pneumonia, and hepatic encephalopathy (Thompson, 1978). The patient may need to be examined further medically despite the profound CNS derangement. Symptoms of the latter are quite dramatic. The patient is panic-stricken, profoundly confused, disoriented, and responds to vivid, frightening, and often persecutory visual and auditory hallucinations. The patient is hyperaroused and intensely restless but largely only in response to internal stimuli or products of deranged consciousness in relation to external cues. Speech is fragmented and changeable, often slurred, and the patient is highly suggestible.

Treatment of Severe Withdrawal.

Treatment of severe alcohol withdrawal consists of parenteral hydration, often 4–10 L on the first day (Thompson et al., 1975) with correction of electrolyte imbalance, especially hypokalemia and hypomagnesemia. Exceptions to vigorous hydration applies to patients with head trauma and edema. Correction of vitamin deficiency, especially of thiamine, pyridoxine, folic acid, and B_{12} is necessary.

Drug therapy in alcohol abstinence syndromes is still a bit controversial, but a closely argued, logical approach has been presented (Thompson, 1978). A few principles and cautions are worth noting. The replacement substance must be cross-tolerant with alcohol. If one encounters severe alcohol withdrawal in a setting where no drugs are available, alcohol itself can be given in diminishing quantities (Funderburk and Allen, 1977; Schmitz, 1978). Propranolol, while helping tremor, will not stop progression of other withdrawal symptoms. Phenytoin, because of its slow onset of action, has no role unless status epilepticus develops and anticonvulsant medication is needed (Victor, 1966). Phenothiazines and butyrophenones, because of their ability to lower seizure threshold, do not belong in the treatment regimen. Nine of ten deaths among 786 patients in six studies occurred in patients given phenothiazines (Thompson, 1978). Furthermore, high doses carry the risk of atropine-like delirium. Paraldehyde, thought to be a good drug for withdrawal, has problems. Given intravenously, it may cause pulmonary edema and death, or given intramuscularly, sterile abscesses may occur. It is excreted partially by the lung, but hepatic function is still required for an estimated 70–80% of its metabolism (Harvey, 1975).

Beyond the guidelines just described, data from well-controlled studies are scanty. Barbiturates, benzodiazepines, chloral hydrate, paraldehyde, and even alcohol itself, all have their proponents for treatment of various phases of withdrawal. There is little data to support using one or the other of these compounds. The guiding principle for treatment is to give regular doses of medication sufficient to calm the patient, while carefully observing the patient and titering medication over the first 24 hours. With care and early identification, delirium tremens need not develop. Various drug and adjunct therapies are summarized in Table 15–6.

Treatment of Sedative-Hypnotic and Alcohol Abuse.

Where significant drug *and* alcohol abuse is suspected and a newly admitted patient is showing the rather nonspecific signs of withdrawal described earlier, the following procedure has proven useful. On the premise that mild symptoms of intoxication (particularly nystagmus, slurred speech, and slight ataxia) are a specific end point, the patient is given 100 mg of an intermediate-acting barbiturate (pentobarbital or secobarbital) every hour by mouth during an initial 6-hour test period until mild symptoms of intoxication appear. This total dose given in the test period is then multiplied by three to approximate the amount that will be needed over the rest of the first 24-hour period. That amount is then divided and given in equal doses every 4 hours during the remainder of the initial 24 hours. Vital signs, behavior, nystagmus, and ataxia are observed. If the patient shows signs of intoxication after this period, the dose is adjusted downward in the second and, if needed, the third 24-hour period, until the patient is calm and showing only mild signs of intoxication. Conversely, if the patient remains agitated, sleepless, diaphoretic, tachycardic, and shows signs of continuous arousal, dosage is adjusted upward after the first 24-hour period (Detre and Jarecki, 1971). Serial EEGs may be used to determine if increasing cerebral irritability is occurring. Intermediate-acting barbiturates ensure rapid adjustment of the medication, especially downward, if increasing intoxication signals accumulation of effect. By contrast, doses of long-acting benzodiazepines are more difficult to adjust over time.

This method removes guesswork about when the patient had a last drink or pill prior to admission, what effect stress of hospitalization may have on anxiety, or how a history of hypertension may alter the vital signs. It is designed primarily to forestall the development of seizures or delirium tremens by erring on the side of intoxication. Close attendance is needed for a patient who is ataxic and is in danger of falling during the first 24 hours. Proper hydration and workup for complications is also begun. Withdrawal can begin after the first 5 days or so, by decreasing the dose by 10% daily or every other day.

TABLE 15–6
Therapies for alcohol abstinence syndromes*

	CROSS-TOLERANCE DRUG	ADJUNCTIVE THERAPY[†]
Tremulousness phase—note if any vomiting or diarrhea	Chlordiazepoxide 50 mg orally Diazepam 5 mg orally Secobarbital or pentobarbital 50 mg orally Paraldehyde 5 mL orally All every 4–6 hr	Monitor intake and output, oral hydration, correct potassium and magnesium (2 mL 50% solution magnesium sulfate IM every 6 hr for 24 hr is typical) IM thiamine 100 mg first day, then 50 mg multivitamins orally
Seizure phase	Chlordiazepoxide 50–100 mg orally, IV or IM[‡] Diazepam 10 mg IV, orally, or IM[‡] Secobarbital or pentobarbital 100 mg IM Paraldehyde 10 mL rectally or IM[‡] All every 3–4 hr	IV fluid therapy—may be 4–6 L/24 hr[†] Potassium needed? Magnesium as noted above or more if needed; check calcium levels with seizures Thiamine 100 mg IM every day until taking food, then 50 mg orally Multivitamins—folate, pyridoxine, B_{12} after hematology studies
Delirium tremens	Total 24-hr dose may be: 800 mg—chlordiazepoxide 50–100 mg IV, orally, or IM[‡] 250 mg—diazepam 5 mg IV initially, then 5–10 mg IV, orally, or IM[‡] 175 mg—paraldehyde 10 mL rectally or IM[‡] 1 g—secobarbital or pentobarbital 100 mg IM All every half hour until patient is calmer; after several doses, monitor peak action time, vital signs, especially respiration, and lengthen dose interval to 1–4 hr over the next 2 days	IV fluids—may be 4–10 L/24 hr Note above adjunct therapies[†]

From Knott and Beard, 1974; Victor, 1974; Greenblatt and Shader, 1975; Thompson, 1978.
* Doses are considered to be a guide and do not substitute for monitoring the patient.
[†] Others: acute hypoglycemia—50 mL of 50% glucose, IV; prolonged prothrombin time—vitamin K, 5 mg IV.
[‡] For benzodiazepines, IM route of administration results in slower and less reliable absorption than oral doses or IV routes. If parenteral administration is justified, benzodiazepines should be given carefully IV.

Alcohol and Psychosis. ICD-9 (see Table 15–3) describes the customary group of four psychoses associated with acute alcoholism. The distinctions made are as follows: *delirium tremens*—with clouding of consciousness and simple delusional and hallucinatory experiences; *alcoholic psychosis*—clouding of consciousness, but with more complex delusions and hallucinations; *alcoholic hallucinosis*—little or no clouding of consciousness with prominent threatening auditory hallucinatory experiences; *alcoholic paranoia*—a state of chronic delusional jealousy with alcoholism. Cutting (1978) noted that this classification continues in use despite observations that these phenomena in patients cannot be so neatly categorized. Furthermore, there have been only a few follow-up studies that indicate whether any of the conditions tend to repeat in a similar manner in a given patient, or whether they were of any prognostic significance, and the data have been largely conflicting.

The *DSM-III* (1980) maintains three categories—*delirium tremens*; *alcoholic hallucinosis* (characterized by auditory hallucinations continuing after any withdrawal syndrome has subsided); and *dementia* in association with alcoholism (primarily chronic brain syndrome without a clear statement that alcohol is causative).

Cutting (1978) reviewed the problems with the *ICD-9* classification and retrospectively surveyed 114 patients with alcoholic psychotic diagnoses. He also followed up 57%–89% of patients in each category. Age and sex differences and problems with diagnostic categorization were noted. Older patients and women tended to present more with clouding of consciousness. Alcoholic paranoia was seldom diagnosed, and delirium tremens could not always be satisfactorily separated from alcoholic hallucinosis. Alcoholic hallucinosis, when it repeated itself, was likely to end up resembling chronic schizophrenia. Some patients in all categories of alcoholic psychosis, except hallucinosis, stayed well and on follow-up some presented with affective illness or paranoia. Thus, at present, it would appear that phenomenologically well-worn classifications work, to some degree, but are not particularly helpful prognostically except for hallucinosis and schizophrenia.

Two other psychotic states associated with alcoholism are rather more clear-cut. The first is *pathologic intoxication*. In this condition marked behavior change and amnesia are associated with drinking an amount of alcohol too small to produce such an extreme effect. The clinician must look for other CNS conditions such as temporal lobe epilepsy, encephalitis, or trauma. The other is the *Wernicke-Korsakoff Syndrome*. This is an amnesic syndrome with confabulation, peripheral neuropathy, ophthalmoplegia, and encephalopathy, which may be reversible to some extent by parenteral administration of thiamine.

For the examiner, the major implications in relation to acute management are preventing and treating alcohol abstinence syndromes and concurrent conditions. Being alert for continuing hallucinosis (signaling schizophreniform illness) or signs of affective illness beyond the acute period are necessary. If found, definitive psychiatric consultation is in order. A diagnosis of pathologic intoxication requires referral to a neurologist.

It should be remembered that homicide, robbery, automobile fatalities, and suicides occur when people have been drinking (Waller, 1972; Goodwin, 1973; Tinklenberg, 1973; Nathan and Turnbull, 1974). A history of these factors added to the presenting medical problems should change the nature of referral for aftercare. Definitive referral becomes mandatory and, if necessary, certification to an inpatient psychiatric setting must occur.

Subacute Stage

The management and evaluation of the subacute stage usually continues over a period of 1–4 weeks after an acute drinking episode. After a week, the danger of delirium tremens is over (unless there are concurrent medical or neurologic complications), yet the overall effect on the alcohol-using individual has yet to be assessed.

The transitional period is a complicated and rather critical time. The examiner's task is to determine the need for a type of aftercare and the patient's motivation and functional mental state. If the alcohol problem is at an earlier stage, morbid psychiatric or organic brain syndrome symptoms, or history of significant aggressive or suicide risk may not be present. In this case, the clinician needs to share his or her concern about the extent and potential of the patient's drinking habits. Having done this with the patient and family, the examiner may wish to consult with and ask someone from Alcoholics Anonymous or another program, to visit the patient. It is important to do this while the patient is in the hospital. If the patient is being seen on an outpatient basis, a joint session with someone from an alcohol program to facilitate referral is in order. Even so, attrition is likely to be as high as 40% (Smart et al., 1977).

There are other important aspects to assessment in the subacute stage. Is there a question of affective illness? Are there persisting signs of psychosis of organic brain syndrome? Who is involved with the patient and what attitudes are present in significant others? Does the examiner regard his or her task, after treating the acute phase, as being over?

In the following section, assessment of the patient's mental status and defensive postures and motivation in all participants in the treatment task is addressed.

Mental Status Examination. A full formal mental status examination should be performed after all acute symptoms have subsided. (See also Chapter 2.) The first reason for doing so is that it provides a basis for assessing future mental functioning. Second, it can help define the need for full psychometric examination by a psychologist. And third, it provides a structure

for the examiner to note presence or absence of neurologic or psychological signs in the present.

Where withdrawal signs and symptoms are short-lived, the examiner's tasks are relatively few. Organic brain syndrome will not likely be present. The examiner needs more history about the context of drinking. Was the acute episode one of pathologic intoxication? If so, this probably indicates the simplest continuing assessment. Is there history of previous CNS insult, or history or evidence of temporal lobe epilepsy? Was the individual unusually stressed or fatigued? Are there any concurrent debilitating medical conditions? If the examiner is certain that the episode was pathologic intoxication, full explanation of the alcohol intake-response problem to the patient and family or significant others is necessary. This may be sufficient intervention.

It is suggested that ancillary sources of information about the patient's drinking be obtained by the examiner early in treatment. If preliminary results from one study hold, computers may be helpful in identifying problem drinking. In 36 men referred to an alcohol program, extent of drinking was found to be similar by two psychiatrists and self-disclosure to the computer, but the men admitted higher quantities of drinking to the computer (Lucas et al., 1977)! Extent and pattern of drinking are key to identifying early patterns of problem drinking, yet, as addressed next, denial and minimization are fixed facets of the defensive posture of alcoholics.

Alcoholic Defensive Postures. Denial and minimization are well-known concomitants of alcohol abuse and elements of this posture need to be understood. The first problem concerns the double-bind situation of the alcoholic. Alcohol is widely regarded and accepted as a social facilitator yet there is social stigma cast on alcohol abuse. As Wuthrich (1977) has noted, in society's definition, breaching accepted social behavior is as important as drinking itself, obviously reeducation in general is needed. Excusing the person who has had one too many drinks occurring over an extended period may not really do that person a favor. After all, in order to become alcoholic, someone must continue to drink and drink.

As for "self-disclosure" about drinking, it appears that among abstainers and moderate drinkers, history of alcohol intake is accurately given by both men and women. Heavy drinkers and alcoholics score low in self-disclosure about their alcohol intake (Miller et al., 1977). Denial is also thought to be a major factor in early dropout from treatment (Altman et al., 1978). Early in the subacute stage, the examiner must be prepared to work with the self-disclosure problem. The most critical factor is accurate knowledge about the patient's drinking patterns, and having the person know the examiner has that knowledge. Involving the family, employer, or any significant others and talking over with them the negative effects alcohol has had on the patient is advised. Involving alcohol program outreach consultants may also be beneficial.

The examiner must also be aware of the dissociative effects of alcohol. This is a later stage problem in alcohol abuse and signals that "denial" has neuropsychological components. Alcohol addicts often do not recall negative emotions while drunk, and also recall drinking only in terms of predrinking expectations when they become sober (Diethelm and Barr, 1962; McGuire et al., 1966; McNamee et al., 1968; Tamerin et al., 1970). Over time, with continued drinking, this amounts to state-dependent learning and clearly different drug and nondrug behavior. It can be reproduced experimentally in normal people and alcoholics (Goodwin et al., 1969; Parker et al., 1974). Again, the examiner, the patient, and the family must be aware of this split phenomenon, which, when clarified, may help to prompt the patient's being receptive to treatment. Psychomotor examination both when sober and after administration of alcohol helps to document this process. Particularly early in the course of abuse, fragments of recollection may aid the patient's recognition of the problem.

Family Defensive Postures.   Defensive postures are taken by significant others of alcoholics as well. The examiner must be aware that denial may operate in family members who choose not to perceive the extent of the alcoholic's drinking. The family member may collude in hiding the drinking, feel unable to confront the alcoholic, or lack the strength to seek treatment in the face of the alcoholic's refusal to do so. Nonetheless, effort must be made in the case of this chronic relapsing illness to confront denial and to support the significant other's desire to encourage the alcoholic to seek treatment. A later section will elaborate some aspects of alcoholism and the family.

Defensive Postures in Caregivers.   Negative attitudes also exist in health care personnel (Lisansky, 1975; Cornish and Miller, 1976). Teaching programs on alcoholism in medical school are scant. Typically, alcoholism goes undiagnosed, especially when the person involved is deemed in some fashion respectable. Physicians themselves, for example, have high rates of alcoholism, and often successful executives who have three-martini lunches are diagnosed as having something other than alcoholism. Patients' alcoholism may also go undiagnosed because of fear of compromising their positions. The whole pattern of avoiding diagnosis of alcoholism among clinicians is typically characterized by a spoken humanistic, knowledgeable approach contrasted with actual behavior that selectively avoids, denies, or ridicules the possibility of alcoholism (Wolfe et al., 1965).

Gerard and Saenger (1966), Allen et al. (1971), Pisani (1977), and Smart et al. (1978) examined the nature of initial treatment and referral patterns. They strongly suggest that an initial comprehensive medical approach to the alcoholic patient be taken and that referral contacts be built in to a subacute period in which definitive contact with follow-up care facilities is accomplished. Too often health care personnel do not see their task as a bridging one for aftercare. The patient, as previously discussed, reacting and remembering differently when sober than drunk, may all-too-willingly and seemingly agreeably "yes" his or her way out of the "quick detoxification" situation. Full medical assessment in a medically oriented facility with a comprehensive approach is most likely to reduce the dropout rate in the relapsing condition of alcoholism.

Loss of Control and Craving. Operant myths in alcoholism are the concepts of craving or loss of control (Mello and Mendelson, 1975) and relapse. These myths help create the helplessness that families and examiners of alcoholics, and indeed alcoholics themselves, feel about their condition. As with many myths, there is a germ of validity to the concepts of craving but it has been overgeneralized. That relapsing drinking is directly associated with craving for alcohol and loss of control is only partly true, and the effect may be minimal. The typology of relapse is more complicated and contains definitive themes. Both pleasant and unpleasant affects can lead to drinking as can both success and failure. Social anxiety and diminished conscious vigilance also seem to be important factors (Litman et al., 1977). But studies repeatedly show that even chronic abusers can control intake even with alcohol freely available (Allman et al., 1972; Bigelow and Liebson, 1972; Sobell et al., 1972). Apparently no overwhelming upsurging physiologic or psychologic desire need occur when an alcoholic takes the smallest sip of a drink. The added ingredients of a cognitive label that alcohol will be the only source of satisfaction must also be present and social context taken into account.

The examiner should not merely apply the label "craving" or "loss of control" and feel comfortable about nothing more being done. Rather, inquiry might proceed taking partial and different phenomena into account as follows. Binge drinkers and steady drinkers have different behaviors. Steady drinkers are more likely to respond to external social cues (Ludwig et al., 1977). Examining and interrupting social cueing is in order here. The dipsogenic effect of alcohol at peak blood levels may result in further intake, therefore, assessing sipping versus gulping patterns of drinking is critical. The alcoholic can be made sharply aware of this (Lawson, 1977). If there is true craving, alcoholics who experience it are more likely to be anxious about drinking, be at later stages of drinking, have somatic symptoms, and impairment in integrating ambiguous situations, suggesting cognitive deficit (Tarter and Sugerman, 1977). Thus, the presence of craving, as such, is a poor prognostic, later-stage sign. Here the notion of total abstinence is useful since the least interoceptive discomfort triggers more drinking.

Acute Neuropsychological Deficits. Psychometric examination is indicated if mental status examination reveals deficits in short-term memory or abstraction. Studies indicate that there is an acute "zonk" effect of alcohol (Page and Linden, 1974; Goldman et al., 1978) in which the first 1–2 weeks for deficits after drinking is an acute recovery period, therefore psychometric examination is best done after the first fortnight. Abstract reasoning, sequencing, coding, and short-term memory recover in about a week. Motor skills and motor coordination recover in 2 weeks. Unfamiliar tasks involving new information, processing visuospatial and cutaneospatial learning may take several weeks to recover.

Assessment of Psychological Symptoms. For drinkers who drink more than moderately, the concept of continuing inpatient assessment for 4 weeks followed by outpatient treatment is quite valid. Presence of the following neuropsychological conditions increase the need for inpatient treatment first: presence of continuing cognitive deficit; present or past affective illness (manic or depressive symptoms); present or past aggressive behavior or suicidal ideation or act with or without alcohol; presence of psychotic symptoms, such as paranoid or nonparanoid delusions or hallucinosis.

Assessment of affective illness and alcohol abuse presents a vexing problem. Is the patient's mood altered because of drinking or did a mood disorder precede drinking? Answers are not much clearer since Mello's review (1968). The problem in assessing affect and alcohol remains that anxiety, dysphoria, and euphoria are generated by alcohol, and more drinking produces more such symptoms. Assessment of the degree of affective illness is confounded by alcohol's effect on other symptoms such as energy, fatiguability, general interest, sleep, appetite, and libido. A similar difficulty arises with persisting psychotic symptoms. Paranoid jealousy, for example, resembles paranoid states in general, and alcoholic hallucinosis resembles schizophrenia. If a family history of psychiatric illness uncomplicated by alcoholism exists, this may help with diagnosis. (See also Chapters 6, 7, 8, 9, 10, and 11.)

The examiner needs to become familiar with morbid psychological symptoms. Rating scales such as the Brief Psychiatric Rating Scale (Overall and Gorham, 1962) for affective illness and psychosis, and the Hamilton Scale for Depression (Hamilton, 1969) are useful. These scales are shown in Tables 15-7 and 15-8. The examiner may choose to obtain psychiatric consultation.

Inpatient psychiatric referral may be desirable when it is apparent that severe symptoms can be assessed more clearly if the patient remains off alcohol; when the need for definitive pharmacotherapy will then be more certain; if the potentiation of neuroleptics by alcohol presents a risk; and/or if compliance with proper medication use seems feasible.

SUICIDE AND ALCOHOLISM

Most suicides are known to have either affective illness or alcoholism (Robins et al., 1959; Dorpat and Ripley, 1960; Barraclough., 1974). These are overlapping categories, since many alcoholics, variously estimated as 24%–59% of them, are depressed (Woodruff et al., 1973; Robins et al., 1977; Weissman et al., 1977). Schneidman (1969) classified motive in completed suicides into three groups: "egotic" or intrapersonal; dyadic—in relation to a significant other; and "ageneric"—fallen out of a place in society. Alcoholics may practice denial and rationalize succesfully, thus may be less subject to "egotic" suicidal motive. However, interpersonal dyadic motives and particularly "ageneric" ones—being isolated and out of place in society—operate significantly. In fact, alcoholism ranks second behind age in discriminant power for predicting suicidal behavior (Litman et al., 1974). (See also Chapter 10.)

In addition, a highly significant specific factor increasing suicide risk in alcoholics is a history of a loss of a close interpersonal tie within the last 6 weeks (Murphy et al., 1967). Drinking alcohol may result in suicide in three ways. First, it may produce confusion and the attempt is undertaken while the person does not have full mental faculties. Second, alcohol is drunk to increase "nerve" enough to attempt suicide, or, third, alcohol is deliberately ingested to potentiate drugs (Beck et al., 1974).

ALCOHOLISM AND AGGRESSION

Belligerent behavior during intoxication and acute withdrawal is common. Further than that, assessment must include history of extent of dangerousness to others. During the subacute phase this history must be obtained in order to plan treatment referral. Small amounts of alcohol inhibit and, with greater intake, facilitate

TABLE 15-7
Brief psychiatric rating scale (BPRS)*

PATIENT'S NAME _____

DATE _____

ITEMS	MARK THE COLUMN HEADED BY THE TERM WHICH BEST DESCRIBES THE PATIENT'S PRESENT CONDITION	NOT PRESENT	VERY MILD	MILD	MODERATE	MODERATELY SEVERE	SEVERE	EXTREMELY SEVERE
Somatic concern	Degree of concern over present bodily health; rate the degree to which physical health is perceived as a problem by the patient, whether complaints have a realistic basis or not	0	1	2	3	4	5	6
Anxiety	Worry, fear, or overconcern for present or future; rate solely on the basis of verbal report of patient's own subjective experiences; do not infer anxiety from physical signs or from neurotic defense mechanisms	0	1	2	3	4	5	6
Emotional withdrawal	Deficiency in relating to the interviewer and to the interview situation; rate only the degree to which the patient gives the impression of failing to be in emotional contact with other people in the interview situation	0	1	2	3	4	5	6
Conceptual disorganization	Degree to which the thought processes are confused, disconnected or disorganized; rate on the basis of integration of the verbal products of the patient; do not rate on the basis of patient's subjective impression of his own level of functioning	0	1	2	3	4	5	6
Guilt feelings	Overconcern or remorse for past behavior; rate on the basis of the patient's subjective experiences of guilt as evidenced by verbal report with appropriate affect; do not infer guilt feelings from depression, anxiety or neurotic defenses	0	1	2	3	4	5	6
Tension	Physical and motor manifestations of tension "nervousness," and heightened activation level; tension should be rated solely on the basis of physical signs and motor behavior and not on the basis of subjective experiences of tension reported by the patient	0	1	2	3	4	5	6

CATEGORIES AND RATINGS

TABLE 15-7—Continued

ITEMS	MARK THE COLUMN HEADED BY THE TERM WHICH BEST DESCRIBES THE PATIENT'S PRESENT CONDITION	NOT PRESENT	VERY MILD	MILD	MODERATE	MODERATELY SEVERE	SEVERE	EXTREMELY SEVERE
					CATEGORIES AND RATINGS			
Mannerisms and posturing	Unusual and unnatural motor behavior, the type of motor behavior which causes certain mental patients to stand out in a crowd of normal people; rate only abnormality movement; do not rate simple heightened motor activity here	0	1	2	3	4	5	6
Grandiosity	Exaggerated self-opinion, conviction of unusual ability or powers; rate only on the basis of patient's statements about himself or self-in-relation-to-others, not on the basis of his demeanor in the interview situation	0	1	2	3	4	5	6
Depressive mood	Despondency in mood, sadness; rate only degree of despondency; do not rate on the basis of inferences concerning depression based upon general retardation and somatic complaints	0	1	2	3	4	5	6
Hostility	Animosity, contempt, belligerence, disdain for other people outside the interview situation; rate solely on the basis of the verbal report of feelings and actions of the patient toward others; do not infer hostility from neurotic defenses, anxiety or somatic complaints. (Rate attitude toward interviewer under "uncooperativeness.")	0	1	2	3	4	5	6
Suspiciousness	Belief (delusional or otherwise) that others have now, or have had in the past, malicious or discriminatory intent toward the patient; on the basis of verbal report, rate only those suspicions which are currently held, whether they concern past or present circumstances	0	1	2	3	4	5	6
Hallucinatory behavior	Perceptions without normal external stimulus correspondence; rate only those experiences which are reported to have occurred within the last week and which are described as distinctly different from the thought and imagery processes of normal people	0	1	2	3	4	5	6

	0	1	2	3	4	5	6
Motor retardation — Reduction in energy level evidenced in slowed movements: rate on the basis of observed behavior of the patient only; do not rate on basis of patient's subjective impression of own energy level	0	1	2	3	4	5	6
Uncooperativeness — Evidence of resistance, unfriendliness, resentment, and lack of readiness to cooperate with the interviewer; rate only on the basis of the patient's attitude and responses to the interviewer and the interview situation: do not rate on basis of reported resentment or uncooperativeness outside the interview situation	0	1	2	3	4	5	6
Unusual thought content — Unusual, odd, strange, or bizarre thought content; rate here the degree of unusualness, not the degree of disorganization of thought processes	0	1	2	3	4	5	6
Blunted affect — Reduced emotional tone, apparent lack of normal feeling or involvement	0	1	2	3	4	5	6
Excitement — Heightened emotional tone, agitation, increased reactivity	0	1	2	3	4	5	6
Excitement (cont.) — Confusion or lack of proper association for person, place, or time	0	1	2	3	4	5	6
Elation — Overtalkative through overtalkative and overactive; then restless, purposeful activity impaired; then continuous flow of speech with outbursts, activity disorganized; then is destructive at 6 and totally exhausted/disturbed at 7	0	1	2	3	4	5	6

*From Overall, J.E., and Gorham, D.R. 1962. The brief psychiatric rating scale. *Psychol. Reports* 10:799–812.

TABLE 15–8
Hamilton psychiatric rating
scale for depression

PATIENT'S NAME _____

DATE _____

FOR EACH ITEM SELECT THE "CUE" WHICH BEST CHARACTERIZES THE PATIENT

ITEM	CUE
Depressed Mood (Sadness, hopeless, helpless, worthless)	0 Absent 1 These feeling states indicated only on questioning 2 These feeling states spontaneously reported verbally 3 Communicates feeling states nonverbally—i.e., through facial expression, posture, voice, and tendency to weep 4 Patient reports virtually only these feeling states in his spontaneous verbal and nonverbal communication
Feelings of guilt	0 Absent 1 Self-reproach, feels he has let people down 2 Ideas of guilt or rumination over past errors or sinful deeds 3 Present illness is a punishment. Delusions of guilt 4 Hears accusatory or denunciatory voices and/or experiences threatening visual hallucinations
Suicide	0 Absent 1 Feels life is not worth living 2 Wishes he were dead or any thoughts of possible death to self 3 Suicide ideas or gesture 4 Attempts at suicide (*any serious attempt rates 4*)
Insomnia early	0 No difficulty falling asleep 1 Complains of occasional difficulty falling asleep—i.e., more than $\frac{1}{2}$ hour 2 Complains of nightly difficulty falling asleep
Insomnia middle	0 No difficulty 1 Patient complains of being restless and disturbed during the night 2 Waking during the night—any getting out of bed rates 2 (*except for purposes of voiding*)
Insomnia late	0 No difficulty 1 Waking in early hours of the morning but goes back to sleep 2 Unable to fall asleep again if gets out of bed
Work and activities	0 No difficulty 1 Thoughts and feelings of incapacity, fatigue or weakness related to activities; work or hobbies 2 Loss of interest in activity; hobbies or work—either directly reported by patient, or indirect in listlessness, indecision and vacillation (*feels he has to push self to work or activities*)

TABLE 15–8—Continued

ITEM	CUE	
	3	Decrease in actual time spent in activities or decrease in productivity; in hospital, rate 3 if patient does not spend at least three hours a day in activities (*hospital job or hobbies*) exclusive of ward chores
	4	Stopped working because of present illness. In hospital, rate 4 if patient engages in no activities except ward chores, or if patient fails to perform ward chores unassisted
Retardation (*Slowness of thought and speech; impaired ability to concentrate; decreased motor activity*)	0	Normal speech and thought
	1	Slight retardation at interview
	2	Obvious retardation at interview
	3	Interview difficult
	4	Complete stupor
Agitation	0	None
	1	"Playing with" hands, hair, etc.
	2	Hand-wringing, nail-biting, hair-pulling, biting of lips
Anxiety psychic	0	No difficulty
	1	Subjective tension and irritability
	2	Worrying about minor matters
	3	Apprehensive attitude apparent in face or speech
	4	Fears expressed without questioning
Anxiety somatic	0 Absent	Physiological concomitants of anxiety, such as:
	1 Mild	Gastrointestinal—dry mouth, wind, indigestion, diarrhea, cramps, belching
	2 Moderate	Cardiovascular—palpitations, headaches
	3 Severe	Respiratory—hyperventilation, sighing Urinary frequency
	4 Incapacitating	Sweating
Somatic symptoms gastrointestinal	0	None
	1	Loss of appetite but eating without staff encouragement; heavy feelings in abdomen
	2	Difficulty eating without staff urging; requests or requires laxatives or medication for bowels or medication for G.I. symptoms
Somatic symptoms general	0	None
	1	Heaviness in limbs, back or head; backaches, headache, muscle aches; loss of energy and fatigability
	2	Any clear-cut symptom rates 2
Genital symptoms	0 Absent	Symptoms such as: Loss of libido; menstrual
	1 Mild	disturbances
	2 Severe	0 Not ascertained

TABLE 15–8—Continued

ITEM	CUE
Hypochondriasis	0 Not present 1 Self-absorption (bodily) 2 Preoccupation with health 3 Frequent complaints, requests for help, etc. 4 Hypochondriacal delusions
Loss of weight	A. When Rating By History: 0 No weight loss 1 Probable weight loss associated with present illness 2 Definite (according to patient) weight loss B. On Weekly Ratings By Ward Psychiatrist, When Actual Weight Changes Are Measured: 0 Less than 1 lb weight loss in week 1 Greater than 1 lb weight loss in week 2 Greater than 2 lb weight loss in week
Insight	0 Acknowledges being depressed and ill 1 Acknowledges illness but attributes cause to bad food, climate, overwork, virus, need for rest, and so on 2 Denies being ill at all
Diurnal variation	AM PM 0 0 Absent If symptoms are worse in the morning or 1 1 Mild evening, note which it is and rate severity of 2 2 Severe variation
Depersonalization and derealization	0 Absent 1 Mild Such as: Feelings of unreality; nihilistic ideas 2 Moderate 3 Severe 4 Incapacitating
Paranoid symptoms	0 None 1 2 Suspicious 3 Ideas of reference 4 Delusions of reference and persecution
Obsessional and compulsive symptoms	0 Absent 1 Mild 2 Severe
Helplessness	0 Not present 1 Subjective feelings which are elicited only by inquiry 2 Patient volunteers his helpless feelings 3 Requires urging, guidance and reassurance to accomplish ward chores or personal hygiene 4 Requires physical assistance for dress, grooming, eating, bedside tasks or personal hygiene

TABLE 15–8—Continued

ITEM	CUE
Hopelessness	0 Not present 1 Intermittently doubts that "things will improve" but can be reassured 2 Consistently feels "hopeless" but accepts reassurances 3 Expresses feelings of discouragement, despair, pessimism about future, which cannot be dispelled 4 Spontaneously and inappropriately perseverates, "I'll never get well" or its equivalent
Worthlessness	Ranges from mild loss of esteem, feelings of inferiority, self-depreciation to delusional notions of worthlessness 0 Not present 1 Indicates feelings of worthlessness (loss of self-esteem) only on questioning 2 Spontaneously indicates feelings of worthlessness (loss of self-esteem) 3 Different from 2 by degree: Patient volunteers that he is "no good," "inferior," and so on 4 Delusional notions of worthlessness—that is, "I am a heap of garbage" or its equivalent

From Hamilton, M. 1969. Standardized assessment and recording of depressive symptoms. *Psychiatric Nevrologia, Neurochirurgia,* 72:201–205.

increasing aggression (Shuntich and Taylor, 1972). Using alcohol as an excuse, therefore having an expectant set for aggressive display, also contributes powerfully to the mix of alcohol intake and aggressive behavior (Lang et al., 1975). History of intrafamilial violence, criminal behavior, and aggressive use of the automobile while drunk should be sought.

TREATING ALCOHOLISM AS AN ONGOING CONDITION

The problem of alcoholism is as diverse as the types of persons suffering from it. The examiner must remember that alcoholism is likely to be both a polymorphous illness and a chronic relapsing condition.

Studies show that *alcoholics who stay in treatment longer have higher rates of abstinence* (Baekland and Lundwall, 1975). No general stable predictors of good treatment outcome (Gibbs and Flanagan, 1977), or particular treatment modalities more successful than others (Emrick, 1975) have been found. Indeed, there is not even general agreement about reliable prognostic indicators at this time! Abstinence, a commonly used criterion, is not a good indicator, for example, of social/interpersonal functioning, and is not easily verified. Inasmuch as there are practical classification systems for diagnosing alcoholism, general agreement on desirable criteria for successful treatment outcome needs to be developed.

Currently, there are shadowy outlines of partial *prognostic indicators* that can be culled from 45 studies of treatment outcome (Gibbs and Flanagan, 1977). These are: higher *social class*, good *work history*, higher level *job*, *employment* at time of treatment, *married* or cohabiting with the relationship stable, *previous AA contact*, little or no *arrest history*, and diagnosis of *psychoneurosis*. There is little that is specific to alcoholics in these criteria, except previous contact with Alcoholics Anonymous, to

distinguish them from people with favorable prognosis in any sociobehavioral problem.

It is no surprise that ongoing treatment modalities are diverse at present with an individual by individual approach or tailormade treatment. The first goal is to get the person to acknowledge the problem and to have the family supporting treatment. Then treatment must be directed toward long-term management and *individualized and geared to the polymorphous aspects of the habit.* It is possible even with the current incomplete state of knowledge to define whether the patient is at risk because of family history; to assign a stage to the alcohol use, abuse, or dependence state with corroborative history from family, friends, and patient; next, to define whether underlying psychopathology exists and contributes to the alcohol problem, especially earlier; and treat coexisting psychological illness even in intermediate stages; and, finally, to determine whether one of a variety of posttreatment drinking patterns may result. Complete abstinence is not necessarily the only good result.

The pattern of the habit must be examined. Examination of the habit is educational for the patient's and family's own knowledge as well, since cooperation in therapy is all-important. This is more easily done in the earlier stages of abuse, before the patient withdraws to the solace of the bottle with every stress and drinking becomes continuous. The significance of *earlier case findings cannot be overemphasized.* Is the drinking intermittent or constant? What major factors prompt drinking? Is it internal states of discomfort, or is it dependent on external cues? What is the nature of these cues? Can they be broken up or repatterned? What is the pattern of actual drinking? Does the patient drink slowly and in prolonged fashion or does he or she gulp drinks? The overall goal is to question every aspect of taking alcohol and to delay or diminish use. To become alcoholic, a person must drink to excess over time. Any strategy that results in retardation of this will help immeasurably, regardless of relapses. Various approaches to treatment of alcoholism are briefly summarized next.

Psychological Therapies

Individual, group, and family therapies have all been used for ongoing treatment of alcoholism (Emrick, 1975). Although there are no predictors for selection of patients, there is agreement about the nature of the therapeutic attitude in all these modalities. Establishing a relationship of rapport with the alcoholic is central. Alcoholics commonly anticipate rejection, and passivity on the part of the therapist may be interpreted as rejection. Likewise, frequent and regular sessions must be scheduled, and the therapist must be prepared to be active. Denial of the condition must be addressed, and resultant maladaptive mismanaged behavior identified. The individual must be supported through the initial phases in a kindly but firm manner, yet must soon be prepared to take some responsibility for identification of factors that promote drinking (Chafetz, 1975). Especially when there are significant medical or neuropsychological problems, the early phase of treatment and the attempt to involve the patient should be on an inpatient basis for the first few weeks. Alcohol programs with medical and neuropsychological expertise, which have outpatient follow-up studies provided for within their program, are ideal.

Some patients dread and cannot initially use group therapy. Group therapies, when appropriate, help de-isolate patients, and enable them to examine their own and other group members' ways of reacting (Yalom, 1974). Family therapy is particularly useful when conflicts leading to drinking arise primarily out of the family environment.

Self-Help Support Systems

Alcoholics Anonymous, that caring fellowship, has a valuable and central place in the therapy of alcoholism. It is the one organization that has maintained a support system in its 7000 chapters when treatment within the medical community has been, at best, fragmented. Furthermore, when the alcoholic refuses therapy, family members can get helpful support within AA.

Major problems that the examiner might find with AA are that some patients are put off by an evangelistic, confessional approach and are unable to bring themselves to speak in a group setting. Also, many AA chapters find adjunctive pharmacotherapy incompatible with the AA philosophy, and wittingly or unwittingly the patient will use this contradiction in goal orientation as an excuse for noncompliance.

Aversion and Conditioning Therapies

Aversion and conditioning therapies have a better outcome when there is a sustaining patient-therapist relationship. Patients who respond to these therapies are also likely to be of a higher socioeconomic status (Chafetz, 1975). The keystone of these therapies is that the wish to drink is a learned habit. Depatterning consists of juxtaposing the drinking of alcohol and (a) an unpleasant effect such as mild electric shock, or (b) taking apomorphine and inducing vomiting. In addition, relaxation techniques are also taught so the patient may overcome anxiety and focus on issues related to drinking and the therapy. As mastery progresses, the patient is asked to merely take alcohol into his or her mouth and spit it out when a signal light or sound occurs. Finally, rejecting alcohol is linked only to the patient's own thought constructs (Slater and Roth, 1970). Reinforcement or reconditioning are done when the patient again craves drink, or otherwise at half-yearly to yearly intervals thereafter.

Deterrent Drug Therapy

Disulfiram (Antabuse) therapy, given orally or via subcutaneous implants, depends upon the alcoholic's fear of a disulfiram-ethanol reaction (DER, described later) occurring especially among impulsive drinkers. As reviewed by

Kitson (1977), however, both the positive effect of disulfiram on maintaining abstinence is controversial, and its mechanism of action is rather more complex than originally thought.

Especially with infrequent oral doses or subcutaneous implants, pharmacologic effects of disulfiram are not thought to be enough to be other than a psychological deterrent. Placebo/double-blind studies are needed to resolve this issue. Human studies of mechanism of action are ethically problematic, and animal studies have produced controversial results. Disulfiram presumably impedes action of acetaldehyde dehydrogenase which results in accumulated acetaldehyde when ethanol is drunk. Increased acetaldehyde produces symptoms of uneasiness, weakness, flushing, nausea, vomiting, hypotension and tachycardia, headache, tracheal irritation, coughing, and stridor. This is the DER effect. After examining the evidence, Kitson concluded that the proposed mechanism is largely correct, but with modifications: (a) that a metabolite of disulfiram, diethyldithiocarbamate or DDC, is more likely the active principle, and further studies need to consider the action and plasma levels of both; and (b) that other effects of disulfiram or DDC are likely. One effect is that acetaldehyde releases serotonin stores. Notably, DER symptoms are very much like those in patients with carcinoid tumor. The second effect is that disulfiram and/or DDC inhibit dopamine-β-hydroxylase, thus decreasing production of norepinephrine. However, without norepinephrine production, acetaldehyde alone produces vasodilatation, thus creating hypotension.

Disulfiram or DDC results in reduction of the rate of metabolism of some medications (isoniazid, paraldehyde, and phenytoin). Use of these drugs as well as cough mixtures, vinegar; and even aftershave lotion in combination with disulfiram should be cautioned against. DDC may also prolong prothrombin time, thus anticoagulant doses would need to be adjusted.

Medical contraindications of disulfiram are: history of heart disease, psychosis, epilepsy, hepatic or nephritic conditions, asthma, or diabetes mellitus. Use of disulfiram includes fully instructing the patient, being certain there are no medical contraindications, gaining his or her consent to prescribe the drug, and making sure the patient knows what substances to avoid. The initial dose is 500 mg per day given as a single dose. This is reduced after a week to 250 mg per day or less. Unpleasant side effects that might occur at higher doses are fatigue, tremor, metallic taste, mild gastrointestinal disturbances, dermatologic problems, and impotence. Reduction in dose usually clears up these problems. The patient is instructed that the DER will be in effect $1-1\frac{1}{2}$ weeks after ingesting disulfiram (Ritchie, 1975).

Lithium Therapy and Alcoholism

There is placebo/double-blind evidence from two studies that suggests that lithium is of benefit in alcoholism (Kline et al., 1974; Merry et al., 1976). In the first study, manic-depressive and depressive patients were excluded. Half of the patients completed the 48 weeks of the study: 75% of the alcoholics significantly reduced disabling drinking and benefited from use of lithium. In the second study, spanning over a year, lithium enabled patients with depression and drinking to greatly reduce their alcohol consumption. Alcoholic patients without depression benefited little or not at all. In both studies, plasma lithium levels maintained were doses of 900–1200 mg per day of lithium carbonate, with plasma levels in the usual therapeutic range for effective illness, that is, 0.8–1.2 mEq/L.

More data and longer-term follow-up studies are needed but these studies highlight the importance of inquiring about affective illness in cases of alcoholism. It also remains to be established whether lithium acts directly or indirectly on alcohol consumption. It may be that the primary benefit may be on the affective, or depressive component, underlying alcoholism.

CHRONIC STAGE OF ALCOHOLISM— NEUROLOGIC DEFICITS

Alcoholic Dementia

Decline in tolerance to alcohol signals that heavy drinking has taken its toll and cerebral atrophy may be present (Ron, 1977). Since the 1950s, evidence has accumulated that atrophy may be more common, even among "heavy drinkers," than is ordinarily supposed (Pluvinage, 1954; Tumarkin, 1955; Courville, 1955; Haug, 1968). Furthermore frontal lobe atrophy in particular is apparent. This makes a significant impact in terms of loss of control behavior, repeated inability to abstain, and, therefore, at this stage, poor rehabilitation potential (Lemere, 1956). Persons with frontal lobe damage display poor judgment, are fatuous, deteriorate in ability to modify behavior despite consequences, and cannot change to new patterns. Standard tests of intellectual functioning often don't reveal problems with frontal lobe function, in fact, if administered may give a misleading impression of the patient's capacities (Fitzhugh, 1960 and 1965; Goldstein, 1965; Jones, 1971; Brewer and Perritt, 1971; McLachlan and Lovinson, 1974).

The clinician must first determine whether there has been any decline in alcohol tolerance even if, for example, the patient appears well-dressed and well-kept. If so, observations need to be made about appropriateness of behavior and judgment. Specialized psychometric examination should be requestd after a minimum of two, or, better, several weeks of abstinence The computerized tomographic (CT) scan has supplanted pneumoencephalogram since the previously mentioned studies were done. This should be ordered and the examiner should ask specifically for assessment of anterior horn enlargement as shown on CT scan, and cerebral atrophy in general.

All in all, alcohol is thought to be the most significant factor in cerebral atrophy occurring in patients in the fifth and sixth decades of age (Courville, 1955; Haug, 1968) even for those with adequate nutrition. Presently, it is not known whether any degree of atrophy secondary to alcoholism is reversible, or whether alcohol produces a premature aging effect (Blusewicz and Dustman, 1977). Prolonged study of reformed alcoholics (more than a year of follow-up observation) is necessary.

Even at the chronic stage, the clinician must identify the problem, which may yet be hidden. Sometimes a very presentable younger patient will come in with only a history of difficulty working. The examiner needs to look for deficits in a full mental status examination, then order and look for atrophy on CT scan. If cerebral or cerebellar atrophy is found, alcohol abuse should immediately be suspected. Even if it is not reversible, the other terrible consequences of profound social alienation, isolation, disintegration, and social instability might yet be prevented. These factors contribute strongly to the last stages of deterioration in alcoholics (Williams, 1977; Gosselin, 1977).

Every effort should be made to enforce abstinence. Good nutrition and vitamin therapies should be instituted. Carney and Sheffield (1978) believe that macrocytosis even without anemia may be a potentially reliable indication of alcohol abuse. Vitamin B_{12} and folate levels in serum should be obtained and replacement therapy instituted.

Wernicke-Korsakoff Syndrome

In this disorder, the Wernicke aspect refers to an encephalopathy that results in extraocular nerve palsies, usually affecting the seventh nerve, or palsy of conjugate gaze, or nystagmus, and ataxia. Doses of 30 mg thrice daily of thiamine are given parenterally since gastritis may inhibit absorption. Wernicke's syndrome is considered to be an emergency requiring prompt effective treatment to avoid permanent deficit (Greengard, 1975).

The Korsakoff component, a deficit in retentive memory along with confabulation, is treated similarly, but is unlikely to be reversible.

Peripheral Neuropathy

Acute compression palsies result from the alcoholic patient lying for a long time in certain positions. Wrist and foot drop (radial and peroneal nerves respectively) result from such pressure injuries. Distal extremity neuropathy producing pain and extreme tactile sensitivity also occurs. Peripheral neuropathy may respond to thiamine administration, usually given slowly (Patten, 1977). Thiamine, 50 mg daily parenterally and later orally should be administered.

Cerebellar Degeneration

Severe, irreversible degeneration of the anterior lobe of the cerebellum is also a concomitant of alcohol abuse. Stance and gait ataxia are common; upper extremities are affected less, and articulation little if at all.

Treatment

Little that is hopeful can be said when alcoholism reaches a chronic stage of neurologic deficits and/or the schizophreniform alcoholic hallucinosis state. Obviously, drinking alcohol will continue to add to the deficit and is contraindicated. The examiner can only attempt to ensure abstinence and good nutrition, and give vitamin supplements. Symptomatic treatment of hallucinosis with low-dose neuroleptics may help with the worst of chronic hallucinations. In the absence of a supportive, protective family, these patients may need to be chronically institutionalized for their own protection.

ALCOHOLISM AND THE FAMILY

Parental Drinking

Problems at school and delinquency, truancy, and dropping out of school are strongly associated with paternal alcoholism (Robins et al., 1962, 1968, 1978; Rosenberg, 1969). Male alcoholics are more inclined to be impulsive, to be arrested, and to be sexually active at a younger age and prone to produce illegitimate offspring. However, while verbal abuse might be common, it remains to be established that alcoholic fathers are more prone than others to physically abuse their children (Mayer et al., 1978). It may be that they withdraw more quickly from the parental role when drinking, and, unlike alcoholic mothers, can do so more easily. Abuse of spouses, however, is a more significant problem.

Alcoholic women who are responsible for care of young children are prone to abuse their children. Dependency and low self-esteem are characteristic of alcoholic women (Beckman, 1977). Furthermore, alcoholic women also are likely to get depressed, which adds a compounding factor in their ability to function as mothers.

In addition to these facts are the different gender patterns of alcohol abuse. Men, who usually develop an alcohol problem earlier in life, would have a considerable effect on young children in the family. The alcoholism of mothers, since women tend to develop alcoholism later, and have a shorter downhill course, may not affect the young children so much as the older ones. Contextual patterns of drinking also need to be taken into account, since alcoholic women drink more alone or with their families, and men drink in a wide variety of circumstances.

Clearly more studies are needed in this area. Comparisons between families with young alcoholic parents and families with older alcoholic parents, and scrutiny of distinct gender-related patterns of drinking and their effect on children are important. History of familial alcoholism, the effect of early losses, being an abused child of an alcoholic parent, familial criminality, and history of affective illness are all important variables in the study of alcoholics' families. And, learning from survivors of alcoholic parents is a potentially important methodologic approach to incorporate into future studies.

Spouses of Alcoholics

Alcoholism is a large factor in divorce (Woodruff et al., 1972) since frequent fights, financial difficulties due to absence from work and job losses, sexual problems, and infidelity are common in alcoholic marriages. Some data suggest that wives of alcoholics who remain in such marriages have a similar pattern in their families of origin. More data are needed, clearly, and the dearth of studies about men with alcoholic wives needs to be corrected (Tomelleri et al., 1977).

Adolescent Alcoholism

Problem drinking in adolescence is growing. Estimates are that 5% of teenagers in the United States show preproblem pattern drinking. The 5% figure comes from the criterion of getting drunk at least once weekly (DHEW, 1975).

The concept of self-derogation is central to the understanding of alcoholism in adolescence (Kaplan, 1975, 1976, 1977). For some teenagers, alcohol becomes a way of managing negative feelings about themselves, feelings very common in adolescence. Unfortunately, alcohol drinking is a poor means of self-enhancement. The problems of alienation from peers, family, school, from society's values at large are not resolved by drinking. Rather, a cycle promoting avoidance of the primary problem and reenforcing the pattern of drinking occurs.

Segal (1975) postulates that adolescents who are problem drinkers have "a guilt-ridden or hostile/aggressive daydreaming style." They also have more contempt for the illegality of substance abuse in general (Stokes, 1974). Feelings of powerlessness, frustration, and dissatisfaction, low expectation for academic advancement, linked to low expectations for acceptance by a desirable peer group, are powerful determinants of college-level adolescent problem drinking. When such a linkage occurs, problem drinking is more likely than if only a single determinant is present. This finding holds for both male and female college students.

However, male preproblem drinkers are more like control males than female preproblem drinkers are to control females among younger people (Jones, 1968; 1971). These differences may exist because, in young males, the desire for power, the alcohol-induced enhancement of aggressive, macho display is incongruent behavior for young females. However, it is unlikely that this alone accounts for later age of onset for drinking problems in females. However, it seems probable that young female problem drinkers are deviant from their female peer group in a way that could be identified sooner. Delineating this will be extremely important, since early identification of potential alcoholics is very important. So far, studies of adolescent alcoholism have been primarily of males since their problem is visible earlier.

Early identification of problem drinking among adolescents is paramount, since opportunities at school for redirecting and influencing achievement are many. Also, the pattern of seeking self-aggrandizement from a bottle is not so fixed or long-standing. Questions about alcohol and drug abuse should be standard in taking a history from an adolescent. Questions about alienation from peer group, family, and school should follow, as should questions designed to assess the extent of self-derogatory thinking. Counseling begun early may prevent grievous patterns of drinking and their sequelae.

Fetal Alcohol Syndrome

No presentation about alcoholism and the family is complete without consideration of the effect of alcohol on prenatal development—it is the most primary prevention possible. There are, at present, data that suggests that alcohol (or its metabolites) is a specific teratogen. Though obviously, abuse of other substances, such as nicotine, caffeine, other drugs, or poor diet may also be contributory factors (Ouellette et al., 1977; Clarren and Smith, 1978). Timing of heavy drinking during pregnancy is important. In general, most maldevelopment is associated with first trimester, while size and nutritional status of the neonate is determined in the last trimester (Little, 1977).

The primary features of fetal alcohol syndrome (FAS) are dysmorphism, especially of facial structures; growth deficiencies both in length and weight, with reduced adipose tissue; and CNS dysfunction. Mental retardation, microcephaly, irritability, and hyperactivity have been seen in over 80% of affected children.

Alcohol intake during pregnancy should be sharply curtailed whenever possible. Appeal to the woman's maternal instincts should be attempted. Interestingly, in Ouellette's study, over a third of heavy drinkers are able to reduce drinking or even stop during the third trimester, but characteristics of those women who reduced their alcohol intake could not be differentiated from those who did not (Rosett et al., 1978). The clinician must inquire about the drinking and substance-using habits of every pregnant woman as early as possible. Since it is not presently known how much alcohol intake is too much in pregnancy, lowering intake of any drug as much as possible is good preventive medicine.

REFERRAL

Several important premises to guide the primary care physician in considering psychiatric referral for persons with alcohol problems are:

1. There is no unitary etiology to clinical presentations of alcohol dependence

2. Any or all of psychosocial, cultural, gender, and genetic variables are important

3. There is no one approach to assessment or treatment

4. Early identification of a problem with alcohol dependence is extremely crucial

5. Scrutiny of emotional adaptation; occupational adaptation; sociofamilial adaptation, and physical health

6. Continued drinking of alcohol is the single worst problem for an alcohol-dependent person

7. The primary clinician must broaden his or her concept of referral for treatment beyond hospitals and physicians

From the premises listed one can derive indications for referral. First, the clinician should be prepared to inquire about various facets of the individual's life adaptation to some extent. Tipoffs, however subtle, of alcohol dependence include: stated concerns by employer, friend, or relative; subtle but notable decline in one or more areas listed in number 5 in the list just given; unexplained physical problems existing in organ systems usually affected early by alcohol; requests for sedative-hypnotic or substitute "minor tranquilizers"; unexplained, usually minor, motor vehicle or household accidents.

Early identification of a problem with alcohol cannot be overemphasized. For the psychiatrist and/or alcohol treatment caregivers, it is frustrating to receive a referral when the person is in some stage of deterioration and usually fixed into a pattern of denying or hiding his or her problems.

The primary care clinician should be prepared for some resistance on the person's part. There may be resistance to acknowledging the problem. Protests such as, "But I go to work everyday," or "I don't drink in the morning" are common. Family members may be helpful but initially may collude with the patient's excuses or deny the problem. Resistance to psychiatric referral such as, "What, do you think I'm crazy?" or "Oh, my problem isn't that bad, I can cut down," or a passive-aggressive stance wherein the person appears to accept referral, but never follows through, are common also. The primary physician must be prepared not for just single simple session, but a process of discussion over time with the alcohol-dependent person. Seeking leverage, from cooperative family members, an enlightened employer, or industrial alcohol program, seeing the patient with a counselor from the local chapter of AA or alcohol treatment center may be desirable. If the patient is uncomfortable about seeing a psychiatrist, a clergyman or psychiatric social-work counselor may be acceptable. The primary intervention, finally, is that the continuing problem pattern of drinking be broken up as much as possible.

Definitive referral to a psychiatrist is necessary when the primary care physician suspects an individual and/or family history of affective disorder, whether primarily depressive or manic-depressive, since alcohol abuse is commonly associated with these conditions. Definitive psychiatric referral should also be sought whenever psychotic symptoms, such as persisting hallucinosis, delusions, or paranoid jealousy syndromes necessitate special intervention and pharmacotherapy and perhaps prompt psychiatric hospitalization. Psychiatrists who are subspecialists in behavior therapies may also be helpful for a subgroup of patients with alcohol dependence.

The primary clinician should be familiar with local AA and Al-Anon Chapters, unaffiliated acute alcohol treatment units, industrial alcohol counseling centers, alcohol treatment units at Veterans Hospitals, and local mental health centers for sources of referral to behavior therapists, marital counselors, and counselors who are members of the clergy. Knowledge of these potential treatment resources plus an attitude of vigilance toward early identification of an alcohol-dependence problem are central aspects of a primary clinician's practice.

LEGAL ISSUES

Tests for Intoxication

If the physician is examining a patient under suspicion for driving while intoxicated, the police may demand that a blood alcohol, urine, or breath test be obtained for their use. There are several guidelines to be noted (Holder, 1971; Eisner, 1979.)

First, the physician is not an agent of the state and is not obliged to practice medicine under duress, in this case acquiesce to the police request that a test be done.

In the second place, on a national basis to date, only two cases have come before the U.S. Supreme Court (*Schmerber vs California*, 383 U.S. 757 1966 and *Breithaupt vs Agram*, 352 U.S. 432 1957). Neither of these has addressed the issue of the physician-patient relationship in this situation, rather, the issue before the court was the ***admissibility of the evidence.*** In *Schmerber vs California*, the patient refused to give the police consent, but the blood alcohol was drawn anyway. Because the patient as a driver was subject to lawful arrest, the blood was found to be evidence subject to seizure without a search warrant. In *Breithaupt vs Agram*, blood was taken from an unconscious patient after an automobile accident, and the court held that no constitutional right to a fair trial was violated by admission of the evidence. Thus, there is yet no precedent case on a national level that addresses either (a) the physician's liability in civil suit; or (b) whether the need for the patient's informed consent to the physician is removed by the police lawfully taking the test result.

In general, however, the physician must not participate in the forcible removal of blood from an actively resisting, clearly not consenting patient. Such action leaves the physician open to charges of brutality and assault and battery regardless of police participation or demand.

The physician should consult with the hospital attorney for statutory guidelines in the state in which he or she practices medicine. For example, in Connecticut and New York, statutes require that no blood sample be taken without the patient's informed consent, despite police request. If the police wish to have a blood test done, a physician employed by the police should obtain it, if the patient is under suspicion.

Medically indicated tests, of course, should be performed as needed by hospital personnel. A medical emergency dictates that necessary tests be obtained even without the patient's consent. However, results of such tests, in order to be made available for legal use, must then be obtained by subpoena. In a conscious or unconscious person, when blood is drawn for ***therapeutic purposes,*** the doctrine of physician-patient privileges applies. However, if a person is unhurt and is brought to the emergency room by the police for the sole purpose of obtaining a blood alcohol level, physician-patient privilege does not apply, and the doctor is not required to obtain a blood alcohol level over the person's objections.

Informed Consent

Informed consent requires: (a) that a patient is in such a state of mind that he or she understands the purpose of the test; (b) that the *physician* and not the police determines this; and (c) that signed consent is then obtained. For a sample of a consent form for "chemical analysis of blood" used in the Yale-New Haven Hospital Emergency Room, see Table 15–9. In Connecticut, for example, refusal to submit to a test of intoxication results in automatic revocation of license to drive.

In many states the doctrine of "implied consent" is used in situations where the patient is unconscious and can neither consent to nor refuse a test. The physician should again consult with the hospital attorney to define procedure in each state. Again, though, it should be noted that the consent is to the police, and not to the physician.

Danger to self or others

Since both suicide and dangerous aggression are important tragic facets of alcohol abuse, the examiner must routinely inquire about both in the process of assessment. This history should be obtained from the patient *and* relevant others.

If the patient has significantly endangered himself or herself or persons close to him or her, particularly if there has been a recent increase or persistence in such behavior, or the alcoholic has suffered a personal loss very recently, the examiner should obtain psychiatric consultation. It must be determined whether either of these problems is severe enough to warrant voluntary admission or, if the patient refuses, legal certification to a psychiatric facility for more specialized evaluation. Furthermore, failure to foresee significant danger to self or others may constitute medical negligence (Holder, 1978). "Due care" must be given to protect the patient. In general, the more obvious and acute the threat, the more likely is the risk of medical liability for negligence. Certification and commitment statues vary from state to state. The psychiatrist and/or the hospital attorney should be consulted for clarification of the state procedure for commitment for psychiatric examination.

TABLE 15–9
Consent to
chemical analysis
of blood

I _____ hereby consent to the drawing of a sample of blood for the purpose of an alcohol or drug content analysis and further authorize the Hospital to turn over the results of such analysis to the police or other authorities.

I understand that I may refuse to submit to the drawing of such a sample, and understand that the Hospital will not draw the sample without my consent whether or not the police request that it be drawn.

_____   _____
Date   Patient

_____
Witness

APPENDIX: CASE HISTORY—THE POSTOPERATIVE MONSTERS

At first glance, the patient may seem to be suffering from a toxic psychosis. A review of the chart and medications, however, did not reveal the presence of toxic state. Careful history taking from the patient's wife (the patient was not in any state to provide coherent history) revealed that the patient had been drinking rather heavily for many years. An alcoholic withdrawal state (delirium tremens) was diagnosed. The patient improved dramatically on a regimen of chlordiazepoxide and vitamin–B complex.

This case illustrates several important aspects of alcoholism:

1. Alcohol withdrawal can occur in individuals who have not been considered to be alcoholic.

2. In evaluating any acute psychotic episode in the general hospital, alcohol withdrawal state should be one of the foremost in differential diagnoses.

3. Careful history taking from significant others can be extremely helpful in the diagnostic process.

PATIENT EVALUATION GRID

DIMENSIONS	CONTEXTS		
	CURRENT (**Current States**)	**RECENT** (**Recent Events** **and Changes**)	**BACKGROUND** (**Culture, Traits,** **Constitution**)
BIOLOGICAL	Diaphoretic, tremors, <u>heart rate 120/min</u>, temperature 101F No medications other than codeine for pain	<u>Strangulated hernia</u>— 4 days ago Excision and herniorrhaphy— 4 days ago General anesthesia— 4 days ago Postoperatively, meperidine 100 mg every 4 hr IM, <u>discontinued</u> after 2 days	Father died of cancer of liver (<u>father was alcoholic</u>) Usual childhood illnesses
PERSONAL	<u>Fearful, visual hallucinations</u> of bugs and monsters Agitated Does not recognize family Mental status: <u>disoriented to time and place; severely impaired recent and immediate memory</u>, uncooperative for other tests	No mood or habit changes reported Appetite: OK Sleep: OK (drinks a "<u>nightcap</u>" every night)	A "domineering" but very outgoing person according to wife <u>Drank several cocktails and one or two bottles of wine at dinner</u> "<u>when he ate home</u>"
ENVIRONMENTAL	In a single room <u>Wife</u> visits	<u>No recent changes</u> reported at home and work Lives with wife (age 50 years) who is socially active Two grown children (ages 29 and 26 years) Patient's mother (age 74 years) living and well	Lower middle class, Catholic background College in hometown Was salesman for several years before being promoted in company—worked his way up to an executive position Married at age 24 years Father died age 55 years when patient was 35 years old One older brother

Demographic data: 53-year-old married male, executive of large company.

RECOMMENDED READINGS

Mendelson, J.H., and Mello, N.K., eds. 1979. *The diagnosis and treatment of alcoholism.* New York: McGraw-Hill. This book has an excellent review of diagnostic criteria for alcoholism, hepatic and gastrointestinal complications, gender and genetic determinants, and five chapters on aspects of treatment of alcoholism.

Pattison, E.M.; Sobell, M.B.; and Sobell, L.C., eds. 1977. *Emerging concepts of alcohol dependence.* New York: Springer Publishing Co. This book compares old and evolving concepts about alcoholism. A new model of alcoholism that challenges traditional ideas, especially about treatment, is emerging. This book helps the practitioner examine ideas (and possibly myths) about the alcoholic.

REFERENCES

Allen, R.P.; Faillace, L.A.; and Wagman, A. 1971. Recovery time for alcoholics after prolonged alcohol intoxication. *Johns Hopkins Med. J.* 128:158–64.

Allman, L.R.; Taylor, H.A.; and Nathan, P.E. 1972. Group drinking during stress: Effects on drinking behavior, affect and psychopathology. *Am. J. Psychiatry* 129:669–78.

Altman, H.; Evenson, R.; and Cho, D.W. 1978. Predicting length of stay by patients hospitalized for alcoholism or drug dependence. *J. Stud. Alcohol.* 39:197–201.

American Psychiatric Association. 1980. *Diagnostic and statistical manual of mental disorders.* (*DSM-III*). Washington, D.C.: American Psychiatric Association.

Baekland, F., and Lundwall, L. 1975. Dropping out of treatment: A critical review. *Psychol. Bull.* 82:738–83.

Barraclough, B.; Bunch, J.; and Nelson, B. 1974. A hundred cases of suicide: Clinical aspects. *Br. J. Psychiatry* 125:355–73.

Barrymore, D., and Frank, G. 1961. *Too much, too soon.* New York: Holt.

Bates, R.C. 1965. The diagnosis of alcoholism. *Appl. Ther.* 7:466–69.

Beck, A.T.; Schuyler, D.; and Herman, I. 1974. Development of suicide attempt scales. In *The prediction of suicide*, eds., A.T., Beck; H.L.P., Resnick;

and D.J. Lettieri, pp. 45–56. Bowie, Md.: Charles Press Publishers, Inc.

Beckman, L.J. 1977. Psychosocial aspects of alcoholism in women. In *Currents in alcoholism—IV*, ed., F.A. Seixas, pp. 367–80. New York: Grune & Stratton.

Bigelow, G.E.; and Liebson, I. 1972. Cost factors controlling drinking. *Psychol. Record* 22:305–14.

Blusewicz, M.J.; Dustman, R.E.; Schenkenberg, T., et al. 1977. Neuropsychologic correlates of chronic alcoholism and aging. *J. Nerv. Ment. Dis.* 165:348–55.

Bourne, P.G. 1975. *Developments in the field of drug abuse. In National drug abuse conference*, eds., E. Senay; V. Shorty; and H. Alksen pp. 197–207. Cambridge, Mass.: Shenkman Publishing Co.

Boyatzis, R.E. 1977. Alcohol and interpersonal aggression. In *Advances in experimental medicine and biology, alcohol intoxication and withdrawal*, ed., M.D. Gross, pp. 345–75. New York: Plenum Press.

Brenner, M.H. 1975. Trends in alcohol consumption and associated illnesses: Some effects of economic changes. *Am. J. Pub. Health* 65:1279–92.

Brewer, C.; and Perrett, L. 1971. Brain damage due to alcohol consumption: An air-encephalographic, psychometric and electroencephalographic study. *Br. J. Addic.* 66:170–82.

Burns, M.; and Moskowitz, H. 1978. Gender-related differences in impairment of performance by alcohol. In *Currents in alcoholism*, vol. 3, ed., F.A. Seixas, pp. 479–92. New York: Grune & Stratton.

Cahalan, D.; 1970. *Problem drinkers*, San Francisco: Jossey-Bass, Inc.

Cahalan, D.; Cisin, I.H.; and Crossley, H.M. 1969. *American drinking practices: A national study of drinking behavior and attitudes.* Monograph no. 6, Rutgers Center of Alcohol Studies, New Brunswick, N.J.

Carney, M.W.P.; and Sheffield, B.F. 1978. Serum folic acid and B-12 in 272 psychiatric in-patients. *Psychol. Med.* 8:139–44.

Chafetz, M.E. 1975. Alcoholism and alcoholic psychosis. In *Comprehensive textbook of psychiatry*, 2nd ed., eds., A.M., Freedman; H.I. Kaplan; and B.J. Sadock, pp. 1331–48. Baltimore: Williams & Wilkins Co.

Clarren, S.K.; and Smith, D.W. 1978. The fetal alcohol syndrome. *N. Engl. J. Med.* 298:1063–67.

Cornish, R.D.; and Miller, M.V. 1976. Attitudes of the registered nurse toward the alcoholic. *J. Psychiatr. Nurs.* 14:19–22.

Courville, C.B. 1955. *Effects of alcohol on the nervous system of man.* Los Angeles: San Lucas Press.

Curlee, J.A. 1970. A comparison of male and female patients at an alcoholism treatment center. *J. Psychol.* 74:239–47.

Cutting, J. 1978. A reappraisal of alcoholic psychoses. *Psychol. Med.* 8:285–96.

Delint, J.E. 1964. Alcoholism, birth rank and parental deprivation. *Am. J. Psychiatry* 120:1062–65.

Department of Health, Education and Welfare. 1975. Young people and alcohol, alcohol health and research world. DHEW publication no. 75–157, p. 4.

Detre, T.P.; and Jarecki, H.G. 1971. *Modern psychiatric treatment*, pp. 296–301. Toronto: J.B. Lippincott.

Devenyi, P.; and Wilson, M. 1971. Abuse of barbiturates in an alcoholic population. *Can. Med. Assoc. J.* 104:219–21.

Diethelm, O.; and Barr, R.M. 1962. Psychotherapeutic interviews and alcohol intoxication. *Q.J. Stud. Alcohol.* 23:243–51.

Dorpat, J.L.; and Ripley, H.S. 1960. A study of suicide in the Seattle area. *Compr. Psychiatry.* 1:349–59.

Dreher, K.F.; and Fraser, J.G. 1967. Smoking habits of alcoholic outpatients. *Int. J. Addict.* 2:259–70.

Efron, V.; Keller, M.; and Gurioli, C. 1974. Statistics on consumption of alcohol and on alcoholism. Rutgers Center of Alcohol Studies, New Brunswick, N.J.

Eisner, J.M. May, 1979. Personal communication.

Emrick, C. 1975. A review of psychologically oriented treatment of alcoholism. II: The relative effectiveness of different treatment approaches and the effectiveness of treatment versus no treatment. *Q. J. Stud. Alcohol,* 36:88–108.

Fisher, G.; and Brickman, H.R. 1973. Multiple drug use of marijuana users. *Dis. Nerv. Syst.* 34:40–43.

Fitzhugh, L.C.; Fitzhugh, K.B.; and Reitan, R.M. 1960. Adaptive abilities and intellectual functioning in hospitalized alcoholics. *Q. J. Stud. Alcohol.* 21:414–23.

Fitzhugh, L.C.; Fitzhugh, K.B.; and Reitan, R.M. 1965. Adaptive abilities and intellectual functioning in hospitalized chronic alcoholics: Further considerations. *Q. J. Stud. Alcohol.* 26:402–11.

Freed, E.X. 1973. Drug abuse by alcoholics: A review. *Int. J. Addict.* 8:451–73.

Funderburk, F.R.; and Allen, R.P. 1977. Assessing the alcoholic's predisposition to drink. In *Advances in experimental medicine and biology*, ed., M.M. Gross, pp. 601–20. New York: Plenum Press.

Gerard, D.L.; and Saenger, G. 1966. Outpatient Treatment of Alcoholism. Toronto: Univ. of Toronto Press.

Gibbs, L.; and Flanagan, J. 1977. Prognostic indicators of alcoholism treatment outcome. *Int. J. Addict.* 12:1097–1141.

Goldman, M.S.; Whitman, R.D.; Rosenbaum, G., et al. 1978. Recoverability of sensory and motor functioning following chronic alcohol abuse. In *Currents in alcoholism—III,* ed., F.A. Seixas. New York: Grune & Stratton.

Goldstein, G.; and Chotlos, J.W. 1965. Dependency and brain damage in alcoholics. *Percept. Mot. Skills* 21:135–50.

Goodwin, D.W. 1979. Alcoholism and heredity. *Arch. Gen. Psychiatry* 36:57–61.

Goodwin, D.W.; Crane, J.B.; and Guze, S.B. 1969. Alcoholic blackouts: a review and clinical study of 100 alcoholics. *Am. J. Psychiatry* 126:191–98.

Goodwin, D.W.; Schulsinger, F.; Hermansen, L., et al. 1973. Alcohol problems in adoptees raised apart from biological parents. *Arch. Gen. Psychiatry* 28:238–43.

Goodwin, D.W.; Schulsinger, F.; Knop, J., et al. 1977. Alcoholism and depression in adopted-out daughters of alcoholics. *Arch. Gen. Psychiatry* 34:751–55.

Gosselin, N. 1977. Social disintegration and alcoholic behavior. *Toxicoman.* 10:5–22.

Greenblatt, D.J.; and Shader, R.I. 1975. Treatment of the alcohol withdrawal syndrome. In *Manual for psychiatric therapeutics: practical psychiatry and psychopharmacology*, ed., R.I. Shader, pp. 211–39. New York: Little, Brown.

Greengard, P. 1975. Water-soluble vitamins. In *The pharmacological basis of therapeutics*, eds., L.S. Goodman, and A. Gilman, pp. 1549–52. New York: Macmillan Publishing Co.

Griffiths, R.; Bigelow, G.; and Liebson, I. 1976. Facilitation of human tobacco self-administration by ethanol: a behavioral anaylsis. *J. Exp. Anal. Behav.* 25:279–92.

Gross, M.M.; and Hastey, J.M. 1976. In *Alcoholism: interdisciplinary approaches to an enduring problem*, eds., R.E. Tarter, and A.A. Sugarman, pp. 257–307. Reading, Mass.: Addison-Wesley Publishing Co.

Gross, M.M.; Lewis, E.; and Hastey, J. 1974. Acute alcohol withdrawal syndrome. In *The biology of alcoholism, vol. 3: clinical pathology*, eds., B. Kissin, and H. Begleiter, pp. 191–263. New York: Plenum Press.

Hamilton, M. 1969. Standardized assessment and recording of depressive symptoms. *Psychiatr. Neurol. Neurochir.* 72:201–5.

Haug, J.O. 1968. Pneumoencephalographic evidence of brain damage in chronic alcoholics. *Acta Psychiat. Scand. (Suppl.)* 203:135–43.

Holder, A.R. 1971. Liability for administering a blood test. *J.A.M.A.* 217:119–20.

———— 1978. *Malpractice: Medical malpractice law*, 2nd. ed. pp. 21–22. New York: John Wiley and Sons.

Horn, J.L.; and Wanberg, K.W. 1973. Females are different: On the diagnosis of alcoholism in women. Proc. 1st Ann. Alc. Conf. NIAAA, pp. 332–54.

Irgens-Jensen, O. 1978. The epidemiology of alcohol usage. In *Currents in alcoholism* ed., F.A. Seixas, pp. 277–86. New York: Grune & Stratton.

Isbell, H.; Fraser, H.; Wikler, A., et al. 1955. An experimental study of the etiology of "Rum Fits" and delirium tremens. *Q. J. Stud. Alcohol.* 16:1–33.

Jellinek, E.M. 1960. *The disease concept of alcoholism.* New Brunswick, N.J.: Rutgers Center of Studies on Alcohol.

Jones, M.C. 1968. Personality correlates and antecedents of drinking patterns in adult males. *J. Consult. Clin. Psychol.* 32:2–12.

Jones, M.C. 1971. Personality antecedents and correlates of drinking patterns in women. *J. Consult Clin. Psychol.* 36:61–69.

Kaplan, H.B. 1975. The self-esteem motive and change in self-attitudes. *J. Nerv. Ment. Dis.* 161:265–75.

Kaplan, H.B. 1976. Self-attitude change and deviant behavior. *Soc. Psychiatry* 11:59–67.

Kaplan, H.B.; and Pokorny, A.D. 1977. Alcohol use and self-enhancement among adolescents: A conditional relationship. In *Currents in alcoholism —IV*, ed., F.A. Seixas, pp. 51–76. New York: Grune & Stratton.

Kitson, T.M. 1977. The disulfiram-ethanol reaction: A review. *J. Stud. Alcohol.* 38:96–113.

Kline, N.S.; Wren, J.C.; Cooper, T.B., et al. 1974. Evaluation of lithium therapy in chronic and periodic alcoholism. *Am. J. Med. Sci.* 268:15–22.

Knott, D.H.; and Beard, J.D. 1974. Diagnosis and treatment of acute withdrawal from alcohol. In *A treatment manual for acute drug abuse emergencies*, ed., P.G. Bourne, pp. 118–23. Dept. of Health, Education and Welfare public. no. 16 (ADM), pp. 75–230. Washington, D.C.: U.S. Govt. Printing Office.

Koch-Weser, J.; Sellers, E.M.; and Kalant, H. 1976. Alcohol intoxication and withdrawal. *N. Engl. J. Med.* 294:757–62.

Kojic, T.; Dojcinov, D.; Stojanovic, O., et al. 1977. Possible genetic predisposition for alcohol addiction. In *Advances in experimental medicine and biology, alcohol intoxication and withdrawal—IIIb*, ed., M.M. Gross, pp. 7–24. New York: Plenum Press.

Lang, A.R.; Goeckner, D.J.; Adesso, V.J., et al. 1975. Effects of alcohol on aggression in male social drinkers. *J. Abnorm. Psychol.* 84:508.

Lawson, D.M. 1977. The dipsogenic effect of alcohol and the loss of control phenomenon. In *Advances in experimental medicine and biology*, ed., M.M. Gross, pp. 547–68. New York: Plenum Press.

Lemere, F. 1956. The nature and significance of brain damage from alcoholism. *Am. J. Psychiatry* 113:361–62.

Lieber, C.S. 1977. Cytotoxic effects of alcohol on the liver. In *Advances in experimental medicine and biology, alcohol intoxication and withdrawal—IIIa*, ed., M. Gross, pp. 359–98. New York: Plenum Press.

Lindenbaum, J. 1977. Cytotoxic effects of alcohol on hematopoietic and interstitial cells. In *Advances in experimental medicine and biology, alcohol intoxication and withdrawal—IIIa*. ed., M. Gross, pp. 415–28. New York: Plenum Press.

Lisansky, E.S. 1957. Alcoholism in women: social and psychological concomitants. *Q. J. Stud. Alcohol.* 18:588–623.

Lisansky, E.T. 1975. Why physicians avoid early diagnosis of alcoholism. *N.Y. State J. Med.* 75:1788–92.

Litman, G.K.; Eiser, J.R.; Rawson, N.S.B., et al. 1977. Toward a typology of relapse: a preliminary report. *Drug Alcohol Depend.* 2:157–62.

Litman, R.E.; Faberow, N.L.; Wold, C.I., et al. 1974. Prediction models of suicidal behaviors. In *The prediction of suicide*, eds., A.T. Beck; H.L.P. Resnik; and D.J. Lettieri. Bowie, MD.: Charles Press Publ., Inc.

Little, R.E. 1977. Moderate alcohol use during pregnancy and decreased infant birth weight. *Am. J. Public Health* 67:1154–56.

Lucas, R.N.; Mullin, P.J.; Luna, C.B.X., et al. 1977. Psychiatrists and a computer as interrogators of patients with alcohol-related illnesses: a comparison. *Br. J. Psychiatry* 131:160–67.

Ludwig, A.M.; Cain, R.B.; Wikler, A., et al. 1977. Physiologic and situational determinants of drinking behavior. In *Advances in experimental medicine and biology*, ed., M. Gross, pp. 589–600. New York: Plenum Press.

McGuire, M.T.; Mendelson, J.H.; and Stein, S. 1966. Comparative psychosocial studies of alcoholic and non-alcoholic subjects undergoing experimentally induced ethanol intoxication. *Psychosom. Med.* 28:13–25.

McLachlan, J.F.; and Levinson, T. 1974. Improvement in WAIS block design performance as a function of recovery from alcoholism. *J. Clin. Psychol.* 30:65–66.

McNamee, H.B.; Mello, N.K.; and Mendelson, J.H. 1968. Experimental analysis of drinking patterns of alcoholics: concurrent psychiatric observations. *Am. J. Psychiatry* 124:1063–69.

Mayer, J.; Black, R.; and MacDonald, J. 1978. Child care in families with an alcohol addicted parent. In *Currents in alcoholism—IV*, ed., F.A. Seixas, pp. 329–38. New York: Grune & Stratton.

Mello, N.K. 1968. Some aspects of the behavioral pharmacology of alcohol. In *Psychopharmacology: a review of progress, 1957–1967*, PHS pub. 1863, ed., D.H. Efron, pp. 787–809. Washington, D.C.: U.S. Govt. Printing Office.

Mello, N.K. 1978. Behavioral pharmacology of human alcohol, heroin and marijuana use. In *The bases of addiction*, J. Fishman, pp. 133–55. Berlin: Abakon.

Mello, N.K.; and Mendelson, J.H. 1975. Alcoholism: a biobehavioral disorder. In *American handbook of psychiatry*, ed., M. Reiser, pp. 371–403. New York: Basic Books.

Merry, J.; Reynolds, C.M.; Bailey, J., et al. 1976. Prophylactic treatment of alcoholism by lithium carbonate. *Lancet* 2:481–82.

Miller, P.M.; Ingham, J.G.; Plant, M.A., et al. 1977. Alcohol consumption and self-disclosure. *Br. J. Addict.* 72:296–300.

Moskowitz, H.; and Murray, J.T. 1976a. Alcohol and backward masking of visual information. *J. Stud. Alcohol.* 37:40–45.

Moskowitz, H. and Murray, J.T. 1976b. Decrease of iconic memory after alcohol. *A. J. Stud. Alcohol.* 37:278–83.

Mulford, H.A. 1964. Drinking and deviant drinking. *A. J. Stud. Alcohol.* 25:634–50.

Murphy, G.E.; Armstrong, J.W.; Hermele, S.L., et al. 1979. Suicide and alcoholism. *Arch. Gen. Psychiatry* 36:65–69.

Nathan, H., and Turnbull, J. 1974. Psychiatrist's role in combating drunken driving. *Can. Psychiatr. Assoc. J.* 19:381–85.

National Council on Alcoholism, Criteria Committee 1972. Criteria for the diagnosis of alcoholism. *Ann. Intern. Med.* 77:249–58.

Ouellette, E.M.; Rosett, H.L.; and Rosman, N.P. 1977. Adverse effects on offspring of maternal alcohol abuse during pregnancy. *N. Engl. J. Med.* 297:528–30.

Overall, J.E.; and Gorham, D.R. 1962. The brief psychiatric rating scale. *Pscyhol. Reports* 10:799–812.

Page, R.D., and Linden, J.D. 1974. "Reversible" organic brain syndrome in alcoholics: a psychometric evaluation. *Q. J. Stud. Alcohol.* 35:98–107.

Parker, E.S.; Alkana, R.L.; Birnbaum, I.M., et al. 1974. Alcohol and the disruption of cognitive processes. *Arch. Gen. Psychiatry* 31:824–28.

Patten, J. 1977. *Neurological differential diagnosis*, pp. 117, 279. New York: Springer-Verlag.

Pisani, V.D. 1977. The detoxication of alcoholics—aspects of myth, magic or malpractice. *J. Stud. on Alcohol.* 38:972–85.

Pluvinage, R. 1954. Les atrophies cérébrales des alcooliques. *Bull. Mem. Soc. Hop. Paris* 70:524–26.

Rathod, N.H., and Thomson, I.G. 1971. Women alcoholics: a clinical study. *Q. J. Stud. Alcohol* 32:15–52.

Raynes, A.; Patch, V.D.; and Judson, B. 1975. In *Developments in the field of drug abuse conference* eds., E. Senay; V. Shorty; and H. Alksen, pp. 250–53. Cambridge, Mass.: Schenkman Pub. Co.

Ritchie, J.M. 1975. The aliphatic alcohols. In *The pharmacological basis of therapeutics*, eds., L.S. Goodman, and A. Gilman, pp. 137–51. New York: Macmillan Publishing Co.

Robins, E.; Gentry, K.A.; and Munoz, R.A. 1977. A contrast of the three more common illnesses with the ten less common in a study, and 18-month followup of 314 psychiatric emergency room patients: II Characteristics of patients with the three more common illnesses. *Arch. Gen. Psychiatry* 34:269–81.

Robins, E.; Murphy, G.E.; Wilkinson, R.H., Jr., et al. 1959. Some clinical considerations in the prevention of suicide based on a study of 134 successful suicides. *Am. J. Public Health* 49:888–99.

Robins, L.N.; Bates, W.M.; and O'Neal, P. 1962. Adult drinking patterns of former problem children. In *Society, culture and drinking patterns*, eds., D.J. Pittmans, and C.R. Snyder. New York: John Wiley.

Robins, L.N.; Murphy, G.E.; and Breckenridge, M.B. 1968. Drinking behavior of young urban men. *Q. J. Stud. Alcohol.* 29:657–84.

Robins, L.N.; West, P.A.; Ratcliff, K.S., et al. 1978. Father's alcoholism and children's outcomes. In *Currents in alcoholism—IV*, ed., F.A. Seixas, pp. 313–27. New York: Grune & Stratton.

Ron, M.A. 1977. Brain damage in chronic alcoholism: a neuropathological, neuroradiological and psychological review. *Psychol. Med.* 7:103–12.

Rosenberg, C.M. 1969. Determinants of psychiatric illness in young people. *Br. J. Psychiatry* 115:907–15.

Rosett, H.L.; Ouellette, E.M.; Weiner, L., et al. 1978. Therapy of heavy drinking during pregnancy. *Obstet. Gynecol.* 51:41–46.

Sarles, H. 1977. Alcohol and the pancreas. In *Advances in experimental medicine and biology—Illa*, ed., M.M. Gross, pp.429–48. New York: Plenum Press.

Schmitz, R.E. 1978. The prevention and management of the acute alcohol withdrawal syndrome by the use of alcohol. In *Currents in alcoholism—III*, ed., F.A. Sexias, pp. 575–90. New York: Grune & Stratton.

Schneidman, E. 1969. Prologue, *On the nature of suicide.* San Francisco: Jossey-Bass.

Schukit, M.A.; Goodwin, D.A.; and Winokur, G. 1972. A study of alcoholism in half siblings. *Am. J. Psychiatry* 128:1132–36.

Schukit, M.A.; and Morrissey, E.R. 1976. Alcoholism in women: some clinical and social perspectives with an emphasis on possible subtypes. In *Alcoholism in women and children*, eds., M. Greenblatt, and M.A. Schuckit. New York: Grune & Stratton.

Schut, J.; File, K.; and Wohlmuth, T. 1973. Alcohol use by narcotic addicts in methadone maintenance treatment. *Q. J. Stud. Alcohol.* 34:1356–59.

Segal, B. 1975. Personality factors related to drug and alcohol use. In *Predicting adolescent and drug abuse: a review of issues, methods, and correlates*, ed., D.J. Lettieri, pp. 165–91. Washington, D.C.: National Institute on Drug Abuse.

Selzer, M.L. 1961. Alcoholism: diagnostic considerations. *Industr. Med. Surg.* 30:457–60.

Sereny, G.; and Kalant, H. 1965. Comparative clinical evaluation of chlordiazepoxide and promazine in treatment of alcohol-withdrawal syndrome. *Br. Med. J.* 1:92–97.

Shuntich, R.J.; and Taylor, S.P. 1972. The effects of alcohol on human physical aggression. *J. Exp. Res. Personal.* 6:34–38.

Slater, E.T.V.; and Roth, M. 1969. *Clinical psychiatry*, 3rd ed. pp. 399–400. Baltimore: Williams & Wilkins.

Smart, R.G.; Finley, J.; and Funston, R. 1977. The effectiveness of post detoxification referrals: effects on later detoxification admissions, drunkenness and criminality. *Drug Alc. Depend.* 2:149–55.

Smart, R.G.; and Gray, G. 1978. Multiple predictors of dropout from alcoholism treatment. *Arch. Gen. Psychiatry* 35:363–67.

Sobell, L.C.; Sobell, M.B.; and Christelman, W.C. 1972. The myth of "one drink." *Behav. Res. Ther.* 10:119–23.

Stokes, J.P. 1974. Personality traits and attitudes and their relationship to student drug-using behavior. *Int. J. Addict.* 9:267–87.

Tamerin, J.S.; Weiner, S.; and Mendelson, J.H. 1970. Alcoholics' expectancies and recall of experiences during intoxication. *Am. J. Psychiatry* 126:1697–1704.

Tarter, R.E.; and Sugerman, A.A. 1977. Role of drinking pattern, psychosocial history, cognitive style, motor control and personality variables. In *Advances in experimental medicine and biology—IIIb*, ed., M.M. Gross, pp. 569–87. New York: Plenum Press.

Tec, N. 1973. A clarification of the relationship between alcohol and marijuana. *Br. J. Addict.* 68:191–95.

Thompson, W.L. 1978. Management of alcohol withdrawal syndromes. *Arch. Intern. Med.* 138:278–83.

Thompson, W.L.; Johnson, A.D.; and Maddrey, W.L. 1975. Diazepam and paraldehyde for treatment of severe delirium tremens: a controlled trial. *Ann. Intern. Med.* 82:175–80.

Tinklenberg, J.R. 1973. Alcohol and violence. In *Alcoholism: progress in research and treatment*, eds., P. Bourne, and R. Fox, pp. 195–210. New York: Academic Press.

Tomelleri, C.J.; Herjanic, M.; Herjanic, B.M.; et al. 1977. The wife of an alcoholic. In *Currents in alcoholism—IV*, ed., F.A. Seixas, pp. 29–38. New York: Grune & Stratton.

Tumarkin, B.; Wilson, J.D.; and Snyder, G. 1955. Cerebral atrophy due to alcoholism in young adults. *U.S. Armed Forces Med. J.* 6:57–74.

Victor, M. 1966. Treatment of alcoholic intoxication and the withdrawal syndrome. *Psychosom. Med.* 28:636–49.

Victor, M. 1974. Treatment of alcohol intoxication and the withdrawal syndrome: A critical analysis of the use of drugs and other forms of therapy. In *A treatment manual for acute drug abuse emergencies*, ed., P.G. Bourne, pp. 105–77. DHEW Publication No. (ADM) 75–230. Washington, D.C.: U.S. Govt. Printing Office.

Victor, M.; and Adams, R.D. 1953. The effect of alcohol on the nervous system. *Proc. Assoc. Res. Nerv. Ment. Dis.* 32:526–73.

Waller, J.A. 1972. Factors associated with alcohol and responsibility for fatal highway crashes. *Q. J. Stud. Alcohol.* 33:160–70.

Waller, S.; and Jorch, B.D. 1977. First drinking experiences and present drinking patterns: A male-female comparison. *Am. J. Drug Alc. Abuse.* 4:109–21.

Wanberg, K.W.; and Horn, J.L. 1970. Alcoholism symptom patterns of men and women: A comparative study. *Q. J. Stud. Alcohol.* 31:40–61.

Weissman, M.M.; Pottenger, M.; Kleber, H.; et al. 1977. Symptom patterns in primary and secondary depression: a comparison of primary depressives with depressed opiate addicts, alcoholics and schizophrenics. *Arch. Gen. Psychiatry* 34:854–62.

Williams, R.J. 1977. Social stability on admission and success of inpatient treatment for alcoholism. *Drug. Alc. Depend.* 2:81–90.

Winokur, G., and Clayton, P.J. 1968. Family history studies. IV. Comparison of male and female alcoholics. *Q. J. Stud Alcohol.* 29:885–91.

Wolfe, I.; Chafetz, M.E.; Blane, H.T., et al. 1965. Social factors in the diagnosis of alcoholism in social and nonsocial situations. II. Attitudes of physicians. *Q. J. Stud. Alcohol.* 26:72–77.

Wolfe, S.M.; and Victor, M. 1971. The physiologic basis of the alcohol withdrawal syndrome. In *Recent advances in studies of alcoholism*, eds., N.K. Mello, and J.H. Mendelson, pp. 188–99. Washington, D.C.:U.S. Govt. Printing Office.

Woodruff, R.A.; Guze, S.B.; and Clayton, P.J. 1972. Divorce among psychiatric outpatients. *Br. J. Psychiatry* 121:289–92.

Woodruff, R.A.; Guze, S.B.; Clayton, P.J., et al. 1973. Alcoholism and depression. *Arch. Gen. Psychiatry* 28:97–100.

World Health Organization. 1977. International classification of diseases. Manual of the international statistical classification of diseases, injuries, and causes of death, 9th rev. ed. Geneva: WHO.

Wuthrich, P. 1977. Social problems of alcoholics. *Q. J. Stud. Alcohol.* 38:881–90.

Yalom, I. 1974. Group therapy and alcoholism. *Ann. N.Y. Acad. Sci.* 233:85–103.

Zilm, D.H.; Sellers, E.M.; MacLeod, S.M.; et al. 1975. Propranolol effect on tremor in alcohol withdrawal. *Ann. Intern. Med.* 83:234–36.

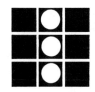

CHAPTER 16

Drug Dependence

Herbert D. Kleber, M.D.

Drug dependency and substance abuse have reached epidemic
proportions in recent years. In addition to such "classical" addictive
drugs as heroin and morphine, numerous new drugs, which were not
initially recognized as addictive or dangerous, are turning out to be both.
Meperidine, benzodiazepines, and phencyclidine are but a few examples. A
drug dependent person often poses complications in medical treatment,
especially when contemplating surgical procedures and analgesia. In
some toxic states due to substance abuse, differential diagnosis from
schizophrenia may be essential for successful outcome. This chapter,
written by a leading authority in the field of drug abuse treatment and
research, deals with these issues in depth, and provides practical
guidelines for management in the appendices.

INTRODUCTION

Mark Twain once said, "Nothing so needs reforming as other people's habits." Drug abuse is an example of a habit usually viewed as needing changing. Sometimes an individual is engaging in behavior that others, such as the family or society, find disagreeable or consider dangerous but the individual wants to continue anyway. The physician may be sought out as the agent responsible for evaluating and initiating the process of change of the individual's bad habit. At other times, the physician may be called upon to treat one of the side effects of the drug use, for example hepatitis secondary to injection of heroin with nonsterile needles or multiple abscesses from frequent injection of barbiturates. Or the physician may be called upon to treat a client who is attempting to hide drug use and is contacting the physician to obtain drugs to carry on the use. Finally, and probably least often, the physician may be confronted with an individual who openly talks about drug use and asks for help in dealing with the problem. This chapter offers information to help in evaluating the type and extent of drug problems and suggests methods for management and referral. It is best that the physician carry out these functions with a nonjudgmental attitude, since a sense of moral condemnation is not conducive to a satisfactory physician-patient relationship. The physician should also always be alert to signs that suggest the possibility of drug abuse, otherwise the diagnosis may be missed.

Definitions

To avoid confusion, it is useful to introduce definitions of certain commonly used terms which have so many different connotations and are often so value-laden as to make discussion difficult. These definitions are from the World Health Organization (Eddy et al., 1965).

1. *Drug:* "Any substance that, when taken into the living organism may modify one or more of its functions." In this chapter, the term will refer specifically to psychoactive substances used primarily for the purpose of altering one's psychological state.

2. *Drug use:* The purposeful taking of any psychoactive substance.

3. *Illegal drug:* In this chapter an illegal drug refers either to a drug that may not be purchased legally in this country except for research (for example, heroin or LSD) or to a drug that can be purchased legally with a prescription but has not been so obtained by the individual in question. Thus, if a teenager's friend takes some prescribed barbiturates from the teenager's medicine cabinet, the friend possesses an illegal drug while the teenager possesses a legal one.

4. *Drug misuse:* The use of legitimately obtained drugs in a manner or amount other than

---

CASE HISTORY 16–1

A 29-year-old, single woman, who works as a secretary in the hospital, was admitted with a fracture of the humerus caused by an automobile accident. During physical examination, it was discovered that the patient had "tracks" on all her veins. The patient's pupils were constricted, and she seemed to be stuporous. Her colleagues had noted that the patient seemed to be often "dozing off" at work. (See Appendix D at the end of this chapter for further discussion and PEG.)

prescribed in order to produce a certain psychological state (for example, using cough preparations containing codeine to get "high" rather than to suppress cough) is drug misuse.

5. *Drug dependence:* As defined by the World Health Organization, drug dependence is "a state, psychic and sometimes also physical, resulting from the interaction between a living organism and a drug, characterized by behavioral and other responses that always include a compulsion to take the drug on a continuous or periodic basis in order to experience its psychic effects and sometimes to avoid the discomfort of its absence. Tolerance may or may not be present. A person may be dependent on more than one drug." The characteristics of the dependent state vary depending on which drug is involved. The term, "drug dependence" has been used to replace the earlier terms, addiction and habituation, which had proven unsatisfactory and had acquired too many negative connotations.

6. *Psychological or psychic dependence:* A state in which a drug produces "a feeling of satisfaction and a psychic drive that require periodic or continuous administration of the drug to produce pleasure or to avoid discomfort."

7. *Physical dependence:* A condition that "manifests itself by intense physical disturbances when the administration of the drug is suspended...these disturbances, i.e., the withdrawal or abstinence syndromes, are made up of specific arrays of symptoms and signs of a psychic and physical nature characteristic for each drug type."

8. *Drug abuse:* The phrase, "drug abuse," is one of the most value-laden and confusing ones in the whole lexicon of medicine. Many writers have, therefore, urged that it not be used. It has been used to mean the taking of any psychoactive drug in any quantity not under medical auspices and/or not for a medicinal purpose. The concept of abuse lies in the *intention* of the user. Thus, an individual who takes an amphetamine-type drug under a physician's direction to help lose weight is a drug user; if the same individual takes the drug to promote

not weight loss but a "speeding" feeling or to stay up all night to study for exams, the person is a drug abuser. By this definition, any use of an illegal drug equals abuse.

A different definition of drug abuse is employed in this chapter. Drug abuse here implies the *nonprescriptive* use of psychoactive chemicals to alter the psychologic state; and, as a result of such alteration, the individual, others around him or her, or society incurs some *harm*. In this definition, the occasional use of a drug, legal or not, in which no harm occurs is not drug abuse. It should be recognized that this is a *medical type* definition rather than a legal one; legally, any use of an illegal drug could equal abuse.

As pointed out so well by Musto (1973), the term "drug abuse" in this country was apparently first applied to cocaine use especially by Southern blacks, then later to the smoking of opium by the Chinese immigrants. It was not until the passage of the Harrison Narcotic Act in 1914 that the use of heroin and morphine was recognised as drug abuse and it was much later that marihuana and the other drugs condemned today were included. For a fuller discussion of the issue of definitions of drug abuse, the reader is referred to Zinberg et al. (1978).

Theories of Etiology

Theories about the etiology of drug abuse abound. While at times the theories are complementary to each other, they are often contradictory and leave unclear the best course of action to follow for treatment or prevention. Several etiologic theories are discussed next (Kleber, 1974).

Availability. In one sense availability can be viewed as the primary cause of drug abuse since without access to suitable drugs, there can be no drug abuse. (Of course, it has been noted that where drugs are not available, individuals may resort to other means of altering consciousness, such as sensory deprivation, self-flagellation, or fasting.) The high incidence of drug abuse in certain populations—inner-city areas or among medical personnel—is mentioned to emphasize the importance of availability to explain individual drug abuse, while sudden easy access to drugs (as with amphetamines in Japan after World War II) is an explanatory concept for epidemics of drug abuse.

Psychological Deficit.

After availability, the most . common theory of the cause of drug abuse relates to psychological problems in the user. Personality disturbances, especially in the handling of aggressive or sexual impulses or conflicts around dependency strivings, are frequently seen in individuals with drug problems. Depression is quite common and much illicit drug use may represent an attempt at self-medication. Some personality types described for drug abusers include: alienated, aggressive, psychopathic, emotionally unstable, immature, hedonistic, cyclothymic, narcissistic, and passive-aggressive. Epidemics are explained by postulating the existence in the population of many disturbed individuals and that when availability of a particular drug increases, an epidemic may then follow. It is, of course, often quite unclear whether a certain psychological picture preceded or followed the drug use.

Pharmacologic Disturbance.

Early in this century narcotic addiction was seen by some medical personnel as due to autotoxins. About 50 years later the concept of metabolic deficiency was popularized by the founders of the methadone maintenance approach to treatment and most recently the discovery of opiate receptor sites and the endogenous opiate-like substances (endorphins and enkephalins) in the brain gave impetus to the proponents of a primary pharmacologic disturbance. Receptor sites have also been found for nicotine and diazepam, two other substances massively used. Like the psychologic theories, however, it is unclear which comes first in the nature of the physiologic changes observed.

Socioeconomic Factors.

Certain kinds of drug use are much more common in ghetto areas—regardless of which minority group predominates in the ghetto at that time. This idea has focused attention on the role of poverty and its frequent concomitant, hopelessness, in the etiology of drug problems. Epidemics may be explained by noting that the drug use in these areas is usually very high but ignored by society in general until something happens to bring it to their attention, at which point it is labeled an epidemic. The "something" may be crime spilling out of the ghetto into the affluent suburbs or drug use occurring in middle-class youngsters.

Social Factors.

To find a single explanation for drug use by individuals as diverse as the housewife using tranquilizers, ghetto residents using heroin, and middle-class adolescents using psychedelics, some theorists have invoked the evils of American society. Issues such as economic inequality (or capitalism per se), excessive emphasis on materialism, sexism, racism, the Vietnam War and its aftermath, and governmental hypocrisy and mendacity have all been put forward as causing drug abuse. These social evils are seen as providing a breeding ground for disturbed individuals who then use drugs to cope with or escape from the disturbing environment. Difficulty with this theory arises from the existence of drug abuse of various kinds in every society where abusable substances exist regardless of the social or economic structure of the country. Socialist Sweden has major problems with amphetamine abuse, while Communist Russia has an alcohol problem.

Summary.

Even a superficial examination of the various theories makes it clear that no one or two theories or their combination can explain all or even most cases of drug abuse. While each may highlight an important causative element, there are too many cases that are not so explained and become exceptions. There are also too many individuals who are *not* drug abusers whose socioeconomic status, family background, and personality structure all indicate they *should* be. It is most practical, therefore, to view drug abuse as a "final common pathway," which results from the coming together of a variety of disparate factors any one or two of which might be insufficient to bring it about. A traditional explanation of drug addiction viewed the causes as an addicting drug, a susceptible person, and some mechanism to bring the two together. While we can currently understand to a moderate extent (though the new discoveries about endorphins, opiate receptors, benzodiazepine receptors, and so on raise new questions) the first and third factors of that explanation, it is still a mystery what makes a person susceptible.

EVALUATION

For a detailed discussion of evaluation of drug abusers, the reader is referred to O'Brien et al. (1976).

Interview

Drug History. In those cases where the use or abuse of drugs is the overt reason the client is seeing the physician, the interview should begin with a discussion of why the patient is coming *now* rather than earlier. Some reasons may be legal pressure, family, peer, or job pressure, medical problems, or self-decision. For the patient's history of drug use, the following information for each drug provides necessary data for evaluation. Whether the physician needs to obtain a drug history as detailed as outlined here depends on the nature and circumstance of the evaluation.

In asking about current use, the physician should ask for the name, length of time used, frequency of use, route of administration, amount, cost, and purpose (to get high, to relieve boredom, to sleep, for energy, socialization, to relieve depression or nervousness, and so on) for each drug used by the individual. To determine previous use, the physician asks for the

name, the age the drug was started, length of time used, any adverse effects, and previous treatment experiences (where, what kind, and outcome) about each drug used in the past.

As mentioned before, in obtaining this information, it is important to maintain a nonjudgmental attitude. This means neither words nor facial expression should indicate disdain toward the individual. Such behavior on the part of a caregiver would either drive away the patient or lead to the giving of false information. It is also best in the early stage of the relationship not to inquire in detail how the individual obtains drugs or money for them. Questions in this area immediately arouse the client's suspicion that the physician may be planning to involve the legal authorities and his or her answers, therefore may be false. It may be useful at this point in the interview to stress the confidentiality of all the information obtained in the interview. If the interview is one in which confidentiality is *not* going to be maintained, for example, when an interview is for legal purposes or if the clinician plans to discuss findings with parents, spouse, or others, the clients *must* be informed *before* any information is obtained so they can decide how much they want to divulge. It should never be taken for granted that the patient is aware that confidentiality is not guaranteed. In terms of gaining the patient's trust, it is far preferable to maintain total confidentiality. Any discussions with parents or spouse about the patient should preferably take place with the patient present and after there has been discussion and agreement by the patient as to what kinds and amount of information will be shared.

Social Situation. After obtaining a picture of the current and past drug use, the interview should move into the area of social functioning. Information about the following material should be elicited: living arrangements (alone, with family, or other), marital status, sexual orientation and functioning, employment and/or educational status, family members (parents, siblings, spouse, other key members), occupation, education, psychological state, friends, and recreational activities. The physician should try to understand not only the factual aspects of these areas but also the emotional ones—thus the *quality* of the patient's relation with his or her parents or spouse should be probed as well as the attitude toward a job or schooling. Does the patient have close friends, hobbies, or sports interests? The nature and degree of the patient's social supports should become clear—is the drug use jeopardizing them or is it taking their place because of their meagerness? The presence of adverse family conditions, currently or in the past, such as alcoholism, mental illness, brutality, compulsive gambling, or the like, should be looked for and noted. Recent changes in the patient's behavior should be taken as clues to either antecedents or sequelae to the drug abuse. Did a divorce precede or follow the increased use of barbiturates? Did the heavy marihuana use precede or follow a grade drop and decision to drop out of school? Did the amphetamine use occur after or before taking up with a new group of friends? Although it is tempting to associate calamitous occurrences as a result of drug abuse, careful questioning may reveal they were prior events.

Psychological Status.   Elsewhere in this book there is a detailed description of comprehensive psychological evaluation of patients. In dealing with drug abusers, such evaluation has several purposes. It aids the nonpsychiatrist in deciding who may need to be referred for specialized help as opposed to being seen for counseling by the physician. It may highlight the existence of conditions for which there is appropriate psychoactive medication. Of course, in dealing with a drug-abusing population, the physician must be very cautious in prescribing such drugs, but they need not be withheld where appropriate. Certain drugs, such as lithium and MAO inhibitors, may be risky to use because a careless life style or haphazard approach to dosage can

create serious hazards when these substances are being taken. Other drugs, such as the minor tranquilizers and certain tricyclic antidepressants, are often abused for their psychoactive effects. Certain categories, such as the phenothiazenes, on the other hand, are rarely abused by these patients and the problem more often is how to get the patient to keep taking such agents when they are prescribed.

As in the preceding section on social supports, it is important to ascertain whether detectable psychiatric conditions predate or postdate the drug abuse. Certain people take drugs on a self-medicating basis to deal with unbearable states of loneliness, depression, or anxiety, or to control unacceptable aggressive or sexual drives. Conversely, continued use of certain drugs may lead to or exaggerate psychiatric states not evident before, for example, chronic amphetamine use may lead to paranoid feelings and even frank psychosis. Personality factors play a role in determining which drug will be used, the pattern of use, and even to some extent psychoactive effects. While, in general, experimental or occasional use of drugs may not indicate any psychopathology, heavy or compulsive use is usually associated with serious problems. However, at present there is no good way to predict whether or not a person with certain characteristics will become a compulsive user or which people will use a particular category of drugs. As one example, although a number of heroin addicts may have passive-aggressive personality features, most passive-aggressive people are not heroin addicts (or even drug abusers) and most heroin addicts are not passive-aggressive.

Physical Examination

Although there is no special physical examination for drug abusers, it is useful to keep in mind certain conditions which can be either direct or indirect sequelae of drug abuse. While many of them can be found in non-abusers and many abusers may have few or none of them, the presence of certain signs should raise one's index of suspicion.

Some **cutaneous signs** directly or indirectly associated with drug abuse are needle **puncture** marks—usually found over veins especially in the antecubital area, dorsum of the hands, and forearms, but they can be found anywhere on the body where a vein is reachable, including the neck, tongue, and dorsal vein of the penis.

"**Tracks**" are one of the most common and readily recognizable signs of chronic injectable drug abuse. They are scars located along veins and are usually hyperpigmented and linear. They result both from frequent unsterile injections and from the deposit of carbon black from attempts to sterilize the needle with a match. Tracks tend to lighten over time but may never totally disappear. Because tracks are such a well-known indication of drug abuse, addicts may hide them by having a **tattoo** over the area. Tattoos in general are not uncommon among certain groups of drug abusers.

When addicts run out of antecubital and forearm veins they often turn to veins on the finger and dorsum of the hand, which can lead to **hand edema**. Such edema can persist for months.

Thrombophlebitis is commonly found in addicts on arms and legs because of the unsterile nature of the injections and the irritating quality of some of the adulterants mixed with the active drug. **Abscesses** and **ulcers** are particularly common among individuals who inject barbiturates because of the irritating quality of these chemicals. These abscesses are often secondary to narcotic injection and are more likely to be septic and around veins.

Ulceration or **perforation** of the **nasal septum** is a frequent effect of inhalation or "snorting." Heroin can lead to ulceration of the septum while similar chronic use of cocaine can cause perforation secondary to vasoconstriction and loss of blood supply.

Cigarette **burns** or scars from old burns are another sign of possible drug abuse. They can occur due to drug-induced drowsiness. Fresh burns are usually seen between the fingers while old scars are often seen on the chest as a result of the cigarette falling out of the user's mouth. It has been estimated that over 90% of addicts and alcoholics smoke.

Piloerection ("gooseflesh") is an opiate withdrawal sign, usually found on the arms and trunk. **Cheilitis** (cracking of skin at corners of mouth) is especially seen in chronic amphetamine users and in opiate addicts prior to or during detoxification. Contact **dermatitis** is observed around the nose, mouth, and hands, in solvent abusers. Sometimes it is called "gluesniffer's rash." In other drug abusers it may occur around areas of injection secondary to use of chemicals to cleanse the skin. **Jaundice**, due to hepatitis, in drug abusers is usually attributable to use of unsterilized shared needles and syringes.

Certain medical conditions, such as cardiovascular, hepatic, pulmonary disorders, and neurologic disturbances are associated with drug abuse. A complete list is found in Table 16–1.

Narcotics

For more detailed description of the signs and symptoms related to drug intoxication, withdrawal, and overdose, the reader is referred to Inaba et al. (1978).

Intoxication. Narcotics such as heroin, morphine, meperidene, codeine, methadone, and so on, are usually taken by injection—either subcutaneous, intramuscular, or intravenously. Nicknames for narcotics include "horse," "scag," "junk," and others. The signs and symptoms of intoxication from narcotics are as follows:

Symptoms

- Euphoria

- Drowsiness (an addict may be "on the nod"— the head falls to chest and then snaps back up as the user tries to stay awake and enjoy the high rather than sleep)

- Scratching (usually a slow sensual scratching)

Signs

- Decreased respiratory rate and depth
- Decreased blood pressure and pulse
- Miosis (contracted or pinpoint pupils)

Although the effects of the drug may last a number of hours, often the only sign visible after the first 30–60 minutes is pinpoint pupils. Except for contracted pupils, the narcotic addict may talk and act in a seemingly normal fashion.

Overdose. While there is some controversy over whether the usual picture of heroin overdose is actually due to an excessive amount of

TABLE 16–1
Medical complications associated with drug abuse

CARDIOVASCULAR	PULMONARY	HEPATIC	REPRODUCTIVE SYSTEM	NEUROLOGIC
Endocarditis	Multiple microinfarcts	Serum hepatitis	Menstrual irregularities	Seizures, usually grand mal but can also have focal seizures and status epilepticus
Myocarditis	Chronic pulmonary fibrosis	Cirrhosis		Acute delirium
Cardiac arrhythmias	Foreign body granulomas			Blindness
Thrombophlebitis	Pulmonary edema			Acute transverse myelitis
Arteritis	Bacterial pneumonia			Peripheral nerve lesions
Necrotizing angiitis	Aspiration pneumonia			Acute rhabdomyolysis
Hypertension and hypotension	Tuberculosis			Chronic fibrosing myopathies
				Bacterial meningitis
				CNS abscess
				Tetanus

HEMATOPOIETIC	GENITOURINARY	SKELETAL	GASTROINTESTINAL
Bacteremia	Nephrotic syndrome	Septic arthritis	Chronic constipation or diarrhea
Bone marrow depression, rarely aplastic anemia		Osteomyelitis	Pancreatitis

heroin or to an acute hypersensitivity or allergic reaction, or other causes, there is no question the condition is an extremely serious one with a possibly fatal outcome. Overdose can occur so swiftly that the addict may be found with the needle still in the vein. More often, the patient is brought to the emergency room in a comatose state with pinpoint pupils; pale, cool, damp skin with a cyanotic hue; severe respiratory depression ranging from apnea to a few shallow gasping breaths per minute; and arreflexia. Frothy pink-tinged sputum indicative of pulmonary edema may be noted. The most apparent sign, pinpoint pupils, may not be present because of either anoxia or the use of certain drugs (for example, atropine or glutethimide). Conversely, pinpoint pupils may be secondary to drugs (pilocarpine) or pupils may be small in a far-sighted individual.

Withdrawal. The appearance of the first signs and symptoms of narcotic withdrawal, their peak and remission depend on the duration of action of the drug. Thus, signs and symptoms of heroin or morphine withdrawal begin approximately 12 hours after the last dose, peak at 36–72 hours, and have mostly gone away by the fifth day. With methadone, withdrawal begins at 24–48 hours, peaks at 96–120 hours, and symptoms may still be evident as long as 3 weeks later. In general, with addiction to equivalent doses, the longer acting the narcotic, the less intense the withdrawal but the longer it lasts.

A common classification of narcotic withdrawal signs and symptoms is described next using a grade system to express increasing severity.

Grade 0—craving for drugs, anxiety, drug-seeking behavior

Grade 1—yawning, perspiration, lacrimation, rhinorrhea, "yen" (light, restless, broken sleep), irritability

Grade 2—mydriasis with progressive decreased reaction to light. At peak of withdrawal, pupils are dilated and unreactive to light; muscular twitches (hence the term "kicking" the habit); piloerection or "gooseflesh" (hence the term "cold turkey"), hot and cold flashes, abdominal cramps, aching joints and muscles, anorexia, chills, lack of energy

Grade 3—insomnia, low-grade fever; increased respiratory rate and depth, increased pulse rate and increased blood pressure, nausea, vomiting, diarrhea, weight loss

The grades outlined are arbitrarily selected and not all signs are necessary to diagnose each grade. In some individuals signs overlap the grades to some extent and individuals differ as to which signs and symptoms they will display. There is a tendency for individuals to have repetitive patterns of withdrawal, that is, to manifest similar signs and symptoms each time they withdraw. Thus, one individual may have predominant gastrointestinal symptoms while another is most bothered by musculoskeletal problems.

Convulsions are not characteristic of opiate withdrawal or intoxication with the exception of meperidene intoxication. If a patient has a seizure, therefore, it usually signifies undiagnosed barbiturate-sedative withdrawal; another medical condition such as epilepsy; hysteria; or a faked convulsion in an attempt to obtain drugs. Since mixed addiction is quite common, the possibility of abuse of barbiturate-type drugs should always be kept in mind when dealing with any narcotic addict.

Even after most withdrawal signs and symptoms have passed, aching muscles, irritability, insomnia, and lack of energy may persist for weeks. A "protracted abstinence syndrome" has been described in which as late as months after the last dose, some subclinical signs of withdrawal can still be found.

Sedatives

Sedatives, such as barbiturates, glutethimide, methaqualone, and minor tranquilizers such as diazepam are usually taken orally or by injection. Since there is a tendency for these drugs to scar the veins, intravenous injection is usuallly replaced by intra muscular in regular users. Some nicknames for sedatives are "ludes," "downers," "reds," among others.

Intoxication.   Signs of progressive barbiturate intoxication are as follows:

- Depression of superficial skin reflexes

- Horizontal nystagmus—first present only on extreme lateral gaze but as intoxication deepens will eventually be found on forward gaze

- Decreased alertness

- Ataxia

- Slurred speech

- Positive Romberg sign

- Excitement followed by depression and drowsiness

Overdose.   The signs of sedative-hypnotic overdose include the signs of intoxication just described accompanied by:

- Thick speech

- Marked ataxia with falling

- Confusion

- Sleep with difficulty in arousing

- Semicoma with constricted pupils

- Marked respiratory depression

- Shock with dilated pupils

Overdose of sedatives can lead to death, if untreated.

Withdrawal.   Unlike narcotic withdrawal, which can be painful but is not medically serious except in the presence of complicating physical illness, sedative withdrawal has a significant fatality rate if untreated. Because of this, it is important to have a high index of suspicion, especially if any of the following features are present.

- Present or past history of excessive use of any of the drugs in the sedative-barbiturate hypnotic class

- Present or past history of excessive use of alcohol

- Signs of barbiturate withdrawal

- History of recent seizure

- Any patient who is a physician

- Multiple drug use

- Complaint of chronic insomnia

Minor signs and symptoms of sedative withdrawal appear within 24 hours and last 3–14 days. They are:

- Anorexia

- Anxiety

- Insomnia

- Muscular weakness

- Nausea

- Orthostatic hypotension

- Tremors of upper extremities

- Twitching movements

The major signs and symptoms appear within 48–72 hours and may last 3–14 days. They are:

- Confusion

- Convulsions (usually grand mal type seizures, which may be single or status epilepticus)

- Delirium—includes disorientation, delusions, hallucinations (usually visual)

- Formication

- Hyperthermia—fever as high as 105–106F is possible

- Paranoid ideation

Convulsions usually do not occur before 16 hours of withdrawal and psychotic behavior usually not before 36 hours after abrupt withdrawal. If these symptoms become severe, they may not be reversed simply by giving barbiturates, but may follow the pattern of many toxic psychoses in which death may occur.

It is important to keep in mind that diazepam withdrawal may not occur until 3–5 days after abrupt withdrawal. The symptoms of mild withdrawal—irritability, anxiety, trouble with sleeping—may be confused with the initial reasons for which the patient took the drug. This may lead both patient and doctor to believe that the drug needs to be continued. These withdrawal symptoms may occur even at relatively low-dosage levels, for example, 40–60 mg per day, while the more serious conditions of seizure and delirium usually do not occur below doses of 80–100 mg per day.

Stimulants

Stimulants, such as dextroamphetamine, methamphetamine, cocaine, methylphenidate are usually taken by inhaling, or by intramuscular or intravenous injection, or by ingestion. Some nicknames are "uppers," "speed," or "black beauties."

Intoxication. Low doses of stimulants produce elevated mood with mild euphoria; increased alertness and self-confidence; increased concentration; decreased appetite, talkativeness; decreased awareness of fatigue, sometimes with enhanced performance; increased pulse and blood pressure; and increased respiration.

High doses can produce irritability, restlessness, insomnia, tremors, hyperreflexia, palpitations, paranoid ideation with or without confusion, dry mouth with frequent licking of lips and cheilosis, cardiac arrhythmias, and dilated but reactive pupils. Chronic high doses may lead to the symptoms just listed, along with paranoid or toxic psychosis, at times very difficult to distinguish from paranoid schizophrenia. Visual and tactile hallucinations may occur as well as auditory ones. The combination of paranoia with the physical hyperactivity may lead to the occurrence of violent behavior. Chronic stimulant use may also be associated with compulsive behavior in which the individual engages in an activity for hours at a time. These range from simple acts like tying and untying shoelaces, to complex ones like taking apart and putting together alarm clocks. Chronic inhalation of cocaine may lead to necrosis of the nasal septum and eventually perforation. Other physical side effects of chronic stimulant abuse may include necrotizing angiitis and cerebral vascular damage.

Overdose. Overdose of stimulants includes the signs of high-dose intoxication along with hyperthermic convulsions, circulatory collapse, and cerebral hemorrhage. Coma may occur, and death can quickly follow.

Withdrawal. Until recently it was believed that stimulants were not physically addicting and that there was no true withdrawal syndrome. It is now felt there is some degree of physical dependence. Typically when the chronic abuser abruptly stops, there is a period of profound fatigue that may manifest itself in sleeping for 24 hours or more. Upon awakening, the individual is still fatigued and in addition, may be quite depressed. The severity of depression may be such that suicide is a possibility and withdrawing patients must be watched for this. The worst fatigue and depression is over within a week but may persist for months at a lower level.

Hallucinogens

Hallucinogens (LSD, mescaline, psilocybin, 2,5-dimethoxy-4-methylamphetamine [DOM, or STP], dimethyltryptamine [DMT], 3,4-methylene dioxyamphetamine [MDA, or "love drug") are usually taken orally. "Acid," "magic mushrooms," are two nicknames for psychedelic substances.

Intoxication. The psychedelic experience brought on by hallucinogenic drugs includes changes in perception, mood, consciousness, and judgment. An initial period of giddiness and euphoria is followed by profound alterations in consciousness. Synesthesia—a phenomenon in which stimulation of one sensory modality leads to changes in another, for example, seeing music, hearing colors—is a common experience. Physical signs include hyperreflexia, dilated pupils, increased pulse and blood pressure, and increased temperature. Anxiety, anorexia, rambling speech, increased suggestibility, and changes in body image may be noted. Illusions and hallucinations are common. Fear of death is often markedly diminished and the whole attitude towards dying significantly altered so that "inadvertent" suicide attempts may occur. Paranoia is not uncommon.

The most common serious untoward event associated with hallucinogenics is a panic reaction or "bad trip." This is usually temporary, lasting less than 24 hours, but can persist, worsen, and become a full-blown psychotic episode. It is controversial whether a prolonged psychotic state is due to the drug's toxicity or to the unmasking of already existing traits. The relation to dose is also unclear. Flashbacks, the recurrence of part of the psychedelic experience days, weeks, or even months after the last use of the drug, usually occur in an individual who has had multiple experiences with hallucinogens, but occasionally happen after only one experience. They usually fade over time if the drugs are no longer used, but marihuana use can apparently stimulate flashbacks. At times, the flashbacks are viewed as pleasant but more often they are frightening and raise fears in the individual that he or she is "going crazy."

Overdose. In hallucinogenic overdose, all of the signs mentioned, plus grand mal seizures, delirium, nausea, and vomiting can take place. Whether the psychotic state is an overdose phenomenon or an uncovering of a preexisting personality trait is debated. Unlike narcotics or sedatives, overdose is usually not associated with a fatal outcome unless delusions of grandeur (for instance, belief in ones ability to fly) lead to a mortal accident.

Withdrawal. Tolerance develops rapidly to psychedelic drugs so that daily usage for only 3–4 days will markedly diminish the effect of the same dose. Tolerance is lost just as rapidly. Since use is usually episodic rather than continuous, physical withdrawal is not commonly seen.

Phencyclidine

Phencyclidine or PCP is nicknamed "angel dust," "*PeaCe* Pill," "hog," "rocket fuel," or "monkey dust." Sometimes classed as a CNS depressant and sometimes as a hallucinogen, PCP has enough special features to warrant its own section. Developed as a general anesthestic for man, the frequency and seriousness of side effects led to its being used only in veterinary medicine under the brand name, Serynlan. Apparently PCP first emerged as a drug of abuse in 1967 under the name "*PeaCe Pill*," but the frequency of adverse effects soon decreased its popularity. In the early to mid 1970s, it began to be used again, often sold under false pretenses. It is sold as tetrahydrocannabinol (THC) or substituted for LSD or mescaline or sprinkled on marijuana PCP is easily and cheaply manufactured from easily obtained chemicals and today is often taken knowingly in spite of or even because of its bad reputation. It is related chemically to the anesthetic, ketamine.

Phencyclidine may be ingested, injected, snorted, or smoked. A common method is to sprinke it on parsley and smoke it. Other forms of PCP besides powder include tablets, capsules, rock crystal, and liquid.

Intoxication. Signs and symptoms of PCP intoxication include:

- Horizontal and vertical nystagmus
- Analgesia

- Tachycardia

- Increased deep tendon reflexes

- Muscle rigidity

- Ataxia

- Flushed skin

- Sweating

- Blank stare

- Calmness and apathy *or* agitation and excitement

- Body image distortion

- Floating feeling

- Hostility and possible violence

- Fever

Overdose. Besides the signs of intoxication, the indications of PCP overdose are:

- Coma or stupor with fluctuating levels of consciousness

- Eyes may be open in coma or closed

- Pupils miotic but reactive

- Hypertension

- Convulsions

- Decreased or absent reflexes

- Hypersalivation, drooling

- Sweating

- Opisthotonic posture

- Inability to speak

- Labile affect

- Disorientation

- Hallucinations

- Amnesia

- Fever

The PCP-intoxicated individual may mimic a schizophrenic reaction. Symptoms typically include several days of confusion, paranoid ideation, insomnia, and restlessness with intermittent aggressive or violent behavior and delusion of grandeur but no systematized delusional system. Although recovery after days or weeks is usually complete, patients may have recurring episodes of schizoid behavior not drug-induced. Chronic PCP users may show memory gaps, some disorientation, visual and speech difficulties even when not using the drug.

In addition to the psychological and physical dangers associated with PCP, there is a significant risk of what has been called ***behavioral toxicity***. Because of impaired perception or delusional beliefs, PCP users have died by fire, falls from heights, burns and drowning even in quite shallow water. PCP-intoxicated persons have been known to show extraordinary strength which, when combined with the loss of pain sensation, may mean that three or four persons may be needed to control a person under the influence of PCP.

Treatment of PCP Overdose. In acute intoxication and early stages of PCP-induced acute psychosis, patients need to be isolated from environmental stimulation with care taken that they do not harm themselves or others. Because of the analgesia and distorted body image, patients have been known to severely mutilate themselves. The propensity to violence against others is also well known. Sedative drugs may be helpful in controlling seizures, violent behavior, agitation, muscle rigidity, and insomnia. Diazepam, 10–30 mg, given intravenously, is often preferred for these states. "Talking down," which can be useful in treating "bad trips" that result from LSD and other hallucinogens, is likely to make matters worse and should not be used in cases of PCP overdose. Phenothiazines should be avoided while the patient is still acutely intoxicated.

If ingestion of PCP was recent, gastric lavage is a worthwhile procedure. Acidification of the urine with ammonium chloride, 2-3 mEq/kg every 6 hours, or ascorbic acid, 2 g every 6 hours, apparently greatly increases urinary PCP excretion. As the urine pH is decreased from 7 to 5, PCP clearance is increased by as much as 100 to 300 times. Acidification is contraindicated in the presence of severe liver disease, renal insufficiency, or when the patient has ingested large amounts of drugs, such as barbiturates or salicylates, and excretion of them would be adversely affected by acidification.

Depression can occur several weeks after the acute PCP episode—and has been associated with suicide attempts. It is important to be aware of this possibility. Any hospital discharge should include a follow-up treatment plan that provides for on-going contact and support.

Marijuana

Marijuana's main mode of ingestion is smoking. At times it is taken orally and very uncommonly injected intravenously. "Pot," "grass," "weed," and "reefer" are some nicknames for marijuana. For more details, see Petersen (1979).

Marijuana comes from a hemp plant called **Cannabis sativa**, cultivated in many parts of the world. Although the principle active ingredient is tetrahydrocannabinol (THC) there are over 400 chemicals in the plant. The THC content is determined by the plant strain, climate, soil conditions, and harvesting. Typically the marijuana used in cigarettes, or "joints", is made from particles of the whole plant, especially the leaves and flowers at the top. Potency may vary considerably. For example, in 1975, the average THC content of confiscated marijuana was 0.5%, in 1978 this had increased to 3% as the source shifted from Mexico to Columbia; California **Sinsimmela** may contain as much as 7% THC. Hashish (hash) is a dark brown or black resin extracted from the plants and smoked to produce a high. Its average THC content is about 2%. Hash oil, an even stronger extract of the plant, may contain up to 35% THC. Hash looks like a tarlike substance and usually is smoked in small amounts on tobacco or marijuana

cigarettes to enhance the effect, or may be smoked in pipes, sometimes called "bongs."

Intoxication. The most common effects of smoking marijuana are feelings of euphoria and relaxation. Users may also experience an increase in pulse rate, reddening of the eyes, dryness of the mouth and throat, and a mild decrease in body temperature. There is also often an associated increase in appetite, called "the munchies." High doses may result in image distortions as well as hallucinations. Marijuana has been claimed by users to enhance tactile, auditory, and visual sensations. Research studies have indicated that marijuana may interfere on a temporary basis with memory and may alter the sense of time, making time seem to pass slower. It also may decrease the ability to perform tasks requiring concentration, swift actions, and coordination such as driving.

The most common adverse reaction to marijuana is a panic anxiety state sometimes accompanied by paranoia. The symptoms are more common in novice users, generally wear off in a few hours, and respond well to reassurance. Marijuana has been reported to exacerbate psychotic symptoms in schizophrenic patients in remission, and especially in the Eastern literature has been noted to produce a psychotic state. Such states are apparently very rare in the United States. Because of the sedative and euphoric effects of marijuana, frequent use may be associated in some individuals with decreased interest in academic and occupational achievement, a situation that has been labeled the "amotivational syndrome." It is likely that heavy daily use of sedative drugs other than marijuana would produce a similar situation. The "burn-out syndrome" is used to describe a situation in which an individual who has been smoking marijuana, usually for 5 years or more, appears to have symptoms suggestive of a chronic brain syndrome. Individuals with this syndrome appear dull, slow-moving, and inattentive. There are memory and attention deficits and the effects may not disappear after marijuana is discontinued but may last for weeks or months. It should be noted in this regard that the active ingredient of marijuana, THC, is fat-soluble and can be stored in the body for up to 30 days.

The major physical effect demonstrated to date has to do with the pulmonary system, since many users inhale the smoke deeply and hold it in their lungs as long as possible. Signs of airway obstruction in chronic users have been noted. Certain animal tests raise the possibility of lung cancer, but as yet the results have been inconclusive. As for the effects of marijuana on the immune system and on chromosomes, test results are inconclusive. Although marijuana has been shown to decrease the testosterone level in males to low-normal levels and to increase the number of defective cycles in women, the implications of these findings are not yet clear.

Withdrawal. The increased potency of marijuana being used today along with increased frequency of use has been associated with more individuals reporting problems in stopping marijuana. There is, however, little evidence in humans that there is physical dependence or physical withdrawal from marijuana in the usual doses used.

Overdose. Although injected marijuana extract has been associated with cardiovascular collapse, it is more difficult to overdose by the inhalation route and more possible but still uncommon via the ingestion route. High doses of THC given orally in laboratories have been shown to produce an acute psychotic syndrome.

Laboratory Tests

Many laboratories are able to do a "toxicologic screen" of urine or blood for the presence of many of the drugs of abuse. Such tests can be useful both because of what they may show and because patients may become more truthful when they know that such tests are being done. It is important to keep in mind the following points: positive test results for the presence of drugs indicate use but cannot indicate how long or how often the individual may be using that drug—they can define use but not abuse. Negative test results may mean the individual is not using or that the drug is no longer detectable in the urine. For example, traces of cocaine last a relatively short period of time, heroin (in the form of morphine) can be detected in the urine often up to 48 hours after use, and quinine, a diluent often used with both these drugs, can last 5–8 days. Since quinine is also found in soft drinks and cold remedies, its presence is at best suggestive. While the presence of a drug in the urine may be helpful in deciding on an overall treatment approach (for example, PCP in the urine of an acutely psychotic patient), such findings usually are not available soon enough to aid in the management of acute situations such as coma. In these cases, diagnosis on the basis of signs and symptoms, and symptomatic management is usually necessary.

To uncover possible medical complications of the drug use, studies of blood constituents, including a complete blood cell count (CBC); SMA 12/60 (Sequential Multiple Analyzer [by Technicon], 12 constituents per specimen per minute); serology and Australia antigen should be done. A positive serologic finding (VDRL) should be further evaluated with a Fluorescent Treponema antibody (FTA) test because of the frequency of false-positive results. Chest roentgenograms and ECG are done when medically indicated, the former especially if one has not been done in the past 6–12 months and the latter especially in patients over 35 years. Because of the deleterious effect of many drugs on the fetus and because drug use may lead to irregular menstrual cycles, a pregnancy test should be performed on any female patient with missed or irregular periods where drug use is suspected. A history of seizures that has not been previously investigated calls for an EEG. Additional laboratory tests may be suggested by the history or physical examination.

Managing Physical Aspects

The diagnosis and treatment of illicit drug use is often complicated by the ignorance of the individual concerned as to exactly what was taken, the dose, and whether contaminants are present. This happens more often with certain drugs than with others but even a similar physical appearance of an illicit drug may have little to do with its exact composition. Heroin is usually white or brown and usually mixed with quinine and lactose. Cocaine is also often mixed with quinine and procaine is a common substitute or filler. Hallucinogenic drugs are commonly mislabeled. Sometimes what is called mescaline or psilocybin actually contains LSD or methamphetamine or PCP. PCP may be passed off as THC, and sometimes is sprinkled on marijuana. Because of these factors, the physician usually has to rely on presenting signs and symptoms while at the same time trying to elicit some history from the client or accompanying individuals.

For a detailed description of the management and treatment of acute drug states, the reader is referred to Bourne (1976).

MANAGEMENT AND REFERRAL

Roles of the Family

Not infrequently the first complication in the treatment of the substance abuser is convincing the individual to seek help. A spouse, parent, or offspring often appears in the office and asks for help in getting the person to seek assistance. The individual who is abusing drugs may deny or minimize the existence of any substance abuse problem and may refuse to see a physician. While this is a difficult situation, there are definite steps family members can take to increase the chances of encouraging the individual to seek help.

First, the clinician should have the family members describe in detail the behavior that leads them to suspect substance abuse and the duration of time over which this has taken place. Despite the prevalence of chemical use in our society, one cannot assume that the family has always made the correct diagnosis. A sharp drop in an adolescent's grades may have more to do with depression or unrequited love than with drugs, for example.

Second, family members should be encouraged to do some reading about the problem. Drug and alcohol treatment centers usually have literature about the nature of substance abuse. (Some examples of useful reading are listed at the end of the chapter.)

Third, the nature of the confrontation that may have to occur is fully discussed. Role-playing may offer a rehearsal for what is usually a very difficult and painful time. The meaning of the ultimatum should be very clear and related to the situation. With a spouse, it may be, "See the doctor or leave the house" or "I'll leave if you don't see the doctor." With an adolescent the threat may have to do with loss of privileges or even the ultimate threat, "See the doctor or get out of the house." It is important not to have the confrontation until the family member is ready for it and has rehearsed ways of handling the usual replies. It is also important that they only make threats that have been fully thought through and that they are prepared to carry out. Idle threats worsen communication and may markedly prolong the period of time before the individual seeks treatment. Finally, when the family member is ready, a date is set for the appointment. This should be a realistic date that takes into account any other circumstances in the individual's life.

Role of Drugs in the Family

When the physician meets with the family member or the drug-abusing client, it may be useful to think first about the role drugs may play in that particular family. Although almost always the family overtly condemns the drug or alcohol abuse, the covert processes may tell a different story. The drug use may serve as a problem that unifies the family and keeps it together. The drug user may be viewed as helpless and dependent, unable to live on his or her own. This attitude may keep adolescents home long beyond the time when they should leave. The parents may intuitively know that if he or she left, their marriage would break up. In the marital situation, a husband or wife may covertly encourage the drug or alcohol use in a spouse because it gives them the dominant role while at the same time they are able to portray themselves and think of themselves as the helpless victim. Physicians have been known to encourage their spouses' heavy use of sedative drugs or even narcotics as a way of forestalling complaints about the amount of time the physicians are out of the home and the lack of attention they give to the family. The sedated elderly parent may be easier to have around than the whining, querulous, unsedated one. These factors may lead the family to sabotage treatment if the physician is not alert to what may be going on in the family constellation. Before expending much effort on treatment, therefore, it behooves the physician to try to understand the particular dynamics for each family in question. For a full discussion of the role of the family in drug-abuse situations, see Chapter 3, and Stanton (1979).

No matter what the role of the family may be, without their help referral or treatment may fail. Thus, it is important for the therapist to involve the family in the treatment process to the extent possible. While the primary physician may not have the time or the training to get involved in specialized therapy such as marital or family counseling, he or she is often in a better position than a therapist to know the family member and to make recommendations about what kind of treatment should take place and what type of therapist should be involved. The physician may also be in a position to provide short-term crisis-oriented service to families and focus on improved communication skills, family negotiations, setting and achieving of realistic goals, and reasonable limit-setting.

Parents are usually confused about how to react to and handle adolescent drug use. This confusion has led them to avoid taking stands or to pretend not to notice obvious drug-related behavior so as not to have to take a position or have a confrontation. This has been true about tobacco and alcohol as well as marijuana and other drugs. The younger adolescent is especially vulnerable to the effects of drug abuse and here parents may have to be especially forceful in their negative statements and limits.

Referral

The decision about referral is the final step of the management process. It involves taking into consideration the drug of abuse, degree of involvement, the presence or absence of serious psychological problems, the existence and role of supporting networks (such as the family), and last, but certainly not least, the time, interest, and skill of the practitioner himself. While certain situations almost always call for referral and others may not, many of the cases the primary practitioner sees fall into a gray area, in which the decision can be made only after a careful evaluation of all of the factors discussed previously. The individual addicted to heroin, or the individual in a chronic psychotic state from frequent hallucinogenic use will almost always need to be referred to a specialized treatment center. On the other hand, the polydrug abuser not habituated to any one drug, or someone using excessive amounts of diet pills may at times be handled without referral.

If referral is to be a useful part of treatment, it must not be merely an avoidance maneuver on the part of the physician. Instead, certain crucial elements need to be considered. First, the practitioner should have some knowledge of the specialized treatment resources available in the area. While almost all communities have AA chapters, specialized drug treatment centers are most likely to be found in larger urban areas. Psychiatrists who are willing and able to work with chemically dependent individuals may be difficult to find. Psychologists and social workers often have more practical experience with substance abuse.

The attitude of the individual toward the referral needs to be explored to increase the likelihood of acceptance and compliance. It is helpful to remember that psychiatric help is often viewed as a stigma to be avoided; this needs to be discussed gently rather than just giving the person the name of a psychiatrist or social worker. Drug treatment programs may be seen as only for the most desperate of criminals—assurance is often necessary to convince people that this is not always the case. The cost of private psychiatric or other psychotherapeutic treatment may be a problem that the patient is reluctant to talk about and needs to be addressed openly by the physician. Many drug and alcohol treatment programs charge no fee or have a sliding scale and many communities have mental health care centers that provide psychiatric assistance on a similar sliding fee basis. The possibility of insurance to defray some of the costs may also be explored as well as the availability of public funds such as Medicaid.

Referrals should be viewed as a positive step rather than as a way for the practitioner to get rid of an undesirable client. Given the current treatment outcomes, it is not unreasonable for the practitioner to express some cautious optimism about the favorable outcome of treatment if the individual is willing to get involved. In certain cases it may be necessary, as with the initial appointment with the primary practitioner, for the family to exert coercive pressure to get the individual to follow through on the recommended approach.

When patients are abusing drugs to the extent that intellectual functioning during counseling is being affected or when their time and energy is almost wholly taken up with obtaining and using drugs, it is obviously unrealistic to continue treating such persons on an outpatient basis. Outpatient treatment may become possible again after a short period of hospitalization. If

patients, however, revert back quickly to such heavy use, it is probably necessary to refer them for longer treatment in a controlled drug-free environment. Adolescent polydrug users, although not addicted to any one drug, may need a brief period of hospitalization to become drug-free prior to beginning counseling.

Counseling.   Psychoanalytically oriented approaches in which the therapist is relatively passive are usually not successful with chemically dependent clients. They are used to rapid relief of distressing emotional states by means of chemicals and usually have little tolerance for the slow, often frustration-evoking process, of the insight-oriented therapeutic approach. Counseling techniques are usually more successful if they are reality-oriented and focus on the here and now for substance abusers. Insight-oriented approaches if they are to be used at all, can await the development of a therapeutic relationship and achievement of control of the drug use. The initial therapeutic goals are more involved with limit-setting and ascertaining areas in which help is needed. Such areas may relate to relations with peers or family or aspects of school or job. It is important to remember that some patients may not do well initially and at first it may be useful to think of the condition as a chronic one in which immediate cure is unlikely to take place. While the therapist cannot condone the drug abuse, a stance as an adversary is likely to either drive the patient away or lead to lies and distortions. The difficult middle ground of accepting the patient but questioning the need for the destructive behavior is more likely to lead to a useful alliance.

Finally, the importance of the family if it figures in the patient's life should not be underestimated. They should be involved if possible in some aspect of the counseling as noted earlier. The frequency and duration of counseling sessions depend on the patient's need and resources and the practitioner's time. In general, however, meeting at least once a week should be sufficient especially in the early stages of treatment.

Specialized Treatment Approaches

Detoxification. Although in the past detoxification was often considered treatment in and of itself, most experienced clinicians now regard withdrawal from drugs as pretreatment or as the first step in treatment. Withdrawal from narcotics without medical help is painful but rarely life-threatening. With medical support it becomes relatively easy to do. It can take place on either an inpatient, residential, or outpatient basis. Outpatient withdrawal is usually difficult without strong family support if the individual remains in more or less the same environment and is able to obtain drugs. The first signs of discomfort under such circumstances are often enough to send him or her searching for more chemicals. On an inpatient or residential basis, through methadone substitution for the heroin, and then withdrawal, detoxification becomes a relatively simple procedure lasting 5–10 days (see Appendix A, p. 286, for this technique). Methadone can also be given on an outpatient basis.

More recently, clonidine, an alpha-adrenergic agonist, has been shown to be effective in the rapid detoxification from opiates (see Gold et al., 1978; 1980). As clonidine is an antihypertensive agent, blood pressure should be monitored carefully during withdrawal, especially in medically ill patients (see Appendix B for clonidine detoxification schedule).

Withdrawing an individual from barbiturates, or similar sedative drugs, on the other hand, carries with it the possibility of a fatal outcome. Because of this withdrawal should be carried out on an inpatient basis. Detoxification from barbiturates is usually carried out by initially giving the individual an intermediate-acting barbiturate such as pentobarbital, stabilizing them for a few days, and then withdrawing usually no faster than 10% of the dose a day. Some clinicians prefer the longer-acting drug, phenobarbital, to provide a smoother withdrawal pattern. However, in the earlier stages, until the proper dose is determined, the longer-acting properties of the phenobarbital may complicate patient management (see Appendix C, p. 290, for detailed techniques).

Patients who are addicted to the benzodiazepines should be withdrawn using those drugs rather than using barbiturates. The mechanics of gradual withdrawal remains the same.

Abrupt cessation of amphetamines and other stimulants can lead to severe depression and suicide and, therefore, should be done on an inpatient basis. There seems to be relatively little success in getting stimulant-dependent individuals successfully detoxified on an outpatient basis. There is some controversy over whether stimulant dependency should be handled by abrupt or gradual withdrawal. The former has been the preferred approach for years but the latter has recently come into favor in some centers and is increasing in popularity.

Individuals dependent on multiple drugs usually need to be detoxified on an inpatient basis as outpatient withdrawal usually means the individual switches over or intensifies the use of one drug while he is being medically withdrawn from another. Individuals with serious medical problems should almost always be detoxified in an inpatient setting.

The Therapeutic Community. Residential therapeutic communities have been used to treat drug abusers in the past few decades. Key elements of their program usually include emphasis on confrontation, group therapy, a relatively rigid hierarchial structure, a reward and punishment system based on fairly strict value code which emphasizes honesty, openness, family feeling, and accepting responsibility, and prohibitions against violence or drug use. Although originally they were operated exclusively by ex-addict staffs who had themselves gone through the program, more recently there has been an increase in the number of mental health care professionals taking an active role. There has also been an increase in educational and vocational training during the residential stay. The programs seem to be especially useful for substance abusers who do not have serious psychiatric problems. Since many adolescent and young adult abusers have serious psychiatric difficulties, however, and probably would not do well in an environment that is confrontation-oriented and where mental health care professionals are not available, the practitioner making a referral must be aware of the program and staff in each facility to be considered. Such patients may do better in programs where the approach is more supportive rather than confrontational.

Outpatient and Day Programs.

Outpatient and day drug-free programs often have little in common with each other than the fact that they do not use methadone or narcotic antagonists and are not residential. They represent the largest number of drug treatment programs in the country today and differ enormously in the kinds of services and quality offered. Their approach may be most appropriate for four groups of clients: people seeking their first treatment experience; those who have successfully completed other treatment modalities; clients who have relapsed following other treatments; and, finally, drug abusers requiring treatment after prison or hospital stays. Approaches used include group therapy, individual counseling, vocational training, family therapy, job counseling, and in some cases specialized programs such as transcendental meditation, art therapy, music therapy, and yoga. If there are medical consultants available to the program, at times psychotropic drugs such as antidepressants may also be used. Group therapy is often more effective than traditional one-to-one counseling because of the peer pressure that can be exerted on the individual and because the group may more effectively cut through many of the denials, rationalizations, and manipulations employed by the drug abuser.

Methadone Maintenance.

Methadone maintenance involves the use on a daily basis of the synthetic narcotic, methadone, as a replacement for heroin. At the usual dosage range, 50–100 mg once daily, it reduces or eliminates drug-seeking behavior, blocks the effect of the average street amounts of heroin, and permits the individual to function without undue drowsiness or euphoria and with a minimum of other side effects. Since its introduction in the mid 1960s it has become one of the more widely used treatments for narcotic addicts and one of the most controversial.

In general, programs that employ ancillary supports such as counseling or vocational and educational help seem to do better than those that provide methadone alone. Individuals who start on methadone maintenance should have been using heroin on a more or less regular basis for at least 2 years and have tried other methods of treatment before being placed on a maintenance drug. Minimum age under federal regulations is 18 years and in some programs age 21 years is required. Once started on methadone, clients usually should continue for at least 12 months before detoxification is attempted. Detoxification appears to be most successful when done on a slow, gradual basis over a 3–6 month period. Because even this gradual withdrawal is at times associated with low-level symptoms that addicts do not tolerate well, many patients who otherwise seem ready to be drug-free have been unable to stop taking methadone.

Recently, the use of the alpha-adrenergic agonist, clonidine, to aid patients withdrawing from methadone has made it possible to detoxify such individuals in 2 weeks instead of many months and with a minimum of symptoms. If it lives up to its initial promise, it may make it possible for individuals to be more successful in discontinuing methadone and remaining drug-free.

Narcotic Antagonists. These are agents which for the most part block the effects of narcotics without producing any substantial problem of addiction themselves. Although they have been used to treat narcotic dependence since the late 1960s, it is only recently that their promise looks likely to be fulfilled because of the development of an agent that is both long-acting and has a minimum of side effects, namely naltrexone. Naltrexone can be given on a Monday, Wednesday, Friday basis and blocks the euphoric effects of street doses of heroin. The groups of patients who may do best on naltrexone are those who are coming out of a drug-free environment such as prison or a hospital and need some help in remaining drug-free; those who are leaving other treatment programs such as methadone or therapeutic communities; and, finally, individuals who may be "chipping" but not addicted to narcotics or who have not been taking them for a long time. However, in order to start on naltrexone, individuals must be free of narcotics for at least 5–7 days.

The last two methods, methadone maintenance and narcotic antagonists, are clearly for the individual with an opiate-abuse problem. Stimulant, depressant, and polydrug abusers need to be treated within the therapeutic community or any of the outpatient approaches. Alcoholics Anonymous, while useful for alcoholics, has not been shown to be particularly helpful with adolescent polydrug users or with adult heroin users. Recently, some AA groups have formed that specialize in working with pill abusers and "Pills Anonymous" groups have begun to appear around the country.

Pain Management in Narcotic-Dependent Patients

Opiate-dependent patients are sometimes in need of acute narcotic analgesics for injuries,

cardiac pain, and the like. In such cases, it is a good idea to maintain the patient on methadone for the opiate addiction, and consider analgesia as an additional issue. The following discussion, then, applies to patients who have been acutely placed on methadone maintenance in the hospital as well as to patients who are in a chronic methadone maintenance program.

Methadone maintenance in the treatment of chronic narcotic dependent individuals has been in existence since the 1960s, however, confusion remains on how to medicate such patients when they require medical or surgical intervention. Individuals on methadone maintenance rapidly develop tolerance to the analgesic and most other pharmacologic effects of methadone. Therefore they perceive pain and require analgesics just the same as nonaddicted individuals. Altering the maintenance dose of methadone to provide analgesia can result in inadequate pain control, may complicate the clinical situation, and hinder future detoxification efforts. Complaints of pain may be ignored and requests for additional medication are often refused, being ascribed to the drug craving and attempts to receive more drugs rather than the anguish of a human being in distress. The following regime is recommended.

First, the hospitalized methadone-maintained patient should be given the normal daily dose of methadone, either as a single or divided dose. If oral administration is not possible, the methadone can be administered intramuscularly at a dose one-half of the oral dose.

In the second place, a different narcotic than methadone, preferably the one the physician usually uses in such circumstances, should be given for pain control. The dose may need to be 25–50% higher than normal because of cross-tolerance, but no change is necessary in frequency of administration.

Next, the duration of such analgesia should be based on the pain symptoms of the patient using the physician's experience with similar conditions as a guide. Although the addict patient may try to prolong the period of analgesic prescription, more often the physician stops the dosage prematurely for fear he or she is being manipulated.

Finally, if other analgesics are used, care should be taken to avoid those with mixed agonist-antagonist action. These drugs can precipitate acute withdrawal symptoms in methadone-maintained patients. Some examples include: pentazocine (Talwin), nalbuphine (Nubain), and butorphanol (Stadol).

Alterations of the methadone maintenance dose can lead to several problems. Raising the patient's dose to achieve analgesia usually results both in inadequate pain relief and patient-physician hostility. Physicians used to giving low doses of narcotics assume that a patient receiving 60 mg of methadone is getting an enormous dose of a painkiller and should have ample pain relief. However, if the patient is on a methadone-maintenance dose of 55 mg, he or she is, in effect, only receiving the equivalent of 5 mg of methadone or less as an analgesic dose. Likewise, when the need for analgesia has passed, physicians will often lower the methadone dose too rapidly and to a very low level because of assumptions about the relatively large dose the patient is getting. All these problems are avoided by using a different narcotic for pain control and simply keeping the patient on the normal methadone dose as if it were a different category of drug. Viewed as one would view a daily insulin or thyroid dose, better medical care can be achieved and inappropriate moralizing or patient-staff hostility avoided.

SUMMARY

It is unlikely that drug abuse will soon vanish from the scene. More likely are the changes in popularity of various chemicals and their social acceptance. New drugs such as PCP, cheap and easy to make illicitly, come into favor and then are replaced by others that promise new sensations or are easier to get onto the clandestine market. The psychological and physical manifestations or complications of these agents, whether old or new, require the primary physician to maintain an index of suspicion about drug abuse. This chapter's purpose is to lay a foundation for an alert and careful assessment, with practical suggestions for procedure once a diagnosis has been made.

APPENDIX A: TECHNIQUE OF NARCOTIC WITHDRAWAL THROUGH METHADONE SUBSTITUTION

Initiation of detoxification

If the patient is receiving narcotics for medical purposes and the physician is reasonably sure about the strength and amount the patient is taking, the following table can be used to convert the dose into milligrams of methadone:

1 mg methadone is equivalent to:

- heroin 1-2 mg

- morphine 3-4 mg

- dilaudanum (Dilaudid) 0.5 mg

- codeine 30 mg

- meperidine 20 mg

- paregoric 7-8 mL

- laudanum 3 mL

- levorphanol (Levo-Dromoran) 0.5 mg

- opium alkaloids (Pantopon) 4 mg

- anileridine (Leritine) 8 mg

In the situation of illicit drug use, it is less likely that the patient will be able to give an accurate picture of the amount used since even with the best of intentions and lack of any desire to deceive, the amount of narcotics in an illegal "bag" varies from dealer to dealer and week to week if not day to day. Under these circumstances, the physician must guess at the initial dose. Usually 10-20 mg of oral methadone is a sufficient starting dose. It is large enough to control the majority of illicit habits and small enough not to be very dangerous unless the individual has little or no tolerance. The patient should be kept under observation to judge the effect of the dose. If withdrawal symptoms are present initially, this dose should suppress them within 30-60 minutes. If not, an additional 5-10 mg of methadone can be given. If withdrawal symptoms are not present, the patient should be observed for drowsiness or depressed respiration. Except in cases where there is documented evidence of use of narcotics in excess of 40 mg methadone equivalent a day, the initial dose should never exceed 30 mg and the total 24-hour dose should never exceed 40 mg. Where 10-20 mg was given as the first dose, a similar amount may be given 12 hours later if deemed necessary. This is usually not practical in outpatient detoxification but is not uncommon in inpatient or residential settings.

There is disagreement as to whether to start the withdrawal regime without the actual presence of withdrawal signs and symptoms. It is usually difficult to know with certainty that an individual is currently physically addicted. With the exception of either waiting for symptoms to develop or giving naloxone to provoke withdrawal, all other indicators point to use rather than tolerance and addiction. In order to prevent nonaddicts from being given narcotics, some clinicians insist on the presence of symptoms either naturally occurring or precipitated. A good case for the opposite position has been made by Newman (1979):

> Generally, however, there is no need to go to such lengths if the history is credible and consistent with the findings on physical examination ... certainly, there is no justification for insisting on observing objective signs of withdrawal as a prerequisite to admission. The withdrawal syndrome, after all, is what the treatment regime is designed to *prevent*. Heroic measures to preclude admission of an application who is not physiologically dependent imply that there is an incentive for non-addicts to seek such admission. There is no evidence to suggest that this is the case, and intuitively the possibility seems remote indeed. ... The notion that non-addicts would submit to the comprehensive intake evaluation (interview, medical history, physical examination, and laboratory testing) which is part of any approved program, merely in order to obtain 'free' methadone for a few weeks, is highly implausible....

Length of Withdrawal

The total dose necessary to stablize the patient in the first 24 hours should be repeated on the second day either in one dose for outpatients or two for inpatients, and corrections made up or down if the dose either excessively sedates the patient or fails to sufficiently suppress the abstinence syndrome. After the patient is stabilized, the dose can then be gradually withdrawn. One common pattern is to decrease the dose by 5 mg per day. A second method is to decrease by 5 mg a day until 10-15 mg is reached and then decrease more slowly. Typical daily patterns may then look like this:

Day	1	2	3	4	5	6	7	8			
Dose	30	30	25	20	15	10	5	0			

Day	1	2	3	4	5	6	7	8	9	10	11
Dose	30	30	25	20	15	12	10	8	5	3	0

In general, inpatient/residential withdrawal takes place over 5-10 days while outpatient withdrawal may be stretched out longer in order to minimize any symptoms. The role of the patient in helping to regulate the duration and speed of his or her withdrawal should continue to be explored. However, methadone cannot be given for longer than 21 days and still be considered part of a detoxification program. Under Food and Drug Administration (FDA) regulations, use of methadone beyond 21 days is considered maintenance and a drug treatment unit needs appropriate governmental approval for such a program.

Other drugs and supportive measures

Even with gradual withdrawal all symptoms may not be totally suppressed and after withdrawal is completed certain symptoms may persist, albeit in a rather mild form. There is no consensus as to the use of other drugs during these periods. The use of tranquilizers and/or bedtime sedation can help allay the patient's anxiety and minimize his craving for morphine-like drugs. On the other hand, nonnarcotic medications are ineffective in relieving the specific symptoms of narcotics abstinence. They add stupor and depression but do not bring restful sleep. If insomnia and other withdrawal symptoms are unusually severe, especially in older patients, relief can be provided by an increment in the next dose of methadone and, therefore, a slower withdrawal schedule.

Experimentors who tried a variety of drugs in combination with methadone-aided withdrawal noted that chlorpromazine, for example, caused patients to complain of feeling "spaced out" and did not relieve their severe depression, cramps, nausea and fear. On the other hand, doxepin proved extremely effective and made the patients less restless and more amenable to group therapy.

Insomnia is one of the more debilitating withdrawal symptoms since it is not only difficult to tolerate in and of itself, but it also weakens the addict's ability to deal with other withdrawal problems. There is general agreement that barbiturates, because of their addicting nature, should not be used to treat insomnia. Drugs that have been advocated included chloral hydrate, flurazepam, diphenhydramine, and the tricyclic antidepressants such as amitriptyline and doxepin. All of these have been used in withdrawal and although objective comparisons are difficult as far as actual efficacy, flurazepam appears most preferred by the patients, and its continuation was more often requested than the others. Because of its cumulative nature, it should not be continued for longer than 3 weeks.

Nonpharmaceutical supports can also play an important and useful role during the detoxification period. Most helpful is a warm, kind, and reassuring attitude of treatment staff. As noted elsewhere in the chapter, involvement of patients in their own detoxification schedule has been found to be of positive value and usually is not abused. It is, therefore, not necessary most of the time to have an adversary role develop around the issue of medication dose. Staff members do need to take a firm stand about visitors, however, since it is not uncommon to have them attempt to smuggle in drugs. Visitors should be limited to only immediate family (parents or spouse) who are not known to be drug abusers themselves. However, even parents have been known to smuggle in drugs under the pressure of entreaties from patients who claim that the staff does not understand their needs and distress. A watchful presence may be necessary, therefore, for all visitors. Such attempts at deception are less likely to occur if there are family meetings and patient involvement.

Other measures that have been advocated include warm baths, exercise when the patient feels up to it, and various diets. Unless there are specific nutritional deficiencies, there is no evidence of the usefulness of one or another dietary regime. However, since addicts are often malnourished, general vitamin and mineral supplements should be given.

Mixed addictions

Unrecognized concomitant sedative dependence can produce serious hazards. Not only can seizures occur, but in addition toxic psychosis, hyperthermia and even death can take place. Abrupt withdrawal from stimulant-type drugs is much less of a physical hazard but can be associated with severe depression and even suicide. If sedative dependence is present, it is often useful to maintain the patient on methadone, withdraw the sedative gradually, and then withdraw the methadone.

APPENDIX B: TECHNIQUES OF RAPID WITHDRAWAL FROM OPIATES WITH CLONIDINE HYDROCHLORIDE

Clonidine is an alpha-adrenergic agonist, which binds to the alpha-2 auto-receptors in the locus ceruleus in the pons. Locus ceruleus is a concentration of presynaptic noradrenergic neurons, which supplies most of the noradrenergic fibers in the brain. Opiate withdrawal states have been associated with an activation of the locus ceruleus. Both opiates and clonidine reduce the activity of locus ceruleus by binding to the specific receptors in the neurons. Thus, clonidine can prevent the excessive activation of locus ceruleus associated with opiate withdrawal states.

On the day before clonidine detoxification is started, the usual dose of opiate is given. And then, on day one, the opiate is withdrawn completely, and clonidine is given in divided doses as in the following outline. Clonidine is to be used with caution in patients with hypotension, patients receiving antihypertensive medications, and patients with previous history of psychosis. As clonidine can cause sedation, patients should be cautioned about driving and operating equipment. In addition, usual precautions concerning prescribing medications should be observed.

Schedule for methadone maintained patients (20–30 mg day methadone):

Outpatients	Total dose per day (mg) in three divided doses
Day 1	0.3
2	0.4–0.6
3	0.5–0.8
4	0.5–1.0
↓	Maintain on above dose
10	Reduce by 0.2 mg a day; give in three or
11	two divided doses, the night time dose should be reduced last

Inpatients	
Day 1	0.4–0.6
2	0.6–0.8
3	0.6–1.0
4	Maintain or increase if any withdrawal
↓	signs occur
10	
11	Reduce 0.2 mg a day

Schedule for heroin, morphine, oxycodone HCL, meperidine HCL, and levorphanol patients:

Outpatient/Inpatient	
Day 1	0.4–0.6
2	0.6–1.0
↓	
5	Maintain above
6	Maintain above
7	Reduce 0.2 mg/day; give in divided doses, the night time dose should be reduced last

Precautions for outpatients:	Do not give more than 1 day's supply
	Patient should not drive the first few days
	Monitor blood pressure when the patient is seen
	If dizziness occurs, instruct the patient to cut back on dose or lie down

APPENDIX C: TECHNIQUE OF BARBITURATE—SEDATIVE WITHDRAWAL

Pentobarbital or secobarbital have the advantage of short intermediate action (4–6 hours) making therapy for barbiturate-sedative withdrawal both flexible and smooth. They are, therefore, the preferable drugs for barbiturate-sedative withdrawal. From the point of view of abstinence symptomatology they appear to have a good cross-tolerance with alcohol, meprobamate, and glutethimide. The initial and essential goal in handling patients suspected of addiction to these drugs is to determine their tolerance as rapidly as possible.

For withdrawal purposes pentobarbital (100 mg) is approximately equivalent to:

- meprobamate 400 mg
- glutethimide (Doriden) 500 mg
- most barbiturates 100 mg
- whiskey 3–4 oz

Initial estimate of tolerance

At the time patients are first admitted to the ward an approximate estimation of their 24-hour barbiturate tolerance should be made as well as their immediate status in regard to their tolerance (just right, intoxicated, or showing withdrawal). The estimate should be based on history, physical findings, and addiction pattern. If the patient becomes intoxicated or shows withdrawal on this dose it should be adjusted accordingly.

Test dose. The morning following admission the patient should be given a test dose of 200 mg pentobarbital about 50 minutes to an hour before the physician is to make rounds. (This test dose presupposes a habit in the range of 400–1,100 mg pentobarbital a day and assumes a "normative" state not showing withdrawal or intoxication.) Below 400 mg/day the withdrawal syndrome is not significant; above 1,200 mg/day a 300 mg test dose is better. (A 100 mg test dose is only used in the elderly or very debilitated patient.) In general it is better to err on the side of intoxicating the patient although keeping intoxication to a minimum greatly facilitates nursing management.

Test dose evaluation. A patient tolerant to 900 mg or more of pentobarbital would show no intoxication one hour after a 200 mg test dose given in a normative state. A tolerance to 700 mg–800 mg would show only nystagmus; a tolerance to 500–600 mg would show nystagmus, mild ataxia, and perhaps some dysarthria. Below this level coarser nystagmus, positive Romberg sign, pseudoptosis, gross ataxia, somnolence. With no tolerance to pentobarbital this test dose would put a patient soundly asleep but they would be responsive. One may extrapolate the interpretations of a 300 mg test dose in this same manner from a tolerance level of 1,200 mg rather than 800 mg.

Several modifying factors must be considered in evaluating test doses. If the patient has some intoxication or withdrawal prior to the test dose (in other words, the patient is not in a normative state), the interpretation must be adjusted. One must be sure that the patient received and retained the entire test dose. States of severe anxiety and agitation seem to elevate the tolerance.

Barbiturate orders

After the test dose evaluation and a more critical estimate of tolerance is made, orders are written to give pentobarbital in divided doses during the day to total (including the test dose) the tolerance level. Usually divided doses follow a four times daily schedule but if the habit is very large (greater than 1,200–1,400 mg tolerance) additional doses at 2:00 PM and 2:00 AM should be ordered for a smoother overall effect and to avoid excessively large individual doses. If the estimate of tolerance still is within a wide range, orders may be written flexibly to adjust to the situation (for example, "omit a dose if intoxicated," or "decrease any dose by 1 g if intoxicated," or even by ordering 100–200 mg of pentobarbital every 1–2 hours until intoxicated if tolerance does not seem nearly approached yet and the patient shows barbiturate withdrawal).

Each day the patient is checked for intoxication and withdrawal. When tolerance is reached the patient is withdrawn from that level at a rate of 100 mg per day modified by the findings on daily examination. A few patients (debilitated, epileptics, and so on) will tolerate a reduction of only 50 mg per day. Doses are reduced in succession with the bedtime dose maintained the longest and to a lesser degree the 6:00 AM dose maintained. (Reduce the 10:00 AM dose first and then the 5:00 PM usually). Any doses after bedtime should be eliminated as quickly as possible as patients may tend to keep themselves awake waiting for their medicine. Whereas large amounts of phenobarbital are to be avoided because of the cumulative effect, small amounts (30 mg of phenobarbital four times daily substituted for 100 mg of pentobarbital) at the end of withdrawal are advantageous in selected cases. It smooths the final drug effect and particularly is supportive to the clinging dependent patient who is anxious, angry, and depressed when the medicine cart passes him or her by.

APPENDIX D:
CASE HISTORY—THE WOMAN WITH TRACKS

At the time of admission, there were presumptive signs of opiate addiction, including miosis, venipuncture tracks, and "dozing off" at work. The patient's roommate provided valuable information concerning the patient's background, as shown in the PEG. The unfortunate early history of child abuse, alcoholic father, foster homes, and so on, probably contributed to the drug abuse problem. Her chronic depression, and perhaps, exposure to various drugs in the hospital added to the problem. It appears, however, that intravenous heroin use seems to have been only of 2 years' duration.

On the basis of the PEG, the following possible diagnoses had to be considered:

1. Fracture of left humerus
2. Opiate abuse/addiction
3. Dysthymic disorder (chronic depression)
4. Possible suicidal attempt (auto accident while driving alone)

On the basis of interview with the patient (as she became more lucid with emergency treatment in the hospital), it was decided that the patient was not suicidal, but that she had taken an accidental overdose of heroin before driving. Following an open reduction of the fracture of the humerus, the patient was detoxified from heroin with clonidine during hospitalization and referred to an outpatient therapist. This course of action was taken in view of the patient's willingness to be involved in therapy, work pressure, and relatively short-term history of addiction. (She was to be examined periodically by the hospital employee health service for evidence of addiction. She was told that her continuing employment was contingent on her being addiction free.)

PATIENT EVALUATION GRID			
	CONTEXTS		
DIMENSIONS	**CURRENT** (Current States)	**RECENT** (Recent Events and Changes)	**BACKGROUND** (Culture, Traits, Constitution)
BIOLOGICAL	Fracture left humerus "Tracks" on all superficial veins Miosis Blood pressure 110/60, Pulse rate 100 beats/min	Dysmenorrhea—1 yr	Father died of alcoholic cirrhosis Patient had many fractures as a child (see below)
PERSONAL	Stuperous but responding to stimuli on admission	Prescriptive heroin addiction—2 yr "Dozing off" at work—2 yr	A "long-suffering" rather "helpless" personality Chronically depressed
ENVIRONMENTAL	Brought to the emergency room by police The patient was driving alone	Broke up with boyfriend—4 wk ago Introduced to drugs by boyfriend—3 yr ago Works in the hospital as a secretary for 3 yr	Lower-class, Catholic background; father alcoholic Father left home when patient was 5 yr old; father died shortly afterwards Mother physically abused patient (causing fractures 3 times); many foster homes; diploma nursing school; lost contact with mother since age 11 yr
Demographic data: 29-year-old, single, female nurse			

RECOMMENDED READINGS

Bair, G.O.; Elder, C.; and Wallsmith, P. 1978. *When it's your kid: The crisis of drugs.* Kansas City: Lowell Press.

Bourne, P.G., ed. 1976. *Acute drug abuse emergencies. A treatment manual.* New York: Academic Press. This is a detailed description of the physical management of drug abuse problems.

Brecher, E. 1972. Licit and illicit drugs: The consumer's union guide to drug abuse. Boston: Little, Brown and Co. This is an excellent source for a general background on drug abuse.

DuPont, R.I.; Goldstein, A.; O'Donnell, J., et al., eds. 1979. *Handbook on drug abuse.* Washington, D.C : National Institute on Drug Abuse. This is a comprehensive guide to current treatment methods.

Manatt, M. 1979. *Parents, peers, and pot.* National Institute on Drug Abuse. (Single copies may be ordered free from the National Clearinghouse for Drug Abuse Information Room 10A56, Parklawn Building, 5600 Fishers Lane, Rockville, Md. 20857. Bulk quantities may be purchased from the Superintendent of Documents, U.S. Government Printing Office, Washington, D.C. 20402. A Family Response to the Drug Problem, National Clearinghouse for Drug Abuse Information (see above for address). Teen drug use: What can parents do? Hazelden Foundation, Consultation and Education Services, Box 176, Center City, Minn. 55012. These sources are suitable and useful for parents concerned about drug abuse.

REFERENCES

Eddy, N.B.; Halbach, H.; Isbell, H., et al. 1965. Drug dependence: its significance and characteristics. *Bull. WHO* 37:721–33.

Gold, M.S.; Redmond, D.E., Jr.; and Kleber, H.D. 1978. Clonidine in opiate withdrawal. *Lancet* 1:929–30.

Gold, M.S.; Pottash, A.L.C.; Sweeney, D.R., et al. 1980. Clonidine: a safe, effective, and rapid nonopiate treatment for opiate withdrawal. *J.A.M.A.* 243: 343–46.

Inaba, D.I.; Way, E.L.; Blum, K., et al. 1978. Pharmacological and toxicological perspectives of commonly abused drugs. *National Drug Abuse Conference Medical Monograph Series*, vol. 1, no. 5.

Kleber, H.D. 1974. Drug abuse. In *A concise handbook of community psychiatry and community mental health*, ed., L. Bellak. New York: Grune & Stratton.

Musto, D.F. 1973. *The American disease: Origins of narcotic control.* New Haven: Yale University Press.

Newman, R.G. 1979. Detoxification treatment of narcotic addicts. In *Handbook on drug abuse*, eds. R.I. Dupont, A. Goldstein, and J. O'Donnell. Washington, D.C. U.S. Government Printing Office.

O'Brien, C.P.; Wesson, D.R.; and Schnoll, S. 1976. Diagnosis and evaluation of the drug abusing patient for treatment staff physicians. *National Drug Abuse Conference Medical Monograph Series*, vol. 1, no. 1.

Petersen, R.C., ed. 1979. *Marijuana and health 1977.* 7th annual report to the U.S. Congress from the Secretary of Health, Education and Welfare. Rockville, Md: National Institute of Drug Abuse.

Stanton, M.D. 1979. Family treatment of drug problems: a review. In *Handbook on drug abuse*, eds., R.I. Dupont, et al. National Institute of Drug Abuse.

Zinberg, N.E.; Harding, W.M.; and Apsler, R. 1978. What is drug abuse? *J. Drug Iss.* 8:9–35.

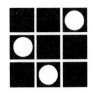

CHAPTER 17

Violence

Daniel C. Moore, M.D.

The practice of medicine can be a dangerous endeavor. Careless exposure to infectious agents and toxins, which are abundant in the hospital, can be lethal to the physician. No less dangerous are patients who are violent. Although it is important to recognize violent behavior as a symptom of psychosis, intoxication, or a personality disorder, it is *crucial* for the physician to recognize and avoid unnecessary exposure to dangerous situations in dealing with a violent patient. As the aseptic technique in surgery protects both patient and physician, so does a judicious approach to the violent patient.

Violence is such an emotion-laden topic that it is often difficult for primary care physicians to keep their own experiences with and reactions to violent behavior from spilling over into the evaluation of the patient. Indeed, the mention of violence in a patient often causes a temporary paralysis of the clinician's usual differential diagnostic logic. A psychiatrist may be immediately called as the only one capable of dealing with "violence," or the police may be seen as the only solution, each without considering what actions on the part of the patient were referred to as "violent."

There is a wide spectrum of behaviors that people lump together as being "violent." Sometimes the term "violence," refers to an alcoholic who went on a rampage in a bar and is still threatening and assaultive. At other times, the patient was destructive hours ago and is now calm and contrite. In still other cases, the violence consists of threats to others, especially family members, but a violent act per se has not taken place. Obviously, any complaint of "violence" must be evaluated and understood before action can be taken. For our purposes here, the term violence will not refer just to completed assault or rape, but rather to the broad spectrum of *aggressive behaviors*, whether verbal or physical, threatened or actual.

Since the term violence encompasses such a broad range of behavior, it is not surprising that there are many theories of causation. Postulated etiologies range from genetic to organic, neurologic, toxic, developmental, psychological, family systems, and social (Kolb, 1977). They all have as a final common denominator the breakdown of regulatory mechanisms for aggressive drives. While certain specific cases have only one causation, it is more common for a number of factors to interact in eliciting the violence. Thus, a patient with temporal lobe epilepsy may continuously have a seizure pattern which could erupt into violence, but it is unlikely to occur except in reaction to emotionally stressful situations. Similarly, a sociopathic patient with a developmental history predictive of future violence will become homicidal only when provoked by his wife around some significant family issue. Careful evaluation sometimes makes it possible to establish the relative importance of

---

CASE HISTORY 17–1

This was Dr. Z's first night on call in the emergency room. After several cases of minor lacerations, drunkenness, and suspected myocardial infarctions, he was informed by a nurse that a patient had come into the examining room holding a gun, demanding to see the doctor. Dr. Z immediately went to the examining room where he found the patient sitting in the physician's chair, screaming that he had been mistreated when he had been an inpatient at the hospital several weeks ago. Dr. Z said calmly, "Please don't yell like that—you will upset other patients. Now, why don't you get off that chair—that's mine, you know—and lie down here on the examining table; I'll see what I can do for you". The patient responded to this with further invectives. Dr. Z then slowly approached the patient, put his hand over the patient's shoulder, and said "Now, why don't you get up. Here, I will help you." The patient, who was visibly startled when Dr. Z's hand touched him, shot Dr. Z through the heart.

certain causative factors in specific cases. In a study of episodic dyscontrol, Bach-y-Rita and his coworkers (1971) identified cases of violence as predominantly psychogenic—predominantly brain dysfunction, or mixed. They went on to describe a large number of organic, psychological, and social factors common to their aggressive patients and which interacted to release violence.

SAFETY PRECAUTIONS

The inconsistent use of the term "violent" by the people who bring patients to physicians requires that the approach and symptomatic management be discussed first. For the patient to be diagnosed, it is necessary for the physician to be able to get near enough to evaluate the patient and still be safe. This statement may seem obvious, but many clinicians either remain too remote out of fear or recklessly disregard the dangerousness of certain patients. Both extremes can lead to unfortunate results.

Before seeing the patient, the primary care physician should gather whatever information is available about the patient. This may be information from relatives or the policemen who brought the patient, from the nurse's or receptionist's observations, or from the chart. Though often limited, this information will give a feel for the potential violence of the patient at present and may even make it clear that the patient is not a real danger to the clinician at this point. As the patient is approached, it is important to remember that with the exception of frankly criminal activities, most *violence occurs when the patient is afraid*, and not just randomly or malevolently. Often the patient has a great desire to retain control and is looking to the physician to help him or her deal with uncontrollable impulses. It is therefore essential that both patient and clinician feel as comfortable and unthreatened as possible during the initial parts of the interaction. For the physician, this means showing respect for the patient's difficulty and not

approaching him or her in an angry or hostile manner. These emotions often appear unexpectedly in the physician because he or she feels threatened in such tense situations. Anger or hostility on the part of the clinician should be watched for so that they do not escalate the situation. Likewise, the patient should be allowed greater than usual personal space so that he or she does not feel cornered—a situation which invites a defensive attack.

Respecting the patient's need for distance is sometimes difficult since close personal contact and the "laying on of hands" is a basic part of medicine, but this aspect of the evaluation must be delayed until there is clear agreement that the patient will allow herself or himself to be touched. Confrontations should be avoided, which means that the physician may have to give up temporarily some usual prerogatives such as telling the patient to go here or to sit there. Insisting that a patient follow a particular order from the doctor in the early stages may escalate the behavior of a threatening patient into actual violence. For example if a belligerent patient provocatively sits down in what is obviously the doctor's chair and begins to fire questions, the physician should not order the patient to get out of the chair. Though acting aggressively, patients often act this way because they are frightened and want to assume a position which makes them feel more powerful. Forcing such a patient to give up the chair may further frighten and push the patient to attack. Instead, the clinician should accept the situation for the moment and use this stabilizing factor to his or her advantage in proceeding with the evaluation. The clinician should show respect for the patient's difficulty and express a willingness to help. Statements like these will further defuse the situation since it is harder for the patient to remain aggressive in a situation where the other has clearly indicated he or she would like to help rather than hurt. The patient can then feel more free in expressing concerns and thus give a more useful history.

It is also true that some patients remain potentially physically violent despite all these measures to make him or her feel more comfortable. For this reason, the physician must decide, within the first minute of meeting the patient in the waiting room or examining room, where and how he or she will feel most comfortable examining the patient. If the clinician immediately has the uneasy feeling that this patient may act violently, he or she should respect that feeling. It is an easily recognized sensation, since it is the same feeling that we have all experienced in possible or actual physical confrontations in our own private, nonprofessional lives. In this clinical situation, the goal is to choose a location that will make physician and patient feel as comfortable and unthreatened as possible. From the patient's point of view, it will lower the likelihood of physical attack. From the physician's point of view, it will allow him or her to work in the most efficient and professional way.

A physician cannot think clearly about diagnosis if he or she is afraid of being assaulted at any moment. In addition, if the physician is afraid, the patient will sense this and either become more aggressive or fearful. Going into a small examining room together and closing the door can be very dangerous. A better approach is to begin examining the patient wherever the doctor feels most comfortable. In some cases, this may mean the waiting room with lots of space for both to move about. In other cases, it might mean nurse or guard is present, or that the examining room door is open with help within earshot. Whatever the initial choice, the location can be changed as the interview proceeds. If a rapport is established after a few minutes, the interview can be moved from the waiting room to the office. If the patient is becoming more aggressive, the clinician can simply leave the room, and reestablish the interview a few minutes later in a safer location. The physician should never stay in a dangerous or deteriorating situation. Such foolhardy courage will not help the patient and may lead to injury for either one or both.

Use of Restraints

With a small number of patients there is no safe way for evaluation to proceed other than to put them in restraints. This is necessary when the patient feels so threatened that all approaches, no matter how peaceful, are perceived as attacks, or when a patient exhibits continuing physical aggressiveness to everyone around him or her. This latter situation is particularly common with alcoholic and other kinds of intoxications which will be discussed later. Many physicians feel uncomfortable about having patients placed in restraints, feeling that his infringes on the patients' personal freedom or civil rights. Indeed it does, but with an actively violent patient there is greater risk to others' rights, including the staff, and the action, though regrettable, is justified. In addition, restraints often cause a paradoxical calming of violent patients since their own violent impulses have been controlled for them, and they no longer have to struggle with themselves.

Large hospital emergency rooms usually have security guards trained in restraint of patients, but physicians may find themselves in smaller emergency rooms or clinics where there are no guards or no restraints. Under no circumstances should a physician try to restrain a patient alone. Such a one-on-one situation will almost inevitably lead to injury. When there is inadequate support or no restraints, it is better to allow the patient to leave and then call the police than to attempt to restrain him or her with inadequate backup. As a rule, a minimum of four and preferably six people are needed to restrain a patient. In one-on-one or two-on-one situations the small number of people often stirs up a desire in the violent person to fight harder in the hope of winning. The larger number of people itself has a calming effect on the patient since he or she cannot win and often will put up only a token struggle to save face.

A leader should be chosen to approach the patient with the five others just behind and ask the patient to lie on the bed voluntarily to be restrained. If the patient refuses, he or she should then be approached by the six people together. Two ways of approach are possible. In the first, the group walks toward the patient from all sides. As the patient turns to strike in one direction, that person retreats and the others grab the arms and wrestle the patient to the floor. The legs can then be grabbed, and the patient carried to a bed with leather restraints.

The second approach is especially useful when the patient has picked up a weapon such as an ashtray or chair. The six people pick up a mattress together and hold it in front of them as they approach the patient. If the patient strikes out or throws anything as they approach, they are protected. When they are about 5 feet away, they throw the mattress on the patient. The weight of the mattress will knock the patient down, and he or she can then be restrained.

Medication of Violent Patients

If the patient is cooperative enough, it is better to avoid medication until a diagnosis for the violent behavior has been established. However, under some circumstances, the degree of agitation may preclude evaluation or even approach. In these cases, control can sometimes be reestablished without the use of restraints by medicating the patient and allowing him or her to sit alone for 30–60 minutes. Sedating medications such as barbiturates or benzodiazepine tranquilizers (diazepam or chlordiazepoxide) should be avoided since they may interact with alcohol or other intoxicants to cause respiratory depression. They may also hide the obtundation of an advancing CNS lesion such as a subdural or epidural hematoma which may be the cause of the violent behavior. Instead, it is advisable to use *haloperidol*, 5 mg, preferably in the elixir form, in cases where the agitated patient's di-

agnosis is not yet known. The elixir begins to act in 20–30 minutes, almost as fast as the intramuscular form—which should be avoided because injections are always perceived as assaults by such patients. If the patient is in restraints, the intramuscular form can of course be given in the same dosage. Haloperidol in tablet form takes up to an hour to work and so is less desirable. Haloperidol has the advantage of causing tranquilization without marked sedation and having little effect on cardiovascular and blood pressure status. When haloperidol is not available, chlorpromazine, 50 mg, or thioridazine, 50 mg, can be given in tablet, elixir, or injectable forms, but both these medications are more sedating, cause lower blood pressure, and can interact with alcohol to cause dangerously low blood pressures. All three medications recommended here may have to be used in greater or lesser amounts depending on body size, medical status, and degree of agitation. If repeat doses are needed, they should be given the same dose at hourly intervals with pulse and blood pressure monitoring prior to each dose. The only contraindications are that they should not be used in conjunction with epinephrine or in patients intoxicated with phencyclidine (PCP). In both situations there can be a paradoxical lowering of blood pressure to a significant degree. The physician should be alerted to the fact that any of these three medications can cause pseudoparkinsonian reactions, oculogyric crises, or acute dystonias, even in single doses. Though dramatic, these side effects are easily treated by an anticholinergic such as benztropine, 1 mg, intramuscularly or by mouth.

EVALUATION OF VIOLENCE

Once rapport has been established, the evaluation can proceed. Recognition of violence or threats of violence is rarely a problem except in two cases. Occasionally patients will become afraid of losing control of their impulses and appear at an emergency room or clinic with some other complaint or, more frequently, without any obvious complaint at all. They may seem highly tense or suspicious of what is happening. As the interview unfolds, the doctor must rethink where and how to continue the interview with the patient. The second case is when the patient has been using an automobile as an outlet for angry, aggressive feelings. Weapons or physical threats stand out as potential violence, but misuse of a car as a means of impulsively avenging an offense or trying to calm down through reckless driving may be missed. In their study of violent patients, Bach-y-Rita and colleagues (1971) found that 72% used automobiles in highly dangerous and self-destructive ways.

In evaluating violent patients, certain items of history are useful for diagnostic purposes. It should be kept in mind that in more imminently explosive patients, long or probing questioning may lead to greater agitation and may have to be left until later. As part of the present illness, a careful description of the violent episode, including inciting events, degree of provocation, any intoxicants, relationship to the target of violence, memory of the actual assault, and present emotional reactions to it are important. Information from family or friends may be valuable here, since violent patients often do not remember, or claim they do not remember, the episode. In addition, the clinician should assess the possibility of delusional ideas or hallucinations associated with the violence as well as the degree of present impulsivity and involvement in violent thoughts.

A history of other violent episodes should be obtained, with particular attention to repetitive patterns such as violence following alcohol abuse, stereotyped behavior suggestive of a seizure disorder, diffuse versus focused violence, or specific psychodynamic issues touching off the violence (Bach-y-Rita et al., 1971). Typically, a male patient with a mainly psychodynamic cause for his illness is very dependent with a hypermasculine facade and a need to defend his

masculinity against other men. Events that cause such a person to feel helpless and inadequate often precede the violent episode which can be seen as a sudden aggressive outpouring in reaction to their feeling of impotence (Bach-y-Rita et al., 1971).

Past history should include any information on childhood deprivation or family disruptions. Many adults with trouble controlling their aggression were battered as children or witnessed repetitive family violence (Bach-y-Rita and Veno, 1974). Histories of childhood hyperactivity, head injury, febrile seizures, and epilepsy are significant (Bach-y-Rita et al., 1971), as are enuresis, fire-setting, and cruelty to animals (Hellman and Blackman, 1966). Also important is a history of juvenile delinquency, multiple arrests, and frequent unemployment or job changes. The symptoms of any psychiatric episodes or hospital admissions, including especially suicide attempts or other self-destructive acts should be elicited. Studies show that a subgroup of violent patients are often *both* self-destructive and other-destructive when they lose control (Bach-y-Rita et al., 1971, Bach-y-Rita and Veno, 1974). A drug and alcohol use history should also be elicited.

Medical history should focus on symptoms of epilepsy, past or recent head injuries, and any other serious medical condition which might affect the central nervous system enough to cause an organic brain syndrome. The confusion and disorientation associated with this syndrome can sometimes lead to violence when the patient misinterprets his or her surroundings or others' intentions and fights to protect himself or herself.

The mental status exam is a more formal approach to the patient's psychiatric presentation (see Chapter 2). Emotional state should be observed for depression or elation or continuing signs of anger or hostility. These affects will be important in the differential diagnosis soon to be discussed. Likewise, the clinician should note the pattern of the patient's speech.

Is it clear and coherent, or illogical, vague, rambling, perseverative, or round-about? The physician should also watch for bizarre or improbable statements which may suggest the presence of delusions or hallucinations. Finally, the patient's intellectual functions should be tested. Is the patient clear and oriented, or confused and disoriented? The precise manner in which intellectual capabilities are tested is outlined in Chapter 6 on the evaluation and management of confusion.

Other specific tests are of use in the evaluation of violent behavior but are better discussed in relation to specific diagnostic possibilities since they do not serve as part of a general screening battery.

DIFFERENTIAL DIAGNOSIS OF VIOLENCE

With the exception of frankly criminal acts done for gain, violent behavior has three general categories of causes. These are violence secondary to intoxicants, psychiatric "functional" disorders, and organic illnesses (Table 17–1). In many cases, there is overlap between these categories, with a particular patient losing control as a result of the interaction of two or more possible causes.

Intoxicants

Alcohol.   Intoxicants of all kinds cause dulling of inhibitions and allow the release of all sorts of behavior, including aggression. Acute alcohol intoxication is the best-known cause for violence, and we are all familiar with the slurred speech, fuzzy thinking, and staggering gait which accompany it. However, some physicians are not aware that not all patients manifest these more obvious signs despite significant alcohol intake and loss of control. For this reason, a blood alcohol level should be drawn whenever alcohol intoxication is suspected, even when the patient does not show obvious signs of drunkenness. Blood alcohol levels are also particularly useful in diagnosing so-called pathologic intoxication. Unlike most alcoholic violence, which occurs under the influence of high blood alcohol levels, the violence of pathologic intoxication is provoked in certain individuals by small

---

TABLE 17–1
Differential diagnosis of violent behavior

INTOXICATION	PSYCHIATRIC DISORDERS	ORGANIC DISORDERS
Acute alcohol intoxication	Paranoid schizophrenia	Mental retardation
Pathologic intoxication	Depressive syndrome	Acute organic brain syndrome
Chronic alcoholism	Manic-depressive illness	Chronic organic brain syndrome
Phencyclidine	Personality disorders	Temporal lobe epilepsy (partial
Heroin addiction	Passive-aggressive	complex seizures)
Other intoxicants	Antisocial (sociopathic)	
	Histrionic	
	Paranoid	
	Borderline neurotic	
	Marital and family problems	
	Spouse and child battering	

amounts of alcohol not usually sufficient to cause drunkenness. Typically, the patient has only one or two drinks followed by a sudden onset of rage and destructiveness. The violence may be diffusely directed or relatively specific. Often it is accompanied by confusion, hallucinations (usually visual), transient delusions, and the patient may appear temporarily psychotic. Following a period that can range from a few minutes to a day, the rage subsides, usually followed by sleep and amnesia on awakening (Bach-y-Rita et al., 1970).

Some patients with pathologic intoxication have abnormal EEG findings in the frontal or temporal lobe, and in some cases administration of alcohol has even induced an abnormal EEG pattern (Thompson, 1963; Bach-y-Rita et al., 1970). However, some authors point to the patients with normal EEG results and suggest that a hysterical or borderline psychotic may decompensate temporarily under the effects of small amounts of alcohol and become impulsively rageful and destructive (Chafetz, 1975). Probably both types exist and therefore every patient with repetitive episodes of pathologic intoxication deserves to have a sleep EEG test. Some physicians empirically treat the patients with abnormal EEG readings with diphenylhydantoin, although the effectiveness of this regimen has not been verified (Bach-y-Rita et al., 1971; Pincus and Tucken, 1974).

Chronic alcoholism does not show a direct one-to-one relationship to violence as does acute intoxication, but it is clearly strongly associated. In his study of 30 patients admitted for violent behavior, Tuason (1971) identified 12 definite and 6 probable cases of chronic alcoholism, but he could establish clearly alcohol-influenced violence in only two of them. It may be that chronic alcohol abuse reinforces a personality style of acting impulsively which can lead to violence. For chronic alcoholism, inpatient detoxification followed by outpatient treatment, group therapy, or AA involvement is necessary. (See Chapter 15.)

Phencyclidine. Lately, a drug of abuse, phencyclidine, has gained popularity in the drug culture. PCP, also known as "angel dust," is often sold as a higher-status drug such as mescaline, psilocybin, or LSD, or used to lace weak marihuana. In low doses (5–20 mg), it causes a "high" with moods ranging from euphoria to depression to violent anger and hostility. It's effect is best described as an acute confusional state with unpredictable mood changes lasting 4–6 hours (Sioris and Krenzelok, 1978). Accompanying physical signs are ataxia, drowsiness, stupor, variable pupil size (usually miotic), blurred vision, horizontal and vertical nystagmus (invariable), tremors, increased deep tendon reflexes, and muscle rigidity. The blood pressure is elevated in some but not all cases (Sioris and Krenzelok, 1978). Some patients develop a phencyclidine psychosis resembling schizophrenia with hallucinations, paranoid delusions, and insomnia lasting as long as 2–4 weeks (Luisada and Brown, 1976). In this state, patients may commit unpredictable or unmotivated homicidal or suicidal acts. At high doses (more than 20 mg), the patient is often comatose or has a zombielike, glazed stare and is unresponsive; the state resembles catatonia. The eyes are open with persistent nystagmus. There is sustained blood pressure elevation, exaggerated deep tendon reflexes, and cardiac arrhythmias, and acute renal failure (Sioris and Krenzelok, 1978). Phencyclidine can be measured in the urine by gas chromatography.

If the overdose has been recent, the stomach may be evacuated with activated charcoal and a saline cathartic (Sioris and Krenzelok, 1978). The excretion of phencyclidine already absorbed can be speeded by as much as 100 to 300 times by administration of furosemide and acidification of the urine with ammonium chloride (Aronow and Done, 1978). Cranberry juice taken orally is another possibility. An antihypertensive is not usually needed, but diazoxide and hydralazine have been used to treat hypertensive crisis. If depression, hostility, hallucination, or paranoid thinking is the presenting symptom, the patient should be hospitalized psychiatrically to assure safety for the patient and others. If agitation must be treated, an antianxiety agent such as diazepam or chlordiazepoxide is preferable to a phenothiazine like chlorpromazine, since the latter can interact with phencyclidine to cause paradoxic hypotension and has not been shown to shorten the duration of a phencyclidine psychosis (Burns and Lerner, 1976) (see also Chapter 16).

Heroin. Heroin addiction is a common cause of violence well known to the clinician. In this case, the violence is not associated with the intoxication since the addict becomes sedated and "nods out." Rather, the patients' desperate drug-seeking behavior as the heroin wears off causes them to commit burglaries, assaults, and other violent crimes in an attempt to get money for their habit. Such patients are more often handled by the police, but the physician may sometimes be confronted in the office or emergency room by an addict who becomes threatening or assaultive in an attempt to get drugs. Such patients are usually only violent when obstructed from obtaining the desired money or drugs. In the absence of adequate security, the physician should retreat and call the police even if this allows the patient temporary access to medical supplies.

Other intoxicants. Other intoxicants are occasionally associated with violence. Barbiturate abuse causes an intoxication similar to alcohol and violence may result when the check on aggressive impulses is loosened. Treatment is by detoxification. Chronic stimulant abuse can cause a toxic psychosis indistinguishable from paranoid schizophrenia, and such patients may become combative as a result of paranoid delusions. The treatment here is admission and detoxification from stimulants, after which the paranoid psychosis will remit.

Psychiatric Disorder

Schizophrenia. After chronic alcoholism, the next most common diagnosis associated with threatened or actual violence is schizophrenia (Tuason, 1971). Usually aggressive behavior occurs in a setting where the patient develops paranoid delusions of attack by others and acts in an attempt to protect him or herself. For example a schizophrenic may believe that he is being slowly poisoned by the food his wife is cooking and repeatedly threatens her with death if she does not stop before finally attacking her. Other schizophrenic patients develop delusional preoccupations with complex systems of persecution that they blame on one particular person who becomes the target of their violence. Less often, patients hear voices telling them to kill someone and express these threats. While violence can occur in all types of schizophrenia, it is more common and more dangerous in the paranoid schizophrenic.

The patient with an acute schizophrenic reaction has extreme disorganization, florid thought disorder, wild hallucinations, and unsystematized delusions as the presenting symptoms. If he or she is violent, it is usually a function of agitation and fear and is not usually planned or carried out effectively. The catatonic schizophrenic may suddenly become excited and attack, but again the aggressive behavior is disorganized and usually easily avoided. By contrast, the paranoid schizophrenic often does not show many of the classic schizophrenic symptoms in day-to-day contact. He or she may seem somewhat easily insulted and oversensitive, with some grandiose or strange ideas, but usually is not obviously psychotic. Instead, the person usually hides paranoid delusional thinking under a mask of apparent calm. Indeed, a paranoid schizophrenic may have developed an extensive persecutory system around a single insignificant incident which insulted him or her. Often the first sign of the paranoid thinking is a threat to kill a particular person, uttered so calmly and unexpectedly that it is taken as a joke. At other times, the first sign may be the homicidal act itself. A number of years ago, a psychiatrist was peripherally involved in the certification and legal commitment of a paranoid schizophrenic patient. Three years later, the patient was released from a psychiatric hospital, apparently recovered, and went straight to the psychiatrist's house where he shot and killed him. This story illustrates another important point in the evaluation of paranoid schizophrenics which is that when presented with a structured situation such as the emergency room and the threat of legal action, they have the capacity to pull together and appear normal, tossing off the threat as a joke. Their ability to minimize the threat or act makes it imperative to question accompanying police or relatives. In patients with a history of paranoid schizophrenia or present paranoid systems of thinking, psychiatric hospitalization should be strongly considered, especially when a person known to the patient seems to be singled out as the focal point of his or her paranoid delusion.

Affective Disorders.   Depression is associated in most clinicians' minds with suicide rather than homicide, but threats of violence are not uncommon in depressed patients. Of 30 patients admitted to a mental health care center following violent behavior, 6 had a diagnosis of depression (Tuason, 1971). The old and well-known concept that depression is anger at others directed inward has relevance here (see Chapter 9).

Depressed patients may alternately threaten to kill themselves or significant others. This is particularly true with separations or divorces, where one spouse cannot tolerate the loss and alternately feels suicidally unworthy about him or herself or homicidally angry at the other. In some psychotic depressions, patients feel so bad and blameful that they cannot contemplate suicide without feeling that it would hurt their family unbearably. Such desperate patients then

hit upon the delusional solution of killing everyone in the family before themselves, thus absolving themselves of guilt for the family's suffering. Murderous ruminations also occur when the depressive develops the delusional idea that he or she can right a wrong for which the depressive is partly guilty by killing a third party. Such depressions are almost always accompanied by the classic vegetative signs of depression: difficulty falling asleep, early morning awakening, decreased appetite, fatigue, and lack of sexual interest. Depression of this severity requires psychiatric hospitalization and treatment with antidepressant medications.

In manic-depressive illness, the manic phase can also result in belligerent or assaultive behavior. Manic patients show increased energy, overactivity, decreased desire for sleep or food, and increased sexual interest. They are euphoric and expansive in mood and often make multiple long-distance phone calls, overspend disastrously, and start projects far beyond their capacity or ability. However, their elation often turns to irritation and anger when thier actions or grandiose plans are questioned. At the extreme, such patients are belligerent, threatening, and assaultive, especially when blocked or confronted. Less ill patients may threaten family members for questioning their expenses, and then manage to appear rational and collected when brought to the emergency room. In these cases, the history of their recent behavior and the assaultive behavior are clues of the need for hospitalization and treatment with lithium carbonate and neuroleptics.

Personality Disorders.   Violence is not limited to psychotic diagnoses. Macdonald (1963) examined 100 patients admitted for threats to kill and found that 50 had non-psychotic personality diagnoses. They were passive-aggressive personality, 23; antisocial personality, 13; histrionic personality, 10; paranoid personality, 2; and neurotic behavior disorder, 2. (See Chapters 4 and 13 for discussion of some of these personality disorders.

The histrionic personality of either sex is emotionally excitable and self-dramatizing and may have irrational, angry outbursts when the helpless, demanding style, and need for reassurance are not gratified. In addition, the patient's exaggerated flirtatiousness, at times with near strangers, can lead to arguments and violence.

The passive-aggressive patient usually expresses chronic anger through covert, passive resistance to normal expectations. Such patients seem to set up situations in which they "accidentally" do something which infuriates the other person. When this leads to a violent argument, the passive-aggressive patient may then become overtly hostile and assaultive. Passive-aggressive and histrionic personality disorders are often attracted to each other and become involved in a sadomasochistic relationship. Typically, there is a constant low level of interpersonal tension which builds at times into a mutually escalating round of "hurts" and "counterhurts," threats and counterthreats. They seek help only when the anger gets out of hand and one partner becomes quite frightened or seriously hurt. Often it may be arbitrary which partner is hurt at that particular time, since both may instigate or attack at different times. Abuse of alcohol by both the aggressor and victim often occurs prior to the violence (DeLeon, 1961). Despite the degree of injury, it is often difficult to separate the partners since the mutually provocative behavior leading up to the violence is so intertwined with their personality and sexual styles. Usually the best procedure is to separate the violent patient physically from the partner until anger and alcohol have worn off. Hospitalization is not usually necessary, but those involved should be counseled to seek outpatient psychiatric help or the violence will recur.

Antisocial personalities have a history of continuous and chronic antisocial behavior with flagrant disrespect for the rights of others beginning before the age of 15 years. Frequently, they come from very deprived childhood backgrounds, with divorce, broken homes, financial instability, and alcoholic parents quite prominent. Often they were physically abused as children with multiple episodes of head trauma and unconsciousness (Bach-y-Rita et al., 1971). Stealing, lying, fighting, resisting authority, and truancy are typical childhood signs, as are the triad of enuresis, fire-setting, and cruelty to animals mentioned before. Hellman and Blackman (1966) compared a group convicted of aggressive crimes against the person to a group with non-aggressive crimes such as theft. They found that the triad of enuresis, fire-setting, and cruelty to animals was present in 75% of the aggressive group and in only 28% of the nonaggressive group. In adolescence, they engage in excessive drinking, use of illegal drugs, and early sexual behavior. These behaviors continue into adulthood with fighting, criminality, alcoholism, and inability to maintain a job as the usual pattern. Antisocial personality characteristics appear in prison populations, but typically prisoners are the unsuccessful criminals whose impulsivity, erratic behavior, and excessive alcohol use make their crimes easy to trace. In all likelihood, their violent behavior has developmental, psychodynamic, and organic aspects to it. In particular, recent studies of prisoners show rates of abnormal EEGs as high as 47% and suggest that seizure activity (possibly pathologic intoxication) may be involved in these violent outbursts (Bach-y-Rita et al., 1971; Bach-y-Rita and Veno, 1974).

Paranoid personalities resemble paranoid schizophrenics in their suspiciousness, oversensitivity, hypervigilance, and narrow, focused searching for hidden motives and special meanings. However, they do not show schizophrenic signs of delusions, hallucinations, or thought disorder. Because they are hypersensitive, excitable, and ready to counterattack against perceived threats, they may instigate violent confrontations in "self-defense." Treatment of both the antisocial and paranoid personalities is very difficult, and they are frequently seen in prison populations, where their habitual violence makes them dangerous to other inmates (Bach-y-Rita and Veno, 1974).

Family Violence. Although martial and family problems are a common cause of aggressive behavior, their occurrence is underreported. In some cases, the pattern will resemble that already described for personality disorders and sadomasochistic relationships, but in many others the problems will be more subtle and less obvious on initial examination, particularly if the violent behavior is threatened or minor. As marital relationships change or dissolve, arguments and sudden violent episodes occur. When adolescents begin to break away from parental authority, arguments and some fights are to be expected, although the more violent or intractable the arguments the more likely the family is to be pathologic. Frequently, a physician is called upon to determine who was right or to chastise the aggressive party. Unless the violence seems likely to continue, the best course is to resist taking sides and refer the couple or family for counseling.

Spouse and childbattering is a much more serious problem involving repeated attacks with little or no provocation. The batterer may have any one of the personality disorders already discussed; battering is mentioned separately to highlight its different presentation. Often there is an attempt to protect the batterer by disguising the injury as a fall or accident. Usually the batterer is not present at the examination, but his or her violent behavior is hidden out of fear, loyalty, or shame. The physician should be alert to injuries that do not match the patient's story, particularly if there are repeated episodes. Most communities now have safe-houses for battered spouses and protective services for children to help them escape the battering situation. Many states now require that the physician report suspected child abuse.

Organic conditions

Organic or physical causes of violence include mental retardation, organic brain syndromes, and temporal lobe epilepsy.

Mental retardation.

In mental retardation, the patient may have a deficiency in the higher cortical controls which usually inhibit direct expression of aggressive or sexual impulses. The lower intelligence makes it difficult to find substitute gratifications or ways around frustrations, so the only outlet becomes a violent temper tantrum. Even so, only a small number of mentally retarded patients are truly violent and other factors such as childhood deprivation or abuse and alcohol intake are equally important.

Organic brain syndrome.

Organic brain syndromes occur when a change in the patient's medical state causes temporary or permanent disruption in the functioning of the brain. The patient cannot bring his or her usual intellectual faculties to bear on the situation and becomes disoriented and confused. Cognitive abilities which may undergo a sudden (acute) or insidious (chronic) deterioration include attention, recent memory, spatial orientation, calculations, logical reasoning, abstract thinking, and orientation to time and place. These primary deficits cause secondary changes including misinterpretations, illusion, and emotional lability with prominent depression, fear and anger.

When the organic brain syndrome is severe, there may be hallucinations (frequently visual) and paranoid delusions. Confused by what is happening to them, such patients may feel they are being attacked and may become violent to others out of fear for their lives. Organic brain syndromes can be clearly differentiated from other psychotic disorders by the impairment of intellectual functions, which is best revealed by the formal mental status examination. Chapter 2 and Chapter 6 on evaluation of confusion in organic brain syndromes outline this test in detail. All psychiatric treatment of organic brain syndromes is only symptomatic. Correct treatment involves medical admission for the evaluation and correction of the underlying medical illness.

Temporal lobe epilepsy. Temporal lobe epilepsy (complex partial seizures) can at times cause seizure behavior which is violent or is interpreted as violent because of the bizarre automatisms and forceful physical activity. Since the manifestations so frequently involve complex behavior rather than simply tonic-clonic movements, temporal lobe epilepsy is often also referred to as psychomotor seizures. Whichever name is used, the seizures are produced by lesions discharging from deep in the temporal lobe. The most characteristic EEG abnormality is an anterior temporal spike focus (Pincus and Tucker, 1974). Unfortunately, EEG diagnosis is often difficult because focal discharges from these deep temporal lesions may be difficult to record with scalp electrodes until after generalization of the abnormal electrical activity has taken place. According to Pincus and Tucker (1974), probably about 50% of temporal lobe epilepsy patients have a normal routine EEG. Recording during sleep and the use of sphenoidal leads will increase the rate of abnormalities found, but nevertheless as many as one third of patients with temporal lobe epilepsy may have normal EEG tracings. As a result, the diagnosis of temporal lobe epilepsy must rest on a combination of clinical and EEG findings.

Clinical symptoms of temporal lobe epilepsy include subjective experiences, chewing movements, and sometimes more complex forms of automatic behavior. Subjective feelings include inappropriate feelings of familiarity or unfamiliarity about a person or place, called *deja vu* and *jamais vu*, respectively. These may be accompanied by more global changes like depersonalization, dreamy states, or "oceanic" feelings. Still other patients may be disturbed by "forced thoughts"—the sudden emergence of repetitive, unpleasant thoughts. They may have sudden mood changes or a sensation of impending doom. Hallucinatory experiences include a wide range of sensory distortions, including visual (macropsia and micropsia), auditory, olfactory and gustatory changes. The most characteristic is an olfactory hallucination consisting of a disgusting smell such as burning rubber (Pincus and Tucker, 1974; Sherwin, 1976).

The most common automatism involves repetitive chewing or lip-smacking movements. More complex behaviors involve repetitive acts which are almost immediately recognizable as inappropriate, such as unbuttoning and buttoning clothes, automatic writing, or running. Aggressive acts have been reported in about 6% of cases, although whether they ever represent truly goal-directed behavior is doubtful. More commonly, they involve hitting, running, or throwing actions, in which bystanders may be accidentally hurt. Sexual disturbances such as hypersexuality, hyposexuality, transvestism, and fetishism have been reported with temporal lobe epilepsy, but are rare (Sherwin, 1976). Some authors have suggested a relationship between temporal lobe epilepsy and pathologic intoxication as causes for violence. Anterior temporal spike focuses have been noted in the EEGs of some people with pathologic intoxication and temporal lobe epilepsy patients on administration of alcohol, but a much larger number of pathologic intoxication patients do not reveal new spike discharges (Thompson, 1963; Bach-y-Rita et al., 1970). Most likely pathologic intoxication involves a more complicated interaction of psychological factors, environmental events, alcohol, and seizure activity (Bach-y-Rita et al., 1970).

Temporal lobe epilepsy patients are usually conscious but confused during the episode. After it terminates, they often fall asleep and are amnestic for the ictal episode on awakening. Friends or relatives may have to describe their bizarre or aggressive behavior to a physician in order to get a complete picture. When temporal lobe epilepsy is suspected, a complete workup including neurologic examination, sleep EEG, computerized tomographic brain scan, and related studies should be performed. Generally, medication of this disorder should be managed by a neurologist.

EMERGENCY CERTIFICATION

Society often calls upon physicians to make legal decisions about physical and mental illness. Most states have emergency certification or commitment laws which allow for involuntary psychiatric hospitalization of mentally ill patients who are dangerous to themselves or others. Many physicians and even psychiatrists are uncomfortable with this power since it violates their convictions about civil rights and has been criticized by some authors as unreliable and arbitrary (Ennis and Litwack, 1974). Nevertheless, threats to kill are a medical emergency since most assaults and homicides are emotionally motivated, unplanned attacks on close relatives or friends (DeLeon, 1961; Macdonald, 1963). The physician needs to act before physical violence leads to disastrous consequences.

Unfortunately, it is true that predictive criteria for other-directed violence are not as well studied or established as for suicide. One author compared patients who had killed, patients who had only threatened to kill, and regular psychiatric patients for eight factors: parental brutality, parental seduction, fire-setting, cruelty to animals, police arrest record, arrests for assault, alcoholism, and attempted suicide (Macdonald, 1967). He found that the incidence of any four of these factors was significantly higher in the homicide offender and homicide-threat group. While these factors may be useful general predictors, a more commonsense notion of violence prediction can be used in the emergency room or clinic. If the psychiatric illness which led to the first threat or act of violence is still going on, it is unlikely that a single visit will stop

the ongoing process. This may be particularly difficult to evaluate in the case of sadomasochistic arguments which may dissipate at the hospital, but begin again at home. Here, it is important to evaluate the degree to which the patient is locked into the rageful thinking which led to the violence. If he or she is still delusional or ruminating about the anger at the other, this is a bad sign. Likewise, if the patient is still intoxicated or has guns at home, the level of danger rises.

Firearms were used in 55% of homicides, and the victims and aggressors were under the influence of alcohol in 36% (DeLeon, 1961). It is a good policy to never let a potentially violent patient go home without first checking about guns at home and having them removed by a friend of the patient. For a patient to be released following an aggressive act, there should be significant indication that the situation that led to the violence has been satisfactorily resolved.

Finally, physicians should be alert to the fact that criminals arrested for violent crimes sometimes try to establish mitigating psychiatric evidence by being evaluated at or transferred to a psychiatric hospital. Unless there is clear evidence of a need for psychiatric hospitalization, it is better for psychiatric evaluation of criminals to proceed through the court system.

SUMMARY

The evaluation of violence is no more difficult than that of other behaviors once the physician's initial resistance to viewing it as a medical and psychiatric disorder is overcome. Proper care and caution must be taken in approaching the patient, who usually has a desire to retain control but may be having great difficulty because of overwhelming anger and fear. The major causes of violent behavior are intoxication, psychiatric functional disorders, and organic illnesses. Assessment of previous violence, ongoing problems, or degree of intoxication if relevant, combined with common sense is the best way of establishing indicators of need for emergency psychiatric hospitalization.

RECOMMENDED READINGS

Bach-y-Rita, G.; Lion, J.R.; Climent, C.E., et al. 1971. Episodic dyscontrol: a study of 130 violent patients. *Am. J. Psychiatry* 127:49–54. Here is a study of the multiple factors involved in patients with explosive violent behavior.

Bach-y-Rita, G.; Lion, J.R.; and Ervin, F.R. 1970. Pathological intoxication: clinical and electroencephalographic studies. *Am. J. Psychiatry* 127:158–63. This is a good review of the pathologic intoxication syndrome, with data on experimental attempts to reproduce the phenomenon.

Macdonald, J.M. 1967. Homicidal threats. *Am. J. Psychiatry* 124:61–68. This paper discusses prognostic factors for violence as well as the role of the victim.

Sherwin, I. 1970. Temporal lobe epilepsy: neurologic and behavioral aspects. *Ann. Rev. Med.* 27:37–47. An excellent review of the diagnosis and treatment of temporal lobe epilepsy is found in Sherwin's article.

REFERENCES

Aronow, R.; and Done, A.K. 1978. Phencyclidine overdose, an emerging concept of management. *J. Am. Coll. Emer. Physician* 7:56–59.

Bach-y-Rita, G.; Lion, J.R.; Climent, C.E., et al. 1971. Episodic dyscontrol: a study of 130 violent patients. *Am. J. Psychiatry* 127:49–54.

Bach-y-Rita, G.; Lion, J.R.; and Ervin, F.R. 1970 Pathological intoxication: clinical and electroencephalographic studies. *Am. J. Psychiatry* 127:158–63.

Bach-y-Rita, G.; and Veno, A. 1974. Habitual violence: A profile of 62 men. *Am. J. Psychiatry* 131:9–11.

Burns, R.S.; and Lerner, S.E. 1976. Perspectives: Acute phencyclidine intoxication. *Clin. Toxicol.* 9:477–501.

Chafetz, M.E. 1975. Pathological intoxication. In *Comprehensive textbook of psychiatry*, 2nd. ed., eds., A.M. Freedman; H.I. Kaplan; and B.J. Sadock, p. 1341. Baltimore: Williams and Wilkins Co.

DeLeon, C.A. 1961. Threatened homicide—a medical emergency. *J. Natl. Med. Assoc.* 53:467–72.

Ennis, B.J.; and Litwack, T.R. 1974. Psychiatry and presumption of expertise: flipping coins in the courtroom. *Cal. Law. Rev.* 62:693–752.

Hellman, D.S., and Blackman, N. 1966. Enuresis, firesetting and cruelty to animals. A triad predictive of adult crime. *Am. J. Psychiatry* 122:1431–35.

Kolb, L.C. 1977. *Modern clinical psychiatry*, pp. 130–31. Philadelphia: W.B. Saunders Co.

Luisada, P.V.; and Brown, B. 1976. Clinical management of PCP psychosis. *Clin. Toxicol.* 9:536–45.

Macdonald, J.M. 1963. The threat to kill. *Am. J. Psychiatry* 120:125–30.

Macdonald, J.M. 1967. Homicidal threats. *Am. J. Psychiatry* 124:61–68.

Pincus, J.H., and Tucker, G.J. 1974. *Behavioral neurology*, pp. 3–40. London: Oxford University Press.

Sherwin, I. 1976. Temporal lobe epilepsy: neurological and behavioral aspects. *Ann. Rev. Med.* 27:37–47.

Sioris, L.J.; and Krenzelok, E.P. 1978. Phencyclidine intoxication: a literature review. *Am. J. Hosp. Pharm.* 35:1362–67.

Thompson, G.N. 1963. The electroencephalogram in acute pathological alcoholic intoxication. *Bull. Los Angeles Neurol. Soc.* 28:217–24.

Tuason, V.B. 1971. The psychiatrist and the violent patient. *Dis. Nerv. Syst.* 32:764–68.

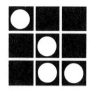

CHAPTER 18

Sexual Dysfunctions

Phillip M. Sarrel, M.D.
Lorna J. Sarrel, M.S.W.

Sex still remains a difficult area for many patients and physicians to discuss openly, in spite of the enlightened social milieu. It is around sexual issues that the patient is at times most anxious but least communicative. Many physicians, while discussing in detail with the patient and family the kinds of activities that might or might not be allowed during convalescence, neglect to even mention sexual activity. Sexual dysfunction may cause strain in family relationships and precipitate stress-related disorders. This chapter, written by a couple who are pioneers in the field of sexology, deals with the practical issues of sexuality and sexual dysfunctions for the primary physician.

INTRODUCTION

The primary physician plays a significant role in the prevention, detection, and treatment of sexual dysfunctions. Many people turn to their primary physician with concerns about sexual function, particularly if the physician communicates that sexuality is a legitimate and appropriate topic. Routinely inquiring about sex as part of regular history-taking is perhaps the best way to give patients permission to bring up questions about sex. But who will give the needed "permission" to the primary physicians? Medical schools have, in the last decade, made major strides toward including sexuality as a regular part of the curriculum. This provides physicians in training with a beginning knowledge base and some sensitivity about talking openly about sex. These courses suggest that people's sexual problems should be of concern to physicians but, too often the basic sex course for new physicians is not reinforced with other courses or in clinical teaching or postgraduate training. As a result, training in this field generally remains incomplete.

The practitioner who graduated from medical school before the late 1960s probably had little or no teaching in human sexuality and may find that the prospect of dealing with patients' sexual problems generates anxiety: Is it really acceptable to ask patients about sex? How should one ask? What should the physician do if the patient *does* present a problem? If the problem is serious, where does one refer a patient?

Problems in the area of sexuality can be thought of as belonging to four categories—behavior, orientation, drive, and response. Exhibitionism, a shoe fetish, promiscuity, or being a rapist are sex behavior problems. Sexual orientation refers to the choice of same-sex or other-sex partners and a person's comfort or discomfort with this fundamental aspect of his or her sexuality. Sexual drive refers to one's level of interest in sexual activity. Sexual response problems include sexual excitement and/or orgasm disturbances. These four categories certainly are not mutually exclusive and, in fact, a problem in one area may lead to problems in any of the other areas; for example problems in sexual response may be associated with concerns about sexual orientation, compulsive and frantic sexual activity, or decreased interest in sex. This chapter focuses on problems of sexual drive and response.

Masters and Johnson (1966, 1970) have evolved a set of basic principles about sexual functioning that form the underpinning in sex therapy. These principles are very important for

---

CASE HISTORY 18–1

A 43-year-old married woman came to a psychiatrist for "marital counseling." She said to the psychiatrist, "I think my husband is having an affair. He used to be a very sexual person, but in the last year, he has touched me about twice." She felt she could not ask her husband directly about his loss of sexual interest because they had never talked about sex, and she was afraid of "learning the truth"—that is, he is having an affair. On further questioning, she told the psychiatrist that her menstruation had been irregular during the past year and her husband had a mild myocardial infarction approximately a year ago. (See the appendix at the end of this chapter for further discussion and PEG.)

all health care professionals to understand; they are summarized as follows:

A first principle is, sex is a *natural* function. This seems an obvious statement, yet many people with sexual problems believe they can learn to force or will their bodies to function sexually. The basic physiologic capacity to respond sexually is present within the healthy body. From birth (and possibly prior to birth) the penis periodically becomes erect and the vagina periodically lubricates. During sleep, erection and lubrication occur during most REM phases throughout life.

"Spectatoring" is the *immediate* cause of most sexual dysfunction. Essentially, spectatoring is the anxious watching of sexual performance of oneself or one's partner. Observing oneself per se is not the problem, it is the anxiety that interrupts the natural flow of sexual feelings, distorts behavior, and causes dysfunction. Telling oneself to "relax and enjoy it" does not usually work. The stepwise program of sex therapy is designed specifically to help the couple deal with the problem of spectatoring. As they progress in the therapy, instances of spectatoring are discussed and the therapists make suggestions that are in line with the person's attitudes and values about sex. It is stressed that sex is not like many other endeavors; it will not yield to a goal orientation. Working at trying to make a sexual response undermines rather than enhances sexual response.

A third principle is, there is no such thing as an uninvolved partner. Many couples tend to see a sexual problem as the partner's problem rather than as *their* problem. A sexual problem has an impact on both partners and they need to work together to reverse the dysfunction. In many relationships dysfunction has been *caused* by interactional patterns or is being *perpetuated* by interactional patterns.

Sexuality is part of personality. Each person has a unique set of life experiences which has molded his or her sexuality. The physician usually needs to understand some of the major influences on a person's sexuality in order to understand the nature and meaning of a sexual problem.

Moreover, sexuality varies throughout the life cycle. The physician must keep in mind the person's age, the extent of previous experience, and the life stage of the patient or couple. Some dysfunctions are very common in adolescence or youth and are part of the normal process of sexual learning. For example, inability to ejaculate during intercourse is not uncommon as a developmental hurdle, but is not usually a problem in adult men. Transitory erectile problems at a stage of becoming committed to a new partner are not uncommon. Some young women need to have months or even years of experience with sexual interaction before they are able to communicate their needs to a partner and trust enough to let go and experience orgasm. Other events with special significance for sexuality are initiation of intercourse, pregnancy and the postpartum period, abortion, marriage or adjustment to a long-term relationship, menopause, and aging. An experience of rape also may affect sexual response.

Another principle to keep in mind concerns the normal patterns of physiologic change in response to erotic stimuli. The physician must understand the normal physiology of sexual response to understand sexual dysfunctions. Masters and Johnson (1966) have described four phases of sexual response—excitement, plateau, orgasm, and resolution. The primary changes are vasocongestive, and there are secondary changes that involve involuntary muscle tension.

It is important to emphasize that not every person experiences all of the physiologic changes described by Masters and Johnson. Kaplan (1974) presents an alternative conceptualization of sex response. In her schema sexual excitement is considered primarily parasympathetic while orgasm is considered primarily sympathetic. At any rate, the same person experiences variations in physiologic response from one time to another. Whether the behavior is homosexual, heterosexual, or autosexual, the physiology of the sexual response is basically the same—except that masturbation tends to produce more intense physiologic responses. Physiology is altered significantly with age but, in healthy persons, sexual response usually continues indefinitely—especially if sexual activity is engaged in on a regular basis. Some changes in the physiology of sex response occur during pregnancy (Masters and Johnson, 1966).

Finally, medical conditions have an impact on sexuality. From the moment of birth, physical illness or injury can be a very important factor in sexuality. Research has shown that an unusually high proportion of persons with severe sexual dysfunctions were seriously ill in the first year of life (18% as compared with a usual rate of serious illness in the first year of 0.2%). The impact of severe illness and prolonged hospitalization on the infant and the family can be profound. Not being held and touched and a failure to form psychological bonds at a crucial life stage appear to be the central issues (Sarrel and Sarrel, unpublished data).

Persons with serious sexual dysfunctions frequently have a history of illness, injury, or marked developmental delay in adolescence. Not infrequently the problems involve the genitals, for example undescended testicle, torsion of the testicle, recurrent urinary tract infections, or genital herpes (Sarrel and Sarrel, 1979). The psychological meaning to the individual of illness or infirmity during adolescence may profoundly affect a person's future psychosexual development. The role of the physician in dealing with adolescent patients may be absolutely crucial to future sexual functioning.

Adults' sexual functioning can also be interrupted by medical problems. While some illnesses or drugs directly alter sexual physiology, illness in itself can lead to anxiety, depression, psychological regression, concern about sexual attractiveness, or fear of sex as causing further illness (for example, in cardiac patients, cancer

of the cervix, or mastectomy or hysterectomy). One's spouse or partner may react to illness in the other. For example, a wife who witnessed her husband's heart attack and thought he was dead could not bear the idea of reinvesting emotionally in the relationship—she was no longer able to relate sexually to him.

DIAGNOSIS

Prior to Masters and Johnson's pioneering research and their evolution of a systematic approach to sexual dysfunctions, physicians had only vague diagnostic categories for sexual problems. Females with almost any kind of sexual problem were labeled "frigid" while all male problems were called "impotence". Even male infertility was sometimes referred to as impotence (impotentio generandi). Now that there is a better understanding of sexual function one can be much more precise in diagnosing which is, of course, a great aid in thinking about treatment. In medicine great stress is placed upon accurate diagnosis. The physician who does not *know* the diagnostic categories currently being used for sexual dysfunctions may tend to avoid discussion of sexual problems because he or she does not know how to proceed from the complaint to a careful diagnosis.

The following discussion of diagnosis will help the physician arrive at an accurate diagnosis. The patient's complaint can reflect anything from a simple misunderstanding of normal sexual function to a very serious dysfunction. For example, when a patient says, "I have a problem of premature ejaculation," he may mean he is worried because he occasionally ejaculates rapidly after a period of relative sexual abstinence without realizing that this is normal. On the other hand he could be describing severe premature ejaculation in which he regularly ejaculates without an erection. Yet another consideration, which is continually stressed in this section, is that the problem cannot be understood apart from the sexual partner. One man's partner may be telling him he is a premature ejaculator because "he doesn't last 40 minutes like her previous lover," while another man's partner may have vaginismus which is triggering his premature ejaculation.

One key to careful diagnosis is the taking of a sexual history. The primary physician ought to think in terms of two different kinds of sexual history. The first is the eliciting of a precise *behavioral* description of the current problem including its duration, the circumstances in which it happens, the patient's feelings about the problem, impact on the current relationship, and previous attempts at dealing with the problem. This may be all the history-taking the primary physician needs to do in order to decide how he or she can help. Many physicians will choose not to go beyond this level of exploration. If the problem seems to call for further exploration the physician may feel that lack of time, expertise, or personal interest in sexual problems calls for a referral (further discussion of referral is included in the later section on interventions). Or, it may be clear that some appropriate reassurance or education is all that is called for.

The second level of sexual history-taking explores the meaning of the problem and involves more time, expertise, and commitment from the physician and is actually a step in the treatment of a problem that cannot be treated more simply. The physician who is interested in pursuing the subject may refer to various guides in interviewing and treating people with sexual problems (see Masters and Johnson, 1970; Annon; 1974; Kaplan, 1974; Green, 1979; Sarrel and Sarrel, 1979; and GAP, 1979).

Who has sexual problems? It is estimated that in about one-half of all ongoing relationships the couple will experience a significant sexual problem at some time. Sexual problems can occur at every point along the spectrum of psychological health, from normal to psychotic, and in couples who are happy in their relationship or in couples who have severe relationship problems.

Classification

Sexual dysfunctions can usually be classified according to the phase of sexual function that is affected—desire, excitement, or orgasm. This classification is becoming standard among professionals and is used in *DSM-III.* A further subcategory of sexual dysfunction is primary versus secondary dysfunction. A primary dysfunction is one which has *always* been present. For a dysfunction to be labeled secondary, the person must have had prior sexual experiences in which the dysfunction was not present.

In males and females the following sexual dysfunctions are the most common (each dysfunction may be either primary or secondary):

1. Desire Phase
   Female
   - low level of interest
   - aversion
   Male
   - low level of interest
   - aversion

2. Excitement Phase
   - female—inability to lubricate, or distractability
   - male—inability to obtain or maintain erection

3. Orgasmic Phase
   - female—nonorgasmic response
   - male—premature ejaculation and ejaculatory incompetence

The primary care physician can expect to hear about problems of sexual desire with some frequency. Although both men and women can experience problems of decreased sexual desire, the problem is much more common in females (Kaplan, 1980). Kinsey and coworkers (1953) described a category of individuals who do not respond erotically to any kind of sexual stimuli and do not have sexual contact with persons of either sex in which there is evidence of any erotic response. Of women in the age group 20–35 years, 14%–19% of the unmarried females and 1%–3% of the married females were classified as unresponsive.

Diagnosing a desire phase problem can be tricky. Many patients express their concern through a statement such as, "I'm not all that interested in sex." They may, in fact, have a problem with excitement or orgasm or vaginismus. As with any sexual complaint, the clinician must help the patient to give an accurate description of the problem—its present manifestations and its history—before arriving at a diagnosis.

These dysfunctions and their phases are detailed in the following sections. Vaginismus, a problem among some females which does not fit into the schema, is also discussed as the major cause of dyspareunia. The occurrence of pain during sexual behavior can be due to the changes of the sex-response cycle or to penetration and movement during coitus. Pain associated with sex is discussed in the various sections to follow. (For a separate and fuller discussion of dyspareunia, see Sarrel, in press.)

Female Desire
Phase Dysfunctions

Low Level of Interest. It is difficult to evaluate problems in the category of sexual drive because so little is known about the nature of sexual desire or libido. Common sense tells us that there is likely to be a continuum of sex drive levels. It is not known to what extent level of sexual interest is biologically influenced through genetic factors or hormones and to what extent it is the product of life experience and learning. However, in cases of primary low sexual interest one usually operates on the assumption that early and/or adolescent life experiences have impaired the "normal" capacity for sexual interest and arousal. An alternative theoretic model is that of "scripting." This sociological view suggests that the individual has failed to learn a "script"

that includes sexual desire and arousal and needs to have an opportunity for such learning.

The histories of both males and females with generally low levels of sexual interest often reveal severe medical problems, hospitalizations, and disruption of parent-child bonding in infancy. The later family history is likely to be one of a sexually repressive environment and one in which affectionate touching was absent or minimal. In adolescence there was usually little dating or sexual interaction. The individual may never have masturbated. Females with a primary problem of this nature usually do not experience sexual arousal or orgasm, although one or both may have happened on rare occasions.

Secondary low levels of sexual interest present completely different considerations. Careful history-taking about the onset of the problem is crucial. In many instances the spouse or sexual partner is able to supply data to round out the picture. There are biophysical factors which can have a direct effect on sexual desire such as fatigue, substance abuse, chronic pain or disability, radiotherapy and medications (Kaplan, 1974). Fear of sex following heart attack, surgery, or even the normal delivery of a baby may present as low libido. Depression can cause sexual interest to disappear entirely. Some current life stresses may have causal significance—a deteriorating marriage, the illness or death of someone close, concern about finance, or investing all of one's energy elsewhere, such as work or studies. Sometimes, too, a person may be reacting to one's partner's sexual dysfunction by surrendering one's own interest in sex.

It is important to remember that sexual interest and frequency normally decline gradually with age in both men and women. Virtually every survey of sexual behavior in heterosexual couples has shown a decade-by-decade decrease in frequency of intercourse regardless of other demographic variables such as income, race, or educational level. Any assessment of a complaint of decreased sexual desire must be viewed against the backdrop of normal changes due to aging.

In all instances of low sexual desire (and in aversion, discussed later), the physician should keep in mind that the patient may be struggling with issues of sexual orientation. The young woman who complains of no interest whatsoever in sex with her boyfriend or husband may not have any lack of desire for a female partner. She may or may not understand her own feelings.

Aversion. Masters and Johnson and Kolodny (1979) have delineated a classification of desire phase dysfunction which they call aversion. Aversion, as they defined it, is a phobia in which sexual interaction or the anticipation of it brings about a fear response. Interestingly, aversion does not necessarily preclude excitement and orgasm and is thus often confusing to patient, sexual partner, and professional alike.

Aversion is more common in females than males. In the female, vaginismus may or may not also be present. The description given by the patient or couple usually focuses on lack of frequency due to the patient's enormous reluctance to *begin* sexual activity with the partner. The patient feels a sense of dread or anxiety usually mingled with guilt about *not* responding. She may be trying every mental tactic she can think of to get past the uncomfortable affect and begin to feel "turned on." Sometimes she can set aside the negative feelings and the excitement and orgasm may be relatively easily achieved. Patients often describe aversion as a very difficult hurdle they must jump in order to get started in sexual activity. The aversive patient may masturbate without difficulty. Some patients have an aversive reaction to only one specific kind of sexual stimulation such as cunnilingus or fellatio. Some women may see the male body or male

genitals as antierotic, and occasionally, repulsive.

The etiologic factors in aversion are diverse and idiosyncratic. Repeated or even isolated sexual experiences in childhood which were frightening and/or painful may be the origin of lifelong aversion. The most common such childhood experiences involve older family members approaching the child in situations where the child feels helpless and complies with the sexual interaction passively. Another history frequently encountered is that of the "promiscuous" adolescent girl whose frequent sexual experiences were sought not for sexual pleasure or the rewards of a close relationship but to meet other needs—a sense of belonging to a group, the skin contact and holding, or to get back at parents. Often past experiences of aversive females include some particularly humiliating scenes, times of painful intercourse, fears of venereal disease, one or more abortions, or rape. Because these events are often difficult to recall, an exploratory-type history is often necessary to uncover what actually happened that led to the aversive state.

Viewed in terms of learning theory, sexual aversion is the outcome of sexual experiences paired (usually over and over again) with negative affect. There are certain personality factors that may predispose one toward such experiences, for example, low self-esteem. Learned values that are very strongly negative about sex may also be important in the background of aversion. The negative influence in such cases usually goes far beyond societal sanctions and negative messages about sex. Generally a significant adult has deeply ingrained in the child or young adolescent the idea that sex is disgusting, degrading, and unpleasant—subsequent life experiences will tend to confirm the already firmly fixed idea.

It is not unusual for women with sexual aversion to be extremely attractive by stereotyped standards. Their sexual history includes their almost constant awareness, since puberty, of males seeing them as sexual objects. They may have spent their high school and perhaps college years fighting off unwanted sexual advances. They often view men as sexual predators and feel alienated from their own bodies.

Women with sexual aversion usually come in for treatment when they enter a long-term or committed relationship. Often their current partner is the first partner they have ever been able to trust. In spite of their feelings of caring and trust, they cannot throw off the anxiety and avoidance pattern they have learned so well in past situations. Their aversion, of course, has a tremendous impact on the partner who usually alternates between solicitousness and frustrated rage. The entire relationship may be threatened and the couple may become bewildered and miserable.

Male Desire Phase Dysfunctions

There is an assumption that all men are interested in sex and have a biological constitution that automatically and continually causes sexual tension. A further assumption is that men who are not interested in sex and/or not aware of sexual tensions are psychologically repressed or abnormal in some very basic ways. These assumptions simply do not hold for all men. There is a difference between lack of interest in sex and lack of sexual tension. Many men, for varying periods (months or longer) choose to withdraw from relating sexually to another person although they may continue to masturbate and be aware of sexual feelings. Others may continue to relate sexually but become aware of decreasing tension.

Low Level of Interest.
Little or no interest in sex, and/or absence of sexual tension can be a primary condition. Kinsey (1948) described a small group of men who gave no evidence of sexual feelings, desires, or behavior. Zilbergeld (1978) has also referred to such individuals. Physicians may encounter men who have never masturbated, are not aware of sexual fantasies and have no sexual experience with others. Kinsey regarded these men as individuals who had not "learned" about sex. Sometimes lack of interest reflects deep-seated feelings about sex, feelings which have not had an opportunity to be changed by positive sexual experiences. The most common time for such a man to present for help is when he has begun a long-term relationship and it has become apparent to the couple that something is missing. Because men are expected to be sexual, when sexual learning is absent, couples fear that the condition is seriously pathologic. Although there may be a serious psychological problem, many men in this category can be helped with a short-term, sexually focused therapy.

Men who have had an active sex life may lose interest in sex for a number of reasons. The biophysical, psychological, and interpersonal factors mentioned in discussing female desire dysfunction also hold for men. Especially common is a loss of interest among men who are overly involved in work or studies. The stress of work and fatigue combine to break the normal bonds between lovers which play such an important role in stiumlating sexual interest and excitement. It is also important to be aware that a change in sexual interest or behavior can be a sign of underlying psychopathology exacerbated by life stresses and of impending nervous breakdown. Recent reports indicate a high rate of sexual dysfunction among psychiatric patients, especially those on neuroleptic drugs (Nestoros and Lehmann, 1979).

Medical conditions in a man's sexual partner may cause him to lose interest in sex. For example, following a spouse's hysterectomy many men stop initiating sexual contact and gradually decline in their sex interest (Vincent et al., 1975). Some of these men, especially if there has been genital cancer, fear catching the disease or harbor guilty feelings about causing the cancer. Conditions that cause heavy vaginal bleeding or pelvic pain or stress incontinence can associate sex with discomfort or lead to long periods of abstinence, which can result in loss of interest on the part of the men. Many men do not understand what a hysterectomy is and are hesitant to initiate sex afterwards because they fear they might hurt their wives or anticipate that their wives will no longer be sexually responsive. This is also true following pregnancy, especially if there has been a long period of abstinence. Any type of painful condition (for example arthritis) in a partner can lead men to avoid sex (to avoid hurting) and eventually to lose interest. Menopausal changes can lead to alterations in sexual physiology, dyspareunia, and failure to respond sexually; this may lead the male partner to lose interest in sexual activity (Sarrel, 1982).

Decreased sexual interest may be secondary to a sense of failure or inadequacy. Men have expectations of how sex should be, for themselves and for their partners. If sex does not meet those expectations they can turn off sexually. For example, many men believe sex response should always lead to orgasm. A single experience of being unable to ejaculate, although a common experience, may cause some men to fear failure or of being "over the hill." Such fears initiate a pattern of complete withdrawal from sex or a gradual decline in interest. Similarly, if their partners are regularly nonorgasmic, some men feel they have failed or feel guilty about having pleasure while leaving their partners unsatisfied.

When sex response has been associated with pain, sexual interest may decline. For example, men with inguinal hernias may experience sharp pain when sexually aroused. Apparently, the testicular rotation and elevation during the plateau phase leads to the painful feeling. Gradually, the association of a disconcerting and interruptive pain results in avoidance of sex response. Other kinds of pain may be associated with male response—pain in the tip of the penis secondary to prostatic engorgement, testicular pain with engorgement and elevation, a feeling of deep internal tenderness after ejaculation, and pain from the foreskin when it is adherent or tight. In any of these situations, what is actually pain avoidance may appear to the physician to be lack of interest in sex (Sarrel and Sarrel, 1979).

When men lose interest in sex with their partners a common assumption (by partners and consultants) is that they are "getting sex elsewhere". As indicated, there are many causes for loss of interest only one of which may be a directing of sexual interest to another person. Apparent low level of sex drive in a heterosexual relationship may indicate a homosexual orientation.

Aversion. Male sexual aversion is much less common than female aversion or male loss of sexual interest. However, the situations just described in which men lose interest in sex may deteriorate into an aversion to sexual behavior. This has been particularly true when sexual dysfunction has been a humiliating experience. Unexpressed anger and feelings of being trapped in a relationship may present as aversion. Certainly, some men who are homosexual are aversive to heterosexual behavior. Aversion in young men may reflect extreme guilt about having sexual experiences. Aversion is also seen in borderline and psychotic patients. Finally, men who have experienced pain as a regular part of their sex response can become phobic, and develop the full-blown syndrome of sexual aversion.

Sarrel and Masters (1982) have reported a series of men who were sexually molested by women. All of the men were seen for sex therapy and presented with different problems of sexual response; aversion, however, was the predominant finding among these men. This rather unusual factor in male aversion is mentioned to offset the myth that a man cannot be sexually abused against his will; physicians should be alerted to a phenomenon that is not widely known.

Excitement Phase Dysfunctions

On a physiologic level, the excitement phase of sexual response is characterized by vasocongestion in specific parts of the body. Vasocongestion in the genital area leads to the earliest physiologic changes of sex response, erection of the penis and lubrication of the vagina. In the younger person this takes 15–30 seconds. The time needed for erection and lubrication gradually increases with age. Past age 60 years it may take 1–3 minutes.

When females bring up a sexual problem they usually do not state it in terms of lubrication. A woman is more likely to describe herself as not liking sex or not being responsive, although a concern with dryness may also be mentioned. The reason for this is fairly obvious; natural vaginal lubrication is not essential for sexual intercourse. However, lack of lubrication becomes a problem if she and/or her partner value her sexual responsiveness and pleasure. Maintaining lubrication is not usually a problem since lubrication occurs almost entirely in the excitement phase and will usually last throughout an entire sexual encounter. (Once in a while prolonged sex play or intercourse may result in decreased lubrication but this is not a dysfunction and can be compensated for with saliva or a lubricating jelly.)

Most problems during the excitement phase are expressed in terms of loss of arousal or distractability by women. Males, on the other hand, are very likely to express their excitement phase dysfunction in terms of the presence or absence of erection since erection is considered essential for intercourse. Not only must the male get an erection, he must maintain it. Many males who complain of erectile dysfunction actually may have a problem generating sexual desire, while some desire phase dysfunctions in females might be seen as excitement phase problems,

for example, the easily distracted female who says she lacks interest in sex.

Lubrication and Distractability.

When a woman complains of vaginal dryness one should *not* assume that lubrication is not present. Many women and/or their sexual partners mistakenly self-diagnose lack of lubrication in the external genital area. In fact, since excitement phase lubrication is produced entirely *inside* the vagina, a woman may have lubricated but the labia and clitoris and even the introitus may be dry. If the woman or her partner will simply insert a finger in the vagina they may well find that there is lubrication. The physician can get a clue about the absence or presence of lubrication by asking whether there seems to be enough lubrication after the penis has moved in and out of the vagina just a few times. If the answer is "Yes" then there probably is no problem of vaginal dryness.

Some women with a moderate degree of vaginismus describe their problem as lack of lubrication. The muscle tension of vaginismus may tend to keep the lubrication inside the vagina so that the introitus remains dry. In other women discomfort caused by penetration is interpreted by the woman as a sign of dryness when she is actually wet. In such instances the partner may have a more accurate view of the nature of the problem.

Vaginal dryness or lack of lubrication may have a biological etiology. Lowered levels of estrogen lead to decreased vascularization in the vaginal walls and thus to decreased lubrication. This is a common syndrome in menopausal women following oopherectomy and occurs in some women taking low-dose birth control pills. Vaginitis may also produce vaginal dryness.

When a woman is not experiencing any sexual excitement she does not lubricate. When lack of lubrication is a primary (rather than secondary) problem the etiologic factors are basically the same as those for absence of desire dis cussed previously. The physician should keep in mind that some women have difficulty accurately perceiving the extent of their own sexual excitement. Careful interviews with the patient and perhaps the couple are called for. Many women who think they are not excited at all actually are producing vaginal lubrication. They may even reach plateau levels of arousal without interpreting the experience as sexually exciting.

If failure to feel aroused and lack of lubrication are presented as a secondary problem the physician must first rule out biological causes and clinical depression. If these can be ruled out then one must assume that some alteration in life circumstance has caused the woman to "turn off." Careful history-taking may reveal clear precipitating events which have affected the woman's feelings about herself, her spouse, or sex. The nature of the causative factors will help determine the approach to treatment. Certain medications may interfere with vaginal lubrication, such as (a) drugs that suppress estrogen production (for example, low-dose birth control pills or cancer chemotherapy agents); (b) major tranquilizers; and (c) antihypertensive medications. These drugs may affect lubrication either directly or indirectly through their effects on the CNS, endocrine system, blood pressure, or liver function.

Ease of distractability during sexual excitement does not cause lubrication to disappear. The distracted woman who is no longer an interested, excited partner may still continue to participate in sexual activity in spite of feeling bored, anxious, or perhaps angry. The ease of distractability may be due to a low level of involvement to start with or it may be the result of anxiety entering the scene after initial enthusiasm and excitement.

Distractability may be caused by concern about something specific. For example, the woman whose husband frequently loses his erection may be nervously watching his response. The mother of young children may have half of her attention alert for a cry. When inter-

course has been painful a woman may begin to anticipate the moment of pain.

The primary physician should be alert to the fact that the subjective experience of sexual excitement may be rather like a roller coaster, with surges of intense feeling followed by moments of seeming lack of excitement. If a woman is anxious about her ability to sustain arousal she can easily interpret a dip in arousal as a sign of having turned off completely. The woman then becomes a *spectator*, anxiously watching herself, and she will indeed turn off.

Impotence.   Inability to have an erection or to maintain an erection are synonymous with impotence. Impotence is categorized as either primary or secondary. The Masters and Johnson (1970) definitions accepted by most therapists in the field, are:

1. Primary impotence—"Never able to achieve and/or maintain an erection quality sufficient to accomplish successful coital connection."

2. Secondary impotence—"There must be ... at least one instance of successful intromission ... [but] an individual male's rate of failure at successful coition approaches 25% of his opportunities ..."

Primary impotence is relatively rare except among adolescents or young adults. Secondary impotence is quite common. Both types may be due to biophysical and/or psychological and/or interpersonal relationship factors. Masters and Johnson (1970), and most other therapists have found primary impotence more difficult to treat than secondary impotence possibly because of the higher incidence of psychopathology when there is primary impotence. However, as better technical means for assessing genital change during the excitement phase are being developed, organic etiologic factors appear to be more common as a cause of primary (and secondary) impotence than was previously suspected. The newer findings indicate vascular occlusive disease and hormonal abnormalities to be significant etiologic factors (Spark, White, and Connolly, 1980; Wagner and Green, 1981). Erectile difficulty may be a transitory problem which disappears on its own. At times the causes are obvious (one-night stand, reaction to stress or fatigue, or fear of hurting or of pregnancy) and reversible. At other times the problem may come and go without any apparent reason. Biophysical, psychological, interpersonal, and cultural factors should be considered when there are erectile difficulties.

Disease in any of the systems which are involved in the changes of sex response (cardiovascular, respiratory, neuromuscular, and genitourinary systems) may lead to erectile problems. For example, a man who has emphysema may become dyspneic during sex response or a man with angina may develop chest pain during sex response. In their cases, stopping during the excitement phase is a protective mechanism. (For fuller discussions of the medical conditions relating to impotence, see Kentsmith and Eaton, 1979; Kolodny, Masters, and Johnson, 1978; Wagner and Green, 1981).

Diabetic men may be impotent secondary to neurologic or vascular changes. One study of men with erectile problems found that 75% of the men had abnormal glucose tolerance tests. (Schumacher and Lloyd, 1976). Unfortunately, there has been so much publicity about sexual dysfunction and diabetes that anxiety over sexual performance has become a significant factor in sexual dysfunction among diabetics.

Any drug that alters blood pressure or blood flow, sensory perception, and response to stimuli and muscle tension can alter the sex response cycle. Careful history-taking to ascertain whether any medications could be causing erectile problems is always important.

Erectile problems may be secondary to a major psychiatric disorder. This sign may be seen in major depressions, schizophrenia, and other affective disorders. For example, a recent study showed that 42% of schizophrenic men had erectile dysfunction (Nestoros and Lehmann,

1979). Erectile problems may be part of milder psychiatric disorders such as minor depression. In such cases the depression may be secondary to the sexual problem. After careful evaluation it may be determined that sex therapy is the treatment of choice.

Psychological factors are often the prime etiologic factors in erectile difficulty. Impotence may be a manifestation of phobia and/or panic over having intercourse. Hurting or being hurt by vaginal penetration may be in the minds of some men. Fear of pregnancy or of catching a disease are not unusual. Fear of loss of control during intercourse is still another concern. For some men, intercourse means commitment to a relationship, making such a commitment can be very anxiety-provoking. These anxieties are often exaggerated in cases of primary impotence but may also be issues when there is secondary impotence.

Pressures to perform sexually are common etiologic factors in erectile failure. Masters and Johnson (1970) feel that actual or perceived female "demand" is perhaps the single most important factor in secondary impotence. The culture or a specific situation may also create intolerable performance pressures, for example a group of friends going together to a local "available" female or even reaching a certain age beyond which virginity seems culturally unacceptable. The physician should be alert to the possibility that erectile problems may be the end stage of a long-standing problem of premature ejaculation or ejaculatory inhibition.

Orgasmic Phase Dysfunctions

Female. In recent literature on women who have never experienced orgasm in any way, the term "preorgasmic" has been used (replacing nonorgasmic) to suggest the future potential for orgasm. The word "frigid" is still used by some patients but it is an imprecise and perjorative term. Before proceeding with the discussion of female orgasmic dysfunctions, it is necessary to restate that there are *not* two kinds of orgasm in women, one clitoral and the other vaginal. Women can reach orgasm in a variety of ways: in sleep, through stimulation of the nipples only, through direct clitoral stimulating, during intercourse, and in other idiosyncratic ways. Orgasm is a physiologic response—or a reflex according to Kaplan (1974) that involves a variety of changes throughout the body. The physiologic response is essentially the same whatever the site of stimulation, although subjective feelings and intensity may vary.

Hite (1976) reported that only one third of women in her study reached orgasm from the stimulation of intercourse alone while two thirds needed to have additional stimulation (usually manual) in the clitoral area. One may argue with Hite's statistics but it is clear that clitoral stimulation is essential to female orgasm for a great many women. This pattern of response should not be classed a dysfunction.

Many women who have never experienced orgasm have simply not yet learned how. The underlying psychological factors causing the problem may be very easily overcome or there may be very powerful inhibitions, fears, or other resistances. The primary physician can gain some sense of the problem's magnitude by asking about extent of sexual experience, current sexual relationship, feelings about sex and orgasm, and techniques already tried to achieve orgasms. Depending on the physician's assessment, the preference of the woman (and her partner) and available resources for treatment, a decision can be made about appropriate intervention.

To be categorized as having secondary orgasmic dysfunction, a woman would describe having orgasms with some regularity in the past but now, despite becoming excited, no longer has orgasms. The primary physician should consider the following factors:

1. Pain during the excitement phase or during intercourse

2. Depression or other psychiatric disorder

3. Significantly lowered estrogen levels, recent reproductive system surgery

4. Chronic fatigue or illness

5. Substance abuse

6. New medications or dosage levels of drugs that could interfere with orgasm (for example, the major tranquilizer thioridazine may have such an effect in some women)

7. A change in a partner's sexual functioning

8. An extramarital relationship

9. Stress or change in life circumstances

10. Deteriorating relationship, particularly if it causes anger or emotional withdrawal on the part of the woman

A great many women who complain about lack of orgasm can and do experience orgasms in masturbation but cannot have an orgasm with their partner. The reasons for this vary considerably. Young women may not have learned enough about sexual exchange with a partner to be really relaxed. The partner may not understand the woman's needs and she may be unable to tell or show him her preferences (Sarrel and Sarrel, 1979).

Some women have learned to reach orgasm in masturbation in one position or with one particular kind of stimulation and cannot have orgasm in any other way. For example, some women masturbate lying face down and using rhythmic thigh pressure. Unless the woman can incorporate at least some of the elements from her accustomed pattern of stimulation into sex with her partner, she may not be able to reach orgasm with the partner.

Some women cannot let go in their partner's presence as easily as they can in masturbation. They may fear that they will look ugly or make sounds or movements that their partner might find offensive. If a woman has ever leaked urine at orgasm she may hold back because of this. Other women cannot let go for more psychological reasons—because they fear orgasms would make them vulnerable or dependent or because they don't trust their partner completely. More deep-seated issues such as an association between orgasm and death or unresolved ties to a father may be involved.

Male. Premature ejaculation is the most common orgasmic dysfunction in men. Ejaculatory incompetence is less common. Other orgasm-related sexual complaints include diminished sensation during orgasm, retrograde ejaculation, and pain at the time of orgasm.

Male orgasm is a reflex response primarily mediated through the sympathetic nerve pathways. It is a two-phase phenomenon. The first part of the reflex is the deposition of seminal fluid in the prostatic utricle at the base of the penis. Described by Masters and Johnson (1966) as the "moment of inevitability," this first phase is irreversible despite the fact that some men try to hold back when it occurs. The second phase includes prostatic, penile, and perineal contractions which serve to expel the fluid, that is, to bring about ejaculation. In physiologic terms, premature ejaculation occurs when the excitement and/or plateau stages are shorter than normal and ejaculatory incompetence occurs when these stages are more drawn out than normal. The Masters and Johnson (1970) definitions of these dysfunctions are based on their work with dysfunctional couples as well as their laboratory investigations of sexually responsive individuals. They define premature ejaculation as follows: "if he cannot control his ejaculatory process for a sufficient length of time during intravaginal containment to satisfy his partner in at least 50% of their coital connections." Ejaculatory incompetence occurs "when the affected individual cannot ejaculate during intravaginal containment."

Premature ejaculation can occur in either the excitement or the plateau phase of sex response. There may or may not be penetration before ejaculation. If ejaculation occurs very early in the excitement phase it can happen with minimal or no erection.

Factors already mentioned that contribute to orgasmic dysfunction include spectatoring, generalized anxiety, phobic states, pregnancy fears, and penetration anxieties. These dysfunctions can be a manifestation of the developmental process of late adolescence and early adulthood. In that context, the condition is usually of a transitory nature. Factors more specific to premature ejaculation include:

1. Conditioning—First intercourse experiences in which premature ejaculation occurred have often been part of the history of men with premature ejaculation (Masters and Johnson, 1970). A masturbation pattern can be established in which ejaculation occurs rapidly, and some men masturbate without an erection.

2. Abstinence—After a period of no sexual activity, most men ejaculate more quickly. Sometimes the build up of sexual tension can be great enough to lead to ejaculation without erection.

3. Extremely erotic stimuli—A rapid response cycle can be triggered by a particular stimulus or set of stimuli of extremely high erotic content.

Ejaculatory incompetence can be primary; that is, no experience of intravaginal ejaculation, or secondary; that is, at least one experience of intravaginal ejaculation. The phrase "ejaculatory inhibition" instead of "ejaculatory incompetence" helps clinicians think of the problem in association with behaviors other than intercourse itself. Some men are unable to ejaculate in masturbation or in petting, while very few men have never ejaculated in their lives. Others develop a secondary ejaculatory inhibition which affects all their forms of sexual behavior. They become arrested in the plateau stage as spectatoring takes over. Anxiety impedes the effects of erotic stimulation. Ejaculatory inhibition can sometimes be traced to first intercourse experiences or to a pattern established in masturbation.

Two psychodynamic issues seem to be in evidence in men troubled by ejaculatory inhibition (Sarrel and Sarrel, 1979). One is inability to express angry feelings. As a result, deep-seated anger and depression can be the most important feelings to deal with in therapy. Another issue is the fear of losing control. The men's fear may represent competition with women and a need to always dominate, or the fear may be of becoming overly aggressive and hurting one's partner. On a more primitive psychological level, the loss of sperm may be felt as a loss of vital body substance rendering a man vulnerable to others both physically and psychologically. In antiquity it was sometimes thought that sperm cells were brain cells and that ejaculation led to brain degeneration.

Ejaculatory inhibition can result when there has been minimal exposure to sexual learning, as in the case of the man who has not masturbated. Sometimes the presence of some facet of behavior perceived as antierotic or repulsive is a factor. Some men, for example, do not experience a woman's vulva as erotic and may find vaginal appearance, secretions or odors distracting or repulsive.

There are biophysical causes of ejaculatory inhibition. Sympathetic blocking agents can block the orgasmic reflex. Antidepressants can also interfere with sex response and the combination of an antidepressant and a sympathetic blocking agent (not a rare combination today) can prove particularly inhibitory. A pituitary tumor is a rare cause of failure to produce an ejaculate. With genitourinary disease, there is often repeated or prolonged catheterization. This can lead to atrophy of the sphincter muscle at the bladder base resulting in retrograde ejaculation or orgasm without very much pelvic feeling. After prostatectomy there can be similar effects.

Premature ejaculation and ejaculatory inhibition can both be precursors of erectile difficulty

as mentioned earlier. When a history of orgasmic dysfunction has been elicited it is important to recognize whether or not there have also been erectile difficulties—if so the approach to treatment is different.

Orgasm-related pain can be associated with premature ejaculation or ejaculatory inhibition or can be a separate entity. The foreskin, as it retracts during the plateau phase, can be a source of pain. With prolonged plateau phase, pain can be experienced in the glans of the penis. It is believed that such pain is referred pain from congestion of the prostate.

Different men react to orgasmic dysfunctions in different ways. Many men who ejaculate rapidly do not think of their response as a problem. Because ejaculation is not an endpoint to their sexual responsiveness, they continue to interact sexually after a brief pause during the hyper-sensitive stage of the postorgasmic refractory period. Others simply stop, feel satisfied and apparently their partners are content as well. For other men however, the pattern can be devastating, leaving them feeling humiliated, inadequate, and depressed. There is also variation in the meaning of ejaculatory inhibition. For some, lasting a long time means more pleasure and superadequacy as a male. For others, inability to ejaculate can be very frustrating, generate feelings of impotence and failure and lead to withdrawal from sexual activity. Inability to ejaculate intravaginally may come to a physician's attention when pregnancy is desired.

The meaning of orgasmic dysfunction to a sexual partner also varies. One woman whose husband was worried about premature ejaculation regarded his response as a compliment, an indicator of how sexy she was. On the other hand, another man with premature ejaculation claimed his wife had left him because she became so sexually tense and dissatisfied. Nonorgasmic response often occurs in women whose sexual partners ejaculate rapidly. Similarly, partners reactions vary from pleasure to dissatisfaction when a man's orgasm is inhibited.

One special problem for a woman when there is prolonged intercourse is recurrent urinary bladder infection.

Vaginismus

Vaginismus is involuntary tensing of the muscles at the vaginal opening when intercourse is attempted or at the time of penetration. It may be so severe that penetration is impossible, but more commonly, penetration can be accomplished but the woman feels pain or discomfort for about a minute (until the muscles relax somewhat). Sometimes pain generating from the tensed muscle persists throughout the time of intercourse.

Just as spectatoring can be considered the immediate cause of most sexual dysfunction, the anticipation of pain with vaginal penetration can be considered the immediate cause of most vaginismus. As with other sexual problems, vaginismus may be primary or secondary, varies in severity, occurs anywhere along the psychologic spectrum from "normal" to psychotic and may have a variety of etiologic factors in the background. Vaginismus is often seen paired with dysfunction in the male partner—either impotence or premature ejaculation being most common.

The most likely etiologic factors in vaginismus are previous experiences of pain with actual or attempted vaginal penetration. The following is a list of the most common such experiences in the histories of women with vaginismus.

1. Childhood injury in the vulva region—usually a minor injury associated with the girl's fear that she may have done serious harm to herself in this mysterious and yet valuable part of her body. Frequently the memory of such an event is repressed and is only remembered in the course of treatment

2. Childhood urogenital problems such as recurrent cystitis involving painful and/or frightening medical procedures

3. Early difficulties using tampons—it is not rare for adolescent girls to have a strand of tissue bisecting the hymeneal opening (Sarrel, 1977). This may make tampon insertion difficult and painful. Many of these girls manage to insert a tampon but when they try to remove it, it gets caught behind the strand of tissue. Tearing the strand causes an early association between vaginal penetration and pain. A thick hymen may also be a factor, making first attempts at intercourse impossible and/or painful.

4. Pelvic examinations which are frightening and/or painful or a history of repeated gyncecologic procedures such as colposcopy, cryosurgery, biopsy, or abortion

5. Sexual experience, particularly involving penetration or attempted penetration which is painful. Rape, of course, is the most traumatic instance of this

6. Probably the most common cause of painful intercourse is vaginitis. Repeated intercourse in the presence of vaginitis and the accompanying pain or burning sensations is a frequent precursor of vaginismus.

Other etiologic factors in the psychological background of vaginismus may include the following:

1. Expectation of pain due to cultural influence or having heard stories from other females of extreme pain or bleeding

2. Having been a girl of small, frail build. The small, frail body image may persist into adolescence and adulthood, and is often paired with a sense of the vagina as small and fragile and the erect penis as too large to fit easily into the vagina

3. Extreme ambivalence about having intercourse the first time—often a feeling of having been coerced by the male followed by rage and guilt on the female's part

4. Fear of men and, more specifically, of the penis. Incest or a frightening experience with an exhibitionist may be the origins of the fear. This fear can be of psychotic proportions, with delusions of penetration by penises

5. A primarily homosexual orientation may be a predisposing factor if it leads a girl or young woman to try to accept heterosexual intercourse which is really not wanted

6. Denial of the genital organs as a part of the body. This is one aftermath of frightening or painful penetration experiences

7. Fear of pregnancy or ambivalence about becoming pregnant either for a first time or after having been through an earlier pregnancy experience which was psychologically and/or physically disturbing.

Vaginismus is not usually confined to sexual situations; that is, a woman with vaginismus will usually have problems with any kind of vaginal penetration by fingers, tampons, and during a gynecologic exam. Some women have vaginismus in some situations but not in others. While vaginismus is often an obvious diagnosis when the woman or couple offer a very clear description of the phenomenon, physicians must be alert to the possibility of vaginismus when the complaint is less obvious, for example lack of lubrication, continuing pain after successful treatment of vaginitis, unconsummated marriage, or sexual aversion. Generally, one can be fairly sure of the diagnosis from history alone but a pelvic exam usually serves to confirm the diagnosis. The physician can see the vaginal opening contract as he or she touches the inner thigh or vulvar area.

TREATMENT

There are four major variables in the decision about how a primary physician should treat a sexual dysfunction: (a) the competence and interest level of the physician; (b) the nature and severity of the given problem; (c) the motivation of the individual or couple; (d) the availability of professional services in the community.

Physicians who are comfortable discussing sex with their patients and who routinely ask about sexual function will hear about more

sexual problems than physicians who avoid the subject (Burnap and Golden, 1967). Physicians may avoid the topic out of personal discomfort and/or because they feel ill-equipped to diagnose and treat sexual problems. If all physicians would take the time and responsibility to become knowledgeable about and reasonably comfortable with the subject of human sexuality, this important dimension of medical care would not be omitted from routine practice.

There are ten types of intervention that might be used, either singly or in combination, by the primary physician in treating sexual dysfunction. Each intervention is discussed in the following sections. They are:

- listening and clarifying the problem

- diagnosing and treating physical causes of dysfunction

- prescribing contraception and discussing its impact on sex

- educating and simple counseling

- encouraging appropriate reading

- encouraging self-help, such as masturbation for preorgasmic women

- encouraging improved communication between patient and sexual partner

- helping to change attitudes and negative feelings

- behavior-modification techniques for specific dysfunctions

- referrals to appropriate specialists

Clarifying the Problem

Clarifying the nature, extent, and meaning of the problem is essential to diagnosis. Listening is a way of telling the patient that his or her question is appropriate, that the doctor takes sexual concerns as seriously as other concerns, and that sex is not a taboo subject. By asking informed questions the doctor demonstrates some capacity to be helpful.

Treating Physical Causes

Medical conditions and drug reactions have been increasingly recognized as the direct cause of sexual dysfunction. Although Masters and Johnson (1970) found this to be true in less than 5% of their cases, recent studies indicate a higher incidence. Most commonly, when a medical problem is present it is only one of the multiple factors contributing to a dysfunction. Still, it is important to recognize medical conditions when they exist for, although they may be but one factor, if left unrecognized and untreated, there may be little or no progress in sex therapy. An example is the woman with vaginismus who has vaginitis or some other gynecologic condition such as endometriosis. If the gynecologic problem is not diagnosed and treated the vaginismus is not likely to be treated successfully.

The diseases and drugs most frequently implicated in sexual dysfunction are those which affect sensory perception, sympathetic and parasympathetic nerve discharge, cardiovascular function, and neuromuscular response. The dysfunction most often associated with disease or drugs is secondary impotence. For that reason, in all cases of secondary impotence a careful and complete medical history with review of systems and accounting of drug intake, including alcohol, is warranted. Masters and Johnson cited 50 diseases and 16 drugs in cases of secondary impotence (Masters and Johnson, 1970). Nonorgasmic response in women and ejaculatory inhibition and primary impotence in men have been related to drugs and diseases, therefore medical history and physical examination is warranted in such cases. Serum prolactin should be measured in all cases of ejaculatory inhibition as elevated levels due to pituitary adenomas have been described in this condition (Masters and Johnson, 1981).

Desire phase disorders may be associated with either endocrine conditions (such as acromegaly, testicular atrophy, menopause) or chronic debilitating diseases. Estrogen replacement therapy is called for in many menopausal women who suffer from inadequate vaginal lubrication and/or negative reactions to being touched. There are usually other signs of inadequate estrogen but the sexual complaint may be the only indicator (Sarrel, 1982).

Impact of contraception

Fear of pregnancy is a common factor in sexual dysfunction. The doctor must always inquire about contraceptive use or nonuse and its meaning for the couple. Sometimes the prescription of contraception, or perhaps sterilization, is all that is needed to reverse a sexual dysfunction.

Specific methods of contraception may be an etiologic or complicating factor in sexual dysfunctions, for example, a condom leading to loss of erection or a low-dose pill causing vaginal dryness. Helping a couple reexamine their contraceptive approach may be crucial to reversing sexual dysfunction.

Sex education and counseling

The primary physician's office should be a resource for correct information about human sexuality. In addition to teaching done directly by the doctor, alternative approaches should be considered. The office could be supplied with pamphlets or other reading material, or audiovisual presentations. There may be a nurse, nurse-clinician, or social worker trained to provide sex education and simple counseling in the office or clinic.

Under the heading of education and simple counseling several functions are appropriate for the primary physician. He or she can help dispel myths—that couples should always strive to have a simultaneous climax, that a woman must have an orgasm in order to conceive, or that men are supposed to ejaculate whenever they become aroused, are three common myths. The physician can also educate patients about normal sexual physiology. Relevant information may be a discussion of vaginal lubrication occurring deep within the vagina or the way erections normally wax and wane during the excitement phase.

The physician may use the physical examination as a time to educate. This may be the clinician's single most valuable contribution to sex education and sexual health. Dicussions of anatomy and physiology, diagrams, photos, and models are all helpful but discussion of the person's own genital anatomy and a chance to view it in a mirror are much more powerful learning experiences. Even highly educated persons have many misconceptions and fears about their own genitals. For example, in a survey conducted of women at Yale, 56 of 100 thought the hymen was a closed membrane deep inside the vagina. Most females have never been able to look inside their vaginas and many harbor fantasies of it as black, bloody, fragile or tiny (Sarrel and Sarrel, 1979). Men, too, have misconceptions and fears about their genitals, for example, being confused about circumcision, thinking the median raphe on the underside of the penis is a scar, or not knowing that it is normal for one testicle to hang lower than the other.

Discussion of spectatoring, even a brief counseling session, may help a patient overcome the feeling of being an onlooker during sexual activity. It isn't possible to stop self-observation by sheer force of will. Since the human mind is never blank (except in meditation, perhaps) the physician may help the patient to learn to focus on something that is not anxiety-provoking and is, preferably, perceived as being sexy. This could be an erotic fantasy, one's own physical sensations, one's partner's body and responses, or doing something a bit unusual to one's partner.

Appropriate Reading

In a busy office practice, the physician may want to encourage a patient or a couple to read books that will provide information or help to change attitudes. Two books we sometimes recommend

are:

1. *Our Bodies Ourselves*, The Boston Womens' Health Collective, Simon and Schuster, N.Y., 1976
2. *Male Sexuality*, B. Zilbergeld, Little, Brown & Co., Boston, 1978

Self-Help

The one dysfunction most often amenable to self-help is primary orgasmic dysfunction in a woman who does not masturbate to orgasm. Many women simply have not learned to have orgasms and can teach themselves to reach orgasm in masturbation. The woman and her partner may need some additional help in order to transfer this learning into sexual interaction with her partner. Obviously the physician must use judgment in deciding to recommend to a woman that she try this approach.

Encouraging Communication

Seeing a couple together to talk about a sexual problem almost always has a salutary effect by alleviating anxiety and encouraging open discussion about sex. The physician must be comfortable talking about sex and able to direct the conversation into the specifics of sexual experience without seeming prurient or intrusive.

When a couple cannot be seen together, the physician can encourage open communication between the partners at home. One may explore the reasons for hesitancy to talk with a partner about sex, make specific suggestions about how to talk about sex, help to provide a vocabulary and perhaps suggest that the couple read one or more books *together*. Couples should be encouraged to communicate what they like and dislike in sexual touching. The hand-on-hand technique described by Masters and Johnson (1970) is often a useful way of communicating in bed and is less interruptive of mood than saying "A half inch lower and to the right."

Changing Attitudes

From the moment the physician or patient raises the subject of sex, everything the physician says and does will be communicating attitudes and feelings about sex. It is important that the clinician not impose his or her idiosyncratic ideas or experience, yet value statements are unavoidable. There is, at present, some agreement among professionals about which attitudes and practices are likely to promote sexual health and which are not, but an individual physician may disagree with some notions. For example, most sex therapists and counselors now believe that masturbation is healthy and can be positively recommended. If a physician finds this idea abhorrent he or she will probably be uncomfortable recommending masturbation to a patient or, if it is recommended, the physician's ambivalent feelings will probably be felt by the patient, who may not follow through on the recommendation. There is no way for the clinician to keep his or her values totally out of the picture.

Reassurance and permission-giving are a chief part of the primary physician's role in helping persons with sexual problems. Reassurance that a particular practice is "normal" or giving permission to explore and experiment with new sexual techniques may be valuable. However, the clinician must guard against imposing his or her values in this area. It is also important to remember that sexual experimentation may be very anxiety-producing and may have a negative effect. The physician must be sensitive to the couple's feelings and help them to set comfortable boundaries. The most important boundary for the doctor to recommend is that each partner say "No" or "I don't like that" when something evokes a negative response.

Behavior modification

Sex therapy is usually a complex and eclectic therapy. Sometimes Masters-Johnson therapy is labeled behaviorist therapy, but in fact behavior-modification techniques are only one part of the overall therapeutic process. However, in some dysfunctions, with some individuals or couples,

behavior-modification techniques can be used alone or in a much simpler format. If the primary physician is willing to learn these techniques carefully and take the time to use them sensitively and judiciously, many sexual dysfunctions could be treated successfully by the physician in office practice.

The two dysfunctions most amenable to behavior-focused treatment are vaginismus and premature ejaculation. Vaginismus can be treated succesfully in almost every case. In perhaps half the cases it can be treated through a fairly simple routine of gradual desensitization to vaginal penetration (Masters and Johnson, 1970). Premature ejaculation can be successfully treated in 90%–95% of cases. Perhaps 15%–20% of premature ejaculation problems can be dealt with easily through techniques such as the "squeeze" (Masters and Johnson, 1970) and the "start-stop" (Kaplan, 1974).

It is not possible to summarize these behavior-modification techniques here. To do so very briefly might encourage physicians to try out these techniques without adequate training. Although much simpler than other forms of sex therapy, these treatment techniques have their own complexities. Primary physicians interested in using such techniques to treat sexual dysfunction should read the books referred to in the Recommended Readings at the end of the chapter *and* have some additional training.

Referral

Referral to a psychiatrist, psychiatric social worker, marriage counselor, or sex therapist is often the best course of action for a physician with limited time in his or her practice. It may seem an easy solution for the physician who prefers not to become too involved in the area of sexual problems, but making a good referral to the right resource, in such a way that the patient (and perhaps the patient's sexual partner) will gladly follow through, requires the clinician's intelligent attention as much as other treatment techniques.

Referral should not be premature. The physician should certainly have a clear picture of the nature of the problem, a history of the problem, and should know whether the patient's partner has a sexual dysfunction and how the partner feels about getting professional help. On the principle that simple methods should always be tried first, the clinician should consider using one or more of the approaches described in this chapter before making a referral.

A few guidelines for referral are suggested. If a patient seems clinically depressed and questioning reveals signs such as sleep problems, loss of appetite, suicidal thoughts, or extreme apathy, then referral to a psychiatrist for evaluation should be considered. If the physician suspects the patient is psychotic or borderline, then individual consultation with a psychiatrist or psychologist is appropriate. If the history of sexual dysfunction seems secondary to marital breakdown and discord, then referral for marriage counseling may be best.

There are many people calling themselves sex therapists in almost every city in the United States, and the physician may need help choosing reliable sex therapists. The American Association of Sex Educators, Counselors and Therapists (AASECT), 600 Maryland Ave. S.W., Washington, DC 20024 publishes a list of certified sex therapists throughout the United States and other parts of the world.

Before making a referral the physician may want to know more about the techniques used by a given sex therapist, fees, or rates of success. Most therapists are glad to discuss their approach with a referring professional.

There are also group therapy approaches to sexual dysfunction which may be useful if they are available in or near the patients' community. The group treatment approach for nonorgasmic women pioneered by Barbach (1975) is a possibility. The Sexual Attitude Restructuring (SAR) programs (Garrard Vaitkus, and Chilgren, 1972) are not designed to treat sexual dysfunction but the positive attitude they convey toward

eroticism and sexual discovery and the opportunity to talk in small groups certainly can be helpful, particularly for people who wish to change their negative views of sex.

If sexual dysfunction in the patient and/or partner seems to be the primary problem and there is no physical cause for the dysfunction, referral to a sex therapist should be considered (unless one of the interventions mentioned above is of sufficient help).

PREVENTION

The primary physician is in a unique position to prevent sexual dysfunction. There are three ways in which this role can be fulfilled. First, the primary physician can serve as a sex-educator to patients throughout their life cycles, offering age-appropriate information *before* misinformation leads to problems: for example, telling parents and/or their 8 or 9-year-old daughters about the normal vaginal secretion girls are likely to experience for a year prior to onset of menses or alerting a 50-year-old man that the time period between ejaculations tends to lengthen with age so that he may sometimes be unable to ejaculate. The value of this kind of education goes well beyond the facts conveyed. It also teaches that sex is an appropriate topic for discussion and opens the way for further physician-patient dialogue about sex in the present or future.

Second, medical examinations can be routinely used as a time to educate and to reinforce positive attitudes toward the human body, including the genitals. The pelvic examination, especially a first one, provides a special opportunity for education about the genitals and for desensitization to genital penetration (Sarrel, 1982). Finally, the primary physician can prevent sexual dysfunction by being alert to the impact of medical illness, handicaps, surgery, medications, psychiatric illness, and substance abuse upon sexual function. The physician may choose to use one drug rather than another based upon the drugs' effect on sexual function. Physicians should alert patients to possible complications, side effects, or common worries associated with the patient's particular condition. It is important for physicians to learn how to bring up these issues without unnecessarily alarming a patient and thereby inducing a problem. This calls for sensitivity and judgment—but these can be learned! The physician should also anticipate any impact of such factors on the sexual partner. Preventive counseling can be invaluable.

SUMMARY

The primary physician should be able to diagnose accurately the range of sexual dysfunctions in men and women. The major areas of sexual disturbances encountered by physicians are desire and excitement phase problems, orgasmic dysfunctions, and vaginismus. Physical illness or medications may play a role in sexual problems but the physician's role should go well beyond that of dealing simply with the biophysical aspects. When the appropriate interventions outlined in this chapter are inadequate, appropriate referral is called for.

APPENDIX: CASE HISTORY—THE FRUSTRATED WIFE

After listening to the wife, the psychiatrist encouraged her to speak with her husband about her concerns related to their precipitously diminished sex life. She decided to speak with him about sex, but not about her suspicions concerning a possible affair. When she spoke with her husband, it became clear that he did not have any instructions about sex when he was discharged from the hospital following the MI; he was also afraid of having sex as he had developed some chest pains following sexual intercourse some time prior to the hospitalization. They decided to make an appointment with the family physician.

The PEG constructed by the family physician indicates that the husband's sexual dysfunction is probably related to his anxiety concerning cardiac function. In addition, diabetes mellitus (considering family history) and drug side-effect (propranolol) had to be ruled out. After a frank session with the family physician concerning sex, the husband was reassured that sexual intercourse was not likely to cause an infarction and advised to take nitroglycerin prior to intercourse as a precaution; full sexual function returned in spite of the propranolol. Laboratory tests did not show any evidence of diabetes mellitus.

This case illustrates how simple discussion on sexual matters can "cure" a sexual dysfunction that caused much anguish in this couple.

PATIENT EVALUATION GRID			
	CONTEXTS		
DIMENSIONS	**CURRENT** (Current States)	**RECENT** (Recent Events and Changes)	**BACKGROUND** (Culture, Traits, Constitution)
BIOLOGICAL	Propranolol 40 mg/day Nitroglycerin prn Has morning erections	Angina pectoris, mild—1½ yr Anterior wall MI, mild—1 yr ago Propranolol Nitroglycerin	Father died MI Mother has diabetes Unusual childhood illnesses Fracture of tibia as a child
PERSONAL	Anxious about heart condition Afraid of sex because angina had developed following sex prior to MI—did not tell wife Mental status: normal except for anxiety concerning MI	Reduced sexual desire—1 yr Some difficulty sleeping through the night—1½ yr Appetite normal Feeling worried and blue at times "without reason"—6 mo	A very "sexual" person, had intercourse at least once a day "Very proud and strong man"
ENVIRONMENTAL	Wife works as receptionist in a law firm Wife concerned about patient's reduced sexual activity—thinks he may be having an affair	Hospitalization for MI—1 yr ago Father died of MI—4 yr ago Mother diagnosed as having diabetes mellitus—5 yr ago Increased competition at work—6 mo	Lower middle-class background One older brother died in accident when patient 12 years of age Athletic in high school Salesman since finishing high school; married at age 25 years, no children

Demographic data: 46-year-old-male, a salesman, Protestant background, not religious.

RECOMMENDED READINGS

Annon, J. 1974. *The behavioral treatment of sexual problems, vol. 1, Brief therapy*. Honolulu: Enabling Systems, Inc. A good summary of interventions that are appropriate for a physician when patients present sexual concerns is presented here.

Kaplan, H.S. 1974. *The New sex therapy*. New York: Brunner/Mazel. This comprehensive text on sexual dysfunction and therapy by a psychoanalyst will be particularly appreciated by psychotherapists. The discussion of premature ejaculation is quite thorough.

Kentsmith, D., and Eaton, M. 1979. *Treating sexual problems in medical practice*. New York: Arco Publishing, Inc. This overview of the subject is a valuable reference for the physician.

Kolodny, R.C.; Masters, W.H.; and Johnson, V.E. 1979. *Textbook of sexual medicine*. Boston: Little, Brown & Co. A comprehensive and valuable basic reference.

Masters, W.H., and Johnson, V.E. 1966. *Human sexual response*. Boston: Little, Brown & Co. Masters and Johnson's report of their pioneering research on the physiology of normal sexual function.

Masters, W.H. and Johnson, V.E. 1970. *Human sexual inadequacy*. Boston: Little, Brown & Co. This is the first description of sex therapy as practice: almost all of sex therapy today derives from this work.

Masters, W.H. and Johnson, V.E. 1979. *Homosexuality in perspective*. Boston: Little, Brown & Co. Masters and Johnson report on recent research comparing homosexuality and heterosexuality.

Archives of Sexual Behavior. For the practitioner who wants to keep up with the latest research in the field of sexology, this journal is very useful.

The Journal of Sex and Marital Therapy. The single best journal in the area of sex therapy is for the physician who is interested in sex therapy for patients.

Medical Aspects of Human Sexuality. This journal is also for the medical practitioner. It has clinically related articles.

Sexual Medicine Today. A monthly magazine-format journal with articles of good quality, this journal is geared to the medical practitioner.

Wagner, G.; and Green, R. 1981. *Impotence—physiological, psychological, surgical diagnoses and treatment*. New York: Plenum Press.

REFERENCES

Annon, J. 1974. *The behavioral treatment of sexual problems, vol. 1, Brief therapy*, Honolulu: Enabling Systems, Inc.

Barbach. L.G. 1975. *For yourself—the fulfillment of female sexuality*. New York: Doubleday & Co.

Burnap, D.W., and Golden, J.S. 1967 Sexual problems in medical practice. *J. Med. Educ.* 42:673–80.

Garrard, J.; Vaitkus, A.; and Chilgren, R.A. 1972. Evaluation of a course in human sexuality. *J. Med. Educ.* 147:772–78.

Green, R., ed. 1979. *Human sexuality*. Baltimore: Williams & Wilkins.

Group for the Advancement of Psychiatry (GAP). 1977. Assessment of sexual function: A guide to interviewing, vol. 3, no. 88.

Hite, S. 1976. *The Hite report*. New York: Macmillan.

Kaplan, H.S. 1974. *The new sex therapy*. New York: Brunner/Mazel.

Kaplan, H.S. 1979. *Disorders of sexual desire*. New York: Brunner/Mazel.

Kentsmith, D. and Eaton, M. 1979. *Treating sexual problems in medical practice*. New York: Arco Publishing Inc.

Kinsey, A.; Pomeroy, W.; and Martin, C. 1948. *Sexual behavior in the human male*. Philadelphia: W.B. Saunders, Co.

Kinsey, A.; Pomeroy, W.; Martin, C.; et al. 1953. *Sexual behavior in the human female*. Philadelphia: W.B. Saunders, Co.

Kolodny, R.C.; Masters, W.H.; and Johnson, V.E. 1979. Textbook of sexual medicine. Boston: Little, Brown & Co.

Masters, W.H., and Johnson, V.E. 1966. *Human sexual response*. Boston: Little, Brown & Co.

Masters, W.H.; and Johnson, V.E., 1970. *Human sexual inadequacy*. Boston: Little, Brown & Co.

Masters, W.H. and Johnson, V.E. 1979. *Homosexuality in perspective*. Boston: Little, Brown & Co.

Masters, W.H.; and Johnson, V.E. 1981. *Sexual physiology: fact and fiction*. Paper presented at Fourteenth Annual Meeting of American Association of Sex Educators, Counselors, and Therapists, San Francisco, April 1981.

Nestoros, J.N., and Lehmann, H.E. 1979. Neuroleptics and male sexual function. *Int. Drug Ther. News.* 14:21–22.

Sarrel, L. and Sarrel, P. 1979. *Sexual unfolding.* Boston: Little, Brown & Co.

Sarrel, P. 1977. Biological aspects of sexual function. In *Progress in sexology,* eds., R. Gemme, and C. Wheeler. New York: Plenum Publishing Co.

Sarrel, P. 1982. Sex problems after menopause: a study of fifty married couples treated in a sex counseling program. *Maturitas* 4(2).

Sarrel, P. 1982. Indications for a first pelvic examination (editorial). *J. Adolesc. Health* 2(2).

Sarrel. P. (In press.) Dyspareunia. In *Signs and symptoms in gynecology,* eds. B.M. Pecklem and S.S. Shapiro. Philadelphia: J.B. Lippincott Co.

Sarrel, P.; and Masters, W.H. 1982. Sexual molestation of men by women. *Arch. Sex. Behav.* 11(2).

Schumacher, S.; and Lloyd, C.W. 1977. Assessment of sexual dysfunction. In *Behavioral assessment: a practical handbook,* eds. M. Hersen and A.S. Bellack. New York: Pergamon Press.

Smith, S. and Carlson, B. 1979. The care of the whole woman. In *Ob-gyn private practice,* paper presented to annual meeting of American Association of Sex Educators, Counselors and Therapists, Washington, D.C., April 1979.

Spark, R.; White, R.; and Connolly, P. 1980. Impotence is not always psychogenic. *J.A.M.A.* 343:750–55.

Vincent, C.; Vincent, B.; Greiss, F., et al. 1975. Some marital-sexual concomitants of carcinoma of the cervix. *South. Med. J.* 68:552–58.

Wagner, G.; and Green, R. 1981. *Impotence— physiological, psychological, surgical diagnoses and treatment.* New York: Plenum Press.

Zilbergeld, B. 1978. *Male sexuality.* Boston: Little, Brown & Co.

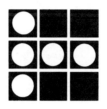

PART III

General Considerations In Management

CHAPTER 19

Chronically Ill Patients—Hemodialysis, Diabetes and Cancer

Jon Streltzer, M.D.

This chapter and Chapters 20 and 21 deal with relatively general issues rather than specific syndromes in psychiatry. In this chapter, we discuss psychiatric issues in the many patients who have chronic medical illnesses. Many of these patients have problems in adapting to the chronicity of their illness and to the implications of the disease, including disability and restrictions in the sphere of activity. Obviously, each chronic illness poses its own unique demands for adaptation, but it is not feasible to discuss even all the important ones in one chapter. Thus, general psychiatric issues applicable to most chronic illnesses are presented; then, three common chronic conditions often associated with psychiatric problems are discussed in detail. Psychiatric issues related to hemodialysis, diabetes, and cancer are presented as models to illustrate how the specific disease or treatment may interact with the patient's psychosocial system.

Although psychiatric conditions of any type may coincidentally occur with chronic medical illness, most of the time psychiatric problems are caused by or influenced by the chronic medical illness itself. A patient's adaptation to chronic illness depends on several factors. These include: the patient's personality style; the patient's life situation and the degree of change of life style imposed by the illness; specific impairments associated with the illness, including degree of pain and suffering; and the demands of the treatment regimen with its side effects and necessity for compliance. In general, a patient's psychological response to chronic illness depends on the meaning that the illness has to the individual in the context of his or her life situation. Awareness of this meaning enhances understanding of psychiatric conditions that may arise in the chronically ill patient and lead to the rational approaches to treatment.

In addition, usual medical approaches to chronic illness can predispose to psychiatric complications. In American society certain behaviors are expected of medically ill patients. With regard to *acute* medical illness, patients are relieved of their responsibilities for work and their duties to family. Patients can rely on sick leave benefits and the help of family and friends to carry out necessary tasks at home. In the hospital the patient is usually expected to passively comply with physicians' and nurses' wishes.

In the case of *chronic* medical illness, however, the situation is very different. Chronically ill patients are expected to continue to take responsibility for most areas of their life. They are encouraged to continue to work, at least part-time if possible, and are expected to continue to assume family responsibilities as much as possible. They are also expected to care for their own illness, which may include complicated diets, giving self-injections, and learning about various aspects of the illness so that they can identify symptoms and periodically initiate treatment. The chronically ill patient knows that the physi-

cian is not perfect and cannot provide a cure. While the disease progresses in severity of symptoms, the physician is seen as subject to human error, making mistakes, and failing to understand the patient's needs at all times. The patient may come to believe that, at times, he or she understands the illness better than the clinician, and may disagree with the treatment plan. Thus, compliance problems are frequent.

In summary, the chronically ill patient receives two seemingly contradictory messages from the physician: (a) "Continue to assume as much responsibility for your life as possible and learn as much about your illness and its treatment as you can"; and (b) "Follow my instructions regarding treatment to the letter." For some patients it is impossible to reconcile these two imperatives. Psychiatric complications may then arise (Alexander, 1976).

PSYCHIATRIC ISSUES

Caregiver-Patient Interactions

To the physician, the chronically ill patient may seem stubborn, hostile, uncooperative, and unappreciative. Patients may see the clinician as uninterested in their problems, unsympathetic, and not fully understanding. Patients often feel anger toward the physician for not being able to cure them and for not understanding them. However, the patient usually will not express this anger directly, for the patient also needs the physician and wants to remain in his or her good graces. The patient often feels the physician has the power to either alleviate or create suffering associated with the illness. Thus, patients may not be totally honest with the physician but may talk to the physician in a way that they expect will please the physician. The physician, likewise, may be frustrated with the patient since the patient does not get better and cannot be cured. The physician is best able to develop a positive relationship with the patient if the physician is aware of these dynamics, and respects the patient as a potential collaborator in the management of the illness. Thus, the physician can allow the patient to help clarify problems and help formulate the proper therapeutic approach.

Chronically ill patients commonly have acute episodes of illness that require hospitalization. During these episodes there may be problems with nurse-patient interactions. Nurses may be uncomfortable with patients who demonstrate extensive knowledge about their illness and attempt to take an active role in the management. Nurses may become caught between physicians' orders and patients' demands which are conflicting regarding treatment. The physician can help to avoid such problems by discussing the particular patient's needs with the nurses and discussing what is expected from the nursing staff.

Behavioral Responses to Chronic Illness

Chronic illness is a stress and a patient's coping mechanisms in dealing with this stress are similar to coping mechanisms in dealing with other

---

CASE HISTORY 19-1

A 19-year-old male became paraplegic as a result of spinal trauma. He always looked forward to visits with his physician. He expressed many fears and concerns that were usually relieved by a discussion with her. During hospitalization the patient continued this pattern with regard to his physician. However, the nurses had great difficulty relating to this patient, finding him manipulative, attention-seeking, and excessively demanding. A psychiatric consultant discovered the existence of a vicious cycle, in which the patient felt anxious that his needs would not be looked after and he would not be cared for properly, and sought frequent attention from the nursing staff. However, he soon found that the nurses were reluctant to come into his room to help him and they became slow to respond when he pressed the call button, which in turn resulted in increased anxiety and need to make sure they were available to him. His constantly pressing the call button for what seemed to be trivial needs caused the nurses to respond more and more slowly; when they did respond, it was abruptly and curtly. This pattern was discussed with the nursing staff, together with an elaboration of the patient's history and needs. A plan was devised whereby a nurse would walk into the patient's room once every hour when he was *not* requesting help and spend a few minutes with the patient to see if there was anything she could do for him. When the nurses began to spontaneously appear in his room and inquire after his welfare, the patient's anxiety decreased. He found less need to call them; as he began to use the call button less and less, the nurses became progressively more comfortable entering his room and interacting with the patient. Thus, the vicious cycle was transformed into a positive one. This patient had been raised in many foster homes and unconsciously feared abandonment. Under stress, his need to be cared for increased and he tended to become overly dependent and demanding.

stresses. These are determined by the patient's personality style. Case History 19–1 describes a patient with a dependent-personality style, and Case History 19–2 is of a patient with an obsessive-personality style.

In summary, flexibility in devising treatment strategies is crucial in the chronically ill patient. A knowledge of the patient's coping or personality style is necessary to understand their response to illness and to plan the most effective therapeutic approaches (Kahana and Bibring, 1964). (See Chapter 4 for a more comprehensive discussion of personality types.)

Dependency. Chronic illness causes increased dependence on family, friends, medications, and physicians. Many patients are able to adjust to this increased dependency successfully, but others have difficulty. Some overcompensate, such as the coronary patient who works increasingly harder and subjects himself to excessively stressful activities (Cassem and Hackett, 1977). For such patients it is sometimes helpful to redefine the meaning of strength and courage. For example, such a patient could be told, "For your health, you must adjust your workload and replace stressful activities with relaxing ones. It

---

CASE HISTORY 19–2

A 24-year-old female sustained severe head and neck trauma, requiring multiple surgical procedures and a tracheostomy. After 2 months in the hospital her condition stabilized and she entered a chronic phase. At this time unusual behaviors began to appear. Dissatisfied with the way her bed was made by the nurse's aide, the patient began to insist on making it herself. In addition, she demanded to suction her own tracheostomy. She did this so frequently and vigorously that the nurses were concerned she would traumatize her trachea. The patient also began to insist that suction catheters, gauze pads, and other supplies be kept in her room in large quantities; she increasingly organized her room and demanded that many details of her care be carried out according to her precise specifications. Unable to talk, she would write long messages, doggedly writing out complete sentences even when the person had already anticipated and verbalized what she was trying to communi-

cate. She had a history of being meticulous, responsible and perfectionistic, but this had caused no difficulties with previous interpersonal relationships. In the hospital, as she passed the acute illness stage, she dealt with her fear, anxiety, and changing body image by becoming very controlling and compulsive regarding the details of her care. When the nursing staff realized that these were coping mechanisms on the part of the patient they negotiated with her regarding what areas she could take care of and what areas would have to be left to the nursing staff. This worked to the comfort of both patient and nurses. In addition, the physicians involved in her care found that explaining aspects of the procedures and other matters in great detail to the patient seemed to be very reassuring and reduced her anxiety. Recognition of this patient's obsessive-compulsive coping style resulted in tailoring treatment for maximum psychological comfort for the patient.

would take great strength and courage for you to make this adjustment. If you are able to do so it will benefit you and your family. Do you think you have the strength to do this?"

For other patients dependency can become a greater problem than the illness itself. This is commonly seen in patients with low back pain or posttraumatic injury (Lishman, 1976; Case History 19–3).

Syndromes following trauma in which the extent of disability seems out of proportion to the actual injury are not uncommon. Often, they are associated with compensation or litigation, but not always. Prognosis for recovery and rehabilitation is difficult to predict, even years after the injury. Unfortunately, there are no good solutions to the problem of overdependency. The best approach would probably be prevention by encouraging independent function as soon as possible after the acute stage of the illness. Although once the dependency reaction has set in it is very difficult to change, one should not give up since in some cases the individual may eventually return to work and assume more independent functioning (Lisham, 1976). The principles that apply to the management of hypochondriasis (see Chapter 13) are often applicable to these patients.

Compliance. Compliance with treatment regimens is a significant issue in management of chronically ill patients. Lack of compliance is associated with complexity of treatment regimen, discomfort associated with the treatment regimen, adverse personal meaning of the treatment regimen to the patient, perceived ineffectiveness of the treatment regimen by the patient, and incompatibility of the treatment regimen with other aspects of the patient's life which may include cultural, family, or personal aspects (Yager, 1975). Personality factors such as low frustration tolerance, acting out of aggression, and lack of obsessive-compulsive traits may also be associated with noncompliance (De-Nour and Czaczkes, 1974). Factors associated with increasing patient compliance include:

1. Physician concern about the issue of compliance including side effects of treatment procedures
2. Simplicity of treatment regimen
3. Maximal understanding of the treatment regimen including its purpose
4. A positive physician-patient relationship in which the patient feels understood and cared for by the physician

---

CASE HISTORY 19–3

A 38-year-old married man with a history of working full-time since his early teens suffered acute trauma to the head which produced a mild concussion and a depressed skull fracture. Following surgery for the skull fracture the neurosurgeon expected full recovery and there were no abnormal neurologic findings. Yet, the patient developed chronic severe headaches, depression, and inability to concentrate. He was unable to work and his social life became greatly constricted. His symptoms had not improved 3 years after the injury. He was involved in litigation related to the injury.

5. A willingness by the physician to discuss and negotiate alternative treatment regimens (Matthews and Hingson, 1977)

Depression. Depression is commonly seen in the chronically ill patient. It is uncommon, however, that this depression becomes the depressive syndrome requiring antidepressant medication or electroconvulsive therapy. Usually depression is a reaction to several phenomena associated with chronic illness, which include physical discomfort associated with the illness and a variety of losses such as inability to perform activities that were previously enjoyable, loss of sexual abilities, and decrease in economic status. Depression may also occur in relation to exacerbation of illness, particularly if a patient had become overconfident in a treatment regimen or nonmedical approach to the illness. Such depressions frequently share aspects of grief and will respond to empathetic discussion and support. Increased support from family, friends, ministers, social workers, physicians, or psychotherapists can be of great benefit. Grief-like depression almost always improves when physical condition improves. Depression may also be a complication of drug therapy, in particular antihypertensive drugs such as reserpine and methyldopa. Depression sometimes occurs in patients taking regular doses of CNS-depressant drugs including narcotics, minor tranquilizers, and hypnotics. Elimination of the CNS-depressant drugs or a change to a different antihypertensive regimen often improves mood.

Pain. Pain is a common symptom associated with chronic illness and in some cases may be the most disabling aspect of the illness. There are many determinants of the pain experience besides the organic lesion involved, such as cultural factors, personality factors, environmental factors, and factors associated with the physician-patient relationships and the treatment milieu (Wise, 1977; Leigh and Reiser, 1980). For many patients treatment with aspirin and acetaminophen is satisfactory; for a few patients special techniques such as self-hypnosis, meditation, biofeedback, acupuncture, transcutaneous stimulation, antidepressant medication, and placebo may be helpful. While acute pain can usually be managed with effective analgesics, chronic pain is much more difficult to treat since narcotic analgesics will lose their efficacy over time due to the phenomenon of tachyphylaxis. Treatment with narcotics is thus hazardous since patients are likely to escalate the dose periodically in order to obtain sufficient relief. Symptoms associated with drug dependence may develop and adequate pain relief may never be achieved. For some patients, the problem of drug dependence becomes more disabling than the original symptoms (Halpern, 1977; Case History 19–4).

The patient with chronic pain is susceptible to taking escalating doses of narcotics in an attempt to achieve relief. He or she frequently is also given minor tranquilizers to decrease anxiety, which is often related to the fear of discomfort associated with the "wearing off" of the narcotic every few hours. He or she inevitably has difficulty sleeping due to the need to maintain regular doses of narcotics through the night; hypnotic medication may be given for complaints of insomnia. All of these drugs are CNS depressants, so as the patient's functioning becomes increasingly restricted, he or she begins to appear depressed. Antidepressant medication may then be added to the patient's pharmacy, which can easily lead to a mental state characterized by a mild organic brain syndrome. Withdrawal from all these medications can often result in remarkable improvements. This is difficult to do, however, for the patient believes the medications are necessary to minimize discomfort and will resist any lowering of dose. Detoxification from narcotics can usually best be accomplished in a hospital setting where controls are complete. The patient requires frequent counseling and support, ideally from a psychiatric consultant. The following guidelines are useful in managing drug-dependent medical patients:

1. The patient usually complains greatly of pain. He or she may therefore be told that the present regimen is not working satisfactorily and there is good reason to believe his or her body has become immune to the beneficial effects of some of the medications. Therefore, another medication regimen will be substituted.

2. Any narcotic may be used for detoxification procedures. Methadone is the longest and smoothest acting narcotic presently available, however, and is the most potent in the oral form. It can be used successfully on a three times a day basis, thus allowing the patient a full night's sleep.

3. The patient will complain initially as the new regimen will not feel the same as the old. Anxiety can be relieved by reassurance, reexplanation of the rationale, and perhaps submitting to demands by giving a benign medication such as diphenhydramine, hydroxyzine, or perphenazine in small doses as needed. These medications have sedative properties and potentiate narcotics but have no addiction liability themselves.

4. It is useful to begin activities such as physical therapy so that the patient can see concretely that he or she is getting stronger and is capable of more activity as the narcotics dose falls. Patients should be lavishly praised for achievements.

5. Significant family members must be counseled regarding the nature of treatment so that they will be cooperative and also praise the patient rather than inadvertently sabotage the regimen.

6. Transition from the hospital to the home is crucial. The tendency to return to old habits when

---

CASE HISTORY 19–4

A 67-year-old man had taken daily narcotics for over 25 years for treatment of pain of the neck and back. He had a history of multiple surgical procedures. For the previous 2 years he had given himself injections of meperidine (Demerol) every 3 hours for pain. This had greatly limited his functioning; he would not leave his apartment for more than 3 hours at a time in order to return for his injection. He was unable to sleep through the night, waking every 3 hours, and had difficulty concentrating. He continued to experience chronic pain, along with chronic anxiety and depression. He took minor tranquilizers for anxiety and for sleep, supplemented by a tricyclic antidepressant. Treatment was instituted with the assumption that the patient was tolerant to narcotics and not receiving significant analgesia from them. The antidepressant medication was discontinued, and the minor tranquilizers were withdrawn on a gradual basis. The narcotic was substituted with methadone which was given in decreasing doses over a 7-day period. Although the patient experienced much anxiety about the change, he responded to reassurance and by the completion of the withdrawal the patient felt more clear-headed, more energetic, had a better appetite, had begun sleeping through the night for the first time in years. He had substantially less pain, which was well controlled with acetaminophen. One year later the patient had remained narcotic-free and his functioning had greatly improved.

the patient returns to his or her own environment must be discussed with the patient. Plans must be made to avoid this happenstance, such as arranging for disposal of all the old medications in the patient's home.

7. If other physicians are involved with the care of the patient, they need to be notified regarding the patient's treatment so that they are not manipulated by the patient into supplying addicting medications.

Further details regarding detoxification procedures will be found in Chapter 16.

Sexual Functioning.   Patients with chronic illness are concerned with all aspects of rehabilitation and this includes sexual functioning. A symptom of the illness or a complication of its treatment may be a sexual dysfunction such as impotence. Many patients, however, are quite reluctant to spontaneously bring up sexual concerns with the physician. A history of sexual functioning should be routinely taken in working with these patients. If the physician is comfortable discussing the subject usually the patient will be also, and will often be relieved to have the opportunity to discuss these issues (Case History 19–5).

The principles discussed in Chapter 18 are generally applicable to chronically ill patients. Attention to their sexual needs may greatly enhance the quality of life.

SPECIFIC ILLNESSES

Many of the psychiatric problems associated with chronic illness have to do with the specific disease process and its treatment. Three examples of chronic illness are looked at in more depth next: end-stage renal disease treated by chronic hemodialysis, cancer, and diabetes.

Hemodialysis

The chronic hemodialysis patient is ordinarily treated for end-stage renal disease by a nephrologist who is active in a hemodialysis program. The primary care physician, however, may be actively involved with these patients in several ways.

1. The primary care physician may be initially involved in diagnosing end-stage renal disease and making the referral to a hemodialysis program.

2. The primary care physician may be consulted regularly by a dialysis patient for other medical

---

CASE HISTORY 19–5

A 58-year-old married man was being treated for cancer with chemotherapy involving multiple drugs. He had become totally impotent, without morning erections and also losing the ability to masturbate. This affected his self-image and he feared the impact on his year-old marriage. When the patient and his wife were interviewed together, each expressed concern about the other's dissatisfaction.

They had not communicated this to each other and discussing the issue seemed to help them both greatly. They were given instructions regarding sexual activity that would not include intercourse but would include massage. They were able to enjoy these activities very much and the patient felt that indeed he was satisfying his wife despite his limitations.

matters or for complications associated with end-stage renal disease.

3. Home dialysis patients may be many miles from the nearest hemodialysis center and may depend on primary care physicians for much of their medical care.

4. The primary care physician may be taking care of family members of dialysis patients.

Prior to 1973 maintenance hemodialysis was not available to all patients with end-stage renal disease and a variety of selection criteria were used in accepting patients at different dialysis centers (Streltzer et al., 1977). These criteria included concurrent medical conditions, age, value of the patient to society, and a variety of psychosocial criteria such as intelligence, ability to cooperate, and family support. Since 1973 federal financing has made this treatment available to all patients and many centers now accept all patients who apply (Streltzer et al., 1977). Because primary care physicians are often in a position to make the initial referral to a hemodialysis program, they should be aware of psychiatric conditions associated with the onset of end-stage renal disease. In particular, organic brain syndrome and depression are common symptoms occurring with uremia (Abram, 1969). Recognition of these conditions should prevent undue delay in making the diagnosis of renal disease. These psychiatric symptoms as well as personality changes that occur with the onset of uremia should not be considered factors that mitigate against referral to hemodialysis programs (Schreiner and Tartaglia, 1978), since they typically clear up after dialysis is begun and uremia is effectively treated. In addition, even if patients do have significant psychiatric disorders prior to the onset of renal disease this does not mean they are inappropriate for maintenance dialysis treatment—many such patients do quite well on chronic dialysis (Streltzer et al., 1977).

Quality of Life. Studies of the quality of life of hemodialysis patients vary greatly in their conclusions. While some studies point out that there is pervasive depression, inability to return to work, and general constriction of functioning (Retan and Lewis, 1966; Bonney et al., 1978); other studies show that most patients are able to adapt well and lead quite satisfactory lives (De-Nour et al., 1968; Bailey et al., 1970). There appear to be significant differences in the manner of assessment of quality of life issues and there also appear to be differences in results among various programs (Czaczkes and De-Nour, 1978). Patients' self-reports and clinical observations reveal that many patients adjust very well, leading active, responsible and happy lives (Colodner, 1973; Oberly and Oberly, 1979), while many other patients have difficulty and their lives become quite constricted (Calland, 1972). For some patients quality of life may be affected by psychological factors associated with the dialysis program.

Treatment Milieu. The typical dialysis patient is on the machine three times per week for 4–6 hours each time. The patient who is treated in a facility regularly becomes very familiar with the habits and idiosyncracies of staff members, and likewise the staff come to know their patients to an unusual degree. For some patients the human contact and social relationships developed in the dialysis unit become the most important relationships in their lives. Thus, nurse-patient interactions can have profound effects on their mood and psychological sense of well-being (Moe and Streltzer, 1981). Patients often become extremely jealous of the attention a nurse may give another patient.

Social relationships among dialysis patients, however, are surprisingly uncommon. While patients seem to be acutely aware of the health status of other patients, particularly with regard to complications and deaths, many patients do not like to identify with the others or be reminded of their kidney disease and its treatment when away from the unit. This trait may be adaptive since survival has been shown to correlate with indifference to fellow dialysis patients

(Foster et al., 1973). Despite the fact that kidney patient groups are common around the country, the sense of fellowship and mutual support that can be found in other patient groups, such as "colostomy clubs," is rare in these organizations. Likewise, group therapy for dialysis patients has been widely attempted but frequently unsuccessful. In one such group of young, single adult dialysis patients who were highly motivated for such a group, it was found that the members were preoccupied with the issue of being "normal" which seemed to mean being different from other dialysis patients. This desire not to identify with other patients led to the group's demise after five sessions.

Compliance.   A major issue in hemodialysis is compliance (Czaczkes and De-Nour, 1978). The dialysis patient must take a number of medications, the most difficult being the antacids to bind phosphates. The large quantities required may cause constipation and bring no apparent immediate benefit. In addition, the patient must be careful with diet, usually restricting potassium and protein. The most difficult restriction, however, is fluid, which needs to be limited to one liter or less per day—including the fluid present in foods such as vegetables. Lack of compliance with diet and fluid restrictions is associated with difficult dialyses, pulmonary edema, and increased mortality (Czaczkes and DeNour, 1978). Nevertheless, compliance is a major problem. Despite the fact that probably only a minority of patients fully comply with their restrictions, the phenomenon has been poorly studied (Case Histories 19–6 to 19–9).

CASE HISTORY 19–6

A 30-year-old single male, on dialysis for 7 years, would periodically become fluid-overloaded. At these times he would report being depressed and was able to discuss his concerns with a psychiatric consultant or a social worker. He would usually then feel better and improve his compliance.

CASE HISTORY 19–7

A 24-year-old single man had been on dialysis 5 years. He was found to have very high phosphorus levels and suffered from anorexia, nausea, and lack of energy. It was discovered that he rarely took his phosphate-binding medication, afraid that because it was constipating, it would cause a bowel obstruction, something he had required emergency surgery for in the past. He believed the antacid phosphate binders congealed in his stomach, forming a hard mass which prevented phosphates and all food from passing. Discussion of his fears and misunderstandings led to compliance with this medication and the patient began to feel better.

A review of these cases reveals that noncompliance may be associated with such factors as depression, personality, habit, misunderstanding, and anger at the treating staff, and it may be intermittent or chronic. The treating physician should be flexible in approaching the problem of noncompliance, tailoring approaches to the dynamics of the specific case.

Home Hemodialysis. Home dialysis has been recommended as the treatment of choice to minimize dependency problems (Blagg, 1972). Home dialysis patients demonstrate superior adaptation compared to center-based dialysis patients, with higher levels of rehabilitation and less morbidity and mortality (Czaczkes and De-Nour, 1978). This may be due, however, to a prior selection factor, namely, the stronger, better adjusted patients are more likely to be chosen for home dialysis. Home dialysis has many advantages for patients: there is flexibility in scheduling time on the machine, there is no time or expense involved in travel to a dialysis center, patients have the satisfaction of knowing that they are in control over their own treatment. Thus, the patient has more freedom, more time, and more control.

CASE HISTORY 19–8

A 25-year-old divorced man had been on dialysis 3 years. He was chronically fluid-overloaded and gained 3–6 kg between each dialysis. He seemed to take pride in not following the restrictions with regard to fluids. The patient had a history of conflict with authority figures from childhood: many methods were attempted to improve his compliance without success.

CASE HISTORY 19–9

A 58-year-old man on hemodialysis developed a compliance problem primarily related to fluids and he regularly became overloaded. Attempts to remove the excess fluid with dialysis led to severe cramping. As he received much criticism about his fluid intake from his wife and from the nurses, the patient became increasingly irritable and his family relationships suffered. When the patient was instructed by a psychiatric consultant to keep a diary of all his fluid and food intake, misunderstandings regarding the fluid content of certain foods were discovered. Changes were made in the patient's diet and the patient continued his self-monitoring by recording his fluid intake. With this method the patient was able to comply very well, leading to increased physical comfort as well as improvement in his marital relationship.

Home dialysis is increasingly stressful for the partner (usually the spouse) of a patient, however (Streltzer et al., 1976). For the spouse home dialysis means less freedom, more responsibility, and less available time. Some couples work well together but others may have difficulty with home dialysis and this may stress their relationship. In general, it appears that if the spouse has been naturally dependent in the relationship prior to home dialysis it will be difficult for the couple to adapt to home dialysis with the patient now depending on the spouse. The relationship may be unable to accommodate changing roles, leading to failure of home dialysis, depression in the spouse, and sometimes divorce (Streltzer et al., 1976). It is helpful to counsel couples during the home training period regarding the psychological aspects of home dialysis. For dependent spouses, special supports will be necessary, such as periodic vacations from home dialysis by having the patient dialyzed in a center and regular counseling sessions with a social worker during times of stress.

Sex.   Sexual issues are very important to dialysis patients (Streltzer, 1981). Loss of sexual abilities is associated with decreased self-esteem. Physiological changes associated with end-stage renal disease have been postulated as causing the impotence and lack of libido commonly noted in male and female dialysis patients (Massry et al., 1978; Antoniou and Shalhoub, 1978; Lim et al., 1978). This is far from being well understood, however, and many patients continue to have satisfactory sexual functioning while on hemodialysis. Anxiety regarding sexual functioning in patients with end-stage renal disease may be an important factor in sexual dysfunction (Case History 19–10).

Most of the literature regarding sexual dysfunction in dialysis patients and regarding sexual counseling techniques refer primarily to couples (Berkman, 1978; McKevitt, 1978; Abram et al., 1975). Dialysis patients who are unmarried, however, are equally concerned with sexual issues if not more so (Streltzer, 1981). A common fear among dialysis patients is loss of sexual attractiveness; they frequently have a poor body image, secondary to growth of vessels where fistulas are placed, surgical scars, and skin discoloration. They also see themselves as weak and fragile. While these concerns are grounded in reality, some patients are able to place them in a satisfactory perspective and continue to socialize, and occasionally even marry. Other patients will be afraid to put themselves in social situations where they have opportunities to meet people of the opposite sex. Attention to these concerns in counseling unmarried patients can

---

CASE HISTORY 19–10

A 40-year-old married male had been on dialysis for 4 months. He was undergoing home training with his wife which was going poorly. He complied poorly to fluid restriction, gaining excessive weight between dialyses, and appeared depressed. A psychiatric consultant who discovered that he was preoccupied about inability to have sexual relations with his wife set up a counseling session with the patient and his wife which resulted in the return of his potency. The patient was no longer withdrawn, his compliance improved, and home training was successfully completed.

be immensely helpful. Dialysis patients have responded well to groups where the focus was sexual issues (Moe and Streltzer, 1981).

Depression. Depression is the most commonly cited psychiatric symptom found in dialysis patients (Czaczkes and De-Nour, 1978). Studies documenting a high incidence of depression have used psychological tests that emphasize somatic symptoms which commonly occur in the dialysis population as a part of the renal disease (Finkelstein et al., 1976; Bonney et al., 1978). Correcting for this factor gives depression scores that approach the normal population (Yanagida and Streltzer, unpublished data).

Depression sometimes begins with the initiation of dialysis. The shock of realizing one is doomed to a life dependent on the machine can be overwhelming. Many patients report confusion, anxiety, and depression at the onset of dialysis. They feel unprepared and they cannot remember what was told to them about their illness; many patients who were well instructed regarding course of dialysis, diet, and medications have to be recounseled and reinstructed after a month or two of being dialyzed.

Most commonly, depression appears later in the course of dialysis when complications begin to arise (Reichsman and Levy, 1972). It appears that when patients fully realize the machine will not solve all their problems, that the treatment is not magical, and they will never feel as healthy as

previously, a more difficult adjustment must be made. Most of the time this depressed mood is not the same as the clinical syndrome of depression which is so often responsive to anti-depressant medication or electroconvulsive therapy. Rather, this general sense of lack of well-being and of facing constant stress is highly modifiable by environmental influences. For example, when a patient's physical condition improves, mood improves also; when complications arise, there is often a setback; when relationships with treating staff are good, the patient's mood improves; when there is conflict, the patient appears more depressed. Vocational and social rehabilitation and sexual counseling all may be helpful in preventing depression.

Suicide. Suicide has been reported to be many times more common in a dialysis population than in the general population (Abram et al., 1971). Suicide appears to account for about 1% of deaths in the dialysis population (Czaczkes and De-Nour, 1978), however, which is the same proportion as in the general population. Thus, the increased rate of suicide matches the increased rate of mortality by other causes. Suicide gestures or attempts also occur among dialysis patients, usually by means of overdose of drugs. Since dialysis patients can easily kill themselves by refusing dialysis or cutting a fistula and exsanguinating, such suicidal attempts are a message that help is needed, and psychiatric

---

CASE HISTORY 19–11

A 27-year-old male dialysis patient did not show up for dialysis. When contacted by telephone he reported that he was very angry at his mother after having an argument with her. He assumed that he would be perfectly safe going 10 days without dialysis and thus was unconcerned about missing one or two sessions. After discussing the matter at length the patient returned for his next scheduled dialysis session.

consultation is certainly indicated. There is evidence that patients with increased suicidal preoccupation are more likely to be noncompliers and have a higher mortality rate than "nonsuicidal" patients (Czaczkes and De-Nour, 1978). On occasion, a patient may express the desire to stop dialysis or they may miss a regularly scheduled dialysis session. These patients often are not suicidal but have other needs as seen in Case History 19–11.

Case History 19–12 describes a patient who sincerely desired to die.

Most of the times when a patient talks about not going on dialysis there is significant ambivalence and the patient is responsive to counseling and support. On rare occasion, however, the decision is carefully thought out with full understanding of prognosis. In these cases it is helpful to provide the patient with whatever is necessary to die comfortably and with dignity. It is also helpful to provide support and counseling to family members in order to minimize any guilt they may feel.

Other Psychiatric Complications. Organic brain syndromes are very common in dialysis patients. They may result from uremia, congestive heart failure, anoxia due to hypotensive episodes, a variety of electrolyte abnormalities,

and other causes. Particularly noteworthy are adverse reactions to medications including too high a dose of tranquilizers or narcotics. The organic brain syndromes may manifest themselves by confusion, personality changes, paranoia, psychotic behavior, and depression and withdrawal. Evaluation and management of these syndromes are discussed in Chapter 6. Other than in connection with organic brain syndrome, psychosis is an uncommon response in the dialysis population. Psychotic reactions have been reported however, most commonly paranoid reactions (Czaczkes and De-Nour, 1978; Case History 19–13).

Violence is an occasional danger with dialysis patients. Some dialysis patients become extremely angry and frustrated when their treatment or disease develops difficulties or complications. Some patients accuse staff of making mistakes, and thinking that their lives are being tampered with they may erupt violently. Support and counseling for the nursing staff is very important in dialysis settings to encourage optimum communication with the patients and provide the most therapeutic milieu. For some patients the dialysis milieu can indeed be therapeutic. Patients with severe preexisting psychiatric disorders, including schizophrenic psychosis, have been effectively managed in

---

CASE HISTORY 19–12

A 22-year-old single female with systemic lupus erythematosus had been on dialysis for 3 years. Her course had been particularly difficult, with frequent hospitalizations for medical complications. Her fistula sites frequently clotted: vascular access was a problem and she was going to need a fistula created across her chest. Because of extreme medical disabilities, dismay with the appearance of her body, and the further mutilation that would be caused by the new fistula, the patient desired to terminate dialysis. A psychiatric consultant confirmed that the patient was rational and that she had developed increasing peace of mind with this decision. She was allowed to return home and she died peacefully.

hemodialysis programs (Streltzer et al., 1977). (Despite a report of cure of schizophrenia with hemodialysis [Wagemaker and Cade, 1977], this has not been replicated and the prevailing opinion is that hemodialysis itself does not influence schizophrenia [Levy, 1979].)

Psychotropic Medications. As a general rule medications need to be used in lower doses in a dialysis population compared with the general population. Antipsychotics such as the phenothiazines and haloperidol are useful in treating psychosis and also in treating agitation associated with organic brain syndrome. Usually the doses needed are quite low. For patients needing maintenance treatment with antipsychotic medication where compliance is a problem,

giving the medication three times a week during dialysis may be satisfactory. These are very long-acting drugs which are metabolized by the liver.

The benzodiazepines or minor tranquilizers are used commonly in dialysis patients for relief of anxiety or induction of sleep. While useful in management of acute anxiety, maintenance treatment on a long-term basis should be avoided if possible, since these are depressant drugs which can contribute to depression and elicit symptoms of confusion. It is preferable to discuss the origin of the anxiety with the patient prior to prescribing one of these medications.

Antidepressant medications are commonly recommended for treatment of depression in the dialysis population. However, case reports

---

CASE HISTORY 19–13

A 63-year-old married male had dialyzed in a self-care unit for 2 years. He began complaining about the treatment rendered him by the nursing staff and threatened to kill the head nurse. Although he had previously refused psychiatric consultation, after he made this threat the consultation was performed anyway. The patient talked readily, describing mistakes that had occurred in his treatment. He felt that his running of the machine himself had been sabotaged by the head nurse when he had closed his eyes, resulting in dangerous errors that were discovered by other friendlier nurses. The patient gave a history of being very independent, suspicious, and mistrustful of other people, believing that he had to take care of himself because no one else would do so. He demonstrated a mild

organic brain syndrome with subtle memory deficits. It appeared that he was losing competence in running his own dialysis, however his fear of dependency would not allow acknowledgment of his own mistakes, and thus he projected the blame onto others. The situation improved when he was transferred to a unit where the nurses were totally in charge of dialysis. One year later the patient's suspiciousness and mistrust of some of the nursing staff resulted in the eruption of violence on two occasions, once striking a nurse with his cane and the other time throwing a dish. Counseling the nurses about their management of the patient by the pyschiatric consultant was helpful. In addition, the patient responded to 2 mg of haloperidol given three times weekly with each dialysis session.

documenting effectiveness are lacking as are adequate studies evaluating their effectiveness. An occasional patient with anhedonia (inability to experience pleasure) responds well to a tricyclic antidepressant in low to moderate doses; however, for the majority of situationally depressed dialysis patients, antidepressants are not effective and have significant medical side effects. With their cardiotoxicity and anticholinergic effects, these medications should not be routinely used in a patient population with multiple medical problems. They may contribute to lability of blood pressure and can block the action of antihypertensive drugs (Solow, 1975). In addition, they are often poorly tolerated by dialysis patients.

Attempting to alleviate chronic somatic symptoms with narcotic analgesics by physicians can lead some patients to become dependent on regular administration of such narcotics as propoxyphene or oxycodone preparations. Dependence on these medications can cause social withdrawal and contribute to mild organic brain syndromes. Moreover, somatic symptoms usually do not decrease but rather increase. The vast majority of dialysis patients can be managed without resorting to daily use of narcotic preparations. An occasional patient, however, may develop renal osteodystrophy with accompanying chronic severe bone pain, which is very disabling and difficult to treat. Methadone, a long-acting narcotic, is useful in helping these patients (Jaffe and Martin, 1975). Giving 15–25 mg orally in two or three divided doses is usually an effective starting dosage. Because of the development of tolerance, the dose will usually need to be raised periodically. At 50 mg or more, side effects such as nausea, sedation, or social withdrawal may occur and effectiveness of the drug becomes unsatisfactory. The patient needs to be detoxified and treatment can begin again with small doses of methadone being effective once more (see earlier section on pain management of chronically ill patients and Chapter 16).

Diabetes

Diabetes mellitus refers to a group of chronic diseases, common both in childhood and adult life. This condition is noteworthy for the degree of self-management required by the patient. Despite the commonality of the disease, literature on psychological aspects of diabetes mellitus is relatively sparse. As with cancer, early investigators concentrated on elucidating psychological factors in the etiology of onset of diabetes mellitus. While stress may be relevant in the onset of some cases, practical concerns have to do more with the psychological ramifications of the illness and the effect of psychological factors on the course of the illness (Treuting, 1962; Kimball, 1971).

Compliance.   Regulation of diet and medication is required for optimum maintenance of blood glucose levels. The issue is complicated, however, by the fact that some authorities believe that mere avoidance of acidosis or hypoglycemia is satisfactory while others feel that it is crucial to keep the blood glucose levels in the normal range (Steinke, 1977). The debate stems from disagreement about the relationship of blood glucose levels to development of long-term complications. Certainly, compliance will be more difficult the stricter the control expected.

Overcompliance occasionally is a problem as well as noncompliance. Some patients with obsessive-compulsive personality styles will manage their diabetes exceedingly strictly. While these patients often please their doctors with their superb control of blood glucose levels, there is the danger that control of their diabetes becomes the dominant theme in their lives, with withdrawal of activity and interests in other spheres. It is important for the physician to help such a patient recognize that management of the diabetes is not the reason for life but rather a means to allow life to be as normal and as enjoyable as possible.

A more common problem facing physicians is noncompliance. Many noncompliant patients deny the significance of their illness and the importance of controlling their diet. In an attempt to allow the illness to influence their life as little as possible they fight it rather than adjust to it. For such patients simple encouragement to comply will not suffice, nor will education alone. The patient's feelings about his or her illness and diet must be explored. It is often helpful when the patient discusses specific reasons and situations that make it difficult for him or her to comply. The physician-patient relationship appears to be a powerful tool in improving compliance (Matthews, 1977). Eliciting fear is generally not useful in helping patients improve compliance; developing rapport so that the patient desires to please the physician is much more likely to be successful (Stearns, 1953).

A small proportion of patients will grossly mismanage their diabetes as a method of dealing with psychological conflict. These patients may have repeated insulin shock reactions of ketoacidosis. Such patients usually have severe psychological problems and psychotherapy is indicated (Levine, 1977).

Obesity. Losing excessive weight and maintaining normal weight are important parts of the management of diabetes. In general, psychological and medical treatments for obesity are notoriously poor, however (Stunkard, 1975). Some new behavioral techniques seem promising and can be effectively used with some patients. For the patient who will not lose weight with diet instructions alone, an appropriate next step is to have the patient keep a diary to record food intake, the time of eating, and the approximate number of calories. Keeping such a diary is by itself often associated with weight loss and for some patients this is sufficient to correct the problem. In addition, aspects of the diet that were not previously known by the physician may be discovered. Other techniques that have been useful in helping people lose weight include restructuring of eating habits, involving such techniques as: instructing the person to take a minimum of 20 minutes to eat each meal; to eat more slowly by swallowing each mouthful of food before putting any more food in the mouth; to limit eating to certain times and place, such as the kitchen; and eliminating all eating in front of the television, in bed, or in the car (Stuart and Davis, 1971).

Hypoglycemia. At times low blood glucose levels may cause psychological symptoms including irritability, tenseness, anxiety, palpitations, and diaphoresis. These symptoms sometimes are mistaken for purely psychological reactions. If they occur commonly, then secondary psychological phenomena may develop, including worry, chronic anxiety, and withdrawal from potentially stressful social interaction (Anthony et al., 1973). Thus, it is important to look for these symptoms and keep the possibility of mild hypoglycemic reactions in mind, since this state is usually correctable. Repeated, severe hypoglycemic episodes can ultimately lead to a chronic organic brain syndrome (Kimball, 1971).

Age of Onset. Children vary greatly in their adaptation to diabetes. Many children appear to adjust quite well without significant psychological complications (Davis, 1965). For example, it appears that diabetes does not predispose to academic difficulties (Swift, 1967). For many children and their families, however, the condition may be chronically stressful (Swift, 1967). Acceptance of the illness by the parents is a crucial element determining the response of the child (Bruch, 1949; Mattsson, 1972). While parental neglect can lead to significant problems with compliance and a brittle diabetic state, more common is an overprotective reaction which develops out of guilt feelings by the parents. This may lead to the child's being excessively dependent on the parents and failing to mature normally (Kimball, 1971; Minuchin,

1975). A parent may seemingly develop more interest in the child's diet and urine glucose content than any other aspect of the child's life, a development that makes it difficult for the child to adapt to the illness. In general, children who accept their illness are able to incorporate management of their illness into a normal life pattern.

The primary care professional can provide parents with the opportunity to ventilate their fears and anxieties about the child's illness and express their guilt if they have it. They should be counseled that it is important to help the child manage his or her own condition and to encourage independent activity as much as possible. Excessive attention should not be focused on children because of the disease state; they need to be appreciated and valued as individuals, not as diabetics. It is often helpful for parents to be able to discuss the psychological management of their child and to be given some direction regarding their interactions with him or her (Mattsson, 1972).

Adolescence seems to be a particularly vulnerable time for a person to develop diabetes and indeed some adolescents act out and rebel against their parents by mismanaging their diabetes (Kimball, 1971). On the other hand, the majority of adolescents seem to cope well and are capable of developing healthy attitudes (Partridge, 1972; Case History 19–14).

Adult-onset diabetics tend to react to their illness with their usual coping mechanisms (Kimball, 1971); there is no common "diabetic personality" (Koch, 1974). Those who had good premorbid psychological adaptation and had been able to cope with stresses effectively will usually adjust well to diabetes. Those with preexisting problems are likely to have them exacerbated. Difficulties tend to be most prominent in the later stages of illness when complications arise.

Sexual Functioning.   Impotence in males and lack of orgasm in females occur commonly in diabetes and are frequently attributed to diabetic neuropathy. It may be, however, that this condition is overdiagnosed — the physician should be aware of the common occurrence of psychological components to sexual dysfunction which are treatable (see Chapter 18). In addition, patients with true organic dysfunctions can also be helped to achieve sexual enjoyment despite their limitations. Early morning impotence may be due to mild hypoglycemia and can be improved by correction of this condition (Myers, 1977).

Complications.   The late complications of diabetes, such as blindness, neuropathy, amputations, and kidney failure are perhaps the most difficult to bear. If such complications develop the patients' adaptational equilibrium is upset

---

CASE HISTORY 19–14

A 17-year-old male developed insulin-dependent diabetes at a time when marital conflict led to separation of his parents. The boy suffered frequent hypoglycemic reactions as a result of his increasing the dose of insulin. At first, he only acknowledged that he misjudged his insulin requirement or that he was changing his diet. Later, he admitted to being depressed and angry at his parents. Because of the severity and frequency of his hypoglycemic reactions the patient was hospitalized on a psychiatric service for several months. Only then did he begin to accept his illness and manage himself more correctly.

and their belief that they are able to control the diabetes is shattered. The physician-patient relationship takes on new meaning as the patient hopes the physician will somehow be able to minimize the effects of the complication or reverse it. When this is impossible, the patient frequently becomes angry at the doctor. It is important for the physician to expect and understand this anger and allow its verbalization if necessary. The patient greatly fears abandonment by the physician at this point and will be very grateful if the physician can tolerate the anger and remain interested and active in treatment. The patient will commonly go through the stages of grief as he or she experiences loss of sight or of another function. The physician must recognize and facilitate natural reaction, and family members may need counseling as well. Rehabilitation, such as for blindness, is often crucial to the psychological well-being of the patient. Some patients are capable of making remarkable adjustments to severe complications (Case History 19–15).

Unfortunately, however, such adjustment occurs less often than one would like, and as complications set in, the qualities of patience, sympathy, and tolerance are of great aid to a physician

Cancer

Cancer is the second leading cause of death in the United States and probably the most feared illness of all. Although some earlier investigators

looked for psychological factors in the etiology of cancer, recent work has more profitably focused on emotional reactions to cancer and rehabilitation (Surawicz, 1976). It is difficult to generalize about psychiatric aspects of cancer since such a variety of conditions are involved. Prognosis varies from excellent to terminal, bodily functions may be prominently impaired or unaffected, and treatment may include surgery, chemotherapy, radiotherapy, or no intervention. The psychiatric aspects of cancer depend on all these factors. For example, a patient with cancer who is symptom-free for long intervals may worry about the possibility of recurrence; this fear may have strong implications for the patient's emotional state and even the conduct of his or her life. The psychiatric sequelae of an active cancer, involving significant physical symptoms and complicated by side effects of treatment, will be quite different. For these patients psychiatric symptoms are generally proportional to somatic symptoms; thus if a patient takes a turn for the worse he or she is more likely to be anxious and depressed and perhaps exhibit other symptoms. If the condition responds to a course of treatment and takes a turn for the better, the patient's mood is likely to improve; he or she will sleep better, eat better, be less irritable and so forth.

Diagnosis of Cancer. The primary care physician is often involved in the initial detection

---

CASE HISTORY 19–15

A 24-year-old juvenile-onset, insulin-dependent diabetic developed blindness at age 21 years and kidney failure requiring maintenance hemodialysis at age 23 years. Despite this, the patient functioned very independently, living in a different city from his family. He effectively utilized resources of several helping agencies and through his intense interest in the antinuclear power movement, had a circle of close friends who provided intellectual and social nourishment.

of cancer. Opinion is not uniform regarding what to tell the newly diagnosed cancer patient and the area is a difficult one for physicians (Oken, 1961; Mastrovito, 1974; Schnaper, 1977). On occasion, the primary physician will not tell the patient with the expectation that the oncology specialist, to whom the patient has been referred, will inform the patient. At the same time, the oncologist may believe that the primary care physician, who has an ongoing relationship with the patient, will reveal the diagnosis. Inadvertently, neither may inform the patient. This situation may occur when more than one clinician is involved in the care of the patient and communication between them is strictly limited to medical aspects of the case (Case History 19–16).

This patient demonstrates two common phenomena seen in cancer patients. First, they usually know what they have even when they are not directly told, and second, some patients exhibit a tremendous amount of denial regarding the implications of the disease (Mastrovito, 1974; Schnaper, 1977). As a result many patients delay seeking treatment (Hackett, 1973). Nevertheless denial can be protective against depression and anxiety (Forester, 1978).

It appears best to inform the patient of the illness but to let the patient be the guide as to how much information he wants to hear

(Abrams, 1966). Listening to the patient may be the most important part of telling (Schnaper, 1977). Some patients ask for details regarding the illness and this must not be withheld: it is important to establish trust at the beginning of the illness (Karon, 1973; Crary and Crary, 1974). Other patients ask no questions, change the subject, and make it clear that there are certain areas they do not want to hear about. For these patients their primary concern is that their doctor will treat them, take care of them, and not abandon them. Some patients, in coping with the initial shock, are unable to retain information regarding the details of their condition (Peck, 1977). At a later stage they may become very interested and information will need to be repeated.

Psychological coping with the illness depends on several factors: (a) the personality of the patient and history of ability to cope with stress; (b) the presence of significant supporting figures in the patient's environment; and (c) the physician-patient relationship. Patients who develop trust and comply closely with the physician's recommendations for treatment adjust better psychologically (Weisman and Worden, 1976–77). Patients must feel that the physician cares about their many concerns, will listen to them, and will stick with them. A little extra

---

CASE HISTORY 19–16

A 46-year-old married woman was interviewed to demonstrate history-taking to a group of first-year medical students. The patient freely talked about her symptoms and social aspects of her history and present life situation. When asked what she thought was wrong with her, she said, "Well, I know I have cancer because the doctors told my husband. I think they are afraid to tell me." The patient indicated she was not afraid of the cancer since she understood she would be receiving radiotherapy treatments for it and she foresaw no changes in her life style as a result. She felt confident that because of the close relationship she had with her husband he would not be particularly upset by her illness.

time spent with the patient in the initial stages of diagnosis is well worth it in the long run. The patient may choose to keep close contact with the primary care physician at this time and throughout the course of illness because of a prior trusting relationship. The primary care physician may be in a uniquely helpful position to explain the course of the illness and treatment which may be managed by specialists.

There are several moving accounts by patients themselves that document the importance of holding out hope for the patients (Harrell, 1972; Harker, 1972; Fiore, 1979). On the other hand, false hope presents a great danger and the patient needs to be realistically prepared for the complications and natural course of the illness.

Psychological Reactions to Treatment.
Treatment of cancer usually involves surgery, chemotherapy, and/or radiotherapy. Each of these has significant complications in themselves. Preparation of the patient for the complications or side effects of treatment is crucial in maintaining a sense of psychological well-being. Particularly noteworthy in this regard is breast surgery. Women facing the loss of a breast are sometimes more concerned about the meaning the event has for their sense of femininity and self-concept than the cancer itself (Asken, 1975). Rehabilitation of the breast-surgery patient, involving cosmetic appearance, and regaining arm function, is crucial for psychological well-being. Rehabilitation programs have reported excellent results in this regard (Winick and Robbins, 1977).

Side effects of radiotherapy and chemotherapy are common and include such symptoms as anorexia, nausea, alopecia, fatigue, and organic brain syndromes (Holland, 1977). It is best to warn the patient clearly of such treatment side effects (Peck and Boland, 1977), since failure to warn the patient may cause fear that the cancer is not responding, that the symptoms are due to the cancer itself, or anxiety about ability to tolerate the treatment necessary to fight the cancer. On the other hand, if patients are prepared for side effects that do not appear, they often take this as a good sign that their treatment is going well and that they are physically responding better than expected.

Depression and Grief.
Depression is frequently noted in association with cancer patients (Craig and Abeloff, 1974), but perhaps even more common is the realization that these patients are vulnerable to depression (Oken, 1961). This may explain why it is so difficult for physicians to fully discuss the implications of cancer with patients. However, objective studies have shown that cancer patients have much less depressive illness than do psychiatric patients and the clinical syndrome of depression probably does not occur much more often in cancer patients than in the general population (Plumb and Holland, 1977). Rather, the depressive elements probably represent variants of grief reactions and specific reactions to events associated with the illness or its treatment. This would explain why antidepressant medication is not often helpful in the cancer patient (Holland et al., 1977).

Grief is a phenomenon experienced by all patients with chronic illness. However, it is particularly pertinent to the cancer patient. Grief reactions occur not only in response to the loss of a close person but also in response to loss of material objects of value, loss of status, loss of self-esteem, loss of parts of the body, loss of abilities that were formerly present. The cancer patient experiences many of these types of losses and in fact, dying itself may be considered the loss of all people and things close to the patient. It is important to recognize the grief process and to allow and facilitate the patient's expression of the pain of these various losses. It is by acknowledging the loss and experiencing the associated grief that the patient can let go and come to terms with his or her new state of reality. The grief reaction has been well described in the classic paper by Lindemann (1944).

Death and Dying. Cancer is associated with the issues of death and dying more than most illnesses. The subject of death and dying has received a great amount of attention in the last decade in both medical literature and public media. This great interest began with the identification by Kubler-Ross (1969) of the natural psychological processes associated with dying. These include phases of denial, anger, bargaining, depression, and acceptance.

While recognition of these phases has been very important in the psychological management of dying patients, it must be recognized that not all patients go through these phases. Expecting the patient to follow the classic pattern may provide a comforting framework for the health care professional, but if the patient does not match expectations this can result in loss of true communication and ability to support the patient (Schnaper, 1975). Of particular concern to dying patients is the fear of the withdrawal of those people close to them, including family and physician (Abrams, 1966; Mastrovito, 1974). The physician must guard against losing interest or avoiding the patient when active treatment is no longer possible. It is the physician's duty to relieve pain and suffering; this includes staying with the patient, and respecting the patient's need to have his or her physician available. Continuing to examine the patient and demonstrate interest is tremendously supportive.

Organic Brain Syndromes. Organic brain syndromes, including fully developed delirium, are commonly seen in cancer patients as a result of the disease or as a complication of treatment (Holland, 1977) (see Chapter 6). In addition, subtle organic syndromes without hallucinations and without disorientation are probably much more common than is generally recognized. Fortunately, such intellectual impairment is often advantageous to the patient and allows the patient to be much less disturbed by the illness. In one study patients with such intellectual impairments survived longer, slept better, were less dependent, less apathetic, and were considered more likeable by treating hospital staff (Davies et al., 1973). For such patients it would be a mistake to insist that they come to some kind of existential acceptance of the process of dying.

Unproven Cancer Treatments. Cancer patients with poor prognoses are particularly susceptible to the claims of those who offer new or unusual treatments outside of scientific medicine (Relman, 1979). The patient who hears of a treatment that claims better results and less side effects than the treatment proposed by the physician is likely to try it in addition to or instead of regular treatment. Thus, despite the total lack of evidence that laetrile has anticancer activity, many patients actively seek its treatment (Jukes, 1976). Another example receiving increasing attention lately is a technique that utilizes "visualization" of white cells attacking cancer cells in one's body (Simonton and Simonton, 1975). Such techniques are often associated with claims of improved survival rates. As such, they give great hope to some patients (Fiore, 1979). These claims are also associated with significant psychological complications, however. When the illness progresses according to its natural course patients may become quite depressed as the reality of their situation has a stronger impact than they had been prepared to accept. In addition, the patient may feel guilty for failing to be successful with the prescribed technique (Case History 19–17).

Counseling Patient and Family. The following recommendations may serve as a guide when counseling the cancer patient and family:

1. Tailor the amount of information relayed to the ability and desire of the patient to understand.

2. When the patient is newly diagnosed, at an appropriate time, ask the patient how he or she plans to discuss the illness with significant others such as spouse, children, and employer.

This will allow the patient to prepare himself for potentially awkward situations.

3. Support the patient who is grieving (Harker, 1972). Allow the patient to express feelings of loss and anguish. It may be appropriate to point out that expressing those feelings takes strength and is healthy.

4. Maintain hope, but do not give false reassurances (Karon, 1973; Dunphy, 1976).

5. Family members may need counseling in regard to their communication with the patient (Schnaper, 1977; Krant and Johnston, 1977–78). Asking how they feel about the patient's illness may allow them to ventilate some of their grief and lead to increased comfort in being with the patient. Asking how they plan to interact with the patient may lead to discussion of their fears and anxieties about what to say and what not to say. Patients can become discouraged by the emotional distance created when family members keep communications light and superficial.

6. Continued contact with the family after death of the patient can be very supportive and help them to resolve their grief (Holland, 1977).

Physician's Reactions. Although it is important for physicians to monitor their own responses to all patients, the patient with cancer is particularly likely to evoke strong emotions in the physician (Schnaper, 1977). A patient who is the same age and socioeconomic class as the caregiver is particularly difficult to come to terms with and manage. Some common defenses include becoming too busy to spend any time with the patient, withholding information or giving the patient falsely optimistic information, and excessive humor or anger at the patient whose "psychiatric problems" seem to take precedence

---

CASE HISTORY 19–17

A 63-year-old married man of high intelligence was shaken when cancer was discovered. He immediately retired from his job and spent a good deal of time reading about cancer and its treatment. He was told that the average survival for his type of cancer was 3–5 years as long as he was on chemotherapy, which itself was associated with significant side effects. The patient read reports about a cancer-prone personality and felt that this applied to himself. Believing the cancer was his fault and that perhaps a change in his approach to life would cure his cancer, he turned to "visualization" techniques with faith that they would improve his prognosis. He learned and practiced them religiously. After a few months when evidence of spread of the cancer was definite, the patient became extremely depressed and sought help from a psychiatrist. At first he attempted to convince the psychiatrist of the validity of the visualization approach, wanting the psychiatrist to help him to practice it correctly. The psychiatrist did not challenge the patient, but simply said he was not familiar with the technique. The patient was then able to discuss at length his feelings about his cancer and to effectively go through aspects of the grief process. In addition, he began to talk about other unresolved conflicts in his life. Within 2–3 months the patient's depression had disappeared; he was much more realistic and prepared for potential complications in his treatment and disease progression.

over the biological aspects of the cancer (Artiss and Levine, 1973). When relating to cancer patients who evoke strong feelings the physician should be aware that such reactions are natural; it is thus important to have colleagues who can help explore such feelings and other concerns about the management of the patient.

SUMMARY

Management of the chronically ill patient includes treatment of the psychiatric aspects of the illness, especially since chronic medical illness predisposes to psychiatric problems not usually associated with acute medical illness. Physician-patient and nurse-patient interactions keenly influence the emotional state of the patient. A patient's personality style commonly determines his or her response to chronic illness. Important issues include dependency, compliance, and sexual functioning. Sometimes, symptoms such as pain may become more disabling than the illness itself.

Frequently the specific disease process determines many of the psychiatric complications. In the case of the hemodialysis patient, burdens imposed by changed physical status; dependency on family, the dialysis machine, and treating staff; and the necessity to comply with strict diet and medication regimens, can all cause psychiatric complications. Psychotropic medications must be used cautiously in dialysis patients. Psychiatric complications in diabetics include compliance problems, management of obesity, psychiatric symptoms produced by hypoglycemic episodes, sexual dysfunction, and emotional reactions to long-term complications. The psychiatric aspects of diabetes vary depending upon the age of onset of the condition. Psychiatric problems associated with cancer include reactions to the diagnosis, reactions to the progression of the disease, reactions to the side effects of treatment, and reactions to loss and to dying. Organic brain syndromes are common. In addition, the physician must contend with his or

her own reactions to severely ill and dying patients.

In general, the physician-patient relationship is extremely important in the management of the chronically ill patient and it has the potential for preventing or alleviating many of the psychiatric problems encountered.

RECOMMENDED READINGS

Abram, H.S. 1977–78. Emotional aspects of heart disease: A personal narrative. *Int. J. Psychiatry Med.* 8:225–33. This is a unique, insightful self-report by a physician on the effects of his chronic cardiac disease and the importance of the doctor-patient relationship.

Czaczkes, J.W., and De-Nour, A.K. 1978. *Chronic hemo-dialysis as a way of life.* New York: Brunner/Mazel. This excellent volume succinctly reviews the medical aspects of the chronic dialysis patient and reviews the literature on psychiatric aspects of dialysis, including a generous portion of the authors' own observations and research. It is thorough and includes recommendations for psychological management of dialysis patients and their families.

Lipp, M.R. 1977. *Respectful treatment: The human side of medical care.* New York: Harper & Row. This is an excellent and very practical book in managing common psychological problems seen in the medically ill patient.

Moos, R.H., ed. 1977. *Coping with physical illness.* New York: Plenum Medical Book Co. This multi-authored book is very readable and covers a variety of topics important in chronic illness, including many in-depth case reports and self-reports. The book emphasizes psychosocial factors associated with coping.

REFERENCES

Abram, H.S. 1969. The psychiatrist, the treatment of chronic renal failure and the prolongation of life—II. *Am. J. Psychiatry* 126:157–66.

Abram, H.S.; Hester, L.R.; Sheridan, W.F., et al. 1975. Sexual functioning in patients with chronic renal failure. *J. Nerv. Ment. Dis.*160:220–26.

Abram, H.S.; Moore, G.L.; and Westervelt, F.B., Jr. 1971. Suicidal behavior in chronic dialysis patients. *Am. J. Psychiatry* 127:1199–1204.

Abrams, R.D. 1966. The patient with cancer—his changing pattern of communication. *N. Engl. J. Med.* 274:317–22.

Alexander, L. 1976. The double-bind theory and hemodialysis. *Arch. Gen. Psychiatry* 33:1353–56.

Anthony, D.; Dippe, S.; Hofeldt, F., et al. 1973. Personality disorder and reactive hypoglycemia. *Diabetes* 22:664–75.

Antoniou, L.D., and Shalhoub, R.J. 1978. Zinc in the treatment of impotence in chronic renal failure. *Dialysis Trans.* 7:912–15; 923.

Artiss, K.L., and Levine, A.S. 1973. Doctor-patient relation is severe illness. *N. Engl. J. Med.* 288:1210–14.

Asken, M.J. 1975. Psycho-emotional aspects of mastectomy: A review of recent literature. *Am. J. Psychiatry* 132:56–59.

Bailey, G.L.; Hampers, C.L.; Merrill, J.P. et al. 1970. The artificial kidney at home. *J.A.M.A.* 212:1850–55.

Berkman, A.H. 1978. Sex counseling with hemodialysis patients. *Dialysis Trans.* 7:924–27; 942.

Blagg, C.R. 1972. Home hemodialysis. *Am. J. Med. Sci.* 264:168–82.

Bonney, S.; Finkelstein, F.O.; Lytton, B., et al. 1978. Treatment of end-stage renal failure in a defined geographical area. *Arch. Intern. Med.* 138:1510–13.

Bruch, H. 1949. Physiological and psychological interrelationships in diabetes in children. *Psychosom. Med.* 11:200–10.

Calland, C.H. 1972. Iatrogenic problems in end-stage renal failure. *N. Engl. J. Med.* 287:334–36.

Cassem, N.H., and Hackett, T.P. 1977. Psychological aspects of myocardial infarction. *Med. Clin. North Am.* 61:711–21.

Colodner, L.J. 1973. Experiences of a surgeon on dialysis. *Md. State Med. J.* 22:35–39.

Craig, T.J. and Abeloff, M.D. 1974. Psychiatric symptomatology among hospitalized cancer patients. *Am. J. Psychiatry* 131:1323-27.

Crary, W.G. and Crary, G.C. 1974. Emotional crises and cancer. *CA* 24:36–39.

Czaczkes, J.W. and De-Nour, A.K. 1978. *Chronic hemodialysis as a way of life.* New York: Brunner/Mazel.

Davies, R.K.; Quinlan, D.M.; McKegney, F.P. et al. 1973. Organic factors and psychological adjustment in advanced cancer patients. *Psychosom. Med.* 35:464–71.

Davis, D.N.; Shipp, J.C.; and Pattishall, E.G. 1965. Attitudes of diabetic boys and girls toward diabetes. *Diabetes* 14:106–9.

De-Nour, A.K. and Czaczkes, J.W. 1974. Personality and adjustment to chronic hemodialysis. In *Living or dying,* ed., N.B. Levy. Springfield, Ill.: Charles C Thomas.

De-Nour, A.K.; Shaltiel, J.; and Czaczkes, J.W. 1968. Emotional reactions of patients on chronic hemodialysis. *Psychosom. Med.* 30:521–33.

Dunphy, J.E. 1976. Annual discourse—on caring for the patient with cancer. *N. Engl. J. Med.* 295:313–19.

Finkelstein, F.O.; Finkelstein, S.H.; and Steele, T.E. 1976. Assessment of marital relationships of hemodialysis patients. *Am. J. Med. Sci.* 271:21–28.

Fiore, N. 1979. Fighting cancer—one patient's perspective. *N. Engl. J. Med.* 300:284–89.

Forester, B.M.; Kornfeld, D.S.; and Fleiss, J. 1978. Psychiatric aspects of radiotherapy. *Am. J. Psychiatry* 135:960–63.

Foster, F.G.; Cohn, G.L.; and McKegney, F.P. 1973. Psychobiologic factors and individual survival on chronic renal hemodialysis—a two year follow-up. Part I. *Psychosom. Med.* 35:64–81.

Hackett, T.P.; Cassem, N.H.; and Raker, J.W. 1973. Patient delay in cancer. *N. Engl. J. Med.* 289:14–20.

Halpern, L.M. 1977. Analgesic drugs in the management of pain. *Arch. Surg.* 112:861–69.

Harker, B.L. 1972. Cancer and communication problems: A personal experience. *Psychiatry Med.* 3:163–71.

Harrell, H.C. 1972. To lose a breast. *Am. J. Nurs.* 72:676–77.

Holland, J. 1977. Psychological aspects of oncology. *Med. Clin. North Am.* 61:737–48.

Holland, J.C.B.; Rowland, J.; and Plumb, M. 1977. Psychological aspects of anorexia in cancer patients. *Cancer Res.* 37:2425–28.

Jaffe, J.H., and Martin, W.R. 1975. Narcotic analgesics and antagonists. In *The pharmacological basis of therapeutics,* eds; L.S. Goodman, and A. Gilman, pp. 245–83. New York: Macmillan Co.

Jukes, T.H. 1976. Laetrile for cancer. *J.A.M.A.* 236: 1284–86

Kahana, R.J., and Bibring, G.L. 1964. Personality types in medical management. In *Psychiatry and medical practice in a general hospital,* ed., N.E. Zinberg, pp. 108–23. New York: International Universities Press.

Karon, M. 1973. The physician and the adolescent with cancer. *Ped. Clin. North Am.* 20:965–73.

Kimball, C.P. 1971. Emotional and psychosocial aspects of diabetes mellitus. *Med. Clin. North Am.* 55:1007–18.

Koch, M.S. and Molnar, G.D. 1974. Psychiatric aspects of patients with unstable diabetes mellitus. *Psychosom. Med.* 36:57–68.

Krant, M.J. and Johnston, L. 1977–78. Family members' perceptions of communications in late-stage cancer. *Int. J. Psychiatry Med.* 8:203–16.

Kubler-Ross, E. 1969. *On death and dying.* New York: Macmillan Co.

Leigh, H., and Reiser, M.F. *The patient: biological, psychological and social dimensions of medical practice.* New York: Plenum Medical Publishing Co.

Levine, R.T. 1977. A phase in the psychotherapy of a juvenile onset diabetic patient. *Int. J. Psychiatry Med.* 7:269–75.

Levy, N.B. 1979. Hemodialysis for schizophrenia, a voice of scepticism. *Dialysis Trans.* 8:86–87.

Lim, V.S.; Auletta, F.; and Kethpalia, S. 1978. Gonadal dysfunction in chronic renal failure. *Dialysis Trans.* 7:896–907.

Lindemann, E. 1944. Symptomatology and management of acute grief. *Am. J. Psychiatry* 101:141–48.

Lishman, W.A. 1976, The psychiatric sequelae of head injury: a review. In *Modern perspectives in the psychiatric aspect of surgery,* ed., J.G. Howells, pp. 162–87. New York: Brunner/Mazel.

McKevitt, P.M. 1978. Role of the nephrology social worker in treating sexual dysfunction. *Dialysis Trans.* 7:928–37; 942.

Massry, S.G.; Procci, W.R.; and Kletzky, O.A. 1978. Impotence in patients with uremia. *Dialysis Trans.* 7:916–22.

Mastrovito, R.C. 1974. Cancer: awareness and denial. *Clin. Bull.* 4:142–46.

Matthews, D., and Hingson, R. 1977. Improving patient compliance. *Med. Clin. North Am.* 61:879–89.

Mattsson, A. 1972. Long-term physical illness in childhood: a challenge to psychosocial adaptation. *Pediatrics* 50:801–11.

Minuchin, S.; Baker, L.; Rosman, B.L., et al. 1975. A conceptual model of psychosomatic illness in children. *Arch. Gen. Psychiatry* 32:1031–38.

Moe, M., and Streltzer, J. 1981. Implications of patient's sexuality for nursing staff. *Dialysis Trans.* 10:912.

Myers, S. 1977. Diabetes management by the patient and a nurse-practitioner. *Nurs. Clin. North Am.* 12:415–26.

Oberly, E.T., and Oberly, T.D. 1979. *Understanding your new life with dialysis.* Springfield, Ill.: Charles C Thomas.

Oken, D. 1961. What to tell cancer patients. *J.A.M.A.* 175:1120–28.

Partridge, J.W.; Garner, A.M.; Thompson, C.W. et al. 1972. Attitudes of adolescents toward their diabetes. *Am. J. Dis. Child* 124:226–29.

Peck, A., and Boland, J. 1977. Emotional reactions to radiation treatment. *Cancer* 40:180–84.

Plumb, M.N., and Holland, J. 1977. Comparative studies of psychological function in patients with advanced cancer—I. Self-reported depressive symptoms. *Psychosom. Med.* 39:264–75.

Reichsman, F., and Levy, N.B. 1972. Problems in adaptation to maintenance hemodialysis. *Arch. Intern. Med.* 130:859–65.

Relman, A.S. 1979. Holistic medicine. *N. Engl. J. Med.* 300:312–13.

Retan, J.W., and Lewis, H.Y. 1966. Repeated dialysis of indigent patients for chronic renal failure. *Ann. Intern. Med.* 64:284–92.

Schnaper, N. 1975. Death and dying: has the topic been beaten to death? *J. Nerv. Ment. Dis.* 160:3.

Schnaper, N. 1977. Psychosocial aspects of management of the patient with cancer. *Med. Clin. North Am.* 61:1147–55.

Schreiner, G.E., and Tartaglia, C. 1978. Uremia: soma or psyche. *Kidney Int.* 13 (Suppl. 8) S2–S4.

Simonton, O.C., and Simonton, S.S. 1975. Belief systems and management of the emotional aspects of malignancy. *J. Transpers. Psychol.* 7:29–47.

Solow, C. 1975. Psychotropic drugs in somatic disorders. *Int. J. Psychiatry Med.* 6:267–82.

Stearns, S. 1953. Some emotional aspects of the treatment of diabetes mellitus and the role of the physician. *N. Engl. J. Med.* 249:471–76.

Steinke, J., and Soeldner, J.S. 1977. Diabetes mellitus. In *Harrison's principles of internal medicine,* eds., G.W. Thorn, R.D. Adams, E. Braunwald, et al. New York: McGraw-Hill Book Co.

Streltzer, J. 1981. Sexual functioning in relation to overall psychological adjustment of kidney patients. *Dialysis Trans.* 10:753–56.

Streltzer, J.; Finkelstein, F.; Feigenbaum, H., et al. 1976 The spouse's role in home hemodialysis. *Arch. Gen. Psychiatry* 33:55–58.

Streltzer, J., Markoff, R.; and Yano, B. 1977. Maintenance hemodialysis in patients with severe preexisting psychiatric disorders. *J. Nerv. Ment. Dis.* 164:414–18.

Stuart, R.B., and Davis, B. 1971. *Slim chance in a fat world: behavioral control of obesity.* Champaign, Ill.: Research Press.

Stunkard, A.J. 1975. From explanation to action in psychosomatic medicine: The case of obesity. *Psychosom. Med.* 37:195–236.

Surawicz, F.G.; Brightwell, D.R.; Weitzel, W.D., et al. 1976. Cancer, emotions, and mental illness: the present state of understanding. *Am. J. Psychiatry* 133:1306–09.

Swift, C.R.; Seidman, F.; and Stein, H. 1967. Adjustment problems in juvenile diabetes. *Psychosom. Med.* 29:555–71.

Treuting, T. 1962. The role of emotional factors in the etiology and course of diabetes mellitus: a review of the recent literature. *Am. J. Med. Sci.* 244:131–47.

Wagemaker, H. Jr., and Cade, R. 1977. The use of hemodialysis in chronic schizophrenia. *Am. J. Psychiatry* 134:684–85.

Weisman, A.D., and Worden, J.W. 1976–77. The existential plight in cancer: Significance of the first 100 days. *Int. J. Psychiatry Med* 7:1–15.

Winick, L., and Robbins, G.F. 1977. Physical and psychologic readjustment after mastectomy. *Cancer* 39:478–86.

Wise, T.N. 1977. Pain: The most common psychosomatic problem. *Med. Clin. North Am.* 61:771–80.

Yager, J. 1975. Cognitive aspects of illness. In *Consultation liaison psychiatry,* ed., R.O. Pasnau, pp. 61–71. New York: Grune & Stratton.

CHAPTER 20

Psychotherapy

Robert L. Arnstein, M.D.

Psychotherapy, together with pharmacotherapy, is one of the major psychiatric treatment modalities. However, it is important for the physician to recognize that almost anything he or she does can be psychotherapeutic. This includes physical examination and bedside conversation with the patient, if it tends to foster the patient's trust and reduce anxiety. The primary concern of this chapter is to provide the physician with a broad appreciation of psychotherapy as a group of techniques and outline indications for their use. Specific indications for psychiatric consultation or referral to a psychiatrist for comprehensive evaluation and treatment are discussed in other chapters dealing with the specific syndromes — for example, anxiety, depression, and so on. In actual referral process, the physician should first consult with a general psychiatrist to discuss the specific syndrome for which referral is being contemplated. The general psychiatrist is usually in the best position to make appropriate referrals to psychotherapists following consultation.

EVALUATION

The indications for psychotherapy are difficult to define in a precise or simple manner. The primary physician must balance a complex mix of information, both negative and positive: symptomatology, history, and duration of difficulties, as well as the feelings of the patient, are all factors to be weighed. Physical signs may be absent and laboratory tests only contributory in that they rule out certain organic or metabolic illnesses. Furthermore, because undertaking psychotherapy requires voluntary and sustained participation on the part of the patient, determining that the indications for psychotherapy exist is only the first step in its successful prescription. The second (and often the more difficult) step is the acceptance by the patient of the need for referral. Although the primary physician may not ultimately control the patient's response, it is clear that the two steps are interlocked if a trial of psychotherapy is to occur.

For the primary physician the assessment phase may be especially difficult because although the negative information may be obtained in a routine visit, the positive information may not. The primary physician is ordinarily interacting with a patient in a context not particularly conducive to eliciting the type of information that might lead to psychotherapeutic referral. The primary physician's training has been to be "efficient" in history-taking, which in view of time pressure is crucial to keeping up with scheduled demands. Information relevant to psychotherapeutic referral, however, is more likely to appear with a more open-ended interviewing technique. Thus, the physician may not be exposed to the relevant information unless his or her style of eliciting information is changed. On the other hand, over time, the primary physician, may come to know a patient so well that the effect of cumulative visits does provide appropriate information for reaching a decision or at least for suggesting the desirability of more open-ended interviewing.

In addition to collecting relevant data, the primary physician must consider the point of reference from which the assessment is made. Is it being made from the standpoint of the patient who is suffering and who is seeking relief? Is it being made from the standpoint of patient's family who feel that the patient's behavior is difficult or inconvenient or worrisome? Or is it being made from the point of view of the physician who has received repeated visits and phone calls from the patient enumerating repetitive complaints for which no physical basis can be found? Obviously, the condition of the patient is the primary consideration, but there may be instances in which the feeling of the family that "something must be done" requires some change in the situation, but this does not mean that referring the patient for psychotherapy is necessarily appropriate. The feelings of the primary physician may also be a relevant factor, but care must be taken that it is not primarily a physician's exasperation, for example, that leads to finding indications for referral.

Indications

In general, patients consult primary physicians for three main reasons: because they have troublesome physical symptoms that they feel should be evaluated and treated by the physician, or because they have symptoms, physical or psychological, that they feel are caused by emotional difficulties, and they feel that the physician is the most available person to turn to for preliminary discussion and possible referral. Sometimes, the patients may not have *symptoms* in the strict sense of the word, but have problems that they feel are caused or aggravated by emotional conflict. In a third situation, occasionally others are concerned about the patient's behavior or psychological state. Under these circumstances, the patient may come with some reluctance.

For the primary physician each situation presents a different problem of evaluation and recommendation in terms of psychiatric treatment.

In the first condition mentioned, the primary physician must initially evaluate possible physical causes for the symptoms. Once this has been accomplished, the physician then considers whether there are emotional factors involved that either partially or totally underlie the symptomatology. If the physician decides that in all probability emotional factors are important, one of two courses may be pursued. The physician may inform the patient of this conclusion and suggest that the patient consult a psychiatrist for a more intensive diagnostic evaluation; or the physician may be so convinced of the importance of psychological factors that an immediate treatment recommendation is made. In either case the physician needs to convince the patient of the validity of these conclusions; this may be less difficult if the initial referral is for further evaluation. An added advantage of the latter approach is that, if the patient has negative preconceptions about psychiatrists and psychotherapy, these preconceptions may be allayed by such a visit. Thus, a recommendation for psychotherapy made by a psychiatrist may be more acceptable than one made by the primary physician when the patient is apprehensive about seeing a psychiatrist even for a single interview.

In the second condition, the patient is already more or less prepared to believe that his or her problems are psychological in nature so that treatment recommendations involving psychotherapy are more easily accepted. In this case the problem is to determine the preferable treatment model.

In the third situation, in which others have initiated consultation and the individual is resisting the idea that he or she is sick, it may be necessary to convince the patient of the need for treatment at all, not to mention the need to consult a psychiatrist for treatment of emotional problems.

The fact that emotional factors have been identified does not, however, immediately mean that referral for psychotherapy is indicated. Part of any primary physician's evaluation involves considering factors that militate against, as well as those that suggest immediate referral. Thus, if emotional problems are of relatively recent origin or if they seem to be evoked by a situation that may be time-limited, the appropriate response may be to temporize and recommend either a return visit or an eventual referral if matters do not improve in a given period of time. A student who feels anxious and tense as graduation nears or who has physical symptoms apparently related to tension may be responding to a buildup of pressures such as academic (finishing a term paper), practical (finding a job and moving), emotional (leaving college friends), or developmental (assuming more adult role) stresses. Once these have been coped with in some manner, tension may diminish.

The question of referral has been made even more complicated in recent years by the rapid development of a series of medications that are used to counteract specific psychiatric symptoms or syndromes. Not long ago the physician had only a few sedatives (barbiturates, chloral hydrate) to prescribe for anxiety or agitation and possibly an amphetamine, for depression. Both types of medication, even in the heyday of their use, were considered relatively ineffective and potentially dangerous, so psychotherapy was almost the only treatment available at the time except for the more dramatic somatic therapies (electroshock or insulin coma), which were generally restricted to the more severe disturbances. Now, there are medications and techniques that may alleviate many psychiatric symptoms, and, if specific symptoms are reported by the patient, the primary physician may be inclined to respond by prescribing a medication, or even relaxation therapies. Thus, because the primary physician has more therapies available, the indications for referral become even more complex than they once were. In addition, as Aldrich (1975) has pointed out, the primary physician may well be able to conduct a type of psychotherapy so the indications for referral to a psychiatrist may be especially difficult to define.

Referral Conditions

Conditions that appropriately warrant referral for psychotherapy cover a variety of symptoms and diagnostic entities. The largest group is within the class of **neurotic disorders**, and the majority of patients will present with underlying *anxiety* and/or *depression*, although the manifestations of these conditions may vary widely. They may include such diverse symptoms as fatigue, insomnia, weight gain, panic attacks, phobias, and sexual difficulties. Some syndromes are essentially reactions to specific events and can be characterized as **adjustment disorders** (see also Chapter 14). These may be reactions to a loss through death or to the breakup of a primary emotional relationship or they may be reactions to broader life situations, such as those characteristic of adult development, such as the transition to adulthood, a midlife crisis, or retirement. In addition to these relatively acute and finite crises, more chronic problems and **personality disorders** may also often warrant referral (see Chapter 4). These are often patterns of behavior that have developed over a long period of time, which seem to have no really indentifiable beginning, and which usually seem to have no clear-cut cause. They range from chronic feelings of depression that severely limit the patient's functioning to personality characteristics which routinely seem to create difficulties in the ability "to work and to love," to quote Freud's dictum of the goals of personal adjustment.

Besides specific symptoms, the presence of **psychological conflict** is the one outstanding feature that should alert the primary physician to consider the possibility of psychotherapy. Although everyone may have some degree of conflict, the quantity of conflict and its consequent interference with the desired functioning of the individual are a useful guide to the need

for psychotherapeutic help. Psychological conflict, as defined by most psychiatrists, exists both consciously and unconsciously. The former is relatively easy to recognize from the patient's account of difficulty; the latter obviously is more difficult to pinpoint, and the primary physician may only get hints of its existence. Conscious conflict usually involves clear but contradictory choices about which the patient is unable to make a satisfactory decision. The importance of the choice will vary from a decision involving marriage to decisions that seem relatively minor, but which create considerable upset for the patient because they seem insoluble. Unconscious conflict, by definition, is not really apparent, but the primary physician may suspect its presence from listening to the patient express certain conscious goals and wishes, which always seem to be frustrated by events. The physician may sense that events are somehow precipitated by the patient, which suggests the possibility of the existence of unconscious wishes in opposition to the conscious goals. Thus, a young adult who states that he or she wants to leave home, but when leaving is effected, somehow always becomes sick or runs out of funds so that a return home seems like a "sensible" move may well be expressing an underlying conflict about independence. Consciously, the individual wishes to be independent, but unconsciously there are strong dependent longings. Unconscious conflict may also underlie difficulty in making conscious choices because the choices may involve significant emotions that do not appear overtly.

Discussion with Patients

In the specific process of assessing indications for psychotherapy, it is perhaps useful to consider again the initial three situations proposed. In the first instance, in which physical symptoms exist, the first task is to seek a physical basis for the symptoms. At some point, however, this may be ruled out, and the primary physician may need to inform the patient that no physical basis can be found. In stating this, the primary physician may explain that such symptoms sometimes have a psychological basis. It then may be useful to conduct a rather open-ended interview to learn more about any psychological difficulties that the patient may be having. If clear-cut problems emerge, it may be relatively easy to suggest referral for psychotherapy as a reasonable next step.

If no psychological problems are clearly manifest, or if the patient resists the suggestion, the primary physician is in a position to say that, acting upon such a referral is obviously up to the patient, but inasmuch as no physical basis can be found, the options are a trial of psychotherapy or a decision to live with the symptoms and whatever impact they may have on the patient's life. In making such a statement it is important for the primary physician to stress the fact that, by suggesting a psychological cause, the reality of the symptomatology is not being questioned because real physical symptoms are often caused by emotions. If the patient remains dubious, it may be helpful to give simple examples of familiar instances of fear or anxiety clearly affecting physiology, such as, "butterflies in the stomach" before an exam, pounding heart when facing a danger situation.

In the second case, when the patient comes with a series of problems that he or she sees as psychological in nature and simply wants to consult the primary physician about the process of referral, communication is less difficult. Here the primary physician may discuss particular psychotherapeutic modalities and either recommend one, or recommend that the individual talk to a psychiatrist who will act as consultant in making a specific recommendation for psychotherapy. Sometimes a patient feels that the problem is clearly psychological but is not sure whether psychotherapy is indicated. This is perhaps the most difficult problem for the primary physician, and aspects of the patient's history or symptomatology that bear on this question will be discussed later.

Another important variant of the second situation is the patient who presents with vague symptoms, such as fatigue, lack of energy, or "just not feeling good." The patient may feel that some "physical" symptom is necessary to justify a visit to the primary physician or may be reluctant to be more forthright in describing the problem as emotional in nature. Presented with this kind of complaint, the primary physician might well ask one or two rather general questions about possible "tensions, stresses, or conflicts" that might be contributing to the symptoms. Given an opportunity to suggest causes for the symptom, the patient may quite quickly cite a problem in some aspect of his or her occupational, social, or family life, which he or she has been uneasy about mentioning. Sometimes with encouragement the patient may be quite explicit about the cause of the difficulty; at other times the patient may not have specific causes in mind but may respond positively to the physician's suggestion that the problem is psychological. At still other times, the patient may have an idea of the cause but may be embarrassed about giving details; in this instance it may be sufficient to establish a psychological base and proceed to referral.

In the third situation the primary physician is consulted because someone is concerned about the patient's behavior and feels that the patient is upset psychologically, but is unable to arrange for the patient to see a psychiatrist initially either because of uncertainty about the proper procedure to follow, or because the patient is willing to visit the primary physician but not a psychiatrist. In this instance it may be fairly clear that the patient needs to see a psychiatrist, but not clear whether traditional psychotherapy is the treatment of choice. The greatest hurdle may be in convincing the patient that there are problems for which psychiatric referral seems appropriate. In general, in this situation it is important to try to find some aspect of the problem that is bothersome to the patient and stress this as the basis for making the referral. This aspect may not be the reason that the patient has been referred by the family member, but a referral is more likely to succeed if the patient's own concerns are addressed. For example, the family may be distressed by the patient's irrational conversation or overspending, neither of which "bother" the patient; the patient, however, may be concerned about insomnia, and referral is more likely to succeed if sleep disturbance is the focus of the primary physician's recommendation. Of course, if the patient is psychotic, one has to be careful not to imply that the psychiatrist is going to help the patient resolve a problem that clearly has an irrational basis, but it usually is important to find some aspect of the problem for which referral "makes sense" to the patient.

Another possible situation involves someone who actually has an acute illness that may be potentially recurrent (for example, regional enteritis) or a chronic illness that is more or less life-threatening (such as diabetes mellitus). In this instance the patient may have emotional problems that are the result rather than a cause of the physical illness (see Chapter 19). Although the primary physician will presumably always provide supportive therapy in such instances, emotional factors are sometimes sufficiently important that referral for psychotherapy is appropriate. For example, patients may have complicated feelings about their illness which require considerable time to clarify and work through, or they may feel that their concerns are irrational, and therefore, they hesitate to "waste" the time of the primary physician or are embarrassed to mention such concerns. In psychotherapy, in which a fixed amount of therapist time is usually available to the patient at a given session and where "irrational feelings" are seen by the patient as the psychiatrist's domain, exploration and clarification of such feelings may seem more acceptable and, therefore, more possible to express.

PSYCHOTROPIC MEDICATION TRIAL OR IMMEDIATE REFERRAL?

One of the most controversial and difficult questions in regard to referral is whether the primary physician should first attempt to alleviate symptoms by a trial of medication. As has already been stated, the development of medication specific for psychiatric syndromes has made it possible for the primary physician to treat certain symptoms successfully by a combination of medication and general support. There is no clear-cut answer as to whether medication should be tried prior to the referral. Factors to be considered include the particular symptomatology, the attitude of the patient, and the experience of the primary physician in the use of the different psychotropic medications.

The physician must also consider whether the problem seems to have developed in response to a somewhat transitory life situation, in which need for medication may be time-limited, or whether there is no reason to anticipate a change in the patient's life situation, in which effects of long-term use of medication must be assessed. If the latter is the case, use of medication may also have the effect of suppressing symptomatology and thereby aiding the patient in avoiding the recognition of underlying conflicts. Furthermore, the physician may wish to consider whether the use of medication is conveying a message to the patient that the conflicts are not resolvable by psychological means. Although there is not necessarily a moral virtue in attempting to resolve such conflicts, there are obviously practical advantages if the failure to do so means a lifetime on medication.

Medications currently in use include minor tranquilizers (mostly benzodiazepines), major tranquilizers (primarily phenothiazines and butyrophenones), antidepressants (MAO inhibitors, tricyclics, tetracyclics), and a cyclothymic leveler (lithium). Some medications are more difficult to monitor than others, and the risks in taking them vary so that the inclination and training of the primary physician may be the determining factor in the decision. However, if a trial of one or another of these medications is successful in dealing with the patient's symptomatology and the patient has no particular interest in psychotherapy, most primary physicians are able to manage matters without referral. On the other hand, if the patient is reluctant to take medication or there seem to be underlying psychological problems that do not appear to be readily modifiable, a trial of medication may be postponed, and a referral made for psychiatric evaluation with the understanding that a decision about the use of medication will be made by the psychiatrist who eventually undertakes treatment.

A more general consideration relates to the broader perspective of the use of medication. Recent popular references have been made to our "overmedicated society," and, while such catch-phrases should not militate against the use of medication when appropriate, medication, if used alone, does tend to create a certain passive attitude in physicians and patients alike. Prescribing drugs may imply that one's emotional problems are beyond influence by any conscious effort. Of course, this may be partially correct, but prescription of medication should not be interpreted as discouragement of active attempts on the patient's part to learn to cope more effectively.

TIMING OF REFERRAL

If symptoms or interaction patterns that interfere significantly with the individual's life or pleasure have existed for a relatively long period and have not been modified by time, life experience, or possibly a trial of medication, immediate referral certainly seems indicated. Thus, if a patient complains of difficulty in forming intimate relationships, it is useful to explore how often this difficulty has occurred. If the patient is

19 years old and has had one unsuccessful love affair, it probably is worth waiting to see what time and additional life experience will accomplish. If, however, the patient is 25 years old and reports four or five relationships which seem to follow a repeating pattern and each ends unsatisfactorily, referral should certainly be considered. If the problem is of relatively short duration, the decision may depend on the assessment of its severity, the past emotional history of the patient, and perhaps its cause, if apparent.

An important factor in the referral process is the motivation of the patient. Motivation includes the patient's attitude toward psychotherapy, belief in the possible efficacy of "talking," and willingness to face unpleasant facts or to reveal embarrassing feelings or experiences. Undertaking psychotherapy also involves having the capability for what may be significant financial outlay, but more importantly, motivation includes accepting the need for this outlay and giving it high priority. Some patients, of course, will not have very specific knowledge about the psychotherapeutic process, and the primary physician may need to outline the general nature of psychotherapy. Sometimes, the patient may feel vaguely uneasy about referral as a result of impressions from television or movies in which psychiatrists are portrayed. Sometimes the patient simply feels that psychiatric referral implies "weakness," and it is important for the primary physician to point out that the patient will be doing most of the work and will be responsible for progress that is made. If these concerns can be dealt with, the patient's motivation may be enhanced.

For problems involving physical symptoms for which no organic basis has been found, a trial of psychotherapy is probably always worthwhile, especially if it is known that the physical symptoms can be caused by anxiety or depression. For conditions involving physical symptoms for which there is a clear organic basis but in which there are also thought to be emotional factors, referral may be more questionable, and will presumably depend on the severity of the symptomatology and the attitude of the patient. It may well be advisable to try psychotherapy although some specialists feel strongly that psychotherapy is contraindicated during the acute phase of such illnesses as ulcerative colitis, in which it is generally agreed that emotional factors can precipitate disease episodes. Because psychotherapy may stir up additional emotional conflicts, acute symptoms may be prolonged. However, psychotherapy is often recommended during remission.

TYPES OF PSYCHOTHERAPY

Although psychotherapy is often assumed to be a monolithic body of treatment, and all psychotherapy does have a common foundation in "talking" as the main mode of activity, the fact is that there are different types of psychotherapy. Many kinds of treatment modes are loosely referred to as psychotherapy, when they differ widely from traditional descriptions (Berlin, 1979). Definitions of traditional psychotherapies may be somewhat cloudy, but they can be categorized along several axes. They may be defined by general intent, that is, analytically oriented psychotherapy or insight therapy, supportive psychotherapy, or behavior modification. Some include psychoanalysis as a special subtype of insight therapy. They may also be classified by general format, namely, brief psychotherapy, long-term psychotherapy, intensive psychotherapy, or psychoanalysis. Even biofeedback is included by some in a catalogue of psychotherapy. There may also be specialized techniques within these general categories, such as transactional analysis, Gestalt therapy, or client-centered therapy. In addition to these modes of individual psychotherapy there are forms of psychotherapy that involve more than one individual as "patient," for example, groups,

couples, and families. There may also be specialized therapies, such as sex therapy and genetic counseling, which deal more directly with focal problems but use some psychotherapeutic techniques.

In regard to format, **brief psychotherapy** is sometimes just that, meaning that an individual will see a therapist a few times, and more intensive or long-term therapy is unnecessary (Langsley, 1978). Sometimes, brief psychotherapy implies a frequency of not more than one interview a week and may be indefinite in the number of weeks that the therapy continues, or it may be clearly time-limited (Mann, 1973). **Long-term psychotherapy** obviously entails a rather extended number of interviews which may or may not be limited to a weekly frequency. **Intensive psychotherapy** by definition usually implies more than one regular weekly meeting.

If referral is decided upon, the primary physician may either refer directly to a psychiatrist or psychotherapist with the idea that the patient will go into therapy with the designated individual, or the primary physician may refer for consultation with the understanding that the psychiatrist will make the final recommendation for the type of psychotherapy appropriate for the patient and the problem. Thus, if a referral for psychotherapy is indicated, it may not necessarily be the task of the primary physician to decide which of the particular psychotherapy modalities is most appropriate. It is important, however, that the physician have some rough understanding of the differences among therapies because thinking only in terms of a narrow definition of psychotherapy may mean that appropriate referrals are overlooked. It should also be recognized that referral for psychotherapy does not necessarily restrict treatment solely to that modality but may be combined with an adjunctive modality, such as the use of medication (Group for the Advancement of Psychiatry, 1975). Brief descriptions of the various types of psychotherapy follow.

Analytically Oriented Psychotherapy

Sometimes called insight therapy, analytically oriented therapy is a method in which the patient talks rather freely about his or her concerns, and the therapist role is primarily that of listener (Offenkrantz and Tobin, 1975). In this role, however, the therapist is not the totally silent figure often portrayed in the stereotype. The therapist may ask questions, encourage the patient to explore or clarify a particular set of feelings or attitudes further, or may make interpretations to help the patient link feelings and attitudes in a new way. The therapist characteristically uses the relationship that develops between the patient and the therapist as a guide to important feelings on the part of the patient, and this may lead to the uncovering of unconscious conflicts which, if brought to consciousness, sometimes can be resolved. Whether brief or long-term or more or less intensive (as defined by the number of interviews per week), this type of therapy is appropriate for many neurotic disorders.

Supportive Psychotherapy

Supportive therapy is less exploratory (or uncovering of unconscious conflicts), although some exploration may be attempted, and it probably is less analytic in its focus than insight therapy (Langsley, 1978). The therapist provides an opportunity for the patient to talk about feelings, to ventilate emotions, and to maintain a relationship with a nonjudgmental, consistent individual. The therapist may make interpretations but more often offers direct reassurances and sometimes even gives advice. Medication is often an adjunct to this type of therapy. Frequency of appointments is highly variable; they may be weekly or at longer intervals, even up to a year. Appointments are rarely made for more than once a week, except possibly in times of acute crisis. Essentially, supportive therapy occurs to an extent in most physician-patient relationships, but may be intensified in psychotherapy. It is especially appropriate in situational disorders and for patients with psychosis in remission or for patients with very isolated lives. For some of the latter, supportive psychotherapy represents a kind of maintenance therapy which may be quite helpful and appropriate (Branch, 1979).

Behavior Modification

Dealing with symptoms by directly conditioning the individual to cope with a particular symptom or anxiety is the thrust of behavior modification therapy (Brady, 1975). It involves careful assessment of the patient's life situation and characteristically consists of a series of graded exposures to the problem situation or a set of directives to modify actions gradually in situations that create anxiety. The patient learns various methods of dealing with the discomfort or the interference in functioning experienced. Behavior therapy may be especially effective with phobic disorders.

Psychoanalysis

In its classic or orthodox form, psychoanalysis is an intensive exploration consisting of four or five interviews a week for a period of at least 2 years. Nemiah (1975) describes its aim as follows: "to bring into conscious awareness the unconscious elements of the psychological conflicts that underlie symptoms and character problems, and to trace these roots to their genesis in the childhood distortions of the normal process of growth and development." Some practitioners practice a modified form of analysis which is not quite so intensive, but almost any form of psychoanalysis represents a major investment of time, money, and psychic energy.

Psychoanalysis usually implies that the patient will lie on a couch and associate freely whereas other forms of psychotherapy tend to have the patient sitting up facing the therapist. Although this may seem like an unimportant distinction, it is considered significant because in the supine position with the therapist not directly in view, the patient is supposedly better able to block out "reality" elements and more easily disclose associations which in turn give greater access to unconscious fantasies; this may help to resolve unconscious conflicts, which may be a major therapeutic goal. Conversely, for those patients whose relationship to reality may be somewhat shaky, it is usually considered unwise to ask them to assume the supine position, and, therefore, classic psychoanalysis is not usually undertaken unless the individual's hold on reality is relatively stable. The indications for psychoanalysis are a whole subject in themselves, and this recommendation should be left to a psychiatrist or psychoanalyst (Aarons, 1962).

Biofeedback

The method of teaching individuals to influence certain physiologic processes by controlling fantasy and inducing certain feeling states is called biofeedback (Gaarder, 1979). It may be especially useful in states of anxiety and tension in which there are prominent physiological symptoms.

Group Therapies

Of the therapies involving more than one patient, *group therapy* is a mode of psychotherapy that deals with a group of individuals and focuses particularly on the relation of the group to the group leader or leaders (Sadock, 1975a). This in some manner frequently recapitulates the relationship of an individual to his or her family. Sometimes groups are formed of individuals with similar problems, but more often they are mixed.

Couples therapy, as the name indicates, involves a couple and usually involves a married couple or a couple who have a primary emotional relationship (Sadock, 1975b). The interactions between the members of the couple and the therapist frequently highlight interactional difficulties that are creating problems for the couple.

Family therapy usually applies to intergenerational members of a family group and may include anywhere from two individuals (parent and child) to an entire family group including parents, siblings, and possibly even grandparents or collateral relatives if the latter are closely affiliated with the family environment (Bowen, 1975). As with couples therapy, an opportunity exists for airing of family interactions and attitudes with the therapist acting as a balance wheel or as interpreter of family interaction. In these three modes of group therapy there may be more than one therapist involved because it is felt that it is useful to have male and female cotherapists in order to understand relationships with individuals of both sexes, or sometimes to simulate the parental dyad.

CHOOSING A PSYCHOTHERAPIST

In making a referral, the referring primary physician should be aware that psychiatrists and psychotherapists may be practitioners and proponents of one or another of the modes of therapy just described. Thus, the referral may determine the kind of therapy that the patient will be offered and it is important to have some knowledge of the practitioner to whom the patient is being referred. Although some psychiatrists may practice more than one modality, not too many practice more than two. Thus, one may find a therapist practicing psychoanalysis and psychotherapy, or brief psychotherapy and group therapy, or family therapy and behavioral therapy, or some other combination. In addition to these general categories, there are some less widely accepted approaches which have particular supporters. In some instances these approaches to therapy have been very successful, but the referring physician should attempt to become aware of who in the community practices such specialized therapies and to be certain that such a referral is appropriate before making it.

It may be especially desirable for the primary physician to find and establish a relationship with a psychiatrist who can function as a consultant (Myers, 1979). This should be someone with whom the primary physician feels comfortable and able to communicate, and someone who has a broad enough view so that all patients will not automatically receive recommendations for identical treatment. Furthermore, the psychiatrist should be capable of recommending, after evaluation, that no psychiatric treatment be undertaken. Obviously, the primary physician can only develop this kind of relationship after experience has been gained through referrals, but some sense of rapport may be gained by a preliminary discussion in regard to referral or even in social interactions.

The primary physician should also be aware that in addition to psychiatrists there are a number of other mental health care disciplines in which a form of therapy is practiced akin to, and sometimes identical with psychotherapy, and practitioners from these disciplines may exist in the community. Most such professionals are clinical psychologists, psychiatric social workers, and psychiatric nurse-clinicians, but there may also be pastoral counselors, marriage counselors, counseling psychologists, vocational counselors, sex therapists, and genetic counselors, all of whom may be appropriate for referral for certain types of problems.

The primary physician should become knowledgeable about individual practitioners in these other disciplines and aware of the advantages and disadvantages of referral to a nonpsychiatrist. Advantages may relate to particular skills of an individual practitioner, the particular proclivity of a patient, possibly reduced expense, and perhaps greater availability of therapeutic time. Disadvantages may include less latitude in treatment approach, for example, medication cannot be prescribed by the therapist, less training in recognizing medical as well as psychological symptoms, and possibly the lack of insurance coverage by third party payment. However, some nonphysician therapists have arrangements with psychiatrists to deal with the need for psychotro-

pic medication, and it may even be possible for the primary physician to manage the medication while the nonphysician therapist works with the patient around psychological issues. This latter arrangement often works very well and may even be preferable when the patient is seeing a psychiatrist, because it keeps issues of medication separate from strictly psychological issues. Furthermore, follow-up visits to the primary physician can guard against overlooking medical problems, and most insurance plans will pay for visits to some nonpsychiatric therapists, if certain conditions are met.

MAKING A REFERRAL

As has already been stated, the primary physician may make a referral to a particular psychiatrist or psychotherapist for psychotherapy, or simply may refer to a psychiatrist for further consultation and recommendation as to the type of therapy, if any, that the psychiatrist feels is appropriate for the patient. There are various opinions about the best way to make a referral. Some psychiatrists feel that the best method is to give the patient two or three names and let him or her select on that basis. Others feel that this is confusing at best, and frustrating at worst. The patient who calls and finds that a psychiatrist has no time open will inevitably feel rejected even though there is nothing personal in the psychiatrist's response. In order to avoid this feeling of rejection and to guard against turning away a patient with an acute problem which needs rapid treatment, some psychiatrists, when called on the phone, will agree to see the patient once even though they have no time open for continuing therapy. The patient may then be required to present the history more often than is really necessary, which in turn may undermine the patient's resolve to pursue therapy as well as constituting an unnecessary cost.

Although it is more time-consuming for the primary physician, it is often helpful for the physician to make a call to a psychiatrist to determine whether the psychiatrist has time open. Sometimes a psychiatrist who knows that time will be opening up in two or three weeks will agree to see the patient when he or she has some idea of the problem and the urgency involved. Very often these considerations can be discussed by the referring physician in a manner that the patient understandably cannot manage in an initial phone call. Without assurance that the problem is not urgent, the psychiatrist may be reluctant to accept the referral. Although it is unwise for the referring physician to try to "sell" a patient, a discussion can often resolve any questions the psychiatrist has about the patient's situation, allowing the psychiatrist to make a decision about the wisdom of delaying the initial appointment, and/or accepting the referral.

Some patients ask whether they should see more than one therapist before making a decision to begin psychotherapy with a particular therapist. This is a reasonable question in view of the investment, both emotionally and financially, that the patient will be making, but it has certain pitfalls. It is true, of course, that no matter how "scientific" the profession would like to make the process of psychotherapy, thereby eliminating the personality of the therapist as a variable, unquestionably some patients do well with one therapist and less well with another. Unfortunately, this is often difficult to predict from an initial interview. There are instances where the patient's initial reaction is negative but therapy has been very successful, and other instances where initial reaction has been positive and therapy has stalled. Thus, the process of "shopping around" may be misleading because it is not easy to find a formula for predicting a good patient-therapist match from an initial interview.

If the primary physician is fairly certain that psychotherapy is indicated, it may be best to refer the patient to one psychiatrist who has time open. It is always wise to tell the patient that if his or her reaction to the therapist is very

negative or if there is some practical difficulty in working out arrangements, such as appointment hours or fees, the patient should not hesitate to discuss the situation again with the primary physician. Even without major difficulties there may be issues that arise in the first visit to the psychiatrist about which the patient may need an explanation or reassurance. Although it is always appropriate, and even preferable, for the patient to take these up with the psychiatrist, not all patients will feel able to do so, and the primary physician may fulfill an important function in facilitating the referral by being available for discussion. If the primary physician is referring the patient to a psychiatrist for consultation only, this should be made clear to the patient. If the patient misunderstands the nature of the visit, he or she may be very disappointed or confused at the end of the interview when the psychiatrist recommends psychotherapy and states that further referral is necessary. Most psychiatric consultants mention at the beginning of the interview if the session is just for consultation, but the patient may be sufficiently anxious about the interview so that the implications of the statement do not register, and understanding the limitation in advance is helpful.

At times the primary physician may be referring the patient to a clinic or an agency rather than to an individual therapist. In this situation it is desirable that the primary physician know the general intake procedures of the clinic or agency and that these be explained to the patient so that he or she is not put off by the application process. Sometimes patients have the mistaken idea that in a clinic they will never see the same therapist twice. On the other hand, they may be surprised and discouraged to find that, after a relatively rapid initial appointment for evaluation, they are placed on a waiting list of weeks or even months for therapy assignment. If the primary physician can explain the referral process relatively thoroughly, the patient is less likely to be disappointed or frustrated, and the referral is more likely to be successful.

Patient Reaction

In discussing the referral with the patient, the primary physician should be aware that the mention of psychiatric referral may evoke from the patient several negative reactions, which result from imprecise interpretations of the physician's statement and may interfere with the referral's success. Croft (1978) states that the patient may feel that the physician thinks he or she is faking or malingering or that such a referral implies that the physician feels he or she is "crazy." He suggests ways of stating the situation to the patient so that these misunderstandings do not occur.

Conversely, some primary physicians may be so concerned about the patient's negative reaction that they are reluctant even to broach the subject of referral. Usually, the physician's concern is exaggerated, since public exposure to psychiatry is extensive enough that most patients will not automatically recoil at its mention. Moreover, if the primary physician's reasons for suggesting a referral are sound and the time can be taken to explain them, the patient usually responds appropriately. A discussion can then ensue about the pros and cons of the referral, and any questions that the patient has can be answered. As has already been stated, this is especially important in referral for psychotherapy, because the voluntary cooperation and motivation of the patient is an important component in undertaking treatment initially and in persevering to a successful conclusion.

Myers (1979) suggests that the primary physician's attitude may greatly influence the patient's reaction. A physician who believes in the benefits of psychiatric treatment and is familiar with the process can usually deal with the patient's resistance; the physician who is sceptical, however, may inadvertently transmit these doubts and increase the patient's reluctance.

Another aspect of referral is the issue of expectations. The problem of the reluctant patient has been mentioned, but there is the opposite problem of the patient who expects too much from psychotherapy and is almost inevitably disappointed. The expectations of the primary physician may also be a factor, particularly if the patient has been difficult or troublesome. The primary physician may feel that referral should essentially shift the responsibility for the patient and the patient's problems to the psychiatrist. If the patient continues to call the primary physician the clinician may feel that the psychiatrist is not handling matters properly, which may lead to poor collaboration between primary physician and psychiatrist. Similarly, the psychiatrist may have inappropriate expectations of the primary physician by anticipating either too much or too little involvement once psychotherapy has begun. Thus, expectations between each pair of the three parties involved should be clarified as early as possible, because unrealistic or erroneous expectations greatly diminish the chance for successful referral and treatment.

Other Referral Considerations

A nonclinical consideration in regard to referral has arisen recently in connection with the development of health maintenance organizations (HMOs), in which financial factors have a direct organizational impact as opposed to a primary impact on the patient. Psychotherapy referral in private practice may be unfeasible or difficult because of the expense involved for the patient. In HMOs, however, there is usually some covered number of visits, and the patient's initial expense, therefore, may be reduced, but there may be organizational pressure to decrease referrals in order to contain operating costs. Administrators may question whether prepaid plans can cover "problems of living," however these are defined, and the primary physician may be under pressure to restrict referrals even though he or she may feel the indications are present. Obviously, within a health care system, there are no absolute or easy solutions to this kind of tension, and a balance must be achieved between the needs of the patient and the financial capability of both patient and health care organization, plus the possible fiscal cost to the organization of *failing* to refer.

SUMMARY

The indications for psychotherapy require an assessment of the patient's physical and psychological state which takes into account a variety of factors including type of symptoms, duration of symptoms, interference with patient's functioning, conscious psychological conflict, evidence of unconscious conflict, as well as the patient's age, and his or her attitude about undertaking psychotherapy. Once the indications have been assessed, a second step in the process for the primary physician is the actual decision to refer. This step involves a decision about a possible prior trial of medication along with considerations about appropriate type of psychotherapy, method of referral, and alertness to patient reactions. Negative reactions may interfere with completion of referral and even influence the effectiveness of therapy, when and if it is undertaken. Despite these complexities, primary physicians should manage the process of psychotherapeutic referral without undue difficulty if they bring their general medical experience and common sense to bear and, in addition, establish a sound working relationship with a psychiatric colleague, to whom they can turn for discussion and advice as well as for patient consultation.

RECOMMENDED READINGS

Frank, J.D. 1975. General psychotherapy: The restoration of morale. In *American handbook of psychiatry*, vol. 5, 2nd ed., eds., D.X. Freedman, and J.E. Dyrud, pp. 117–33. New York: Basic Books. The author states his view of the core problem, namely, demoralization of individuals appropriately referred for psychotherapy. He discusses the common features offered by all psychotherapies and their chances of achieving positive results. The author's eclectic approach is in clear, understandable language.

Malan, D.H. 1976. *The frontier of brief psychotherapy*. New York: Plenum Medical Book Publishers. This book provides a comprehensive review of the development since 1960 of brief psychotherapy including the work of Sifneos and Mann. There is a description of research study and an elucidation of the principles upon which Malan's therapeutic method is based. Clinical material is presented as illustrative examples of therapeutic planning, treatment hypotheses, and course of therapy.

Orne, M.T. 1975. Psychotherapy in contemporary America: Its development and context. In *American handbook of psychiatry*, vol. 5., 2nd ed. eds., D.X. Freedman and J.E. Dyrud, pp. 3–34. New York: Basic Books. This is a broad description of the development of psychodynamic psychotherapy with commentary on its relationship to the medical model, its practitioners, and evaluation of its effectiveness. The book concludes with an assessment of the state of contemporary psychotherapy.

Stewart, R.L. 1975. Psychoanalysis and psychoanalytic psychotherapy. In *Comprehensive textbook of psychiatry—II*, vol. 2, 2nd ed., eds., A.M. Freedman; H.I. Kaplan; and B.J. Sadock, pp. 1799–1824. Baltimore: Williams & Wilkins. The author gives an excellent general account of the beginnings of psychoanalysis, its development, and the main features of the psychoanalytic method. He describes its derivative, psychoanalytic psychotherapy with its various subtypes, and includes a table which compares four types of therapy on items such as goals, basic theory, interpretative emphasis, and prerequisites.

REFERENCES

Aarons, Z.A. 1962. Indications of analysis and problems of analyzability. *Psychoanal.* Q. 31:514–532.

Aldrich, C.K. 1975. Office psychotherapy for the primary care physician. In *American handbook of psychiatry,* vol. 5, 2nd ed, eds., D.X. Freedman, and J.E. Dyrud, pp. 739–56. New York: Basic Books.

Berlin, F.S. 1979. Psychological therapies for anxiety. *Psychiatr. Ann.* 9:51–56.

Bowen, M. 1975. Family therapy after twenty years. In *American handbook of psychiatry*, vol. 5, 2nd ed. eds., D.X. Freedman, and J.E. Dyrud, pp. 367–93. New York: Basic Books.

Brady, J.P. 1975. Behavior therapy. In *Comprehensive textbook of psychiatry—II*, vol. 2, 2nd ed., eds.; A.M. Freedman; H.I. Kaplan; and B.J.Sadock, pp. 1824-31. Baltimore: Williams & Wilkins.

Branch, C.H.H. 1979. Maintenance versus treatment in medicine and psychiatry. *Psychosomatics* 20: 143–44.

Croft, H.A. 1978. When you have to suggest a psychiatrist. *Res. Staff Physician* 24:103–4.

Gaarder, K.R. 1979. Biofeedback and future directions of psychiatry. *Psychiatr. Opinion* 16:29–35.

Group for the Advancement of Psychiatry.1975. *Pharmacotherapy and psychotherapy: Paradoxes, problems and progress*, report no. 93. New York: GAP.

Langsley, D.G. 1978. Brief psychotherapy. *J. Cont. Educ. Psychiatry* 39:17–28.

Mann, J. 1973. *Time-limited psychotherapy*. Cambridge, Mass.: Harvard University Press.

Myers, J.M. 1979. Making a psychiatric referral. *Medical Tribune* (May 2, 1979) pp. 6–7.

Nemiah, J. 1975. Classical psychoanalysis. In *American handbook of psychiatry*, vol. 5, 2nd ed., eds., D.X. Freedman, and J.E. Dyrud, pp. 163–83. New York: Basic Books.

Offenkrantz, W., and Tobin, A. 1975. Psychoanalytic psychotherapy. In *American handbook of psychiatry*, vol. 5, 2nd ed., eds., D.X. Freedman, and J.E. Dyrud, pp. 183–206. New York: Basic Books.

Sadock, B.J. 1975a. Group psychotherapy. In *Comprehensive textbook of psychiatry—II*, vol. 2, 2nd ed., eds., A.M. Freedman; H.I. Kaplan; and B.J. Sadock, pp. 1850–77. Baltimore: Williams & Wilkins.

Sadock, V.A. 1975b. Marital Therapy. In *Comprehensive textbook of psychiatry—II*, vol. 2, 2nd ed., eds., A.M. Freedman; H.I. Kaplan; B.J. Sadock, pp. 1886–91. Baltimore: Williams & Wilkins

ACKNOWLEDGMENT

The author acknowledges the constructive suggestions of Drs. Jay Katz, Ernst Prelinger, Eric Millman, and Hoyle Leigh in the preparation of this chapter.

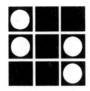

CHAPTER 21

Psychotropic Drugs and Their Interactions

Craig Van Dyke, M.D.

The advent of effective psychotropic drugs has revolutionized our understanding and approach toward psychiatric disorders. Nevertheless, it is essential for the physician to recognize that a good physician-patient relationship is a prerequisite for effective drug treatment. This chapter discusses the practical aspects of commonly used, basic psychotropic drugs and their interactions with other drugs. Since new psychotropic drugs are introduced almost every day, it is not possible to cover all the drugs in one chapter. This chapter is intended to give the practicing physician the basic principles concerning the use of psychotropic drugs. For use of the drugs in specific conditions such as anxiety, depression, psychosis, and so on, the chapters dealing with these syndromes should be consulted for further details.

Although this chapter focuses on psychotropic medication, it should not be forgotten that the time taken by the primary physician to express interest, understanding, and reassurance can have a powerful therapeutic effect on emotional symptoms associated with medical problems. Psychotherapy, discussed in Chapter 20, can also be quite effective in treating anxiety and depression and has fewer side effects than psychotropic drugs. In addition, changes in the patient's social and occupational status can improve emotional outlook.

When used judiciously, psychotropic drugs can be of great benefit in treating emotional problems that so often occur in patients with medical and surgical conditions. These medications are indicated when the psychiatric symptoms are prolonged or severe, interfere with the patient's work or personal relationships, or make appropriate medical treatment difficult or impossible. Their use in a primary care setting requires a special awareness of drug-disease and drug-drug interactions. This is so since most patients in this setting are ill and receive one or more medications to treat their physical problems. In addition, since most psychotropic drugs are depressants of the central nervous system, physicians should caution their patients about combining ethanol with these drugs. This combination can lead to excessive sedation and impaired performance in such complex skills as driving an automobile.

Another consideration is that a significant proportion of patients treated in a primary care setting are elderly. They are susceptible to developing adverse drug reactions because age tends to reduce and delay absorption from the gastrointestinal tract, and to reduce the rate of liver metabolism and renal clearance. Consequently, plasma half-lives of many drugs are prolonged in the elderly. In addition, tissue distribution of drugs may be altered because of decreased cardiac output and low concentrations of albumin in the plasma (Salzman et al., 1970; Bender, 1974; Lamay and Vestal, 1976). The net result of these alterations is that the elderly are more sensitive and more likely to develop drug toxicity (Seidl et al., 1966; Hurwitz, 1969).

This chapter describes the use of antipsychotic drugs, antidepressants, antianxiety agents, and sedatives in primary care medicine. Lithium carbonate, a drug with a low therapeutic index that is used in the treatment of manic-depressive illness, is also discussed since occasional patients on this medication are treated in the primary care setting. Although the risk-benefit factors for the use of these medications are described here, there is no substitute for good clinical judgment, especially in decisions of *whether or not to treat*. Finally, in prescribing these drugs for prolonged periods, therapeutic gain must be weighed against the possibility of long-term side effects.

ANTIPSYCHOTIC MEDICATION

Classes of compounds used to treat psychosis include phenothiazines, butyrophenones, thioxanthenes, and dihydroindolenes. Discussion here will focus on the phenothiazines and butyrophenones since these are the most commonly used. The other classes of antipsychotic drugs (that is, thioxanthenes and dihydroindolenes) are no more efficacious in the treatment of psychosis and are used less commonly. (See Chapters 7 and 8 for discussion of psychosis and drug therapy of schizophrenia.)

There is no sound basis for the selection of one drug over another on the basis of specificity of therapeutic effect. The selection of an antipsychotic medication is determined by the predominant side effects of the particular chemical class. For instance, chlorpromazine may produce severe hypotension before an antipsychotic response is achieved. Chlorpromazine (Thorazine and others), thioridazine (Mellaril), perphenazine (Trilafon), and haloperidol (Haldol), a butyrophenone, will be discussed as representative antipsychotic medications.

Phenothiazines

Chlorpromazine's major side effects are drowsiness and hypotension. Its major advantages (other than being the most extensively studied of the phenothiazines) are that it has a low incidence of extrapyramidal side effects (EPS) and is inexpensive. Chlorpromazine is the preferred drug in psychotic patients who have marked trouble sleeping. However, it is less desirable in patients who have little tolerance for hypotension (for example, older individuals with compromised CNS circulation). Hypotension is particularly prominent following parenteral administration and for that reason chlorpromazine should be given orally whenever possible.

Thioridazine is a sedating phenothiazine with a very low incidence of EPS. It is the preferred drug in patients where EPS would be contraindicated (for example, patients with fractures of the cervical spine). It is also particularly effective in treating psychoses that have an agitated depressive component. However, in males it is less desirable than other antipsychotic medications, because it produces delayed or retrograde ejaculation (Kotin et al., 1976). At higher doses it also produces a pigmentary retinopathy.

Perphenazine is a very well-tolerated phenothiazine that generally can be administered without adverse effects limiting its use. It is relatively nonsedating and one of the preferred phenothiazines for the treatment of psychosis under emergency conditions.

Butyrophenone

Haloperidol is the only butyrophenone currently available in the United States for the treatment of psychosis. Structurally different from the phenothiazines, haloperidol nevertheless has pharmacologic actions and clinical effects similar to the other antipsychotic medications. It does produce EPS but has the advantage over phenothiazines in producing relatively few autonomic effects and little or no weight gain. It

is the drug of choice for treating Gilles de la Tourette syndrome, which is characterized by motor tics and sudden loud expletives. It is also frequently used to treat psychosis under emergency conditions.

Dosage

In treating the acute phase of psychosis relatively higher dosages of medication are required than in the chronic stage. Initially the antipsychotic drug is administered on a multiple dose schedule with the therapeutic endpoint being control of behavior— this may involve controlling agitation or inducing sleep. Oral medications are preferred to parenteral medications, since the latter route is often associated with more severe adverse effects. Elixir preparations are especially beneficial in that they are more effectively absorbed than tablets and insure that the patient has actually swallowed the medication (a common problem with suspicious and paranoid patients). Once behavior is controlled, the daily dose can be given in divided dosages or the total dose given once per day at bedtime to take advantage of any sedative effect and the absence of EPS during sleep. Although the control of behavioral agitation may be achieved over the course of days, elimination of delusions and hallucinations may require weeks or months of treatment (Table 21–1).

In the treatment of acute psychosis, the recommended single dosage can be administered as frequently as every 1–2 hours as needed to control behavior, provided the total dosage in any 24-hour period does not exceed the upper limit of the extreme daily dosage shown in Table 21–1. The patient's level of consciousness and blood pressure should be monitored prior to each dosage. The drug should not be administered if the patient is sedated, hypotensive or is manifesting other serious side effects. Beacuse of the increased likelihood of hypotension, the intramuscular route should not be used unless absolutely required by the clinical situation.

It is not uncommon for patients to be treated with antipsychotic medication for 6–12 months after an acute psychosis. However, the actual duration of treatment is highly variable and must be individualized for each patient. These drugs do prevent relapse in certain patients, yet it is also clear that other patients do just as well without the medications (Davis, 1975). There is also the risk of tardive dyskinesia developing in patients maintained on these drugs for prolonged periods (Baldessarini and Tarsy, 1978). This late-appearing dyskinesia is characterized by involuntary movements, usually of the face or tongue. Occasionally choreoathetoid movements involve the trunk or limbs and can be serious enough to interfere with speaking, swallowing, and breathing. The syndrome often emerges as the dosage of the antipsychotic medication is being lowered or stopped. Although the dyskinetic movements usually disappear within 3 months after the medication is discontinued, there are a few patients in whom the abnormal movements persist indefinitely. Currently, there is no effective treatment and the best approach seems to be prevention or early detection by using these drugs in the lowest possible dosage and for the shortest possible

time. Patients and, whenever possible, their families should be informed about the risk of tardive dyskinesia before they are treated with these medications. Antipsychotics should not be used as sedatives or as a treatment for chronic anxiety. However, they may be used in low dosages to control agitation in patients with organic brain syndrome (see chapter 6).

Antipsychotic medications also are used for the treatment of behavioral agitation and confusion in patients suffering from organic brain syndromes. These agents should be administered temporarily while vigorous attempts are made to determine the etiology of the organic brain syndrome. Common causes of an organic brain syndrome in primary care patients are infections, metabolic disturbances, and drug reactions. Clearly any disease process that affects the central nervous system can be manifested as an organic brain syndrome, and it is imperative that these patients are fully evaluated medically and neurologically. Antipsychotic medications are also used chronically in these patients to control behavioral agitation when the etiology of the organic brain syndrome is not correctable. Control of confusional states and behavioral agitation can usually be achieved with much

---

TABLE 21–1
Drug guidelines for treatment of psychosis

| DRUG | SINGLE DOSAGE (mg)* | | DAILY DOSAGE (mg)† | |
	ORAL	INTRAMUSCULAR	USUAL (ORAL)	EXTREME (ORAL)
Chlorpromazine	25–50	25	200–800	25–2000
Thioridazine	25–50	Not available	100–600	50–800
Perphenazine	4–8	5	8–32	4–64
Haloperidol	1–5	1–5	2–20	2–30

* Dosage for acute treatment.
† Dosage for chronic treatment.

lower doses of these medications than is required for the treatment of psychosis. For example, perphenazine in a daily dose of 1–12 mg or haloperidol, 1–5 mg, is usually effective.

Toxicity. The most troublesome effects of the antipsychotic drugs are the extrapyramidal side effects (EPS). EPS can occur with any of the medications but are more prominent after perphenazine and haloperidol. Most commonly, a parkinsonian syndrome develops with rigidity, akinesia, masklike facies, and a resting tremor. More disturbing for patients is a restlessness and inability to sit still. Known as akathisia, this side effect can be difficult for the clinician to distinguish from the increased activity and agitation observed in psychotic patients. The latter requires more medication, not less. Rarely, patients develop acute dystonic reactions such as spasmodic torticollis or oculogyric crisis. All of these side effects are upsetting to patients and are a major factor in their failing to take antipsychotic medication. Lowering the dosage of the drugs may be helpful. EPS can also be treated with divided doses of benztropine mesylate (Cogentin) in a total daily dose of 0.5–3.0 mg. Acute reactions often require rapid treatment with 1 mg of intramuscular benztropine mesylate or 25 mg of diphenhydramine (Benadryl). Since the medications used to treat the EPS have anticholinergic side effects of their own, they should be used as briefly as possible. For instance, even if EPS do occur, they are frequently time-limited, and the benztropine mesylate can usually be discontinued after 3–6 months of treatment.

Other side effects of antipsychotic medications include: weight gain, galactorrhea, gynecomastia, amenorrhea, peripheral edema, obstructive jaundice, and agranulocytosis. Antipsychotic medications can also impair the thermoregulatory mechanism of the patient and allow body temperature to vary with changes in the environmental temperature. Photosensitivity of the skin occurs especially with chlorpromazine, and pa-

tients may need to wear a sunscreen containing para-aminobenzoic acid (PABA) to protect themselves from this effect (Sunscreens, 1979).

Drug-Disease Interactions. Chlorpromazine and thioridazine have marked anticholinergic activity and commonly produce a dry mouth, constipation, and blurred vision. These drugs should be used with caution in individuals who are at risk for developing urinary retention (for example, males with enlarged prostates) or mental confusion. Antipsychotic drugs produce a number of changes in the ECG including: prolongation of QT and PR intervals, ST segment depression, and blunting of the T waves. They also lower the seizure threshold and should be used cautiously in patients with seizure disorders.

Drug-Drug Interactions. Phenothiazines may block or reverse the pressor effects of epinephrine and alpha-adrenergic medications. This can make management of hypotension in surgical patients more complex and is of special concern in patients having outpatient surgery when a general anesthetic is employed (for example, dental extractions). This effect is much less prominent with haloperidol and is one of the major reasons for using this drug in patients with cardiovascular disease.

ANTIDEPRESSANT MEDICATION

Depression of mood is common in everyday life and does not require psychotherapy or pharmacotherapy. However, when the depressed mood is present for greater than 2–3 weeks and is accompanied by physiologic changes (such as changes in sleep, appetite, or weight), then treatment with antidepressant medication should be considered. It must be remembered that antidepressant medication is not the treatment for suicidal ideation. Rather, these patients should be carefully evaluated and involved in psychiatric care. Usually, they require hospitalization on a psychiatric unit. (Chapters 9 and 10 discuss depression and suicide.)

Tricyclic Antidepressants

Tricyclic antidepressants are the drugs of choice in the treatment of depression. Amitriptyline (Elavil and others) and imipramine (Tofranil and others) are the most commonly prescribed. Although it is clear that certain patients will respond to one tricyclic antidepressant and not to another, there is no reliable method of choosing one or the other of these drugs prior to treatment. If the patient or family member has responded to a specific drug in the past, then it is reasonable to start with this drug. Starting dosages for amitriptyline or imipramine are 25–50 mg orally, gradually increasing to a final dosage of 100–200 mg per day. Once an adequate dosage is achieved, it takes 1–4 weeks for these drugs to have a therapeutic effect. The tricyclic antidepressants are sedating and in patients whose depression is characterized by hyposomnia, it is advantageous to administer the drug as a single dosage at bedtime.

There is now evidence that steady-state plasma levels for a given dosage of these drugs vary by as much as twentyfold within a population of patients (Alexanderson and Sjoquist, 1971). Consequently, dosages of these drugs must be individualized. What is an adequate dose for one patient may be inadequate or excessive for another. Older patients develop higher antidepressant plasma levels than younger patients, and since the elderly are particularly vulnerable to the side effects of the tricyclic antidepressants, the drugs should be prescribed in lower dosages in the elderly (Nies et al., 1977). With the greater availability of assays for tricyclic antidepressant-plasma levels, clinicians will be able to adjust the dosage to maximize therapeutic and minimize adverse effects.

Toxicity.   The most common side effects of the tricyclic antidepressants are dry mouth, seda-

tion, and orthostatic hypotension. Some tolerance to these effects occurs with time; however, orthostatic hypotension may be severe and can limit the dosage of these drugs (Kantor et al., 1978). In approximately 10% of patients, a fine motor tremor develops. The mechanisms responsible for these side effects are not known at the present time, although it is presumed that the sedative effect is secondary to the anticholinergic activity of the drugs. Rarely, the tricyclics cause obstructive jaundice and agranulocytosis.

Prescribing tricyclic antidepressants for depressed patients creates the dilemma of giving a toxic drug to precisely those patients who are most likely to use them in a suicide attempt. Because of this, patients should be given only a one-week supply of these medications. Unlike barbiturate overdoses, the seriousness of a tricyclic antidepressant overdose cannot be judged simply by the level of consciousness of the patient or by the levels of the drug in the blood. The major risk in tricyclic overdoses is from cardiac arrhythmias. Individuals who have ingested large amounts of these drugs should be hospitalized and have their cardiac rhythm monitored for a minimum of 72 hours (Bailey et al., 1978).

Drug-Disease Interactions.   Tricyclic antidepressants are quite anticholinergic and should be prescribed with caution in patients who cannot tolerate increased anticholinergic activity. For instance, males with benign prostatic hypertrophy can develop urinary retention when placed on these medications. Some patients, especially the elderly, have a combination of depression and mental confusion (for example, disorientation or poor memory), and tricyclic antidepressants can aggravate their mental confusion, occasionally leading to a vicious cycle in which the physician prescribes ever-increasing doses of the drugs in an effort to cure toxic confusional effects of the drugs (Prange, 1973). These drugs lower the seizure threshold and should be used cautiously in patients with a seizure disorder. They can also precipitate an attack of glaucoma in individuals with narrow-angle glaucoma. In patients with manic-depressive illness, these drugs may precipitate a manic episode.

The pharmacology of tricyclic antidepressants and their effects on the cardiovascular system have been studied extensively (Jefferson, 1975). They have a number of pharmacologic actions that include anticholinergic activity, direct myocardial depressant activity, and a sympathomimetic activity that is related to their ability to block the reuptake of biogenic amines. All of these actions may contribute to the cardiotoxicity of these drugs. Cardiac arrhythmias and orthostatic hypotension are the most frequent and serious adverse effects from these drugs: patients with underlying cardiac disease are most at risk. For example, those with preexisting bundle-branch disease are at increased risk for heart block when placed on these medications (Kantor et al, 1975; Glassman and Bigger, 1981).

At this time it is not known which of the tricyclic antidepressants is the safest to use in patients with cardiovascular disease or which has the fewest anticholinergic effects clinically. An in vitro study (Snyder and Yamamura, 1977) suggests that amitriptyline has the most anticholinergic activity and desipramine (Pertofrane) the least. Currently, it seems reasonable to choose desipramine when there is concern about conditions that would be aggravated by anticholinergic effects. Glassman and Bigger (1981) recommend the use of nortriptyline in patients with cardiovascular disease because it has a lower incidence of orthostatic hypotension at therapeutic levels. In patients at high risk for adverse effects, the tricyclic drugs should be started at very low doses (10–25 mg) and increased very gradually while monitoring the patients for toxicity (for example, ECGs and plasma levels). Other patients may be too ill physically to warrant even a gentle trial of medication.

Drug-Drug Interactions. The tricyclic antidepressants can have their binding to plasma albumin reduced by phenytoin, phenylbutazone, aspirin, and phenothiazines, thereby increasing their effect (Morselli, 1977). Barbiturates increase the rate of liver metabolism of the tricyclic antidepressants and thereby decrease their efficacy. Because of this and the combined depressant effect on the CNS, these two classes of drugs should not be used together. Methylphenidate (Ritalin), in contrast, inhibits the liver enzymes responsible for the metabolism of the tricyclics and consequently leads to an increase in the steady-state plasma levels of the tricyclics (Hansten, 1979). The antihypertensive effect of guanethidine (Ismelin) and clonidine (Catapres) is blocked by the tricyclics (Briant et al., 1973; Jefferson, 1975). The tricyclics also have a quinidine-like effect on the heart and quickly produce cardiotoxicity in patients taking quinidine. As with quinidine, prolongation of the QRS interval in the ECG is an index of tricyclic cardiotoxicity. Finally, the tricyclics can potentiate the pressor response of intravenous epinephrine, levarterenol, and phenylephrine (Svedmyr, 1968; Boakes et al., 1973).

Monoamine Oxidase Inhibitors

Occasionally, patients being treated with a monoamine oxidase (MAO) inhibitor, such as tranylcypromine (Parnate) or phenelzine (Nardil), are cared for in a primary care setting. These medications can be effective as antidepressants especially for less severe depressions (Quitkin et al., 1979). However, these drugs have many serious interactions with foods and other drugs and should be used only after patients have failed to respond to separate treatment trials with more than one tricyclic antidepressant. Patients using MAO inhibitors must be intelligent and reliable in guarding against the possibility of ingesting foods containing tyramine (ripe cheeses, broad beans, avocado, yeast preparations, chicken livers, beer, sherry, and chianti) or being administered drugs such as L-dopa, amphetamine, phenylephrine, metaraminol, and meperidine (Brownlee and Williams, 1963; Sjoquist, 1965; Hunter et al., 1970). Combining MAO inhibitors with any of these foods or drugs can result in a hypertensive crisis with subsequent headache or cerebral vascular accident. Reactions have also occurred following the use of over-the-counter diet pills or cold remedies that contain sympathomimetic amines. It is important to remember that the effects of MAO inhibitors may last for as long as 2 weeks after the drug is discontinued. Because of their many serious interactions, MAO inhibitors should not be used in patients with serious medical illness, nor should they be used in patients who are not sufficiently vigilant to avoid the many foods and drugs that may precipitate a hypertensive crisis.

Although a hypertensive crisis is the major worry with these drugs, they also commonly produce orthostatic hypotension, weight gain, and constipation. The combination of MAO inhibitor and tricyclic antidepressant is occasionally (and perhaps inappropriately) used to treat refractory depressions, despite there being no evidence that this combination is effective. It is quite clear, however, that these two classes of drugs are extremely toxic when taken in an overdose and may cause excitation, hyperpyrexia, convulsions, and death (Spiker and Pugh, 1976).

Lithium Carbonate

Patients with manic-depressive illness may be successfully treated with lithium carbonate. It is the drug of choice for the treatment of acute mania, and there is now good evidence that maintenance treatment with lithium carbonate is effective in preventing relapses of manic-depressive illness (Davis, 1976). Although the drug has a very low therapeutic index, it can be administered safely because of the comparative ease and inexpense of measuring the serum

concentrations of the drug. The therapeutic range for the treatment of acute mania is 0.8–1.5 mEq/L, while for maintenance treatment the range is 0.8–1.0 mEq/L. Because of its low therapeutic index, the drug is administered in divided doses three to four times per day in order to minimize the toxicity immediately after its ingestion. During the first few weeks of treatment, measurement of lithium levels should be obtained three times per week until a steady state has been attained. After that, measurements can occur every 1–4 weeks. The lithium levels should be obtained 10–12 hours after the last dose is administered (for example, just before the first morning dose). In treating acute mania, antipsychotic medication may be required initially to control behavior, since it requires 4–10 days for lithium to have its therapeutic effect. As the acute episode of mania subsides, less lithium is usually required and frequently the antipsychotic medication can be discontinued.

Toxicity.   Because lithium carbonate is a toxic drug and has many interactions, it is important before ever starting the medication to perform the following laboratory tests: complete blood count; urinalysis; assessment of blood urea nitrogen and creatinine levels; ECG; and thyroid indices. As with other drugs, taking serum levels alone is not a substitute for observing and talking with patients. For example, it is not uncommon for patients to have side effects from lithium carbonate when their serum levels are in the therapeutic (and presumably nontoxic) range. Such patients should have their dose and serum levels of lithium lowered in an effort to minimize the adverse effects.

Common side effects of lithium include nausea, vomiting, diarrhea, weakness, and fatigue. These effects usually occur in the first few weeks of treatment. If the symptoms persist, they may improve when the dosage and serum levels are lowered slightly. A fine motor tremor, thirst, polyuria, edema, weight gain, and leukocytosis may persist for the duration of treatment. When serum levels exceed 1.5–2.0 mEq/L, serious CNS toxicity commonly occurs. Symptoms of CNS toxicity include confusion, slurred speech, ataxia, disorientation, convulsions, and coma Elderly patients or those with an underlying organic brain syndrome are more likely to develop CNS toxicity.

Overdosage of lithium carbonate results in serious CNS toxicity. Several hours may elapse before signs of toxicity occur, with the earliest indications being gastrointestinal symptoms, lethargy, confusion, unsteady gait, and slurred speech. Signs of even more serious overdosage include neuromuscular irritability, abnormal EEG, seizures, delirium, and finally coma. Serum electrolyte levels may also be abnormal. Treatment is supportive with correction of the electrolyte abnormalities. Diuretics are of little use and, in fact, may increase serum lithium levels. However, dialysis may be helpful when serum levels are extremely elevated.

Drug-Disease Interactions. Lithium can induce a mild and transient hypothyroidism. When there is a prior history of thyroid disease, patients have a greater risk of developing a goiter or hypothyroidism (Schou et al., 1968). Since lithium does not affect circulating thyroid hormones, the hypothyroidism can be treated by replacement therapy. The drug produces numerous changes in the ECG (for example, T wave flattening or inversion or widening of the QRS complex) as well as cardiac arrhythmias. If possible, it should not be used in the period immediately following a myocardial infarction. Haloperidol is a better choice for controlling disruptive behavior in a patient with manic-depressive illness after a heart attack. Lithium should not be prescribed during pregnancy because of the increased risk of producing cardiovascular abnormalities in the newborn (Weinstein and Goldfield, 1975).

Lithium usually causes polyuria but in certain individuals a nephrogenic diabetes insipidus syndrome develops (Forrest et al., 1974). In most cases, there is no impairment of renal function. There is evidence that in certain individuals, especially those with increased urine volumes, lithium produces permanent renal damage characterized by loss of ability to concentrate the urine and by sclerotic glomeruli and focal nephron atrophy (Hestbech et al., 1977). In response to this finding, it now seems prudent to monitor renal function every 6 months in patients maintained on lithium. The drugs should be used with exceeding caution, if at all, in patients with preexisting renal disease.

Drug-Drug Interactions. Diuretics, especially thiazide diuretics, or a low sodium diet promote increased reabsorption of lithium by the kidneys and thereby produce increased serum lithium levels (Himmelhoch et al., 1977). This interaction can create a problem when certain patients on lithium develop mild edema and seek treatment for this problem from a physician. Using a diuretic to treat the edema can quickly lead to very high lithium levels and serious toxicity (Hertig and Dyson, 1974).

ANTIANXIETY MEDICATION

Anxiety in response to the vicissitudes of everyday life is a normal reaction that does not require treatment. Anxiety also occurs in association with other major psychiatric illnesses (for example, depression and schizophrenia) or with medical illnesses (such as hyperthyroidism). When this is the case, primary attention should be focused on treating the underlying illness. However, when anxiety is intense and interferes with normal physiological functions or with work and social relations, then brief treatment with antianxiety agents is indicated (for further discussion of anxiety and its treatment, see Chapter 11). Only benzodiazepine compounds will be discussed here, since the other class of antianxiety agents, such as propanediol carbamates or meprobamate (Miltown), offers no therapeutic advantage over the benzodiazepines and may lead to greater toxicity.

Benzodiazepines

Antianxiety drugs are now the most widely prescribed of all drugs in the United States. The two most commonly prescribed benzodiazepines are diazepam (Valium) and chlordiazepoxide (Librium and others). The dosage range for diazepam is 5–30 mg per day while for chlordiazepoxide it is 15–60 mg per day. The dosages are usually given in divided dosages but often two-thirds of the daily dose can be given at night to treat difficulty falling asleep. It should be remembered that although both drugs are absorbed well orally, they have a slow and erratic rate of absorption when administered intramuscularly and may be less effective by this route (Hillestad et al., 1974; Gottschalk et al., 1974; Assaf et al., 1975). The major consideration in using these drugs is that they are most effective when used for short periods (1–3 weeks). Tolerance develops to their therapeutic effects and the drugs may be habituating.

Toxicity. The benzodiazepines have a remarkable margin of safety and are generally much safer than other sedatives (such as barbiturates or chloral hydrate) when taken in overdose, because they depress respirations less. Occasionally, benzodiazepines produce ataxia, skin rashes, nausea and vomiting, headache, impaired sexual functioning, agranulocytosis, and menstrual irregularity. They may increase hostility in irritable and angry patients (Salzman et al., 1974). When the drugs are stopped, tapering the dosage over 2 weeks is preferred to abrupt discontinuation since the latter may be associated with a withdrawal syndrome. It should be remembered that diazepam and chlordiazepoxide have prolonged half-lives and withdrawal symptoms may not be manifest until a week after the drug is discontinued. Typical symptoms of withdrawal include anxiety, dysphoria, tremor, and numerous somatic complaints (Pevnick et al., 1978). Seizures are rare and occur after high doses.

Drug-Disease Interactions.   The antianxiety drugs are extremely well tolerated and have very little effect on the cardiovascular system following oral doses. In patients with chronic obstructive pulmonary disease, the drugs can seriously depress respirations (Lakshminarayan et al., 1976). Since the drugs are metabolized by the liver, their effects can be prolonged in patients with impaired hepatic function (Klotz et al., 1977). Chlordiazepoxide and diazepam should not be prescribed for pregnant women because of the increased risk of the patient giving birth to a child with a cleft lip (Saxen, 1975; Safra and Oakley, 1975).

Drug-Drug Interactions.   Antianxiety drugs are depressants of the CNS, and when combined with other depressants such as alcohol or barbiturates they potentiate the activity of these drugs and can cause decreased respirations, coma, and even death. Ingestion of alcohol may also increase the bioavailability of these antianxiety drugs by increasing their absorption following oral administration (Hayes et al., 1977). Unlike the barbiturates, diazepam and chlordiazepoxide do not induce enzyme systems in the liver and can be used safely with a number of other drugs including oral anticoagulants. There is evidence that heavy cigarette smokers metabolize antianxiety drugs more rapidly and because of this higher doses are required to provide therapeutic effects (Miller, 1977). In contrast, cimetidine (Tagamet) decreases the elimination of benzodiazepines and enhances their clinical effects (Desmond et al., 1980; Klotz and Reimann, 1980).

SEDATIVE MEDICATION

Insomnia requires careful evaluation by the primary physician (Soloman et al., 1979). For instance, depression and schizophrenia are commonly associated with profound disturbances in sleep. Medical conditions that cause chronic pain may also interfere with sleep patterns. In these conditions primary attention should be directed to treating the underlying psychiatric or medical illness.

Benzodiazepines

Flurazepam (Dalmane) is the most widely prescribed benzodiazepine for the treatment of insomnia. This drug has gained popularity over barbiturates in the treatment of insomnia because of its ability to remain effective with repeated use without producing serious adverse effects (Kales et al., 1975; Kales et al., 1976a). Usual dosage is 15–30 mg. Flurazepam does have one complicating effect; it produces active metabolites that may have a sedating effect during the daytime. This may be especially prominent in the elderly who use the 30 mg dosage (Greenblatt et al., 1977). Three other benzodiazepines—oxazepam (Serax), temazepam (Restoril) and lorazepam (Atavin)—do not produce active metabolites and have relatively short half-lives of 5–20 hours (Greenblatt et al., 1976). These drugs may be more beneficial in the treatment of insomnia since there is little feeling of "hangover" the next day (Wang et al., 1976). However, the short-acting benzodiazepines may be associated with more severe rebound insomnia when discontinued.

Toxicity. All of the benzodiazepines that are used as sedatives have the same toxicity and interactions as noted previously for diazepam and chlordiazepoxide in the treatment of anxiety.

Barbiturates

Pentobarbital (Nembutal), secobarbital (Seconal), and amobarbital (Amytal) are the most widely prescribed barbiturates for the treatment of insomnia. Barbiturates have been supplanted as sedative drugs because of the widespread popularity of the benzodiazepines. The barbiturates

accounted for 47% of hypnotic prescriptions in 1971 but for only 17% in 1977. However, barbiturates are effective as sedatives when used for brief periods of time and are an alternative to the use of drugs such as flurazepam. Their effectiveness over prolonged usage is unclear at this time (Kales et al., 1976b). If they have any advantage over flurazepam (but not over the shorter acting benzodiazepines), it is that barbiturates have average half-lives of 14–42 hours; whereas flurazepam and its active metabolites have half-lives of 50–100 hours. Because of the shorter half-lives, barbiturates may create less of a "hangover" than flurazepam.

Toxicity. Barbiturates are more toxic than benzodiazepines and can rapidly produce coma and death when taken in excessive amounts. They should be prescribed in limited amounts since the drugs can be quite lethal when used in suicidal attempts. Initially, barbiturates suppress REM sleep; however, with chronic administration a degree of tolerance develops to this effect. Tolerance also develops rapidly to their therapeutic effects, resulting in patients increasing their dose in order to maintain a uniform level of effectiveness. Habituation may occur from the ever-increasing doses of the drug. Although tolerance develops to their sedative effects, there is no alteration in the lethal dose of barbiturates. Following long-term administration, barbiturates should be gradually tapered in dosage before discontinuing them in order to minimize the risk of withdrawal seizures (see Chapter 16).

Drug-Disease Interactions. The barbiturates have little effect on the cardiovascular system but are profound respiratory depressants and should not be prescribed for patients with serious pulmonary disease. The drugs are contraindicated in patients with acute intermittent porphyria, because they can precipitate severe attacks of the disease. There is also evidence that the use of barbiturates during pregnancy may increase the likelihood of brain tumors in the offspring (Gold et al., 1978).

Drug-Drug Interactions. Following just a few doses, barbiturates increase the activity of the hepatic microsomal enzyme system. The impact of this action is that these drugs actually increase the rate of their own metabolism as well as other drugs. The oral anticoagulants and digitoxin have their half-lives shortened when combined with barbiturates thereby decreasing their effectiveness significantly (Hansten, 1979).

ALTERNATIVE SEDATIVES

There are a variety of other drugs widely marketed as sedatives. Chloral hydrate has many of the properties of barbiturates. For example, it alters the metabolism of oral anticoagulants and may precipitate attacks in patients with acute intermittent porphyria. It has a low therapeutic index with 1 g given orally being only slightly effective as a sedative and with 4 g occasionally producing death. Nausea and vomiting are frequent side effects, and chloral hydrate should not be used in patients with gastritis. In addition, it should be used with caution in patients with liver, renal, or cardiac disease. As with the barbiturates, tolerance to the therapeutic effects develops with chronic usage and there is risk of habituation. Seizures may occur on rapid discontinuation of the drug.

Numerous anticholinergic and antihistaminic drugs are marketed as hypnotic agents, yet their efficacy has been poorly evaluated. Methyprylon (Noludar), glutethimide (Doriden), and ethchlorvynol (Placidyl) are probably similar to the barbiturates (including the risk of habituation) but have not been studied as extensively.

RECOMMENDED READINGS

Drugs in breast milk. 1979. *Medical Letter*. 21:21–24. This article summarizes the effects of drugs that are excreted in breast milk.

Drugs that cause psychiatric symptoms. 1981. *Medical Letter*. 23:9–12. This is a current listing of drugs that cause psychiatric symptoms.

Gilman, A.S.; Goodman, L.S.; Gilman, A., eds. 1980. *The pharmacological basis of therapeutics*. New York: Macmillan. This is the standard pharmacologic reference that contains very useful sections on psychotropic medications.

Hansten, P.D. 1979. *Drug interactions*. Philadelphia: Lea & Febiger. This is an up-to-date summary and discussion of drug interactions.

Kbantzian, E.J., and McKenna, G.J. 1979. Acute toxic and withdrawal reactions associated with drug use and abuse. *Ann. Intern. Med.* 90:361–72. This article is a current summary of intoxicated states and drug withdrawal syndromes associated with drug abuse.

REFERENCES

Alexanderson, B., and Sjoquist, F. 1971. Individual differences in the pharmacokinetics of monomethylated tricyclic antidepressants: Role of genetic and environmental factors and clinical importance. *Ann. N.Y. Acad. Sci.* 179:739–51.

Assaf, R.A.E.; Dundee, J.W.; and Gamble, J.A.S. 1975. The influence of the route of administration on the clinical action of diazepam. *Anaesthesia* 30:152–58.

Bailey, D.N.; Van Dyke, C.; Langou, R.A., et al. 1978. Tricyclic antidepressants: Plasma levels and clinical findings in overdose. *Am. J. Psychiatry* 135:1325–28.

Baldessarini, R.J., and Tarsy, D. 1978. Tardive dyskinesia. In *Psychopharmacology—a generation of progress*, eds. M.A. Lipton; A. Di Mascio and K.F. Killam, pp. 993–1004 New York: Raven Press.

Bender, A.D. 1974. Pharmacodynamic principles of drug therapy in the aged. *J. Am. Geriatr. Soc.* 22:296–303.

Boakes, A.J.; Laurence, D.R.; Teoh, P.C., et al. 1973. Interactions between sympathomimetic amines and antidepressant agents in man. *Br. Med. J.* 1:311–15.

Briant, R.H.; Reid, J.L.; and Dollery, C.T. 1973. Interaction between clonidine and desipramine in man. *Br. Med. J.* 1:522–23.

Brownlee, G., and Williams, G.W. 1963. Potentiation of

amphetamine and pethidine by monoamine oxidase inhibitors. *Lancet* 1:669.

Davis, J.M. 1975. Overview: Maintenance therapy in psychiatry. I. Schizophrenia. *Am. J. Psych.* 132:1237–45.

———. 1976. Overview: Maintenance therapy in psychiatry. II. Affective disorders. *Am. J. Psychiatry* 133:1–13.

Desmond, P.V., Patwardhar, R.V., Schenker, S., et al. 1980. Cimetidine impairs elimination of chlordiazepoxide (Librium). *Ann. Intern. Med.* 93:266–69.

Forrest, J; Cohen, A.; Torretti, J., et al. 1974. On the mechanism of lithium-induced diabetes insipidus in man and the rat. *J. Clin. Invest.* 53:1115–23.

Glassman, A.H; and Bigges, J.T. 1981. Cardiovascular effects of therapeutic doses of tricyclic antidepressants. *Arch. Gen. Psychiatry* 38:815–20.

Gold, E.; Gordis, L.; Tonascia, J., et al. 1978. Increased risk of brain tumors in children exposed to barbiturates. *J. Natl. Cancer Inst.* 61:1031–34.

Gottschalk, L.A.; Biener, R.; and Dinovo, E.C.. 1974. Effect of oral and intramuscular routes of administration on serum chlordiazepoxide levels and the prediction of these levels from predrug fasting serum glucose concentrations. *Res. Commun. Chem. Pathol. Pharmacol.* 8:697–702.

Greenblatt, D.J.; Allen, M.D.; and Shader, R.I. 1977. Toxicity of high-dose flurazepam in the elderly. *Clin. Pharmacol. Ther.* 21:355–61.

Greenblatt, D.J.; Schillings, R.T.; Kyriakopoulos, A.A., et al. 1976. Clinical pharmacokinetics of lorazepam. *Clin. Pharmacol. Ther.* 20:329–41.

Hansten, P.D. 1979. *Drug interactions.* Philadelphia: Lea & Febiger.

Hayes, S.L.; Pablo, G.; Radomski, T., et al. 1977. Ethanol and oral diazepam absorption. *N. Engl. J. Med.* 296:186–89.

Hertig, H., and Dyson, W. 1974. Lithium toxicity enhanced by diuretics. *N. Engl. J. Med.* 290:748–49.

Hestbech, J.; Hansen, H.E.; Amdisen, A., et al. 1977. Chronic renal lesions following long-term treatment with lithium. *Kidney Int.* 12:205–13

Hillestad, L.; Hansen, T.; Melsom, H., et al. 1974. Diazepam metabolism in normal man. I. Serum concentrations and clinical effects after intravenous, intramuscular, and oral administration. *Clin. Pharmacol. Ther.* 16:479–84.

Himmelhoch, J.M., Poust, R.I., Mallinger, A.G., et al.

1977. Adjustment of lithium dose during lithium chlorothiazide therapy. *Clin. Pharmacol. Ther.* 22:225–27.

Hunter, K.R.; Boakes, A.J.; Laurence, D.R. et al. 1970 Monoamine oxidase inhibitors and L-dopa. *Br. Med. J.* 3:388.

Hurwitz, N. 1969. Prediagnosing factors in adverse reactions to drugs. *Br. Med. J.* 1:536–39.

Jefferson, J.W. 1975. A review of the cardiovascular effects and toxicity of tricyclic antidepressants. *Psychosom. Med.* 37:160–79.

Kales, A.; Bixler, E.O.; Scharf, M., et al. 1976a. Sleep laboratory studies of flurazepam: A model for evaluating hypnotic drugs. *Clin. Pharmacol. Ther.* 19:5:576–83.

Kales, A.; Hauri, P.; Bixler, E.O., et al. 1976b. Effectiveness of intermediate-term use of secobarbital. *Clin. Pharmacol. Ther.* 20:541–45.

Kales, A.; Kales, J.D.; Bixler, E.O. et al. 1975. Effectiveness of hypnotic drugs with prolonged use: Flurazepam and pentobarbital. *Clin. Pharmacol. Ther.* 18:356–63.

Kantor, S.J.; Bigger, J.T.; Glassman, A.H., et al. 1975. Imipramine induced heart block: A longitudinal case study. *J.A.M.A.* 231:1364–66.

Kantor, S.J.; Glassman, A.H.; Bigger, T., et al. 1978. The cardiac effects of therapeutic plasma concentrations of imipramine. *Am. J. Psychiatry* 135:534–38.

Klotz, U.; Antonin, K.H.; Brügel, H., et al. 1977. Disposition of diazepam and its major metabolites desmethyldiazepam in patients with liver disease. *Clin. Pharmacol. Ther.* 21:430–36.

Klotz, U.; and Reimann, I. 1980. Delayed clearance of diazepam due to cimetidine. *N. Engl. J. Med.* 302:1012–14.

Kotin, J.; Wilbert, D.E.; Verburg, D., et al. 1976. Thioridazine and sexual dysfunction. *Am. J. Psychiatry* 133:82–85.

Lakshminarayan, S.; Sahn, S.A.; Hudson, L.O., et al. 1976. Effect of diazepam on ventilatory response. *Clin. Pharmacol Ther.* 20:178–83.

Lamay, P.P., and Vestal, R.E. 1976. Drug prescribing for the elderly, *Hosp. Practice* 111–18.

Miller, R.R., 1977. Effects of smoking on drug action. *Clin. Pharmacol. Ther.* 22:2:749–56.

Morselli, P.L., ed. 1977. Psychotropic drugs. In *Drug disposition during development*, pp. 431–74. New York: Spectrum Publications, Inc.

Nies, A.; Robinson, D.S.; Friedman, J., et al. 1977. Relationship between age and tricyclic antidepressant plasma levels. *Am. J. Psychiatry* 134:790–93.

Pevnick, J.S.; Jasinski, D.R.; and Haertzen, C.A. 1978. Abrupt withdrawal from therapeutically administered diazepam. *Arch. Gen. Psychiatry* 35:995–98.

Prange, A.J. 1973. The use of antidepressant drugs in the elderly patient. In *Psychopharmacology and aging*, eds., C. Eisdorfer, and W.E. Fann, pp. 225–37. New York: Plenum Press.

Quitkin, F.; Rifkin, A.; and Klein, D.F. 1979. Monoamine oxidase inhibitors. *Arch. Gen. Psychiatry* 36:749–60.

Safra, M.J., and Oakley, G.P. 1975. Association between cleft lip with or without cleft palate and prenatal exposure to diazepam. *Lancet* 2:478–80.

Salzman, C.; Shader, R.I.; and Pearlman, M. 1970. Psychopharmacology and the elderly. In *Psychotropic drug side effects,* eds., R.I. Schader, and A. Di Mascio, pp. 261–79. Baltimore: Williams & Wilkins.

Salzman, C., Kochansky, G.E., Schader, R.I., et al. 1974. Chlordiazepoxide-induced hostility in a small group setting. *Arch. Gen. Psychiatry* 31:401–5.

Saxen, I. 1975. Associations between oral clefts and drugs taken during pregnancy. *Int. J. Epidemiol.* 4:37–44.

Schou, M.; Amdisen, A.; Jensen, S.E., et al. 1968. Occurrence of goiter during lithium treatment. *Br. Med. J.* 3:710–13.

Seidl, L.G.; Thornton, G.F.; Smith, J.W., et al. 1966. Studies on the epidemiology of adverse drug reactions. III. Reactions in patients on a general medical service. *Bull. Johns Hopkins Hosp.* 119:229–315.

Sjoquist, F. 1965. Psychotropic drugs (2). Interactions between monoamine oxidase inhibitors (MAO) and other substances. *Proc. R. Soc. Med.* 58:967–78.

Soloman, F.; White, C.C.; Parron, D.L., et al. 1979. Sleeping pills, insomnia, and medical practice. *N. Engl. J. Med.* 300:803–08.

Snyder, S.H., Yamamura, H.I. 1977. Antidepressants and the muscarinic acetylcholine receptor. *Arch. Gen. Psychiatry* 34:236–39.

Sunscreens. 1979. *Medical Letter* 21:46–48.

Svedmyr, N. 1968. The influence of a tricyclic antidepressive agent (protriptyline) on some of the circulatory effects of noradrenaline and adrenaline in man. *Life Sci.* 7:77–84.

Wang, R.I.H.; Stockdale, S.; and Hieb, E., 1976. Hypnotic efficacy of lorazepam and flurazepam. *Clin. Pharmacol. Ther.* 19:191–95.

Weinstein, M.R., and Goldfield, M.D. 1975. Cardiovascular malformations with lithium use during pregnancy. *Am. J. Psychiatry* 132:529–31.

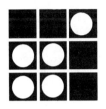

PART IV

Evaluation of Psychiatric Syndromes and Disorders in Children

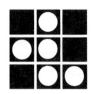

CHAPTER 22

Psychiatric Problems of Childhood

Robert D. Hunt, M.D.
Donald J. Cohen, M.D.

Early childhood often is considered to be a critical period during which the foundations of adult personality (and psychopathology) are established. This chapter discusses in relative detail the basic aspects of development, assessment techniques of psychiatric and behavioral problems, and possible management strategies. Since childhood is an especially dynamic phase of life, the approach taken in this and the next chapter is more developmental and psychodynamic than in other parts of this book.

The primary physician attends not only to the physical and medical development of patients, but also assesses their intellectual, social, and emotional functioning. Therefore, when dealing with children the physician asks not only whether a child is ill, but whether he or she is achieving a sense of identity and self-esteem that will enable the child to progress to subsequent stages of personality development. Under the constraints of limited time and information, the physician must determine whether a child's behavior indicates that there is a problem when this is viewed in the context of the given phase of development. Second, when children are evaluated in the context of family, school, ethnic group, and community, the clinician must decide whether the problem primarily lies within the child or the environment.

In the assessment of a child, the physician attempts to answer several interrelated questions (Cohen, 1976):

1. What are the child's competencies?

2. Does he or she have a significant problem in development, manifested in social, emotional, or intellectual functioning at home, school, or in the community?

3. What are the biological, familial, social, and intrapsychic roots of the difficulties, and what maintains them?

4. What forces facilitate the child's development?

5. Is intervention necessary? If so, of what types?

Primary care physicians use not only their experiences with many other children but their own awareness of the child's family history, often obtained over years of personal involvement with grandparents, parents, and now the child. Who can replace the information, trust, and judgment available to the physician who knows the family through more than a generation of births, toddling, schooling, and working? Primary physicians often have been confidants and counselors through threatening illnesses, crises in parenting, marriage, or work. They may already know the family's role in the community, their aspirations, style of rewarding and punishing, feelings of pride or disgrace, or patterns of drinking, fighting and problem-solving that are the matrix of the child's world. She or he may have prior experience with the family's accomplishments and failures, factors which may help predict the child's strengths, aspirations, competencies, and vulnerabilities.

Since children seldom come by themselves for medical or psychiatric evaluation, the physician is usually dependent upon others to provide additional information about the child's behavior and development. An assessment of the child's personality and emotional competencies

---

CASE HISTORY 22–1

Tom, an eight-year-old boy in the third grade, attends a special education class. Although Tom has always been distractable and overactive, his disruptive behavior became unmanageable recently. In class he is usually out of his seat, makes impulsive movements, and is excessively clownish. He has been fighting almost constantly with his classmates. He is often teased, seems to have no stable playmates, and looks sad, especially of late. The teacher decided to refer him to the pediatrician for a comprehensive evaluation. (See the appendix at the end of this chapter for further discussion of this case and PEG.)

can be achieved only after assimilating information from important contacts such as parents, siblings, school teachers, scout leaders, friends, or even courts, as well as children themselves.

RECOGNIZING PSYCHIATRIC PROBLEMS

Recognition of psychiatric problems demands an understanding of the varying tasks and competencies of children at each developmental stage. A problem or symptom at one stage may be normative at an earlier stage; for example, bedwetting is expected in early childhood but is problematic in a child over 7 years old. There are also phases of psychological development. Separation anxiety in an infant of 10–12 months is a sign of appropriate attachment to mother and ability to differentiate familiar from foreign people. At 8 years, such shyness may reflect diffuse anxiety and insecurity, and impede healthy socialization and learning. Defiant behavior in a 2-year-old may indicate development of a healthy sense of self, an awareness of separateness from parents. Persisting and pervasive defiance in an 8-year-old may be symptomatic of problems in the child or family, ambiguous parental expectations, and inconsistent parental responses to the child's behavior (Lewis, 1982).

Emotional maturity of a child must also be evaluated in relation to intelligence. For example, a bright child may appear prematurely "grown up" because she can articulate ideas fluently but may feel an emotional insecurity and vulnerability belied by her words; an intellectually slow child may be delayed in his emotional maturity.

Emotional development must be assessed against the backdrop of each child's own culture. For example, within many Hispanic families, mother-son ties are normally more protective, possessive, and overtly intense than in many Northern European families. Norms for assertiveness, expressiveness, and tolerance for antisocial behavior are experienced differently by a child reared in an impoverished ghetto in which racketeers and drug dealers have money, power, and women, than by a child reared in a social structure in which the overt rules of success reflect more conformity to education and legality. The process and values of school adjustment are very different for a child attending an inner-city school fraught with fears of bodily harm and lacking individualized instruction than in a school where teachers have time and skill and there is an ambience that fosters individual learning.

In children whose behavior is symptomatic within the context of their development and culture, it is useful to determine whether the problem is a *fixation* —a failure to progress to a more mature level of development—or a *regression*—a loss of a previously acquired skill or level of maturity. A 2-year-old who has learned to tolerate brief separations from mother may be overwhelmed by her extended absence and exhibit regressive behavior. After she returns, he or she may temporarily follow her around, unable to tolerate previously acceptable intervals of separation. A previously continent 8-year-old may become temporarily enuretic after moving to a new neighborhood. By obtaining a careful history, the clinician usually can determine whether the symptom reflects a fixation or a regression and, knowing this, look more specifically for events or precipitants within the environment or within the child (Nagera, 1964; Freud, 1965).

It is also important to assess whether a component of development is delayed or aberrant. While poor fine motor coordination in an 8-year-old may reflect a delay in maturation, frequent motor tics are an abnormality in motor development. Delayed and abnormal factors may coexist; for example, not only may the speech of an autistic child be delayed, but it is usually peculiar.

The biological distinction between **genotype** and **phenotype** provides a useful model for conceptualizing some severe emotional illnesses.

Genotype implies the underlying etiologic process; phenotype refers to the manifestations, symptoms, or clinical presentation of the illness. There are multiple etiologies, subtypes, or genotypes of autism. Similarly, the phenotype of the disorder changes with each developmental phase and with social-environmental influences. The older autistic child may be more aggressive; the well-trained autistic child may have more appropriate social skills (Cohen, 1976).

EVALUATION

Since physicians are so dependent upon other observers to obtain behavioral data about a child, they must be certain that they have enough information from relevant sources to complete the composite. A description of the child's personality depends on the perspective of the informant. The physician can best assess the child's physical development, neurologic status, sensory receptive systems, and motoric coordination (Rutter, 1970; Livingston, 1980). However, the clinician may greatly underestimate the extent of a child's behavioral difficulties (for example, restlessness and distractability) when evaluating him or her in the office setting, where the child presents his best behavior to an authority figure. Teachers may be excellent observers of task orientation, intellectual functioning, behavioral difficulties, and social skills, but may be less aware of a child's mood.

Parents can describe the child's behavior, personality, and compliance at home; but children may behave quite differently outside the home. Unfortunately, the parents of troubled children are often disturbed and embroiled themselves. They may bring the child in for evaluation precisely because the child "is oppositional" and engaged in a struggle with them. In many disturbed families, the child becomes the scapegoat, the deflection, and the symptom of parental conflict. Thus, parents' report of a child's behavior and attitude must be seen in the context of their own needs (see Chapter 3). The physician must obtain and integrate others' observations and facilitate the child's own disclosure of himself or herself (Minuchin, 1974).

Talking with Parents

Generally, if parents initiate referral of a preadolescent child, the physician may choose to meet first with the parents to obtain preliminary information. It is useful to schedule an open-ended amount of time with both parents in order to establish rapport, obtain an adequate history, and jointly assess information. Usually, parents are the physician's strongest allies in promoting the emotional health of their child. Parents may hesitate to discuss their child's difficulties, fearing that they may be blamed or viewed as the source of their child's problems. While they seek assistance in dealing with their child, parents do not wish to lose their authority or autonomy.

Through a demeanor of respect and accessibility, the family physician may inquire annually about the child's progress at home, school performance, moods, interests, behavior (Simmons, 1974). If the physician suspects that a child has significant emotional difficulties which are ignored or avoided by parents, creative tact is required to initiate discussion of their problems. Any evidence of psychophysiologic symptoms, physical abuse, parental neglect, or significant behavioral problems requires a systematic evaluation of the child and family. Parental resistance to such inquiry can be diminished by beginning with a review of areas of the child's strengths. What do they like about their child? What activities do they enjoy together? In what areas is the child doing well outside of the home? With parents who may be reluctant to discuss personal issues, the physician may invite discussion without pressure by saying, "I frequently talk with families about personal difficulties encountered in marriage, parenting, or about problems experienced by their children. In fact, as part of my annual physical exam, I often include a brief review of nonmedical issues that may be important in people's lives. Would it be all right with you if we talk for a few minutes about how things have been going with your child during the past year?"

To recognize psychiatric difficulties in children, it is useful to review their biological, personal, and social development. The PEG provides a useful outline for inquiry (see Chapter 1). The child's environment includes his relationships with family, school, and peers.

What is the employment, education, economic status, and composition of the family? Who are the family's supports; that is who are the relatives, church, clubs, friends, important neighbors, social service or welfare agencies that are involved with the family? To what extent do the parents experience a sense of intimacy, support, stability, enjoyment, and sexuality with each other? Have there been significant life changes in work, relocation, deaths, or births within the family? Is there a family history of psychiatric hospitalization or treatment; excessive use of drugs or alcohol; episodes of depression, mania, or cognitive disorientation; or difficulties with the law?

Regarding the child, the physician secures a clinical data base that includes information about the following areas of the child's life:

1. Medical development: Pregnancy, birth, early developmental milestones, medical/surgical history with review of systems

2. Relationship with parents: How does he or she get along with each parent? Is the child particularly close to, or allied with one parent? What does each parent like and enjoy about the child? Do the parents frequently disagree about discipline, rewards, and expectations of the child? What activities do they share together as a family? Do they have intimate talks, and, if so, about what issues? In what ways is the child developing independence from the parents?

3. Relationship with siblings and friends: Does he or she frequently fight with others? Is the child teased and bullied by siblings and friends? Is he or she comfortable meeting new people and making friends? Does the child always have to get his or her way? Are there special friends with whom the child spends time? Does he or she keep friends? Does the child belong to any clubs, groups, or gangs?

4. Sexuality: How secure is the youngster's acceptance of his or her own sexual role and identity? Are there age-appropriate friends of both sexes? Is the child unusually preoccupied with or avoidant of sex?

5. Task orientation and interests: How well does the child work on his or her own? Are attention span, ability to finish projects, management of frustration, and persistence with difficult tasks normal for the age group? What household chores and duties are performed by the child and how well are they carried out? What incentives are given for good behavior (allowance, special treats, or events)? Is academic performance at school appropriate to abilities? What are the areas of particular strength, ability, and achievement? Are there any special interests, hobbies, or athletic pursuits?

6. Behavior difficulties: Is the child frequently disobedient or destructive? Does she or he lie, steal, set fires, run away from home, abuse animals? Has the child been in trouble with the law or police? Does he or she abuse alcohol or drugs? These difficulties may be preludes to the development of antisocial personality disorders as an adult (see Chapter 4).

7. Mood and neurotic symptoms of childhood: Does the child have irrational fears, nightmares, or seem overly shy and afraid of new people or circumstances? Is he or she unusually anxious, compulsive, obsessional, depressed, sad, or self-blaming? Is enuresis or encopresis a problem? Does the youngster have difficulty separating from parents or being alone?

8. Psychosomatic difficulties: Does the child develop marked physical symptoms under stress? (Freud, 1965; Winnicott, 1971; Cox and Rutter, 1976; Bemporad, 1980).

Talking with School Personnel

Communication with teachers, principals, and counselors can be vital to the recognition of behavior and achievement problems in children and to the coordinated management of subsequent treatment. After obtaining *formal consent* from parents to communicate with schools, the physician may talk directly with the child's teacher. The primary physician can convey interest without alarm about the child's academic, social, and behavioral progress at school.

Teachers often have the most experience in assessing a child's relationship to peers and performance of tasks that require sustained attention and frustration tolerance. They are usually the most sensitive observers of *attentional and behavioral disorders* and may assist with the evaluation for and monitoring of the response to medication. Obtaining an alliance with the child's teacher is often essential to effective assessment and intervention. Discrepancy between a child's abilities and academic performance is frequently a sign of emotional or specific *learning difficulty*. Teachers are usually aware of the child's social behavior, role in the classroom as leader or follower, class clown or class supervisor, social charmer or buffoon, bully or scapegoat. They also observe a child's mood, self-esteem and self-awareness, acceptance of personal difficulties, or projection of blame onto others.

Symptom checklists and parent or teacher report forms can provide systematic, quantifiable behavioral data. These structured reports may assist in preliminary screening and provide a baseline for assistance in monitoring treatment and drug response. The Conners 28-item Teachers Checklist is a useful form for teachers to quantify behavioral disturbance of attentionally impaired children with hyperactivity or conduct disorders (Goyette, Conners, and Ulrich, 1978; Gayton, Thorton, and Bassett, 1982).

Interviewing the Child

No tool is as useful as the diagnostic interview in assessing the child's competence in relating, conceptualizing, tolerating, and sharing the difficulties of his or her life. The effective interview usually begins by making the child comfortable and establishing some personal contact. It is generally helpful to acknowledge and explore the child's expectations of the visit.

The second stage of the interview is usually unstructured. Time and attention are given to let children express their own views of the situation, or talk about themselves in ways which may at first appear only tangential to the specific problem. This unstructured component allows an assessment of children's ability to relate, to deal with problems on their own terms, and to experience the interviewer as someone who does not have a predefined opinion, a quick remedy, or "adult" suggestions or reprimands.

The final portion of the interview may be more *structured* and concrete. One may use this time to make a rough assessment of cognitive functioning in a child referred for developmental delay or school difficulties (McDonald, 1965; Werkman, 1965; MacCarthy, 1974, Winnicott, 1971; Cox and Rutter, 1976).

A child's *fantasies* can be tapped by asking about a favorite television show, movie, or book. A vignette from a recent episode may carry an emotionally relevant theme. Asking a child to describe a segment from a dream may provide another window. The response to a request for three wishes, or the person with whom she or he would go to a desert island, may lead to useful discussion. Many children can describe their own moods, especially if asked, "Do you remember a time when you felt very mad? Unhappy and sad? Lonely? Wanted to be someone else?" Curiosity about friends, shared activities, sports, dolls, pets, hobbies, toys, teachers, siblings, and parents reflects the physician's interest in the child's world. Children can often describe their own moods and *self-esteem* when asked if they think they are "bad," often make their parents mad, "get real down on themselves," hate themselves, or think about dying. Their endings to stories—such as the fate of the baby bird blown from the nest during a storm while the mother bird was away fetching food—may partly reflect their view of their own destiny.

Family Sessions and Physical Exam

Family sessions with all relevant members present may be especially useful in dealing with behavior problems or parent-child or intersibling conflict. While consent for these sessions should not be forced, they are often acceptable to families as a means of "putting our thoughts together" about the problem. The family session can be a way of identifying alliances, communication problems, and deflecting blame from the parents. The session may mobilize support and affection for the child (Lidz, 1970; Anthony, 1973; Rutter et al., 1977; Napier and Whitaker, 1978; Tseng and McDermott, 1979).

From interviews with child, parent, teachers, and others, the physician begins to assemble a composite of the child's functioning and personality. A physical examination includes appropriate assessment of fine and gross motor coordination and the mental status examination (Chapter 2) evaluates appearance, behavior, speech, thought process and content, mood, suicidal potential, intellect, judgment, and insight or understanding about the problem (McDonald, 1965; Rutter, Graham, and Yule, 1970; Cramer, 1980; Lewis, 1982).

Before ending the interview, a brief summary of issues discussed, plans for future sessions, and the need for contact with parents, teachers, or additional testing may be useful. A review of the boundaries of *confidentiality* may help secure trust. Some initial agreement about the physician's role as advisor, consultant, or referring agent may clarify the relationship for the child (Werkman 1965; MacCarthy, 1974; Schaefer, 1976).

Psychological Testing

Psychological testing proceeds from the initial information regarding the child's personality and difficulties to more precise probing by the physician to define the child's general level of emotional, intellectual, and social competence. (Holt, 1968; Cronbach, 1970). Table 22–1 (page 440) lists several types of psychological tests for children—the findings may eventually suggest further exploration of specific questions by an educational psychological, or neuromuscular specialist (Benton, 1980; Gittelman, 1980).

It is valuable for the clinician to be familiar with a few test procedures that he or she can do independently and quickly to obtain reliable standardized information according to age, sex, and cognitive or emotional status of the child. With a pencil and paper, a few blocks, a piece of string, and a few cards with standardized stimuli, one can make reasonable approximations of the child's level of intelligence, and neuromuscular coordination. Familiarity with the basic tasks included in a formal *developmental test*, such as the Denver (Frankenberg and Doddes, 1969) or the Gesell (1940), offers more accurate assessment of neuromuscular integration and maturation (Knobloch and Pasamanick, 1974). In young children, the copying of a line, cross, circle, square, and triangle provide some index of neuromuscular competence. The ability to rapidly alternate aposition of fingers, to tap rhythmically, to rapidly pronate and supinate the hand, and to write or print are indicators of fine motor control. Gross motor competence can be approximated by observing performance tasks such as tandem gait, the Romberg test, standing on one foot, hopping, skipping, catching, and throwing a ball (Solomon, 1975).

In middle childhood, more complex drawings may be requested. The Bender-Gestalt test provides an effective approximation of many parameters: overall organization on the page; neatness; ability to copy segments of a pattern; and perceptual difficulties as evidenced by rotations, transpositions, and disproportional size (Pascal and Suttell, 1951). Task orientation, frustration tolerance, and impulsivity can be assessed by observing speed of work, number of erasures, and obsessive focus on detail versus overall shape (Bender, 1938; 1956).

The Draw-a-Person (DAP) test or the kinetic family drawing offer another index of both cognitive and emotional development. Cognitive assessment is possible by consideration of the complexity, composition, level of detail, and the creativity of the figures drawn (Koppit, 1968). Emotionally significant themes are suggested by the facial expressions, sexual differentiation, spatial relationships, size, position, interactions, and activities depicted. Visual-motor integration is reflected in the quality of shapes and lines. Task orientation and defensiveness are reflected by the eagerness or reluctance with which the child approaches the drawing, the extent to which figures are expressive and revealing, as opposed to constricted and stereotyped. Perfectionism or carelessness is indicated by the level of detail and precision and by the extent of planning or impulsive sketching which precedes the drawing (Koppitz, 1968; DiLeo, 1973).

The physician may invite the child to make up stories in response to a standard set of pictures, such as those of the Thematic Apperception Test (TAT) (Bellak, 1954). Recurrent themes projected into the pictures or obviously omitted from their content may suggest areas of the child's preoccupation or of defensive avoidance. Repeated optimism or despair conveyed in the outcome of the child's stories may reflect the child's expectations and mood. The manner in which characters relate and effect each other may reveal children's perceptions of themselves in relation to others and their expectations for nurturance or abandonment, power or helplessness, competition or cooperation. The degree to which characters are influenced by their environment may convey children's experiences of internal or external locus of control over the destiny of their own lives (Bellak, 1954).

Additional tests that can be administered in the office assess the *perceptual systems* of vision, hearing, and touch. The presence and overall servity of perceptual reversals, visual rotation, reading recognition and comprehension, visual recognition, labeling, and auditory discrimination can all be approximated in response to brief testing in the office (Gardner, 1979). Areas of difficulty can be pursued by specialized tests administered for more accurate assessment of specific areas of intelligence (Wechsler Intelligence Scale for Children—Revised; Stanford-Binet), of academic achievement (Wide Range Achievement Test), or of projected feelings (Rorschach; Thematic Apperception Test; Sentence Completion) (Bellak, 1954; Jastak, Bijou, and Jastak, 1965; Ames, Metraux, and Walker, 1971; Thorndike, 1973; Aronow and Raznikoff, 1976). Areas of specific difficulty can be further dissected into receptive versus expressive language, auditory versus visual discrimination, through tests such as the Illinois Test of Psycholinguistic Ability (ITBA) (Kirk et al., 1965; Rutter, 1972).

FORMULATION

The *formulation* is an integration of the clinical data about the child and his or her environment which serves four purposes. First, the physician states the problem as currently conceptualized from the information distilled from the parents, child, school, psychological testing, and other sources. Next, he or she summarizes the child's competencies and style of managing problems and interacting with others. The third step in formulation is a definition of the relationships between the major events in a child's life and current personality and difficulties. In other words this step describes the child's role in and response to the family. The last step in formulation is an outline of treatment goals and methods (Freud, 1965; G.A.P. Report No. 87, 1973).

In the formulation, the clinician organizes information and observations from all sources into a coherent pattern that describes the child's endowment and development—the interplay between personality and events. In this process, the physician can organize the problem into personality themes or symptom clusters, rather than deal with an unrelated string of complaints (G.A.P. Report 87, 1973).

The PEG system described in Chapter 1 provides a coherent method of integrating clinical information. The axes of biological, personal, and environmental dimensions can be organized along a temporal continuum of current, recent, and background events. The appendix of this chapter describes how the PEG can facilitate diagnosis and treatment in a specific case example.

The *biological dimension* includes current symptoms such as vegetative signs of depression, physical signs of hyperactivity, delay in motoric development, or poor articulation (Gualtieri et al., 1982). Recent illnesses, injuries, or traumas may be the immediate precipitant. Background biological information includes family medical and psychiatric history, prenatal and birth events, and developmental milestones. A reconstruction of the child's early temperament and rhythmicity, may provide some index of his or her intrinsic biological endowment. The biological changes that occur during the formative stages of growth have profound psychological impact. A child's self-concept evolves rapidly when important physical milestones are achieved, such as learning to walk or entering puberty.

The *personal dimension* includes the child's intelligence, mood, and energy level. Does the child organize his or her thoughts and feelings in a manner which effectively contributes to the development of self-esteem and competence? Are there any problems that extend beyond the circumstances and situation of the child's life? How does the youngster view current difficulties? The physician assesses the child's strengths, talents, and capacities for resolving the current difficulty. What are the child's strategies for coping with problems and stress? To what extent does he or she deny, avoid, or distort the realities of life? Are other people or events blamed for most of the child's difficulties, failures, or unhappiness? Does he or she avoid problems or unpleasant feelings by acting impulsively, becoming excessively self-critical, developing physical symptoms, daydreaming, or clowning? Does he or she cope with anxiety by becoming obsessed, worried, or preoccupied with detail? Does the child respond to frustration by becoming anxious, excessively emotional, or overwhelmed? Some children develop disturbances in thought or mood when experiencing failure or disappointment; they become confused or depressed. Persistence of these symptoms is an indication for psychiatric referral (Cox and Rutter, 1976).

Evidence of *mature coping styles* includes age-appropriate capacity to choose one's goals, discipline oneself, tolerate frustration, enjoy achievement, and delay gratification. A sense of humor, commitment, and enthusiasm in pursuit of interests characterize the emotionally healthy child and adult. The child who takes pride and pleasure playing the piano or football is demonstrating the emotional competence in life as does the adult who enjoys and succeeds in his or her work.

The foundation of emotional development is the increasing capacity to form important attachments to others and remain connected to them while developing awareness of their desires and needs. Children's level of emotional maturity is greatly reflected in their ability to engage in and sustain relationships within and outside the family. Their experience of being loved and cared for, and being responsive to relationships with parents, teachers, siblings, and friends reflects and shapes their development as a person. Children react to and contribute to the interpersonal events of their lives (Bowlby, 1958; Ainsworth, 1973; Mahler, 1975; Neubauer, 1976).

The child's present level of functioning is suggested by appearance and behavior during the interview. Does he or she relate to the interviewer in a manner suggesting capacity for warmth and attachment? Does he or she exhibit difficulties in self-control? Is speech coherent and articulate? Is mood and energy level depressed for age and level of development? What is the child's level of cognitive functioning; ability to focus and sustain attention; his memory, ability to abstract? Is performance and judgment commensurate with intellectual abilities? What does the child understand about and expect from problem? How does the child experience herself or himself? What are the levels of self-esteem and self-expectation?

Some children experience themselves as having very little control over the choices and outcome of their lives; they may blame others or feel helpless to effect change. Others perceive themselves at the center of their destinies; they may blame themselves, or feel empowered to alter their "fate." The child's perception of the *locus of control* is an important consideration in prescribing medication or other active interventions. Some children experience taking of medication as a validation of feelings of helplessness and dependency (Rotter, 1975).

Any recent changes in the child's behavior, mood, or functioning should be correlated with any alterations in the child's environment or health (Rutter, 1976).

In the *environmental dimension*, the boundary between personal and environmental influences is often very narrow. It is useful to assess the child's interaction with three major components of the environment: family, school, and peers. Children mirror much of the love, stability, conflict, or trauma within their family. Have there been changes in the family composition through birth, death, divorce, or moving away? What is the affective tone of the family, that is, how are affection, anger, disagreement, and sadness expressed? What activities are shared and enjoyed between each parent and child or experienced collectively as a family? It is also useful to understand the structure and

functioning, the "business side," of the family. What are the rules, expectations, chores, allowances, punishments, and rewards within this home? How are these negotiated, clarified, and executed? Does the child have enough input? Does the parent provide enough control and consistency? How is power expressed and distributed between parents and children? What roles and alliances identify this child within the family? Who is he or she close to? Who is imitated or admired, appreciated or taken care of by the child? Is the youngster identified within the family as "the bright one," "the cute or pretty one," the "problem child," or the "needy" or "sick child?" How flexible is the family's categorization of the child? To what extent does this child receive the family resources of love, time, and money? (Lidz, 1970; Anthony, 1973; Rutter, Quinton, and Yule, 1977; Napier and Whitaker, 1978; Tseng and McDermott, 1979.)

At school the child's academic performance can be considered in relation to apparent intelligence. Task orientation, ability to apply oneself, and toleration of frustration is evident. School also provides a social environment where the child's interactions may be monitored. Whether he or she is respected, teased, shunned, ignored, or liked by peers is an important index of personality. Does this child maintain age-appropriate friendships and loyalties? Have there been recent changes in the educational or social environment such as a shift in neighborhoods, schools, teachers, or academic placement? Have special friends come and or gone? Was the child accepted or rejected for a team, class office, or social group? (Whalen et al., 1979; Beitchman et al., 1982.)

In making a formulation the physician reviews the data gathered and weaves them into a pattern that acknowledges the child's endowment, and reflects important events, changes and traumas in his or her life. The formulation places children and their problems within the context of their life histories and personal resources. What supports and strengths may be mobilized to facilitate growth? In what manner may biology, relationships, or events collude to impair progress? How does the child process the events and difficulties of life? (Eissler et al., 1977.)

The stage of emotional development at which a traumatic event or significant loss occurs greatly colors its psychological impact. Death of a parent before 6 months of age may be less traumatic than the same loss occurring after more individualized attachment has developed. Geographic moves may be very disruptive to an older child who is deeply involved in school and with friends. Sometimes the birth of a sibling may be experienced by a child as a statement that he or she was not "enough" for the parents. The loss of attention incurred as parents invest time and love in a new child may elicit feelings of abandonment and competition.

Diagnosis

The diagnosis of psychiatric disorders recognizes a hierarchy of abilities and disabilities. Patients with pervasive disturbances such as autism, mental retardation, or pandevelopmental delay exhibit multiple deficits in attention, memory, perception, symbolization, modulation of activity, mood, motoric control, and interpersonal relatedness—each of which might merit a specific label or diagnosis. The final diagnosis selected identifies the areas of disability and reflects the overall level of function. While autistic children usually meet the diagnostic criteria for attentional deficit disorder (ADD), the lesser disability is subsumed under the more comprehensive diagnosis. The *Diagnostic and Statistical Manual of Mental Disorders (DSM-III)* (1980) reflects multiple aspects of health through a multiaxial approach. A comprehensive diagnosis addresses categories of *psychiatric* diagnosis, *personality* disorder, *medical* disabilities, psychosocial *stressors*, and assessment of the overall *severity* of the disorder. Some children meet diagnostic criteria for several disorders or approximately equivalent significance, such as ADD or aphasia, which may be diagnosed separately. Children often fall between diagnostic labels and they change with each phase of development (Spitzer and Cantwell, 1980).

Indications for counseling. The physician can often be very useful to the child, adolescent, or family as a counselor. Physician Counseling is most effective and adequate when all the following circumstances apply:

1. The diagnostic issues are clear and indicate that the child and family are basically emotionally healthy. There is no pervasive disruption in functioning and no fixation in development.

2. The presenting problem is a response to an *acute* precipitant, trauma, stress, or a new developmental phase.

3. The setting in which the child is experiencing difficulty is limited to *one area* of the child's life, such as home, school, or with peers.

4. The symptoms are not disrupting the child's *overall functioning* and mood in "conflict-free" areas. The symptoms are not impairing the child's attention, memory, self-esteem, energy level, or attachment to many important interests or people. For example, if bedwetting or sleep disturbance occur without evidence of more pervasive disruption in mood or personal functioning, they may be treated symptomatically.

Psychotherapy. Counseling usually supports and organizes the existing strengths of the child and family, and is often directive and instructive, while psychiatric therapy often includes the development of an intense relationship in which very private feelings can be experienced and expressed. Within the therapeutic process the child may experience the attitudes and feelings which characterize his personal life, but would be unsafe to express within the family and are often painful to acknowledge to oneself. Nonphysician therapists, psychologists, psychiatric nurses, social workers, family therapists, and school counselors can collaborate with the physician in the treatment of the child and family—each providing the particular skills and perspective of their disciplines (Smirnoff, 1971; Krumboltz and Krumboltz, 1972; Schaefer, 1976; McDermott and Harrison, 1977).

Referral for Psychiatric Evaluation. Referral for evaluation by a child psychiatrist should be considered in *any* of the following cases:

1. The child's difficulties are of *long duration* (perhaps greater than 6 months).

2. The child's performance and behavior in *several areas* of life is disturbed, for example, at home, school, and with peers.

3. A specific symptom is indicative of overall more *generalized difficulty* in the child's personality. If basic mood, memory, attention, cognitive organization, or reality testing (the accurate perception of environment, events, or interaction in spite of emotional loading) are disrupted, the child should be referred for therapy. For example, bedwetting may be a presenting symptom of depression, or fear of the dark may reflect pervasive anxiety and global withdrawal.

4. The child has *inadequate social or familial supports*. Severe deprivation or abuse requires intensive intervention in the family or placement of the child outside the family. Most states require the physician to report physical abuse or neglect to child protective agencies.

DEVELOPMENTAL CONTEXT

The principal psychological tasks and focus of emotional energies shift throughout a child's development. As they establish new competencies, children form more complex relationships and develop more sophisticated mechanisms to modulate attention, thoughts, feelings, and behavior. At each major life phase, the interplay of child, parents, and society evolves—each stage brings new strengths and skills and presents new

vulnerabilities and potential problems. There are no sharp lines between stages; movement from one to another is usually marked by slow changes in emphasis, not by totally new life issues. Earlier phases of psychological development anticipate subsequent life issues; personality development and adaptive styles at later stages bear the stamp of earlier experiences. Yet, a child is more concerned with being who he or she *is* than with becoming an adult. Children's competencies should not be evaluated in relationship to adult competencies; they must be viewed in the context of *present life tasks*. The overriding task of development is to meet effectively the challenges and experience the joys of each era of life. Some significant milestones in the evolution of personality are briefly highlighted next, along with suggestions for the physician in identifying important psychiatric difficulties which may emerge in each (Eisenberg, 1980).

Prenatal

Some factors present before and at birth may influence a child's development and place the child at relatively higher risk for psychiatric and emotional difficulties (Winick, 1981). Alcohol consumption can lead to development of fetal alcohol syndrome characterized by minor physical anomalies, mental retardation, and attentional impairment (Ouellette, 1977). Benzodiazepine, meprobamate, and thalidamide taken during the first trimester have been suggested to be teratogenic (Ameer, 1978). Illnesses such as rubella and cystomegalic inclusion can be detrimental to the fetus. *Genetic factors* appear to contribute to vulnerability to major personality and behavioral disorders (for example, manic-depression, schizophrenia, depression, alcoholism, ADD, and others) and probably to general intellectual competence as well. As described in Chapters 8 and 9, there is considerable evidence for genetic contribution to the development of a major psychiatric disorder. The increased vulnerability to schizophrenia of the second twin in a monozygotic twin pair is 86% compared to 15% for dizygotic twins (Kallmann, 1946). The concordance rate varies with the diagnostic method and criteria and the severity and duration of the illness; also, it must be corrected for age. Other studies found a concordance rate of 50% (35% when age corrected) for monozygotic twins and 10% for dizygotic twins (Gottesman and Shields, 1972; 1976). Data from the Danish registry for hospitalized schizophrenics found similar concordance rates (56% for monozygotics; 26% for dizygotic twins) (Fischer, Harvald, and Hauge, 1969).

Adoption studies provide an alternative method for discriminating genetic factors. Heston (1966) found that 16.5% of 47 children, who had at least one schizophrenic biological parent but were adopted in infancy by normal parents, developed schizophrenia themselves (Rosenthal and Kety, 1968). In contrast, children, who had healthy biological parents but were adopted and raised by schizophrenic parents, showed no increase in incidence of psychotic symptomatology (Wender et al., 1974).

Similarly, in manic-depressive disorder, Kallmann (1953) noted concordance rates increasing from 16.7% in half siblings, to 22.7% and 25.5% for siblings and fraternal twins, respectively. Monozygotic twins approached 100% concordance for manic-depression. Of the individuals with manic-depression, 23% of parents have evidence of the disorder. When the diagnosis was based on a standardized interview of patients with bipolar illness and their families, 41% of the parents and 42% of the siblings of manic-depressive probands had evidence of affective disorder (Mendlewicz et al., 1972). The likelihood of illness among relatives increased with the severity of the illness in the proband.

Genetic vulnerability for schizophrenia or affective disorder is well differentiated, suggesting that these are distinct illnesses. Epidemiologic studies suggest genetic contribution to depressive illness, hysteria, alcoholism, Tourette's disease, and perhaps personality disorders. Yet the genetic contribution only explains a small percent of the variance in psychiatric disturbances, suggesting that environmental factors, life events, and the individuals mechanisms of coping all contribute to the vulnerability for psychopathology.

Other prenatal or natal factors that may affect a child's development include maternal illness during pregnancy (for example, rubella); maternal consumption of medications (for example, thalidomide, tetracycline); and excessive ingestion of alcohol, opiates, cigarettes, and caffeine. A child's emotional health is greatly affected at all stages of development by the environment into which he or she is born. Some studies indicate that a child born into lower socioeconomic position families is at greater risk for subsequent psychiatric hospitalization. Yet, regardless of the socioeconomic level, the interplay of personal and life events plays a crucial role in psychological development.

Infancy

At birth, the human infant is equipped with remarkable abilities to perceive stimuli, emit organized patterns of behavior, and regulate its state. The balance of these capacities defines a child's temperament—level of activity, ease of adaptability, frustration tolerance, rhythmicity, attentional span, level of emotional and basic mood (Thomas et al., 1968; Graham et al., 1973; Mahler, Pine, and Bergman; 1975; Rutter, 1976; Greenspan, 1981).

What the infant brings to the family reciprocally affects the care he or she receives. The interplay between child and environment changes both factors. For example, an irritable infant strains a mother's patience, and a passive infant is likely to explore less intently the subtle potentials of the environment. Piaget's (1958) concept of the reinforcing cycle of *accommodation and assimilation* describes the process through which a child's perception of the world is altered by the child's interaction with it. The ability to perceive and explore finer aspects of the environment increases with the child's experience, probing, and manipulating of the world (Jossetyn, 1962; Flavell, 1963; Chess, 1973).

Psychologically, by 3–4 months the competent infant demonstrates interest in, and growing attachment to, the mother and father. This *attachment* is evident from the infant's following the mother with its eyes and brightening when it sees her; later the infant crawls and walks to seek proximity. If a trusting relationship has been achieved, the mother's voice, touch, and presence comfort and calm the infant when it is distressed. The infant experiments with sense of control and helplessness; he attempts mastery of vulnerability to the mother's absence by initiating experiences of brief separation, loss, and restitution. Games of peek-a-boo and hide-and-seek, repeatedly enjoyed, establish this sense of internal control by recreating the comfort reassurance associated with the mother's presence. Such manifestations of attachment and trust are signs of emotional health (Bowlby, 1958; Piaget, 1958; Ainsworth, 1963; Robson and Mors, 1970; Inhelder, 1971; Stone, Smith, and Murphy, 1973; Stern, 1974).

By 1 year of age, normal infants usually walk with support and stand alone briefly. They imitate scribbling, match two simple objects in front of them, utter sounds equivalent to "mama" and "dada," label some objects with expressive jargon, and respond to their own names and simple requests. By the end of the first year, children play simple games, such as pat-a-cake or peek-a-boo, feed themselves crackers and other small foods, and hold their bottles. The attentive, curious, and deliberate play of a 1-year-old infant, secure in its attachment to the mother, reflects the trust and concentration which are the roots of competent *socialization* and *task orientation.* Disturbances in aspects of motoric, adaptive, linguistic, and social behavior require assessment (Brazelton, Koslonski, and Main, 1974; Stern, 1974; Earls, 1976; Schaffer, 1977; Lewis, 1982).

The Toddler

The development of walking and speech signals a process of profound psychological significance and mobilizes a crucial organizing stage. The toddler elaborates awareness of, and mastery of, his or her own body. They delight at their increased ability to explore, manipulate, and play. The world is a toy; the joy of walking and running, of being able to make controlled sounds, fills much of the second year with excitement (Rutter and Bax, 1972; Brown, 1973; Moerk, 1974; Bloom, 1975; Geschwind, 1976; Nelson, 1977).

Locomotion enables *separation.* To be able to walk away from the mother reinforces the internal sense of separateness. At this stage both parents and children express their differences with each other. The child's ability to say "no" enhances his or her internal experience of individuality. Parents become occupied with chasing, limiting, and removing dangerous or valuable objects. Involvement with the father often increases as he and the toddler share more activity, limit-setting, and play (Erickson, 1959; Mahler, 1968; Abelin, 1971; Inhelder, 1971; Mahler, Pine, and Bergman, 1975; Rutter, 1976).

At age 2 years, the toddler can run without falling, kick a large ball, climb stairs, build a tower of six cubes, align cubes to imitate a train, use three-word sentences, follow simple commands, put on a simple garment, imitate simple domestic activities, and refer to him or herself by name (Nelson, 1977).

From about 18 months to 3 years, the dominant psychological issues are connected with mastery of *internal controls*, including the achievement of bowel and bladder continency. Attitudes toward cleanliness, or messiness, toward letting go and giving, withholding and retaining, may, in part, derive from the inner experience of the child's development of greater self-control. Interaction with parents during this period of defiance and limit-setting provides experience with authority which will be expanded through subsequent interaction with teachers and other adults (Kleeman, 1966; Mahler, 1968; Rutter, 1976).

By age 3 years a child is able to ride a tricycle, alternate feet walking upstairs, imitate a three-cube bridge, copy a cross and circle, feed herself or himself, put on shoes, string beads, unbutton buttons, and dress with minimal supervision. They comprehend propositions, opposites, concepts such as "cold," "tired," "hungry," and recognize basic colors. By $3\frac{1}{2}$ years, children can sort buttons. By this age, most children can be apart from their mothers for a few hours or longer and can play simple games with peers. Increased self-awareness is reflected in using first and last names, expressing preferences strongly, and taking pride in achieving. Three-year-olds value their own property and strive for mastery over objects. They demonstrate improved *frustration tolerance*, test limits but accept "no," and are willing to accept a substitute toy or activity. They may strongly express wishes and feelings toward others, and display a range of affective responses, including love, anger, empathy, sadness, surprise, humor, and enjoyment with new people and new situations (Hartmann, Kris, and Lowenstein, 1949; Lourie, 1971).

The child may naturally have mixed or ambivalent feelings about parents, who must frequently limit activity and exploration and from whom he or she experiences longer periods of separation. At one moment, the parents are the source and reflection of joy as they care for the child and delight in their son or daughter's emerging competencies. The next moment, they are saying "no," scolding for knocking over the lamp, or leaving to go to work. As the child perceives herself or himself and the parents as more clearly separate, the child becomes aware of their distinct and changing moods and their ability either to comfort or to thwart the child. The integration of this range of contradictory feelings toward another person is the process of achieving "*object constancy*"—the acceptance, for example, that the same mother who at one moment evokes feelings of comfort and joy can also precipitate anger, fear, or the sadness of loss. The struggle for *autonomy* occurs on the precipice of feelings of abandonment and resentment (Hartman, Kris, and Lowenstein, 1949; Erickson, 1959; Fraiberg, 1959; Feshbach, 1970; Mahler, Pine, and Bergman, 1975; Bornstein and Kesson, 1979).

Preschoolers

By age 4 years, the child's movements are smoother, and he or she demonstrates greater control of acceleration, deceleration, and running. A 4-year-old can stand on one foot for a few seconds, walk a beam, hold a pencil, and throw a ball with an appropriate stance. Improved visual-motor coordination is evident in manipulation of common objects. A 4-year-old can put on shoes and button buttons. With pencil held in adult fashion, they can make vertical and circular lines, trace a diamond, and draw a "picture". Speeding away on a tricycle, or climbing and swinging from the jungle gym, the 4-year-old experiences growing independence and individuality.

Intellectual development is evident in beginning awareness of abstract concepts. The 4-year-old not only knows more words and body parts, he or she can conceptulize analogies, and complete sentences such as "brother is a boy, sister is a ...." Short-term memory is reflected in increased digit span (memory of concrete stimuli), and the 4-year-old can now identify an object missing from a series of previously seen objects (Piaget, 1958; Flavell, 1963; Kagan, 1979).

By age 4 years concepts of size, shape, position, and direction are established. But while 4-year-olds can identify which column of water is higher and which is wider, they do not integrate this into a coherent sense of mass or volume. Hence, they can be fooled into believing that the volume of water or mass of clay increases as its shape changes to produce a larger visual image. The manipulation of internal representations is still centered on one dimension of a stimulus or situation at a time.

In 1969 Piaget and Inhelder described the development of *internal representation* of an object or event which is no longer present. A 4-year-old may spank a doll in the manner reminiscent of a parent's discipline. They may symbolically wash dishes in a dollhouse, or attempt to draw a graphic image of a remembered object. They visually portray objects through drawing and talk about missing objects or toys. This ability to represent and manipulate the external world through symbols underlies the development of object permanence and emotional object constancy. By age 4 years, the capacity to represent actions, sequences, and emotions facilitates an explosion of thematic play (Flavell, 1963).

The speech of a 4-year-old demonstrates increased length of utterance and improved coordination of nouns and verbs. Speech becomes more socially communicative and less egocentric (Rutter, 1971). Much group play at this age contains themes requiring mastery, which includes tolerance of separation, need to care for each other, provision of protection, mutual feeding and cleaning. These play patterns assist the child in the transition from being cared for by parents to taking care of oneself (Rutter, 1971).

The ability to symbolize and remember facilitates the child's move from home to nursery school and enables toleration of separation from the mother (Raph et al., 1968). Separation evokes feelings of anger, abandonment, and rejection; these are abated by feelings of love and comfort from the internalized image of the mother. The 4-year-old's increased ability to modulate aggression reflects identification with parental values, increased control over muscles and sphincters, and improved sense of time, sequence, and consequence (Carmichael, 1970).

Physicians can support and counsel parents to foster their child's emotional development at this stage by meeting physical needs and demon-

strating affection for their child. Parents can encourage a child's curiosity and support development of relationships with peers, babysitters and teachers outside the home. Physicians can assist parents to establish reasonable limits which protect a child's safety and encourage task orientation and the development of social skills (Illingworth, 1970).

Sexuality

The awareness of one's gender identity has roots in "discovery" of and increased interest shown in genital exploration-stimulation at approximately 12–18 months of life. Awareness of sex differences increases during the second and third year of life and enhances identification with the same-sexed parent. By age 3 years, boys and girls are aware of sex groupings and curious about anatomical differences—which they attempt to explain and understand through their own logic (Rutter, 1971). The development of gender identity and gender role becomes organized by age 4 years. The locus of greatest sensual pleasure shifts from the anus to the genitals; more enjoyment is derived from touching or being stimulated there. The genitals are experienced as both a source of pleasure and an object of vulnerability (Newman and Stoller, 1971; Green, 1974, 1979; Zucker, 1982).

While recognition of anatomical distinctions between males and females is a universal phenomenon, the meaning given to one's gender and the level of anxiety or comfort associated with it reflects the child's highly individualized interpersonal life—the degree to which children perceive themselves as men and women to be valued, nurtured, ignored, or rejected in their family. A child who feels loved, happy and secure in other (nongender) aspects of life and whose parents are content in their gender roles is likely to accept his or her own sexuality with minimal childhood conflict. When the child feels insecure, vulnerable, or rejected by parents for reasons quite independent of gender, the child's sense of his or her sexuality may become conflict-ridden.

As a child feels more secure about controlling his or her own body and relying on parents to meet needs, the child begins to integrate the "good and bad" attributes of self and others. This maturing identity allows them to relate to their parents from a new level of individuation. They become aware of their own sexual identity as a male or a female—as a boy destined to become a man who will probably have an important relationship with a woman, or as a girl who will probably have a significant relationship with a man when she becomes a woman. Children experience pride in their own accomplishments which now enable mobility, speech, expression, control of bodily functions, and self-sufficiency to dress, feed, and care for themselves. This new confidence and competence, coupled with increased enjoyment of phallic sexuality, often catalyzes a more intense relationship with the opposite-sexed parent. A boy wants to be admired by his mother; a girl frequently "shows off" for her father.

Family Romance. From age 3–6 years, the child negotiates new relationships with both parents. Toward the opposite-sex parent, the child often feels attraction and excitement. A girl may enter the phase of being "daddy's little girl," while the boy shows his mother masculine toughness and achievements. The same-sex parent is simultaneously both a role model and a competitor. The boy imitating his father, for example, carries a hammer or pretends to "go to work." He attempts to treat his mother as he has seen his father do, perhaps with romantic overtures. In fantasy, his relationship with his mother shifts from being primarily that of a dependent infant in need of nurturance to that of a friend, peer, or suitor. He practices with her whatever skills and charm he can adapt from his father. Yet, he may sense the inherent *rivalry* in using his father's techniques "against him"— for there is fantasized and real competition for

the mother's time, attention, and affection— particularly if a rift in the marriage exists. Symbolically, the danger and competition is experienced in an exaggerated form by the child. And yet, the son needs and loves the father too. The child feels suspended between romantic excitement, fear of discovery and retaliation, and need for love and safety from both parents. A boy may vacillate between clinging and stubborn independence, between feelings of admiration and envy and expressions of jealousy, fear, and contempt for father. Even in a single-parent family, issues of competitiveness and triangulation emerge—as a girl or boy tries to maintain potentially competitive relations.

Girls often begin to idealize and romanticize their fathers, directing charm, coyness, and enthusiasm towards them while they experience more subdued feelings of attachment coupled with competition toward mother. Mother is often "taken for granted" and becomes the respository of negative feelings, while father becomes the object of intense feelings of excitement and fantasy. While girls look to their mothers as role models and as sources of support, they also may blame them for difficulties and vie with them for their father's time and attention. The relationship with mother becomes the platform from which the daughter experiences new feelings of love and delight.

As a son strives to imitate and internalize his father's behavior, mannerisms, and values, he begins to consolidate his own *conscience*. Fear of his father's anger and revenge further buttress the son's desire not to offend him. He gradually learns that his mother shares a unique bond with his father and begins to accept the fact that he will have to wait until he grows up and can love a woman of his own. Similarly, a girl identifies with the values and personality of her mother and accepts the limitations this imposes on the relationship with her father. If parents share similar values and are supportive and respectful of each other, the child can more easily incorporate a congruent sense of self. Intense parental conflict at this time can intensify the child's sense of polarization between the same-sexed parent with whom the youngster identifies or the opposite-sexed parent whom the child may romanticize. Increasingly, a child avoids doing things which would displease the parents, not only out of fear of immediate punishment, but because he or she "knows better"— the child demonstrates an understanding of consequences and an internalization of values based on a desire to please and imitate parents (Konopka, 1973; Stierlin, 1974; Kohlberg, 1978).

The process of gender identity and value formation is greatly shaped by the individual personalities and relationships within the family. An absent or violent father or an alcoholic mother have much different impact on the developing child of either gender than does a parent who is a better role model and more emotionally available.

During the stage of development from 4 to 6 years olds, a child may be brought to a physician because of experiences of anxiety, nightmares, fear of separation, phobias, shyness, secondary enuresis, or excessively defiant behavior. The physician can assess whether this is a transient symptom in a healthy child or reflects more significant disturbance. Negotiation of this phase of a child's development establishes a pattern or template for future experiences of his or her own desires, ambitions, romance, sexuality, self-assertion, and gender identity; the resolution of these issues colors subsequent relations with authority figures, friends, lovers, and competitors.

Difficulties that occur during this "Oedipal phase" may determine a child's later personality development. Patterns of managing anxiety may include: excessive and diffuse emotionality (hysteria); self-protection, fear, worry, and perfectionism (obsessiveness); pervasive avoidance of competition and assertion (passive-dependency, inadequate personality); or excessive guilt and low self-esteem (depression) (Freud, 1965; Kraus, 1973). The physician may assist parents

during this stage of their child's development to confirm the strength of their parental bond and to delineate role boundaries between parents and child. Parents can encourage the child's developing competence rather than treating emerging independence as a threat (Rutter, 1980).

Parents must affirm that they will not exploit the child's sexuality nor undermine achievement and ambition by prematurely withdrawing their caretaking. For example, the successful mother gives her daughter safe permission for her heightened interest in the father and does not withdraw her support or love. The daughter who experiences father's interest and pride, coupled with mother's continued support of this attachment, is best able to feel secure in her femininity and attractiveness. If mother is unavailable and unsupportive, the girl may develop a premature or excessively intense attachment to father. If her overtures are ignored by father, she may feel rejected and depressed; if her romantic and sexual feelings are exploited by father, she may develop profound feelings of guilt and anger. Boys need permission for their interest in mother and their competitive feelings toward father. Their infatuation with mother should not be exploited as a substitute companionship for absent father. Boys also experience emotional vulnerability in relation to both parents; they need approval and enjoyment of new competencies without the expectation of being too assertive or mature. Parental depression or absence at this stage of development may be especially traumatic for a child of either gender (Freud, 1924; Neubauer, 1960; Winnicott, 1965; Anthony, 1970).

As discussed previously, referral for psychiatric evaluation is indicated if a child sustains high levels of anxiety or develops symptoms which persist for longer than 6 months or which impair functioning outside the home. Emergence of significant withdrawal, aggression, or fear during this stage should be monitored. The loss of a parent through death or divorce at this highly charged stage frequently leaves a residual of exaggerated guilt. A child may need special assistance to mourn such a loss (Thomas et al., 1963; Barnes, 1964; Nagera, 1970; Howells, 1971; Neubauer, 1976; Bemporad, 1980).

PSYCHIATRIC PROBLEMS IN PRESCHOOL CHILDREN

Pandevelopmental Delay and Organicity

The distinction between brain damage and disturbed psychological functioning is a central theme in differential diagnosis. In assessing problems of early childhood, the physician often wrestles with this distinction. A child whose perceptual or proprioceptive systems are disorganized—and especially if higher cortical systems are impaired in their ability to integrate, modulate, and interpret experience—is more vulnerable to emotional impairment affecting attachment and attention. Irregularities and inconsistencies in the perception of posture, motion, and orientation in space and time may create profound disruption in the subjective representation of the self. Disruption in neurointegrative systems impairs the internal process of organizing one's experience of the internal and external world. Children with psychiatric difficulties identifiable within the first 18 months of life usually suffer from pandevelopmental disturbances due to organic brain disturbance or profound physical and emotional abuse and neglect (Crandall, 1977; Cytryn and Lourie, 1980).

Prior to beginning school, children with pervasive developmental delay may be identified by their slow or uneven development of motoric, social, and linguistic skills. Given the reciprocity between motoric, cognitive, and psychological experience, children with developmental delay are often slower in achieving a psychological sense of independence and separateness. Such children need referral for special testing, education, and parent counseling. Since physical handicaps frequently accompany cognitive delay, they also may require special medical attention (Grossman, 1977).

In mental retardation there is pervasive delay encompassing multiple aspects of development. Severe impairment may be evident when an infant of 6–8 weeks does not briefly hold up its head, does not follow moving objects to midline, shows no vocalization, or has no regard for the mother's face. A 6–8-month-old child who is unable to sit by itself, grasp, bang, or shake toys, laugh or vocalize, or who does not exhibit the "social smile" or apprehension of strange situations should be carefully evaluated for pandevelopmental delay.

Childhood Autism

Autism is a form of pathologic development often associated with pervasive delays in development. Childhood autism has its onset before age 3 years and is predominantly found in males. The primary disturbances are profound impairment in social relatedness and language development. Autistic children experience and treat people as objects who may be physically manipulated or used as extended tools. Their eye contact is limited; social responsiveness, smiling, laughing, and stranger anxiety are all diminished. In many ways, autisim reflects a disturbance in "meaning," the process of perceiving human relationships and attributing significance to them (Rutter, 1970; Ornitz and Ritro, 1976).

A profound disruption of language development parallels the disturbance in organizing relationships and tolerating changes and inconsistencies. Autistic children do not exhibit the normal development of language. They lack the preverbal understanding of concepts and relationships that is normally evident in the evolution of speech. Instead of their speech evolving from rhythmic babbling to increasingly well-formed words, they may burst from silence into a first word, such as "dandelion." Autistic *speech* tends to be oddly inflected, uninventive, monotonic, and poorly communicative. Nonverbal means of communication, such as socially appropriate facial expressions and gestures are absent or diminished. The autistic child used "canned" phrases without apparent awareness of the syntactic relationship of individual words.

In childhood autism the acquisition of motor milestones is often normal; however, there are frequent suggestions of perceptual-motor dysfunction. The autistic child stimulates and "comforts" himself or herself by such actions as rocking, twirling, head-banging, or spinning. This activity may be directed against himself or herself as self-destructive, even self-mutilating behaviors. Sensory stimuli appear to be inconsistently perceived in autism. Objects that spin and twirl or sounds that hum or swish are of heightened interest to many autistic children. Tops, fans, light switches, and flushing toilets may be enchanting, while the child may appear oblivious to the voices of others, loud sounds, or to his or her own name. Many autistic children demand sameness and routine and resist even minor changes made in their environment or in their rituals. They may remain absorbed in manipulation of a piece of string or a rubber band, and wail if furniture is moved or a new route is taken to a store. Many of these "symptoms" may be autistic children's way of coping with a world they cannot understand and which frightens and perplexes them.

Over 70% of autistic children have a developmental quotient below 70. Seizure disorders are common, especially in the children with the most severe disturbances and at adolescence. EEG abnormalities increase in incidence through adolescence and may include asymmetry, immaturity, or discrete paroxysmal features (Eisenberg, 1956; DeMyer et al., 1973; Lotter, 1974; Hanson and Gottesman, 1976; Ritvo, 1977).

Childhood Schizophrenia

Childhood schizophrenia is the other major psychotic disturbance in childhood. The age of onset is later than in autism, after age 3 years, and the schizophrenic child demonstrates more language ability and greater social relatedness. His or her involvement with others is fragmented, unpredictable, inconsistent, grossly inappropriate, and frequently charged with fear, anxiety, or hostility. The schizophrenic child may at one moment cling dependently and then abruptly withdraw in panic. Their affective life mirrors the confusion and fragmentation of their sense of self and others; their moods may oscillate from passive compliant to angry-hostile-fearful (Kolvin et al., 1971c; Fish, 1977).

Anxiety may be overwhelming, unprovoked, and unresponsive to comforting. Their thoughts are often bizarre and may center on obsessive preoccupations, frequently on morbid or frightening subjects. A psychotic child may suddenly become violent and may destroy toys or lash out against people. At other times they may be so quietly involved with fantasies that it is almost impossible to get their attention. Intense attachment to generally insignificant objects may develop and then disappear. Language is usually more fluent and less characterized by the monotonic, stereotypic echolalia of autism. Speech may be perseverative, melodic, or original—with words created for their unique meanings or sounds. The schizophrenic child may verbalize fears and bizarre beliefs, detailed delusional systems, or focused delusional beliefs. Motoric behaviors may include self-stimulation, twirling, rocking, and self-destructive biting, hitting, and head-banging.

Evaluation and Treatment

Physiologic Evaluation. Children with severe developmental or psychotic problems often receive inadequate physical examinations because they are such uncooperative patients. Hearing, vision, nutrition, and gross motor abilities may be assessed from careful observation. Systematic neurologic testing may require two or more sessions and improvisation. Laboratory studies may add information by discounting certain diagnoses or leading to a new one. At a minimum, a child with psychotic symptoms must be screened for inborn errors of metabolism (such as phenylketonuria) that may produce autism. Other predisposing factors include maternal rubella, infantile spasms, encephalitis, and tuberous sclerosis. A broader range of tests may be indicated—for example, hemoglobin; liver function; levels of blood urea nitrogen, ceruloplasmin, lead, electrolyte balance; calcium, phosphorus, thyroxin; and protein electrophoresis. An EEG, skull X-ray films, and perhaps computerized axial tomography (CAT scan), may provide valuable information. In some cases, examination of the cerebrospinal fluid (for cells, protein, glucose, immunoglobulins, and colloidal gold) is necessary.

Cognitive Evaluation. Formal testing of the cognitive, language, and adaptive skills of severely disturbed children requires patience and special training. Only hours of observation of a child may reveal the full range of competencies. In practice, the most useful diagnostic assessment is that of a child's response to carefully designed educational and therapeutic intervention (Kolvin et al., 1971b).

Treatment. The major modality of intervention in autism is *special education*. Children should be involved in special programs from the time of the diagnosis. Parents require support and specific instruction in dealing with the child. Programs of *behavior modification*,—the use of rewards to encourage specific behavior and discourage others,—can be designed for use at home and in the special education classroom. Usually, by age 3 years, if not sooner, autistic children require intensive, full-day educational programming. The 10% of autistic children with intellectual abilities in the normal range may achieve considerable autonomy and pleasure in useful work (Ritvo, 1976).

Treatment of childhood schizophrenia follows many of the same principles outlined for autism. Special education in a structured environment, and *psychotherapy* for patient and family are the main vehicles of treatment. Hospitalization may be required for diagnostic assessment, obtaining behavioral control and treatment planning. Medication has limited utility in treatment of psychotic disorders of childhood. Neuroleptics may calm anxiety and reduce aggressive hyperactivity and somewhat diminish psychotic thinking, but they do not significantly alter the poor prognosis and course of these disorders (Campbell, 1973; Mikkelsen, 1982).

Aphasia

Language develops initially as a map or symbolic representation of people, objects, events, and relationships which the child has perceived as meaningful during preverbal development. A major function of language is the regulation of self and others. The meaning of the infant's cry, at least by 8 months of age, is tied closely to its function—regulation of the mother's behavior. The infant recognizes and is attached to its mother before identifying her through language and the use of names (Baker and Cantwell, 1980).

Vocalizations such as crying, cooing, and babbling, as well as smiles, frowns, and gestures, share communicative function with the language they precede. Language also secondarily refines perceptions, increases discrimination, and defines new, more abstract relationships. Language then becomes the medium which allows the child to identify, sequence, and interrelate more complex components of the world.

Language difficulties may reflect problems occurring at various levels of cognitive competence. A child with pervasive developmental delay may be unable to conceptualize the phenomenon that language represents. The delayed and aberrant language of the autistic child reflects a failure to ascribe the usual significance to people and events as well as their cognitive rigidity which impairs creative speech (Geschwind, 1976; Paul and Cohen, 1982).

Children with *congenital expressive aphasia* may be identifiable by 18–24 months of age by failure to babble or rapidly acquire speech. Such children appear to correctly perceive and internally represent the world, but they exhibit problems with the process of speech rather than the ability to conceptualize language.

Children with *congenital expressive aphasia* demonstrate meaningful attachment to others; in infancy, they form secure relations with parents and respond to others' actions, moods, and commands. They utilize inner language and verbal representation to symbolize and organize perceptions as revealed by play, social relatedness, and gesture. Aphasic children may comprehend most receptive speech but are often impaired in the encoding and production of expressive speech. They may have difficulty with the perception, discrimination, or production of speech sounds. Aphasic children usually have normal motoric milestones. Their EEGs may demonstrate paroxysmal abnormalities (Rutter, 1972).

Aphasic children have a higher incidence of subsequent difficulties with reading and may have an increased tendency for perceptual reversal of visual stimuli or dyslexia. Academic failure and impaired social relations are common complications of aphasia. As language becomes a central vehicle for developing internal controls and social relations, as well as cognitive understanding, aphasic children often develop serious behavioral difficulties. They become anxious, hyperactive, and more difficult to manage. At age 4 or 5 years, an aphasic child may be anxiously attached to the mother, the only person who can understand the child's communication (Eisenberg, 1975; 1978).

Elective mutism is the conscious or unconscious withholding of speech in which a child becomes virtually silent in a particular setting, as in school, or with a specific significant person (for example, teacher or parent). In other settings these children demonstrate significantly more language competence—although they often have some expressive difficulty. Elective mutism is often a manifestation of emotional conflict rather than language impairment.

Diagnostic distinctions between pervasive delay, autism, and aphasia can be difficult. Many children demonstrate marked variability in symptomatology and competence with age. The infant who appears aloof, nonverbal, and autistic may develop greater interpersonal and linguistic competence or may subsequently exhibit a true thought disorder. The child who initially exhibits an isolated linguistic delay characteristic of aphasia may later exhibit cognitive slippage or lose associations and resemble children with schizophrenia.

Assessment and Treatment.   Children with speech and language difficulties need a careful physical examination including assessment of auditory and visual competence and fine motor coordination. Specialized language and speech evaluation by a speech pathologist or linguist is needed. The keystone of treatment for aphasic children is special education. With maturation, the language of aphasic children may improve, especially with intensive special education; however, articulation and vocabulary may remain impaired forever. Special speech and language training should start at the time of diagnosis and may continue for several years. The prognosis for such children is usually very good.

Aphasic children should have an audiometric exam and an examination of tongue and vocal cord functioning. Additional assessment of visual and auditory information processing is useful in defining an underlying cognitive deficit, which may produce aphasia. Referral for child psychiatric evaluation is indicated if the child demonstrates impaired social functioning or persistent high levels of anxiety. Counseling or brief therapy may be useful in children whose speech impairment creates increased psychological dependency on parents or who are easily frustrated, explosive, or exhibit poor self-esteem. Therapy may be useful when high levels of anxiety or fear impede speech production as may occur in ***elective mutism***, the absence of speech in a specific setting.

Stuttering

Stuttering is a genetically influenced, sex-linked disorder characterized by repetition or prolongation of sounds, syllables, or words, or by unusual hesitations in the flow of speech. The severity of disability may oscillate between periods of relative fluency and periods of extreme difficulty. Stuttering usually is worse when the speaker is under communicative pressure. The difficulty may increase with mounting anticipatory anxiety about speech production. More than half recover spontaneously; prognosis is better for milder cases. Social and behavioral problems may follow from the anxiety or possible teasing experienced by stutterers. Speech therapy and behavioral reenforcement is often beneficial in stuttering. Psychiatric referral is indicated only if stuttering is indicative of high levels of anxiety or other behavioral difficulties.

MIDDLE CHILDHOOD

During middle childhood, roughly from age 6 years until puberty, a child's emotional energy shifts away from the "family romance" and is directed towards *learning*, *mastery*, and intense *exploration* of the world. Biology propels physical growth producing an increase in strength, coordination, and grace. The child's physical and social development intertwine through participation in group activities and sports. Music lessons and recitals, ballet and gym classes may become important vehicles of self-definition and development. Hobbies, skills, and attitudes toward accomplishment bear the more distinctive mark of the individual as he or she establishes a footing outside the home (Thomas and Chess, 1974).

As the child's own personality becomes more differentiated, he or she becomes more selective in the choice of playmates and friends. The nature of play develops through stages of parallel but noninteractive play, to complex games with their shared rules, and includes thematic play in which fantasies are enacted and shared. Children increasingly select companions they trust and enjoy. As a child enters school, teachers become new authorities, role models, and objects of idealization and romance. Some affection and influence previously invested in parents is redirected towards teachers and other adults.

Intellectual development is a major thrust of middle childhood. Most children experience pride and enjoyment in learning the alphabet, numbers, new games, new words, and acquiring skills such as printing and drawing. A child begins to share in the symbols of the adult world. Mastery of fundamental skills of reading, writing, and arithmetic opens new ways of learning about the community and world. Life outside of home and school takes on clarity and significance through exposure to social studies, travel, television, news, and movies.

Emergent intellectual capacities allow for "concrete operations," the cognitive manipulation of symbols instead of objects; properties of objects can be verbally represented and rearranged. Numbers and words that stand for objects in the child's world can be added and transposed to make new relationships. The child becomes able to cognitively comprehend concepts of conservation of volume, mass, length, weight, and area (Flavell, 1963; Wender et al., 1967).

In psychoanalytic theory, this period of middle childhood has been termed ***latency***— reflecting a phase of diminished intensity of sexual drives. Sexual and romantic feelings usually become sublimated into fantasy. The latency-age child has secured the ability to distinguish fantasy from reality (Freud, 1905; Sarnoff, 1976).

A child of this age may create an imaginary companion who helps him or her deal with problems such as the pain of loneliness. Later, religious feelings may become a predominant vehicle of feelings of love, nurturance, importance, and guilt or evil. Fairly tales, myths, and science fiction embody the conflicts and struggles of childhood. They tell of little heroes who successfully fight huge monsters, of ugly ducklings who become beautiful, of ignored and abused Cinderellas who are transformed by love and a touch of magic. Within these tales children find meaning and courage in their own quest for love, recognition, and competence. The elaboration of fantasy assists the latency-age child to develop tolerance of frustration, to delay gratification, and inhibit impulses (Sarnoff, 1971; Bornstein and Kassen, 1979).

As the child becomes increasingly involved with activities outside the home, the relationship with parents alters. While parents are no longer the exclusive source of the child's joys and supporters of accomplishments, they are the major facilitators of the child's investment in the world beyond the home. Children may begin to compare their parents with other children's parents. They become more explicitly aware of familial conflicts and of the status of their family in the community. They learn about bills and budgets and about bickering or cooperation that affect the family. They know where the power and decisions lie in the family and manipulate these for their own purposes. Children may compete actively with siblings for space, toys, attention, and achievement as they consolidate their own role within the family. Effective parents help provide a safe emotional environment for the child's exploration and expression of individuality. The child who fears for physical, sexual, or emotional safety has little energy to invest in the new tasks and relationships of latency (Kestenberg, 1970).

Often a referral for medical or neurologic evaluation stems from a teacher's observations and recommendations. The physician may assist the parents to form a cooperative alliance with the school. Physician counseling may assist par-

ents to moderate excessive performance pressure on the child and to support appropriate social behavior at school. Parents often need assistance to recognize their importance in fostering the child's growth outside the home. The physician may help parents understand that while the *tasks* of parenting shift during school age, the *importance* of parenting does not. Physicians may assist parents in defining age-appropriate rules and workable incentives and punishments for their child. The physician may also help parents to manage their own life transition resulting from the loss of a full-time parenting role.

Most problems arising during middle childhood bridge many developmental stages and are not restricted to "latency" or "adolescence." They will be discussed within the development context in which they predominantly occur.

Physical Abuse

The physician is often the principal detective responsible for recognizing physical and sexual abuse of children. Child abuse may be evident from multiple bruises located in areas of vulnerability, cigarette or symmetrical immersion burns, or hand, finger, or buckle marks. Frequent emergency room visits with stories that are overly elaborate or inconsistent, extended delays from time of injury to seeking of help, apparent resentment or lack of communication between parents—or a sense of guarded, excessive fear in the child, may raise the physician's suspicion. Sometimes, allowing a child or parent to describe in greater detail the events of the trauma, to discuss methods of discipline, or to acknowledge their distress, facilitates a request for assistance from the parents. Referral for parent counseling can provide a relief for families, some of whom have multigenerational patterns of physical violence. In many states, referral to a child's social service agency is mandatory.

PSYCHOSOMATIC INTERACTION

The link between mind and body, between emotional and physical health, is discussed in detail in Chapter 10. However, emotional coping styles and life events affect the vulnerability to and outcome of many diseases. The interaction between environmental demands and supports, personal styles of coping, and one's biological vulnerability to physical disease are significant dimensions of any illness (Prugh, 1963; Minuchin et al., 1975).

The effects of chronic illness, hospitalization and medical procedures on the personality of children are becoming better defined. The impact of physical illness varies with the child's stage of personality development. For example, the toddler with eczema lives in conflict between the impulse to scratch, scrape, and rub the skin to temporarily obtain relief—and the resultant perpetuation of excoriation that scratching produces. When eczema occurs at a stage where mastery of self-control is first being achieved, it may lead to rage directed against oneself and despair at attempts to achieve impulse control.

Orthopedic illness in the toddler that limits mobility can interfere with normal feelings of separation and autonomy. Hospitalization in preschool children may produce abrupt, prolonged, and overwhelming separation from parents, which may be coupled with fears of vulnerability to the illness and to medical procedures. Before a child has internalized a sense of time and sequence, pain, illness, and separation can seem eternal. The young child often fantasizes that illness and suffering are a punishment for "bad" feelings or behavior. Illness in adolescence may threaten the teenager's narcissistic investment in being physically attractive, strong, and emotionally autonomous. Feelings of being defective, inadequate, or dependent may be intolerable to the teenager who wants to be "just like everyone else" and who places high value on strength and beauty.

Children occasionally "use" physical symptoms to avoid unpleasant tasks. What child hasn't had at least one stomachache that made him or her just "too sick" to go to school on the day of a test, only to recover after it was "too late" for school? When such behavior becomes a pattern, it may indicate a pathologic style of avoidance of difficulties buttressed by parental indulgence. It may reflect a child's withdrawal and underlying depression.

It is seldom useful or accurate for a physician to label an illness "psychological or psychosomatic." It is not enough to say that an illness is due to "nerves, stress, or worry" simply because the physician has not uncovered an organic etiology. Rather, the physician's task is to identify the specific interactions between stress, illness, and psychological and interpersonal responses which perpetuate the physical problem.

Clinical and physiologic research usually has not demonstrated a direct link between specific personality traits (such as obsessiveness or hysteria) or specific areas of conflict or styles of parenting, and specific illness or symptoms. However, some individuals are much more prone to psychosomatic symptoms than others. The particular symptoms or organ systems that manifest anxiety may reflect physiologic vulnerability or environmental influence. Rather than attempting to pair personality and physiology or to identify specific illnesses as psychosomatic, it is useful to conceptualize mind-body interactions as universal and to remain alert to emotional reactions to acute and chronic illness. Similarly, the physician acknowledges affective influences that may precipitate and exacerbate a variety of physical illnesses.

For example, the history and observation of child and family may disclose that a child with documented asthma is enmeshed in an alliance of mutual control and protection with the mother. The child may attempt to dominate and intimidate the mother but never directly express anger toward her. The physician may observe that immediately after avoiding the mother's hesitant attempts at limit-setting, the child appears dejected and begins to wheeze. Mother immediately rushes to comfort, apologizing for "upsetting my baby." The wheezing gradually subsides with mother's strokes, and the child is then allowed to do what was previously forbidden. The process may be virtually unconscious— not an attempt at manipulation. The asthma is real and in need of medical treatment. However, the interpersonal and intrapsychic processes also require evaluation and intervention. If the clinical data confirm—and the alliance allows— the child can be assisted to express his or her anger and desires more directly and be assisted to feel less intimidated. Parents can be supported in efforts to withstand confrontation, maintain parent-child boundaries, and to be supportive without being smothering.

Since a child's life is embedded in the emotional and physical matrix of family, medical illness reflects and affects the child's relationships to parents, siblings, and peers. Reaction to illness will be a function of the child's developmental level, temperament, adaptive style, and familial supports. Psychosomatic illnesses or symptoms reflect both a physiologic vulnerability of a specific organ system and the emotional contribution of stress or conflict, which activates the symptoms. In all cases, an appropriate medical workup should be pursued even if emotional contributions to a symptom are evident, since physical illness and emotional difficulty are not mutually exclusive. A psychiatric diagnosis should rest independently on direct evidence of emotional distress or conflict, and not simply be the heir of failure to identify an organic etiology (Minuchin et al., 1975; Apley, 1977; Gauthier et al., 1977).

Hospitalization

Hospitalization presents emotional stress to a child on many levels. The fact of separation from parents, which may be the most prolonged separation of the child's life, activates fears of abandonment and punishment. A young child may be unable to retain the comforting memory of mother—and thus may experience overwhelming abandonment anxiety. The sequence of denial and protest may be followed by an anaclitic depression characterized by severe withdrawal and apparent indifference to pain. The child frequently blames herself or himself and parents for this "rejection" and is angry, aloof, and distant when parents visit. Trust may need to be gradually reestablished; the child may follow his mother around like a shadow for several days upon returning home. In addition to separation anxiety, hospitalization is often accompanied by weakness, pain, unfamiliar and frightening procedures, and dependency on strangers. For the Oedipal-stage child, illness or surgery can become elaborated into fantasies of genital harm and loss of the capacity for pleasure and identity, which is imagined to be a punishment for illicit desires. These fears are often vague and unformed, yet may evoke considerable irrational anxiety.

Many of the child's fears of separation, strangers, and procedures, or the exaggerated images of bodily harm can be diminished by careful preparation. A sensitive and accurate, age-appropriate explanation of the illness, giving the reasons for the child's discomfort, and a rehearsal of the expected procedures increases the child's adaptability. Practicing examinations and injections with dolls or oranges, for example provides the child a sense of mastery (Erickson, 1958). A child can be helped to anticipate feelings and fears so these are not new and unexpected. To know that an injection will hurt for a moment, that mother will be away until suppertime, and that some diagnostic procedures and machines are uncomfortable and intimidating augments trust and coping ability. Falsely promising that "it won't hurt" or that one will go home prematurely, diminishes confidence. With sensitive help, a child and family can be assisted to understand and encounter even grave illness or death with courage, dignity, and feelings of love.

Chronic Illness

As described in Chapter 19, a child's illness affects the entire family, who must rearrange their priorities to offer support and care to the child. A child's prolonged illness changes family roles. The child may regress to a position of physical and emotional dependency as parents provide increased physical caretaking. Patients with chronic pain and long-standing illness exhibit common responses which begin to shape their personalities and alter thresholds of irritability, generate feelings of vulnerability, and increase demands for nurturance. The boundaries of personal autonomy change if a child is unable to exercise self-care. Parents who must assume responsibility for a child's medications or must limit a child's activity and regulate diet, are forced to intrude into areas of the child's emerging autonomy. Struggles for control and independence commonly emerge. This forced regression produces a conflict in the child, who welcomes the safety and comfort of being cared for but feels angry at being infantilized.

The child's resentment at being dependent, or the parents' impatience with the demands of a child's chronic illness, may gradually dominate the relationship between parent and sick child. The anger ignited by this circumstance in both parent and child can easily be projected onto the other—and yet may remain unexpressed and unrelieved. Attempts to control each other or to passively resist the treatment may escalate. This anger may exacerbate an asthmatic's wheezing or a diabetic's refusal of medication. In many chronic illnesses, issues of autonomy, self-care, helplessness, guilt, and inadequacy can plague a child. Parents can be consumed with worry, fear, self-sacrifice, and guilt, which create distorted forms of attachment, confusion of ego boundaries, and a sense of hovering entrapment. A special bond of indebtedness, worry, and resentment may enmesh mother and ailing child and

further impede autonomy. As a child matures, increased responsibility for self-care and management of chronic illness must be delegated to him or her.

Chronic illness may place a child in a special role within the family. Competition for parental attention can divide siblings and couples. Familial fights and confrontation may be overtly avoided in order not to "upset" the child whose symptoms may parallel levels of marital strife or parental distress—and become the cement which binds a fragile marriage. Unfortunately, this position sometimes perpetuates the child's illness as a vehicle of family stability; the child learns that parents may unite and rally as long as he is sick.

Parents often need added support, encouragement, and counseling to manage the complicated demands of having a chronically ill child. Participation in parents' groups with others whose children experience a common disability can be a vehicle of sharing information about the illness, finding and creating community resources, and learning to manage their own and their child's needs.

Children with chronic illness may have difficulty developing a clear sense of their emotional identity separate from their illness. In some cases, their life is so dominated by symptoms (such as wheezing, diarrhea, seizures) that their emotional expression is virtually limited to physical discomforts. They may need assistance to develop an affective awareness—to identify feelings separate from symptoms, and to define themselves as distinct from their illness. This linkage of feelings to symptoms often prompts "hysterical" manifestations such as "pseudoseizures" or "false wheezing" as emotions become indiscriminately discharged through familiar somatic pathways. The physician must remain aware that the child has needs and interests which transcend the illness.

The course and type of illness has specific implications for personality formation, especially if the illness involves the central nervous system. There is an unusually high incidence of emotional difficulties in brain-impaired children. Children with aphasia have emotional difficulties, in part, due to their diminished ability to communicate with others, but also because they may lack the internal comforting and control provided by language, labeling, and verbal concepts. For example, an aphasic child may not be able to tell him or herself, "Calm down; it won't hurt much; it will all be over in just a minute." Children with chronic multiple tics may become obsessed with efforts to control movements and outbursts. Children with generalized seizures may experience difficulty in achieving a sense of self subsequent to the repeated episodes of complete loss of ego functioning attendant to seizures. They may have repeatedly endured the aura, weakness, gradual blurring of consciousness, amnesia, confusion about who they are, where they are, what just happened—and the experienced fatigue, embarrassment, bruises, and somewhat clouded, lethargic sensorium attendant to the medication (Schowalter, 1977).

Chronic pain leaves its own stamp on personality—the mark of irritability, fatigue, resentment, feelings of entitlement, caution, and restriction. Persistent weakness, at a time when strength and energy are symbols of youth, creates inferiority and alienation. The enuretic or encopretic child may experience embarrassment or an intrusion into areas of privacy and modesty that invade sexually charged boundaries of control, retention, and release.

Recent investigations into brain neurotransmitter and neuroendocrine systems suggest another level of psychosomatic interaction. Neurotransmitters such as dopamine, norepinephrine, serotonin, gamma-amino butyric acid, and many others, occur in multiple brain areas and affect modulation of movements as well as of emotions. The impulsivity and inattention of a "hyperactive" child may not just be a physical response to an emotional or attentional disruption. The difficulty in controlling words,

thoughts, and attention experienced by many patients with chronic multiple tics is not merely an emotional reaction to a physical disability. Rather, there may be a substrate or a neurochemical imbalance which modulates movement, attention, thought, and emotion. An understanding of the mechanism of psychosomatic interaction is increasingly being sought through the study of the neurochemical transmitters which are the vehicles of interneuronal communication. Altered regulation of the synthesis, release, and degradation of neurotransmitters may mediate the expression of many serious psychiatric disorders of children. Genetically regulated variability in brain function is further modified by stresses and supports of life experience and the consistency and comfort provided by parents and others (Cohen and Young, 1979).

Enuresis

Enuresis is the persistent, involuntary voiding of urine considered abnormal for the age of the child and for which there is no known organic cause. Enuresis is considered to be *primary* if it has occurred at least once per month since age 4 years, and considered *secondary* if inappropriate voiding returns following a period of greater than 1 year of continence. Nocturnal enuresis occurs only during sleep, while diurnal incontinence occurs either when the child is asleep or awake (Kolvin et al. 1972).

Enuresis is not associated with any specific psychiatric syndrome and may occur in children with no associated symptoms. However, the prevalence of emotional disorders is slightly higher in enuretic than continent children. Enuresis usually remits spontaneously or is self-correcting without subsequent complications; its incidence diminishes with increasing age: 10% of 5-year-olds, 7% of 7-year-olds, and about 5% of 10-year-olds are enuretic (Lewis, 1982). Boys are more commonly enuretic than girls; enuresis is more common in low socioeconomic groups and sometimes has a familial pattern. The major difficulty created by incontinence is social embarrassment and inconvenience to children and their families.

Primary enuresis may reflect a developmental delay of the nervous system (commonly seen in mentally retarded children), whereas secondary enuresis is more likely associated with familial disruption or life stress. Secondary enuresis may suggest a regressive reaction to stress. It can occur as a conversion system and may appear in children with a chronic personality disorder or psychosis. Enuresis may be associated with coercive toilet training in infancy or is occasionally found in a child whose overly permissive parents did not attempt to train him or her. Daytime enuresis may be seen in excessively shy children who are afraid to ask to go to the toilet or are afraid of strange toilets, or in negativistic, oppositional, chronically anxious, or very impulsive and inattentive children.

Nocturnal enuresis may be a manifestation of psychoneurotic disturbance and has been found in passive, inhibited, overly dependent, or phobic children, as well as in children without psychiatric diagnosis. Enuresis may be associated with relaxation of external sphincters in response to terrifying nightmares or passive-dependent dreams symbolizing submission, infantile helplessness, loss of control, and abandonment. In active, independent children, enuresis may occur in association with anxieties about competition and hostile retribution. Diurnal enuresis may occur as a tension discharge phenomenon in impulsive children; it may be one of several manifestations of poor control, immaturity, and high stress, indicative of conflicts about control and punishment. Occasionally, bedwetting has a quality of hostile revenge and may even be volitional. In others it preserves the protective overinvolvement of a hovering, worried parent and dependent child. The family's response to bedwetting may be significant. A parent may use enuresis as an invitation for overinvolvement in a child's self-care and, thereby, maintain a cyclical pattern of attention which inadvertently reinforces the symptom. Some parents, even those who were bedwetters themselves, may shame or insult an enuretic child in a manner that internalizes guilt and perpetuates immaturity (Sperling, 1965).

Treatment. The physician should evaluate the possibility of organic contributions to enuresis which may include urinary tract infection, diabetes, seizure disorder, and structural urinary tract abnormalities. Diagnostic studies should include urinalysis for identification of possible cystitis and urine protein and glucose levels. The sleep EEG, although almost always normal, may reveal a focal episodic disorder. If structural abnormalities are suspected (especially in primary enuresis), an intravenous urogram may be diagnostic. Retrograde cystoscopy is usually not indicated in children with normal urinalysis and can precipitate excessive anxiety.

Treatment of children with evidence of difficulty establishing sphincter control should begin with parental counseling. Parents should encourage the child to void before going to bed and should limit liquids after supper; it is sometimes helpful to awaken the child for voiding during the night. Institution of a chart with rewards (such as stars) for continence is frequently effective. Children over age 7 to 8 years may be encouraged to change their own sheets and pants. Simple guidance and patience is followed by reduction of enuresis in at least 30% of all young children.

Specific behavioral management is useful in older children. Several devices are commercially available, for example, a liquid sensing pad and a bell; when the child wets, the alarm rings. These are quite effective and sometimes lead to lasting control after termination of treatment. Older children may welcome their use. The antidepressant imipramine in low doses (10–50 mg before bedtime) often effectively relieves enuresis, but there are frequent relapses. Imipramine has led to cardiac toxicity and there is a danger of overdose (Martin, 1971). Referral for psychotherapy is indicated in those children for whom previous interventions are not effective and where evidence of conflict anxiety and poor impulse control exists.

Encopresis

Encopresis is the repeated, inappropriate soiling or passage of feces in a medically healthy child of over 4 years of age. Encopresis is considered *primary* if soiling has occurred at least at monthly intervals since infancy; it is *secondary* if the child has been fecally continent for at least 1 year. Encopresis is often associated with or secondary to constipation, impaction, or stool retention with subsequent overflow. One fourth of encopretic children are also enuretic. Encopresis creates social embarrassment, feelings of shame and loss of self-control, and familial conflict in an effort to obtain regulation. Multiple medical procedures may be endured in an effort to clarify diagnosis, rule out organic etiology, and cleanse the bowels.

Primary encopresis may occur subsequent to inconsistent toilet training and poor social skills; it is found with developmental delay or psychosis, in which fecal smearing may be a prominent feature. Secondary encopresis more often reflects intrapsychic and familial conflict over issues of control, retention, withholding, and fears of giving up and letting go. Such children may be inhibited, dependent, compulsive, and immature; they may show excessive concern about cleanliness in other areas. The soiling may be an expression of unconscious hostility and resistance toward parents. It creates both a need for and frequent resentment of continued parental supervision. Mothers of encopretic children are often seen as domineering, overly controlling, intrusive, and compulsive, while fathers are often viewed as passive and disinterested. The child may be the object of anger, punishment, rejection, and humiliation from caretakers and peers. Family conflict may precipitate secondary encopresis (Warson et al., 1953; Bemporad et al., 1971).

Treatment.   Encopresis often remits spontaneously and without serious sequelae. In some cases, it remains a tenacious problem. A physical examination should include evaluation for overall developmental maturity. The abdomen should be examined for evidence of stool retention and megacolon; a rectal examination is performed for evidence of impaction and obstruction. Lower gastrointestinal roentgenographic series usually verifies a patent and intact bowel and help restore colonic tone. Daily evacuation and doses of mineral oil may reestab-sympathetic ganglia to rule out Hirschsprung's disease (absence of myenteric ganglion cells in the large bowel).

A combination of medical and psychiatric treatment is often effective. Hypertonic phosphate or oil retention enemas can cleanse the bowel and help restore colonic tone. Daily evacuation and doses of mineral oil may reestablish regularity. By confirming the child's role in performing and monitoring his or her bowel movements, the cycle of parental overinvolvement can be interrupted. Psychotherapy may be useful in assisting a child to verbalize feelings of anger, withholding, and desire for control. Such children may be assisted to "let go," and to feel less afraid of feelings of anger and helplessness.

School Avoidance

School avoidance may reflect the child's fear of entering new and complex circumstances or may be symptomatic of concern that he or she feels needed at home to provide domestic safety and stability. School phobia may signify a retreat from involvement in the larger world, particularly if the child has not found safety in resolving the issues of competitiveness with and separateness from parents. It is useful to explore with the truant child whether he or she is staying, or being kept, at home to satisfy some real or imagined wish for the child to be there; or whether he or she is afraid of being unable to learn or of being rejected socially at school.

Treatment. School avoidance is an urgent problem requiring rapid intervention to facilitate reentry into school. If allowed to continue, many secondary supports and reinforcements may actually perpetuate truancy; the child's fears of separation and inadequacy may escalate and the family may adapt to the child's remaining at home. The physician can often help the family understand reasons for school avoidance and mobilize the child and family for return to class. Separate counseling sessions for parents and child may be useful in identifying any precipitants to truancy occurring within the family or the home.

Recently, antidepressant medication has been found to be useful in severe cases of school avoidance, especially in those children who experience phobic anxiety in social or learning situations. A referral for psychiatric evaluation is indicated for a child who remains out of school in spite of counseling for more than 2 weeks; who appears symptomatically depressed or severely anxious; or who continues to withdraw from school due to a real or imagined need to be at home. Intervention may include individual therapy, family guidance, and school consultation. Vigilance and support should not end immediately upon the child's return to school since this difficulty may be symptomatic of trouble which can persist in altered form.

Learning Disabilities

School entry frequently leads to identification of problems in learning, attention, and behavior. Selective learning disabilities, in contrast to pandevelopmental delay, are evidenced by difficulty with specific modalities of learning (visual, auditory), or with selected conceptual tasks such as abstraction, sequencing, encoding, or retrieval of information. Reading, spelling, and arithmetic are frequent areas of impaired learning. Because these skills provide the essential foundation for subsequent learning, difficulties in these areas profoundly impede education. Specific reading disorder and specific arithmetical disorder are the most common learning disabilities (Shain, 1972; Gaddes, 1976; Hughes, 1976; Lynn et al., 1978).

Specific reading disorder occurs in children with adequate overall intelligence. It is exhibited by omissions or addition of words, or failure to abstract meaning from words correctly read. Tests such as the Illinois Test of Psycholinguistic Abilities (ITPA) or the McCarthy aid the school psychologist in assessing the mechanism of this learning disorder. Reading disability may reflect impaired visual perception, impulsive response to stimuli, or difficulty organizing and interpreting visual stimuli (Wiig et al., 1977). Some children have difficulty integrating information across sensory modalities (for example, connecting the spoken or printed word to the actual object). Difficulties in sequencing of information may impair a child's organization of chains of events and perception of cause and effect (Rourke, 1978). These children frequently have secondary academic difficulty and may develop low self-esteem and antisocial behavior. Specific reading disorder occurs more commonly in boys, especially those with a family history of reading difficulty (Rutter and Yule, 1975; Silver, 1975; Weil, 1977; Jansky, 1980).

Specific arithmetical disorder consists of difficulty in learning and retaining arithmetic rules and mathematical procedures for computation in children with adequate intelligence and appropriate schooling. It is less common and probably less disabling than reading difficulty.

Treatment. The physician can assess perceptual and neurologic integrity in the learning disabled child. Cognitive difficulties may be the first recognized manifestation of a genetic disorder (Rossi, 1972) (for example Tourette's syndrome or Huntington's chorea), of a metabolic disturbance, or of attention deficit disorder with hyperactivity. The physician can assist parents to understand that learning disorder is not synonomous with low intelligence, and may not be assisted by medication. The physician may assist the parents and child to obtain the best possible remedial services available and then to work cooperatively with the professionals involved (Eaton, Sells, and Lucas, 1977).

Parents and child alike may feel embarrassed by the child's educational difficulty; they may blame each other or the school. The child may begin to feel a loss of self-esteem and confidence due to the learning problem. Parents may need to discuss with the physician their concern about the effect of labeling and segregating their child or the selection of the most appropriate special programs and schools.

Medication has not proven useful in the treatment of nonhyperactive learning disabled children (Gittleman-Klein, 1976). Referral for a child psychiatric evaluation is indicated if anxiety, fear, depression, or family pressures appear to underlie the learning difficulty (Hartlage, 1977; DeQuiros and Schrager, 1978). Special educational techniques for teaching the learning disabled child include emphasis on the sensory modality which is most effective, and reinforcing learning by simultaneous multisensory stimulation. These sophisticated methods have proven quite successful with many learning disabled children (Sulzbacher, 1975).

Attention Deficit Disorder with Hyperactivity

Two clinical syndromes illustrate the interplay between cognition, attention, motor control, and personality: attention deficit disorder (ADD) and chronic multiple tics of Tourette's disease.

ADD is a behavioral syndrome characterized by a triad of inattention, impulsivity, and frequently, hyperactivity. Historically, these children have been described as having minimal brain dysfunction (MBD), hyperactivity, hyperkinesis, hyperactive child syndrome, and other diagnoses. The hyperactivity may be manifested, by excessive running or climbing, difficulty sitting still and staying seated; fidgeting and restlessness may even persist during sleep. Some children experience themselves as being "driven by a motor." Inattention and distractibility may include difficulty concentrating or finishing tasks, especially academic assignments requiring sustained attention. These children often seem not to listen and they typically do not finish projects. Their impulsivity is evident by acting before they think or plan, or by rapid shifting from one activity to another. They have difficulty organizing work and require almost constant supervision. ADD children find it hard to wait, to delay, to take turns, or to avoid disrupting and speaking out of turn (Cantwell, 1976; Hunt et al., 1982).

In the characteristic ADD child, symptoms appear before age 7 years and are of long-term duration. ADD with hyperactivity occurs predominantly in males with ratio estimates of 5–9 to 1 of boys to girls. Attentional disturbance without hyperactivity may be much more evenly distributed. Girls with ADD may create less behavioral disturbance and, hence, be underrecognized. Patients with pervasive developmental disorders such as severe organic brain dysfunction, schizophrenia, autism, or mania, may have many or most ADD symptoms. These lesser symptoms of attentional impairment, however, are automatically encompassed by the more pervasive diagnosis (*DSM III*, 1980).

The phenotypic expression of the attentional deficit changes with developmental phase. Careful history may disclose that the ADD child was an unusual infant, that is, cried a lot, was irritable, and slept less than most infants. The child did not sustain play or exploration with one toy or object, and destroyed and lost even the most "child-proof" toys. The child wore out clothes, playpen, and parents' patience more rapidly than other youngsters.

The problem of modulation usually affects attention to both internal and external events. It stretches across the boundaries of motoric activity, visual and auditory integration (Satterfield, Cantwell, and Satterfield, 1974; Gardon and

Kantor, 1979; Hiscock et al., 1979). Thus, the ADD toddler is likely to be more active than other 2-year-olds. Less attentive to bodily stimuli, such as the need to void, they may impulsively soil or wet themselves. Many ADD children are identifiable during the first 3 years of life—even before the rigors of academic education demand the ability to sit still, to master visual symbols, and to sustain attention on immobile stimuli such as words. Others first become symptomatic at school (Shouse and Lubar, 1978).

By elementary school, the ADD child does not take sufficient time to review and integrate perceptions. ADD children are frequently dyslexic, reflecting perceptual reversals so that the child sees "was" as "saw" and "b" as "d." The impulsive child frequently skips over endings of words thereby missing tense and confusing words that look alike. They may sound out the first syllable and then "make up" the remainder of the word. Integration of part-whole relationships is difficult for the attentionally impaired child. They may strain to sound out individual words or syllables but fail to integrate these into meaningful words, sentences, or paragraphs (Safer and Allen, 1976; Weiss and Hechtman, 1979).

Frequently, these children are delayed in development of fine and gross motor coordination; performance may be slow and awkward. Handwriting is usually sloppy; gross motor coordination is often floppy or loose. Although their bravado and provocativeness lead to frequent fighting, ADD children are usually poor athletes. Whether this coordination difficulty reflects a delay in maturation or aberrant development of integrative mechanisms is unclear. These are nonspecific signs of some difficulty in motor development or a delay in neurologic maturation. Symptoms of decreased motor tone or diminished control and specificity of movement are frequently associated with diminished attentional and behavioral control. Some delay in the development of motoric control may reflect the impulsive child's failure to practice and rehearse

motoric skills. The development of motoric finesse requires patience, tolerance of failure, sustained attention, and the ability to connect segments of learning into useful sequences. For example, one learns to play the piano by concentrated repetition of motor patterns and the eventual connection of stanzas into finished pieces (Gardner, 1979; Hertzig, 1972). Minor physical anomalies such as hyperteleonism, low-set ears, high-arched palate, and interphalangeal webbing may be genetically determined or reflect toxic insult such as occurs in fetal alcohol syndrome.

Lack of attention is often associated with an insensitivity to social cues. ADD children often ignore facial expressions, are unaware of danger, and fail to anticipate the effect their behavior will have on others. Many social difficulties reflect the impetuousness with which they approach relationships. The ADD child intrudes into, and takes over groups, insists on being the "leader," and fails at fairness, reciprocity, and taking turns. Recess provides too many opportunities for fights as these children become bullies or are teased. Although lack of shyness and fear may initially appear to be friendliness, friends are lost as quickly as they are made.

Children with severe ADD create havoc in their environment. They forget obligations, rules, homework, or household assignments. At home, drawers are always open, clothes and toys strewn and disassembled and chores are ignored. The ADD child seems to invent new problems faster than parents can generate responses, thwarting their efforts to maintain consistency in dealing with the child. Babysitters may be quickly defeated by the child's stubborn insistence on "getting into things." Teachers complain of restlessness, failure to finish projects, impulsivity, short attention span, defiance of authority, and distractibility. Schoolwork and appearance are sloppy and disheveled. Teachers must continually remind them to sit down and keep still. Neighbors may complain of fights, negligence, and destroyed property. The ADD child is soon labeled as a "bad influence," and other parents restrict his or her play with their children (Wender, 1972).

By middle childhood, depressive or antisocial personality features may emerge. The ADD child becomes aware of learning difficulties, social isolation, and poor self-control and experiences himself or herself as a failure. The low self-esteem frequently experienced by these children is, in part, a reflection of their lack of accomplishment, social rejection, and feelings of isolation and failure to sustain attachment. Lack of sustained attention or interest leads to feelings of boredom and diffusion of identity. Internal disorganization parallels the symptoms of external or behavioral chaos. The ADD child lacks a sense of commitment, direction, and accomplishment. If these frustrations are camouflaged by avoidance and manipulation, antisocial personality disorder may develop. ADD children are as easily distracted from their own thoughts and awareness of their own feelings as they are from the problems in a math book or the words on a spelling list. It is difficult for them to consolidate any consistent sense of self, since they may lack internal continuity of feelings, interests, and attachments. ADD children exaggerate and deprecate their own abilities and fail to channel efforts into a meaningful sequence of accomplishment. Development of emotional continuity—the internal linking of perception and understanding to feelings—is difficult for children with impaired attention and impulsivity. The experience of attachment, internalization of controls, and, hence development of conscience may be fragmented (Douglas, 1975; Cunningham and Barkley, 1978; Sandberg, Rutter, and Taylor, 1978; Gillberg et al., 1982).

Attentional deficit and impulsivity may persist into adulthood, although motoric hyperactivity usually diminishes to levels of manageable restlessness. Behavioral difficulties may assume more adult forms of impulsive gambling or excessive drinking to calm the agitation. Fragmented attention and effort may lead to a life history of poor judgment and unfinished beginnings. Marriages may be fragmented, friendships brief, parenting inconsistent, and work record unproductive. Some ADD children develop character disorders and have substantial antisocial or legal difficulties as adults. ADD may be a precursor to some later forms of psychosis (Wood et al., 1976; Crabtree, 1981; Horowitz, 1981; Hechtman et al., 1981).

Family studies of attentionally impaired children suggest a genetic contribution to the illness. It predominates in males (approximately 5 to 1 ratio) who may have a family history, usually paternal, of flight of attention, academic underachievement, reading difficulty, restlessness, and impulsivity (Cantwell, 1976). Prenatal factors may contribute to the development of ADD. Prematurity, low birth weight, or maternal ingestion of substantial amounts of alcohol or barbiturates increases the infant's vulnerability to later attentional difficulties. Complications during labor and delivery resulting in fetal distress or anoxia may slightly increase risk of subsequent ADD—though most children who experience infantile anoxia do not develop ADD.

Although frequent anecdotal reports suggest an etiological role for food additives, dyes, and high-carbohydrate or sugar diets, controlled studies have usually failed to find a clear effect of challenge diets on expression of these symptoms. Although diet may affect behavior and concentration of some children with ADD, it does not appear to greatly alter parent and teacher behavior ratings in controlled studies of groups of ADD children (Weiss, 1982).

Psychological development and interpersonal relationships may thwart the development of attentional processes. Children raised in emotionally chaotic or deprived environments may desperately seek contact and reassurance, and themselves perpetuate conflict. The high levels of anxiety or fear in such environments may prompt children to be continuously vigilant and self-protective. They may find it difficult to care about and remain focused on a learning task.

Treatment. The most important aspect of care of ADD children usually is special educational evaluation and intervention, which should start as soon as a learning difficulty is diagnosed. ADD children should receive tutoring, periods in special learning laboratory programs, or the opportunity for full-time special education programs. Special education in a small classroom with few distractions may help improve academic skills, modulate impulses, and sustain more consistent and intimate interpersonal relationships. Early remediation may allow a child to move back into the mainstream of education; specific programs for enhancing motoric skill may improve writing and coordination. (Gittelman et al., 1976; Pelham et al., 1980).

Counseling by a physician may assist parents with behavioral management of their ADD child, enable them to ventilate feelings of anger and disappointment, and select and coordinate an educational program. Parents often need help in maintaining appropriate and consistent consequences for their child's behavior and in avoiding excessive punishing or indulging. The ADD child continues to need some discipline-free play time with parents on a regular basis to prevent the entire parent-child relationship from being problem-focused (Miller, 1975).

Counseling with the child may assist him or her to be more aware of difficulty in concentration, sustaining effort, and organizing behavior. Greater clarity about the difficulty can help a child mobilize conscious resources to maximize attention and increase frustration tolerance. Emotional deprivation, physical abuse, or prolonged familial conflict can contribute to a child's internal disorganization and self-preoccupation. A child, consumed with concern that his or her needs will not be met, may have little energy left for cognitive tasks.

Referral to a child psychiatrist is indicated for children who appear depressed or severely disorganized by their attention disorder and its consequences. Depression may be a primary underlying process for which hyperactivity is the prominent clinical manifestation. In this situation, the child may be overactive in order to release anxiety. Depression and low self-esteem may also result from the failures experienced by a child who has difficulty paying attention and completing tasks. Inattention may be secondary to daydreaming rather than to external distractibility. Extreme disorganization of thought and effort may be an indication of an underlying thought disorder or psychosis. Hyperactive children may lose their train of thought through external distraction, but can usually easily return to the subject. Their manner of symbolization and the type of issues on which they focus are usually age-appropriate and typical, but perhaps skewed towards violence and activity. The psychotic child may lose his or her thoughts in internal ruminations and may have unusual preoccupations or assign unique meaning to words or events.

Long-term psychotherapy can be useful in assisting a child to develop internal controls, to become more aware of emotions which might trigger overactivity, to improve social behavior, and to tolerate unavoidable rejection and criticism. Psychotherapy may change self-concept from that of an inadequate underachiever who has compensated for these deficits by charm, humor, or indifference to one of a more competent and more consistent individual.

Stimulant medication is useful in reducing the motor hyperactivity that frequently accompanies ADD. Methylphenidate or amphetamine narrow the spectrum of attention and reduce impulsivity, thus diminishing distractibility in class and improving persistence in vigilance and memory or associated learning tasks (Conners, 1972; Kupietz and Balka, 1976; Barkley and Cunningham, 1979b; Charles, 1979; Thurston et al., 1979; Hunt et al., 1982). Stimulants frequently improve behavior and ease social interaction at home and school (Barkley and Cunningham, 1979a; Whalen, Henker, and Dolemoto, 1980). Many ADD children experience an increased sense of control and mastery on medication. However, unless coupled with appropriate psychotherapy, family counseling, or focused educational intervention, medications alone usually do not lead to improved academic learning or increase in achievement scores. Stimulants do not appear useful for most learning disabled children who are not also hyperkinetic. Prior to initiating medication, teachers should be asked to complete a behavior rating scale such as the Conners teacher's scale (Spring, Greenberg, and Yellin, 1977; Goyette, Connors, and Ulrich, 1978).

Initial choice of medication is frequently methylphenidate (Ritalin) at doses of approximately 0.1–0.2 mg/kg given before school. Medication dosage can gradually be increased toward a maximum of about 0.5–0.75 mg/kg, which may be given in divided doses, in the morning and at noon. Weekly monitoring and rating of behavior by teacher and parents will assist in determining the optimal dose. The dosage required to produce optimal improvement in attention may be only half of the dose needed to achieve maximal behavioral control. In a child with primarily attentional learning difficulties, a low dose (10–20 mg daily) may yield the best cognitive improvement, although some restlessness may remain. Alternative stimulants include amphetamines, which are about twice as potent as methylphenidate. Pemoline is associated with hepatotoxicity.

The most frequent, acute side effects of stimulants are stomachache, anorexia, weight loss, motor tics, insomnia if given in afternoon or evening, and irritability. Long-range side effects include modest suppression of growth if high doses are administered continuously throughout the school year. Weekend and summer holidays from drugs may diminish growth suppression. Diagnosis of underlying psychosis, multiple tics, and major side effects to previous stimulants are contraindications to stimulant medication for ADD and hyperactivity. While stimulant medications have substantial potential for abuse in nonADD adults who exploit the arousing and anorectic effects—the use of stimulants in latency-aged ADD children does not increase their incidence of subsequent drug abuse. About 20% of children receiving methylphenidate may require a modest increase in dose during the year; however, tolerance to the medication does not develop with the frequency of that which occurs when used illicitly for euphoric or antidepressant purposes. In children with atypical childhood psychosis and multiple tic syndrome, stimulants may lead to dramatic exacerbation of symptomatology. Since these children initially often have attentional problems and hyperactivity, physicians may increase the medications rather than recognizing that the symptomatic exacerbation is a side effect of medication. The results may be disastrous.

Tricyclic antidepressants, such as imipramine, are useful in the treatment of ADD with hyperactivity but have cardiac toxicity and are potentially lethal if taken in overdose. Neuroleptics such as thioridazine and haloperidol effectively quiet much aggressive, overactive behavior but produce greater sedation, and may diminish motivation, attention, and learning. For some children, a combination of a phenothiazine and a stimulant have been beneficial.

Children treated with stimulants should be monitored at monthly intervals by teacher and physician to reassess efficacy of medication. Except in severe cases, drug-free weekend and summer holidays are advisable and allow reassessment of the need for continued treatment. Many ADD children can begin each academic year with a trial off medication or be tapered after their initial adjustment to a new classroom allowing an assessment of the ‘continued need for stimulants. While most ADD children can be withdrawn from medication before adolescence, some require continued treatment into adolescence and later.

Tourette Syndrome

Tourette syndrome of chronic multiple tics typically has a rapid onset around age 7 years, almost always between the ages of 4 and 12 years. Before the onset of the tics there are often pre-existing difficulties in attention and the regulation of activity, diminished ability to inhibit, irritability of mood, and behavioral problems during the early school years (Leckman et al., 1982; Shapiro, 1981).

While benign tics may occur in about 10% of all school children at some time, in Tourette syndrome, eye-blinking and facial tics are followed by an incessant series of other multiform movements. These become increasingly persistent and widespread and may include rapid movements or jerks of the head, abrupt thrusts of hands and shoulders, arm waving and even stomach spasms. These explosive motor discharges become embedded in an array of more troubling behavior difficulties which make the disorder so incapacitating (Cohen et al., 1982).

Compulsive and ritualistic behaviors appear, initially often manifested as the need to keep objects neatly arranged and routines unchanged. Soon, however, the child may touch people and things nearby, snap the fingers, kick, hop, walk one step forward and then back, grimace, or assume odd postures. For many children, this phase may be followed sooner or later by the explosive, sudden outpouring of foul language. The child may interject brief exclamatives while someone else is talking—"OK, sure, of course, you bet"—or immediately echo a phrase or sentence just spoken to him or her.

Such children feel trapped in their own bodies or possessed by a force not under their own control, which compels them to express sexual and aggressive ideas as they occur. Yet the tics and vocalizations are partially under voluntary control and can be temporarily inhibited. At times of developmental transition, such as early adolescence, psychophysiologic structures of self-control may weaken and behavioral or motor symptoms may emerge as increased impulses become more powerful. Most children with this syndrome are more than simply aware of their disorder. They are frightened by it,

pained by their lack of control and eager to behave like their peers.

A biological basis for Tourette syndrome has been supported by the prevalence of abnormalities on neurologic testing, EEG abnormalities, genetic history, occasional association with birth trauma, and consistently higher incidence in males (3 to 1 or higher). A familial vulnerability to Tourette syndrome has been demonstrated recently, suggestive of an autosomal dominant pattern of inheritance with sex-modified penetrance (Kidd, Prusoff, and Cohen, 1980). Catecholamine metabolism has been implicated by the pharmacologic observations that dopamine-blocking medication (particularly haloperidol) reduces the severity of the disorder in many patients, while dopamine-releasing medication (such as dextroamphetamine) leads to exacerbation. Direct evidence of dopaminergic involvement has, however, been lacking (Leckman et al., 1982; Cohen et al., 1979).

Treatment. Haloperidol (Haldol) is initiated in low doses (0.5 mg) for patients with severe symptoms of Tourette disease. The dose is gradually increased until control is achieved, but many patients dislike the attendant sedation, apathy, and weight gain (Shapiro and Shapiro, 1981). Pimozide has the same general range of efficacy and side effects as haloperidol; however, it may be less sedating and appears to be useful for some patients who do not tolerate haloperidol. Preliminary evidence suggests that clonidine (Catapres), an alpha-adrenergic agonist, may diminish aggressiveness, compulsions, and tics, which suggests a possible adrenergic component to this disorder. Double-blind control studies and additional longitudinal follow-up studies are in process to verify the utility and define possible indications for clonidine. No adequate control studies have yet been done to assess the relative benefits of haloperidol, phenothiazines, pimozide, or clonidine (Cohen et al., 1980).

In addition to medication, Tourette syndrome patients often require a range of other treatments including counseling, family guidance, special education, and psychotherapy. It is important for physicians to not simply focus on symptoms and their amelioration through medication; they need to address the whole person. Years of painful and humiliating experience tend to leave emotional scars and learned patterns of behavior which cannot be erased by medication alone.

Referral for child psychiatric evaluation is indicated to assess the child's coping with this psychologically devastating illness. Some children are able to use psychotherapy to clarify the sources and management of their aggression, feelings which emerge frequently and abruptly. Children with Tourette syndrome frequently need to become aware then how much of their personality is affected by their illness without giving in to despair and helplessness. With compassion and firmness, the therapist can help moderate the intensity of aggression and assist the patient to manage the experience of these primitive feelings.

APPENDIX: CASE HISTORY—THE SAD, BAD BOY

Tom had been diagnosed as having a learning disability in the first grade and a specific reading disability with tendency to reverse letters. Although Tom seems to enjoy sports he has been below average in coordination and often is distracted and makes errors during games. (The pediatrician found the following additional information concerning Tom from school and family.)

Family History

Tom is the second of three children whose mother works as a secretary-typist. His siblings are Jennifer, age 11, doing well in the sixth grade and very allied with mother, and Jeff, age 6, anxious and enuretic. Father is a house painter, currently unemployed, with history of intermittent substance abuse and occasional gambling binges.

Parents separated 4 months ago after an explosive argument following the father's loss of $250 betting while drinking with friends. The mother wants Tom's father to participate in Alcoholics Anonymous, but he denies he has a drinking problem. Father lives in a small apartment 4 miles away; sees Tom about three times a week. Tom says he wants to live with his father. Father recalls that he had frequent difficulties in school both in behavior (was often sent to the principal's office and was suspended) and academically (repeated fifth grade, never liked reading). He dropped out of school in eleventh grade, worked as a truck driver for 3 years but was laid off for having too many accidents; he has since been working for a small local painter. He has had episodes of drinking with two arrests for drunken driving and a history of prior drug abuse, primarily amphetamines which he says calms him down. Mother has had recurrent depressions. During these times she is less involved with Tom; his behavior often becomes more disruptive.

Birth and Development

During this pregnancy mother drank to the point of intoxication about once a week. Tom was born 1 month prematurely and experienced some fetal distress. His birthweight was 2.5 kg (5 lb 9 oz). As an infant Tom was described as colicky, irritable, and an irregular sleeper. Developmental milestones were normal; he seemed to run almost as soon as he began to walk. Since age 2 years old Tom has been very active and never remained interested in anything very long. He was easily upset by minor disappointments. He seems happy when things go well, but rapidly explodes when he is excited or anticipates something special such as a birthday party.

Medical History

Past medical history includes allergies to dust, pollen, and ragweed. Mother reports that he "behaves worse" after eating candy or foods high in sugar and preservatives content.

Physical Examination

Physical examination reveals Tom is of normal height and weight for his age. Some minor physical anomalies are noted: slight asymmetry of the ears, and soft cartilage, hypertelorism, moderately elevated, steepled palate, malalignment of maxillary teeth, short fifth finger, increased space between the first and second toes. Gross motor coordination is moderately "floppy." Fine motor skills are poorly developed. He is slow and awkward at rapid finger-thumb alteration and has mild left to right overflow. Laterality remains poorly defined.

Mental Status

Tom is alert and oriented, but appears hypervigilant, overactive, and fidgety. He touched and commented on many objects in the room, noticed outside noises, and was easily distracted. Sitting restlessly in the chair, frequently fidgeting with his fingers and pencil, he interrupted the examiner several times and changed the subject to ask about objects in the room. His mood seemed happy, almost indifferent.

He expressed sadness and fear about his parents' fights and their recent separation. He wishes they would get back together or wants to live with his father. He acknowledged feeling sad at his lack of friends and being frequently teased, but quickly changed the subject. He says that he likes his teachers but feels they pick on him unfairly and his classmates "get him into trouble and blame him for stuff." He and his younger brother fight frequently.

Intelligence testing showed Verbal IQ of 112 and Performance IQ of 92 with a Full scale score of 104 on the Wechsler Intelligence Scale for Children. There was considerable scatter among subtests with low test scores in digit span, digit symbol, and coding. Highest scores were obtained on comprehension and similarities. The ITPA results suggested a specific reading disability with difficulty in visual memory and sequencing. Results of the TAT and DAP and kinetic family drawings suggested themes of helplessness, depression, and anger. Performance on the Bender-Gestalt test was 2 years below age level. The DAP finding was 1.5 years delayed. There was no suggestion of psychotic thought disorganization in spite of his low frustration level.

Teacher's behavior ratings on the Conners 28-item scale obtained for Tom over 3 weeks (no medication) showed high scores for hyperactive items: restlessness, fidgety, hums, and makes noises, fails to finish tasks, demands excess attention and low frustration tolerance. Parents' behavior ratings (Conner's 48-item scale) were high for restlessness, fights, overactivity, makes noises, easily distracted, and needs frequent reminders.

Diagnosis

On the basis of the comprehensive evaluation, a PEG was constructed and the following diagnoses and treatment plans were devised.

1. Biological dimension: Multiple allergies
2. Personal dimension: Attention deficit disorder with hyperactivity; specific learning disability with perceptual reversals; depressed mood associated with parents' separation
3. Environmental dimension: parental marital discord and separation 4 months ago, which in turn increased Tom's hyperactivity, inattention, and depressed mood

Treatment

1. Methylphenidate, 5 mg per day given before school; this was gradually increased (while monitoring of behavior ratings) to 10 mg in the morning and 5 mg at noon on school days only.

2. Behavior ratings obtained from teachers and parents on a weekly basis until the dosage was stable, and then monthly.

3. Special education and use of the school's resource room enabled Tom to receive individual tutoring in reading for 1 hour a day.

4. Parent counseling by physician to see if they could reconcile their differences and resume living together or proceed towards an equitable divorce. Mother begun on Elavil for depression. Counseling also focused on obtaining parental agreement and clarification of behavioral expectations for Tom and with specific rewards for completing tasks on a behavioral checklist. Specific circumstances were defined for which Tom would be grounded for the afternoon or for 1–2 days. The physician also suggested some activities which Tom and mother would do together for about 15 minutes a day and assisted Tom and his father to enrich the quality of their time together. The physician supported Tom and father in discussion of Tom's resentment of his parents' separation, but Tom usually became more restless and changed the subject.

5. After 3 months a psychiatric consultation was obtained because Tom's low self-esteem persisted even after his behavior began to improve with medication. The psychiatrist was able to spend more time alone in play and story-telling activities with Tom. Gradually he used puppets to describe his parents separating and the boy-puppet feeling abandoned and angry. Tom began to connect these feelings with his aloof and distant behavior towards his father during his visits. After talking with his therapist about his feelings of disappointment in his relationship with his father, Tom was able to talk more openly and directly with his father. The

PATIENT EVALUATION GRID

DIMENSIONS	CONTEXTS		
	CURRENT (Current States)	RECENT (Recent Events and Changes)	BACKGROUND (Culture, Traits, Constitution)
BIOLOGICAL	Allergies Decreased fine and gross motor coordination	Multiple allergies Mother thinks sweets make him more hyperactive	Maternal alcohol ingestion during pregnancy; born 1 mo prematurely; low birthweight; mild fetal distress Father had behavior difficulties in school; episodic alcohol and drug abuse, poor employment and school record
PERSONAL	Physically overactive (out of seat, restless) Irregular sleep Short attention span Impulsive, low frustration tolerance Low self-esteem Learning disability	Misses father, visits 3 times weekly, wants to live with father Began saying he was "no good," could do nothing right, "all my fault" Having nightmares 2 mo ago	Overactivity noted—age 2 yrs Impulsive, accident-prone Happy disposition Blames others No regular hobbies, sports, friends
ENVIRONMENTAL	Family: Mother "can't handle him," "doesn't obey" School and work 3rd grade spec. ed. class, reading disability, grad. improvement, restlessness, overactivity, inattention Peers: No stable playmates, frequent fights, teasing, blames others; wants own way—temper tantrums; poor athlete and team player	Family: Parents separated—4 mo ago after fight about father gambling; father unemployed—6 mo; mother, depression for past 2 mo; irritable, loss of energy School and work: Suspended from school—3 mo ago; made some ed. progress last year in spec. ed.; kicked off soccer team for fighting—2 mo ago Peers: Best friend moves—6 mo ago	Family: drinking and gambling focus of marital distress; mother has prior depression School and work: Reading disability noted in 2nd grade spec. ed.; IQ: Verbal = 112, Performance = 94, FS = 104 Peers: Always bossy, demanding, controlling of peers; pushes, shoves excessively; frequently teased, blamed

Demographic data: 8-year-old male, in third grade.

TABLE 22–1
Psychological and developmental tests for children

DEVELOPMENTAL AND INTELLIGENCE TESTS	AGES	COMMENT
Catell Infant Intelligence Scale	3 mo–$2\frac{1}{2}$ yr	Motor and language
Bayley Infant Scale of Development	8 wk–$2\frac{1}{2}$ yr	Motor and social
Denver Developmental Screening Test	2 mo–6 yr	Motor, social, language
Yale Revised Developmental Schedule	4 wk–6 yr	Motor, adaptive, language
Leiter International Performance Scale	2 yr–Adult	Nonverbal intelligence
McCarthy Scales of Children's Abilities	$2\frac{1}{2}$–8 yr	General I.Q.; six subscales
Wechsler Preschool and Primary Scale of Intelligence (WPPSI)	4–$6\frac{1}{2}$ yr	
Wechsler Intelligence Scale for Children Revised (WISC-R)	6–17 yr	Full scale, verbal, perform; ten subscales
PERCEPTUAL-MOTOR ASSESSMENT		
Bender-Gestalt Test	4 yr–12 yr	Standard age-scoring
Draw-A-Person	2 yr–Adult	Koppitz norms
Bruininks-Oseretsky Test of Motor Proficiency	$4\frac{1}{2}$ yr–$14\frac{1}{2}$ yr	Gross and fine motor; eight subtests
Porteus Mazes	3 yr–Adult	Visual-motor, impulsivity
Beery Test of Visual Motor Integration (VMI)	3 yr–16 yr	
LANGUAGE AND EDUCATIONAL		
Illinois Test of Psycholinguistic Ability (ITPA)	2 yr–11 yr	Receptive and expressive language
Peabody Picture Vocabulary Test-Revised (PPVT)	$2\frac{1}{2}$ yr–Adult	Visual-language screening
Wide Range Achievement Test (WRAT)	5 yr–Adult	Reading, spelling, math
Peabody Individual Achievement Test	$5\frac{1}{2}$–18 yr	Language, math, information
Gray Oral Reading Test	1st–12th grade	Reading proficiency
PERSONALITY AND SOCIAL ADAPTATION		
Rorschach Test	3 yr–Adult	Projective patterns
Children's Apperception Test (CAT)	$2\frac{1}{2}$ yr–Adult	Stories from animal pictures
Thematic Apperception Test (TAT)	6 yr–Adult	Stories from pictures
Vineland Social Maturity Scale—Revised	0–Adult	Parental report for motor, social, communication skills

psychiatrist met with the father to help him talk with his son about these feelings. Their relationship improved after these confrontations. The therapist met with the mother and subsequently with Tom and his mother to improve her consistency in limit-setting. As Tom's feelings of blame toward his mother for the divorce abated, he acted less defiantly at home. His attention span, grades, and behavior began to improve at school. He felt calmer and had more self-confidence. His prognosis has improved given his response to these multiple interventions.

RECOMMENDED READINGS

Adams, P.L. 1900. *A primer of child psychotherapy.* Boston: Little, Brown & Co. This is a well written introduction to the goals and process of psychotherapy with children.

Berlin, I. 1976. *Bibliography of child psychiatry.* New York: Human Science Press. This is a guide to references by topic in child and adolescent psychiatry.

Cantwell, D.P. 1975. *The hyperactive child: diagnosis, management, current research.* New York: Spectrum Publications, Inc. This excellent description of the hyperactive child with attentional and learning disturbances, written primarily for physicians, describes issues regarding medication and research.

Eissler, R.S.; Freud, A.; Kris, M., et al. 1977. *Psychoanalytic assessment: the diagnostic profile.* New Haven, Conn.: Yale University Press. This is an introduction to psychoanalytic assessment and formulation in children.

Flavil, J.H. 1963. *The developmental psychology of Jean Piaget.* New York: D. Van Nostrad Co. Flavil gives a readable review of Piaget's concepts of cognitive development in childhood.

Fraiberg, S.H. 1954. *The magic years: understanding and handling the problems of early childhood.* New York: The Scribner Library. This useful overview of child development and the tasks of parenting during the first five years is a good introduction for parents and physicians.

Freud, A. 1965. *Normality and pathology in childhood.* New York: International Universities Press. This is the classic description of psychoanalytic concepts of normal and pathologic libinal and ego development.

Mahler, M.S. 1975. *The psychological birth of the human infant: separation and individuation.* New York: Basic Books. Careful clinical observations of children up to age 5 years that describe the development of intrapsychic awareness of self, separateness from parents, and beginnings of autonomy.

Nicholi, A. 1978. *The Harvard guide to modern psychiatry.* Cambridge, Mass.: Harvard University Press. This is a brief overview and reference for clinical psychiatrists.

Nospitz, J.D. 1979. *Basic handbook of child psychiatry,* 4 vols. New York: Harper & Row. Four volumes that are an excellent reference text in child psychiatry.

Simmons, J.E. 1974. *Psychiatric examination of children.* Philadelphia: Lea & Febiger. This is a practical introduction to interviewing and assessing the emotional state of children.

REFERENCES

Abelin, E.L. 1971. The role of the father in the separation-individuation process. In *Separation-individuation: essays in honor of Margaret S. Mahler,* eds., J.B. McDevitt and C.F Settlage, pp. 229–52. New York: International Universities Press.

Ainsworth, M.D.S. 1963. "The development of infant-mother attachment." In *Review of child development research,* vol. 3, eds. B.M. Caldwell and H.N. Ricciuti, pp. 1–94. Chicago: University of Chicago Press.

Ameer, B. 1979. Teratology of psychoactive drugs. In *Psychopharmacology update: new and neglected areas,* eds. J.M. Davis and D. Greenblatt. New York: Grune & Stratton.

American Psychiatric Association. *Diagnostic-statistical manual of mental disorders,* (DSM–III), 3rd ed. Washington, D.C.: American Psychiatric Association.

Ames, L.B.; Metraux, R.W.; and Walker, R. 1971. *Adoles-*

cent *Rorschach responses*, Rev. ed. New York: Brunner/Mazel.

Anthony, E.J. 1970. The reactions of parents to the oedipal child. In *Parenthood*; eds. E.J. Anthony and T. Benedek, pp. 275–88. Boston: Little, Brown.

Anthony, E.J. 1973. A working model for family studies. In *The child and his family*, eds. E.J. Anthony and C. Koupernik, pp. 3–20. New York: Wiley.

Apley, J. 1977. Psychosomatic aspects of gastrointestinal problems in children. *Clin. Gastroent.* 6:400.

Aronow, E.; and Raznikoff, M. 1976. *Rorschach content interpretation.* New York: Grune & Stratton.

Baker, L., and Cantwell, D.P. 1980. *Developmental language disorders*, pp. 2695–705.

Barkley, R.A.; and Cunningham, C.E. 1979a. Stimulant drugs and activity level in hyperactive children. *Am. J. Orthopsychiatry* 49(3):491–99.

Barkley, R.A.; and Cunningham, C.E. 1979b. The effects of methylphenidate on the mother-child interactions of hyperactive children. *Arch. Gen. Psychiatry* 36(2):201–08.

Barnes, M.J. 1964. Reactions to the death of a mother. In *Psychoanal. Study Child* 19:334–57.

Beitchman, J.H., Patterson, P.; Gelfand, B., et al. 1982. IQ and child psychiatric disorder. *Can. J. Psychiatry* 27(1):23–28.

Bellak, L. 1954. *The thematic apperception test and the children's apperception test in clinical use.* New York: Grune & Stratton.

Bemporad, J.R. 1980, *Child development in normality and psychopathology.* New York: Brunner/Mazel Inc.

Bemporad, J.R.; Pfeifer, C.M.; Gibbs, L., et al. 1971. Characteristics of encopretic patients and their families. *J. Am. Acad. Child Psychiatry* 10:272–92.

Bender, L. 1938. *A visual motor Gestalt test and its clinical use.* New York: American Orthopsychiatric Association.

Bender, L. 1956. *Psychopathology of children with organic brain damage.* Springfield, Ill.: Charles C Thomas.

Benton, A.L., 1980. Psychological testing of children, In *Comprehensive textbook of psychiatry*, 3rd ed. eds. A.M. Freedman, H.I. Kaplan, and B.J. Sadock, pp. 2473–83. Baltimore: Williams & Wilkins.

Bloom, L. 1975. Language development review. In *Review of child development and research*, ed. F.R. Horowitz. Chicago: University of Chicago Press, 245–303.

Blos, P. 1971. *The child analyst looks at the young adolescent. Daedalus* 100:961–78.

Bornstein, M.D.: and Kassen, W., Eds. 1979. *Psychological development from infancy: image to intention.* Hillsdale, N.J.: Lawrence Erlbaum Associates.

Bowlby, J. 1958. The nature of the child's tie to his mother. *Int. J. Psychoanal.* 39:350–73.

Brazelton, T.B.; Koslonski, B.; and Main, M. 1974. The origins of reciprocity: the early mother-infant interaction. In *The effect of the infant on its caretaker,* eds. M. Lewis and L. Rosenblum. New York: Wiley.

Brown, R. 1973. *A first language: the early stages.* Cambridge, Mass.: Harvard University Press.

Campbell, M. 1973. Biological intervention in psychoses of childhood. *J. Autism Child. Schizo.* 3:347.

Cantwell, D.P. 1976. Genetic factors in the hyperkinetic syndrome. *J. Am. Acad. Child Psychiatry* 15:214–23.

Carmichael, L. 1970. The onset and early development of behavior. In *Manual of child psychology*, Vol. 1, 3rd ed., pp 447–563. New York: Wiley.

Charles, L.; Schain, R.J.; Zelniker, T.; et al. 1979. Effects of methylphenidate on hyperactive children's ability to sustain attention. *Pediatrics* 64(4):412–418.

Chess, S. 1973. Temperament in the normal infant. In *Children with learning problems: readings in developmental-interaction approach*, eds. S.G. Sapin and A.C. Nitzburg, pp. 291–301. New York: Brunner/Mazel.

Cohen, D.J. 1976. The diagnostic process in child psychiatry. *Psychiatric Annals* 6:404–16.

Cohen, D.J.; Caparulo, B., and Shaywitz, B. 1976. *Primary childhood aphasia and childhood autism: clinical, biological, and conceptual observations. J. Am. Acad. Child Psychiatry* 15(4):604–45.

Cohen, D.J.; Shaywitz, B.A.; Young, J.G., et al. 1979. Central biogenic amine metabolism in children with the syndrome of multiple tics of Gilles de la Tourette: norepinephrine, serotonin, and copamine. *J. Am. Acad. Child Psychiatry* 18:320–41.

Cohen, D.J.; and Young, J.G. 1979. Neurochemistry and child psychiatry. *J. Am. Acad. Child Psychiatry* 18:353–411.

Cohen, D.J.; Detlor, J.; Young, J.G. et al. 1980. Clonidine ameliorates Gilles de la Tourette syndrome. *Arch. Gen. Psychiatry* 37:1350–57.

Cohen, D.J.; Caparulo, B.K.; and Wetstone, H. 1981. The emergence of meanings and intentions: mother's dialogue with normal and language-impaired children. *Psychiatric Clinics of North America* 3(4):489–507.

Cohen, D.J.; Detlor, J.; Shaywitz, B.A., et al. 1982. Interaction of biological and psychological factors in the natural history of Tourette's syndrome: a paradigm for childhood neuropsychiatric disorders. In *Proceedings of the First International Gilles de la Tourette Syndrome Symposium,* ed. T.N. Chase and A.J. Friedhoff. New York: Raven Press.

Conners, C.K. 1974. *Clinical use of stimulant drugs in children.* New York: American Elsevian Publishing Co.

Cox, A.; and Rutter, M. 1976. Diagnostic appraisal and interviewing. In *Child psychiatry,* ed. M. Rutter and L. Hersov. Oxford: Blackwell.

Crabtree, L.H., Jr. 1981. Minimal brain dysfunction in adolescents and young adults: diagnostic and therapeutic perspectives. *Adolesc. Psychiatry* 9:307–20.

Cramer, J.B. 1980. Pyschiatric examination of the child. In *Comprehensive textbook of psychiatry,* 3rd ed., eds. A.M Freedman, H.I. Kaplan, and B.J. Sadock, pp. 2453–61. Baltimore: Williams & Wilkins.

Crandall, B.F. 1977. Genetic disorders and mental retardation. *J. Am. Acad. Child Psychiatry* 16:88–108.

Cronbach, L.J. 1970. *Essentials of psychological testing,* 3rd ed. New York: Harper & Row.

Cunningham, C.E.; and Barkley, R.A. 1978. The role of academic failure in hyperactive behavior. *J. Learning Disabilities* 11(5):274–80.

Cytryn, L.; and Lourie, R.S. 1980. Mental Retardation. In *Comprehensive textbook of psychiatry,* 3rd ed., eds. A.M. Freedman, H.I. Kaplan, B.J. Sadock, pp. 2484–525. Baltimore: Williams & Wilkins.

Douglas, V.I. 1975. Are drugs enough?—to treat or to train the hyperactive child. *Int. J. Mental Health* 4(1–2):199–212.

DeMyer, M.K.; Barton, S.; DeMyer, W.; et al. 1973. Prognosis in autism: A follow-up study. *J. Autism Child. Schizo.* 3:199.

DeQuiros, J.B.; Schrager, O.L. 1978. *Neuropsychological fundamentals in learning disabilities.* San Rafael, Calif.: Academic Therapy Publications.

DiLeo, J.H. 1973. *Children's drawings as diagnostic aids,* p. 227. New York: Brunner/Mazel.

Earls, F. 1976. The fathers (not the mothers): their importance and influence with infants and young children. *Psychiatry* 39:209–26.

Eaton, M.; Sells, C.J.; and Lucas, B. 1977. Psychoactive medication and learning disabilities. *J. Learning Disabilities* 10(7):403–10.

Eisenberg, L. 1956. The autistic child in adolescence. *Am. J. Psychiatry* 112:607.

Eisenberg, L. 1975. *Psychiatric aspects of language disability, reading perception and language.* Drake, D. and Rowson, R., eds. Baltimore: York Press, p. 215.

Eisenberg, L. 1978. Definitions of dyslexia: their consequences for research and policy. *Dyslexia: An appraisal of current knowledge.* Benton, A. and Pearl, D., eds. New York: Oxford Univ Press, p. 29.

Eisenberg, L. 1980. Normal child development. In *Comprehensive textbook of psychiatry,* 3rd ed., eds. A.M. Freedman, H.I. Kaplan, and B.J. Sadock, pp. 2421–42. Baltimore: Williams & Wilkins.

Eissiler, R.S.; Freud, A.; Kris, M, et al. 1977. *Psychoanalytic assessment: the diagnostic profile.* New Haven, Conn.: Yale University Press.

Erikson, E.H. 1959. Initiative verus guilt. Identity and the life cycle. *Psychol. Issues* 1:74–82.

Feshbach, S. 1970. Aggression. In *Carmichael's manual of child psychology* vol. 2, ed., P.H. Mussen, pp. 159–259. New York: Wiley.

Fischer, M.; Harvald, B.; and Hauge, M. 1969. A Danish twin study of schizophrenia. *Br. J. Psychiatry* 115:981.

Fish, B. 1977. Neurobiologic antecedents of schizophrenia in children. *Arch. Gen. Psychiatry* 34:1297.

Flavell, J.H. 1963. *The developmental psychology of Jean Piaget,* pp. 150–63. New York: Van Nostrand.

Fraiberg, S.H. 1959. *The Magic Years,* p. 305. New York: Charles Scribner's Sons.

Frank, R.A.; and Cohen, D.J. 1979. Psychosocial concomitants of biological maturation in preadolescence. *Am. J. Psychiatry* 136:12.

Frankenberg, K.; and Doddes, J.B. 1969. *Denver developmental screening test.* University of Colorado Medical Center.

Freud, A. 1965. *Normality and pathology in childhood.* New York: International Universities Press.

Freud, A 1969. Adolescence as a developmental disturbance. In *Adolescence: psychosocial perspectives*, eds., G. Caplan and S. Lebovici, pp. 5–10, New York: Basic Books.

Freud, A. 1976. The concept of developmental lines. in *The process of child development*, ed. P. Neubauer. New York: Jason Aronson, Inc.

Freud, S. 1924. The dissolution of the Oedipus complex. In *Standard Edition*. London: Hogarth Press, 1953 (19):173–179.

Freud, S. 1953. *The period of sexual latency in childhood and its interruptions. Standard Edition*. London: Gotarth Press, 7:176–179.

G.A.P. Report No. 87 (1973). *From diagnosis to treatment: an approach to treatment planning for the emotionally disturbed child*, p. 139. New York: Group for the Advancement of Psychiatry.

Gaddes, W.H. 1976. Prevalence estimates and the need for definition of learning disabilities. *The neuropsychology of learning disorders*. Knights, R.M. and Baker, D.J., eds. Baltimore: Univ. Park Press, p.3.

Gardner, R. 1979. *The objective diagnosis of minimal brain dysfunction*. Cresskill, N. J.: Creative Therapeutics.

Gauthier, Y.; Fortin, C.; Drapeau, P.; et al. 1977. The mother-child relationship and the development of autonomy and self-assertion in young asthmatic children. *J. Am. Acad. Child Psychiatry*, 16: 127.

Gayton, W.F.; Thorton, K.; and Bassett, J.E. 1982. Utility of the behavior problem checklist with preschool children. *J. Clin. Psychol.* 38(2):325–27.

Geschwind, N. 1976. Language and the brain. In *Progress in psychobiology*, ed, R.F. Thompson, pp. 341–48. San Francisco: W.H. Freeman.

Gesell, A. 1940. *The first five years of life*. New York: Harper & Row.

Gillberg, C.; Rasmussen, P.; Carlstrom, G., et al. 1982. Perceptual, motor and attentional deficits in six-year-old children. Epidemiological aspects. *J. Child Psychol. Psychiatry* 23(2):131–44.

Gittelman, R. 1980. The role of psychological tests for differential diagnosis in child psychiatry. *J. Am. Acad. Child Psychiatry* 19:413–38.

Gittelman-Klein, R.; and Klein, D.F. 1976. Methylphenidate effects in learning disabilities: psychometric changes. *Arch. Gen. Psychiatry* 33(6):655–64.

Gittelmen-Klein, R.; Klein, D.F.; Abikoff, H., et al. 1976. Relative efficacy of methylphenidate and behavior modification in hyperkinetic children: an interim report. *J. Abnor. Child Psychol.* 4(4): 361-79.

Gordon, N.G.; and Kantor, D.R. 1979. Effects of clinical dosage levels of methylphenidate on two-flash thresholds and perceptual motor performance in hyperactive children. *Percept. Mot. Skills* 3(1): 721–2.

Gottesman, I.I.; and Shields, J. 1972. *Schizophrenia and genetics: a twin study vantage point*. New York: Academic Press.

Gottesman, I.I.; and Shields, J. 1976. A critical review of recent adoption, twin, and family studies of schizophrenia: behavioral genetic perspectives. *Schizophr. Bull.* 2:360.

Goyette, C.H.; Conners, C.K.; and Ulrich, R.F. 1978. Normative data on revised conners parent and teacher rating scales. *J. Abnor. Psychol.* 6(2): 21–36.

Green, R. 1974. *Sexual identity conflict in children and adults*. New York: Basic Books.

Green, R. 1979. Childhood cross-gender behavior and subsequent sexual preference. *Am. J. Psychiatry* 136:106–08.

Grossman, H.J., ed. 1977. *Manual on terminology and classification in mental retardation*. Washington, D.C.: American Association on Mental Deficiency.

Gualtieri, C.T.; Adams, A; Shen, C.D., et al. 1982. Minor physical anomalies in alcoholic and schizophrenic adults and hyperactive and autistic children. *Am. J. Psychiatry* 139(5):640–43.

Hanson, D. R.; and Gottesman, I.I. 1976. The genetics, if any, of infantile autism and childhood schizophrenia. *J. Autism Child. Schizo.* 6:209.

Hartlage, L.C. 1977. Maturational variables in relation to learning disability. *Child Study Journal* 7(1): 1–6.

Hartmann, H.; Kris, E.; and Lowenstein, R.M. 1949. Notes on the theory of aggression. *Psychoanal. Study Child* 3(4):9–36.

Hectman, L., Weiss, G.; Perlman, T., et al. 1981. Hyperactives as young adults: various clinical outcomes. *Adolesc. Psychiatry* 9:295–306.

Hertzig, M.E. 1982. Stability and change in nonfocal neurologic signs. *Am. Acad. Child Psychiatry* 3:231–36.

Heston, L. 1966. Psychiatric disorders in foster home reared children of schizophrenic mothers. *Br. J. Psychiatry* 112:819.

Hiscock, M.; Kinsbourne, M.; Caplan, B., et al. 1979. Auditory attention in hyperactive children: effects of stimulant medication on dischotic listening performance. *J. Abnor. Psychol.* 88(1):27–32.

Holt, R.R., ed. 1968. *Diagnostic psychological testing,* rev. ed., eds. D. Rapaport, M.M. Gill, and R. Schafer. New York: International Universities Press.

Horowitz, H.A. 1981. Psychiatric casualties of minimal brain dysfunction in adolescents. *Adolesc. Psychiatry* 9:275–94.

Howells, J.G. 1971. *Modern perspectives in child psychiatry.* New York: Brunner/Mazel.

Hughes, J.R. 1976. Biochemical and electroencephalographic correlations of learning disabilities. *The neurophysiology of learning disorders.* Knights, R.M. and Baker, D.J., eds. Baltimore: Univ. Park Press, p. 53.

Hunt, R.D.; Cohen, D.F.; Shaywitz, S.E.; et al. 1982. Strategies for study of the neurochemisty of attention deficit disorder in children. *Schiz. Bull.* (8):2,236–252.

Illingworth, R.S. 1970. The predictive value of developmental assessment. In *The development of the infant and young child: normal and abnormal,* 4th ed, pp. 5–25. Edinburgh: Livingstone.

Inhelder, B. 1971. The sensory-motor origins of knowledge. In *Early childhood: the development of self-regulatory mechanisms,* eds., D.N. Walcher and D.L. Peters, pp. 141–55. New York: Academic Press.

Jansky, J.J. 1980. *Developmental reading disorders (alexia, dyslexia),* pp. 2551–57.

Jastak, J.J.; Bijou, S.; and Jastak, S. 1965. *The wide range achievement test (WRAT)* New York: Psychological Corp.

Jossetyn, I.M. 1962. Concepts related to child development in the oral stage. *J. Am. Acad. Child Psychiatry* 1:209–24.

Kagan, J. 1979. The form of early development. *Arch. Gen. Psychiatry* 36:1047–54.

Kallmann, F.J. 1946. The genetic theory of schizophrenia. *Am. J. Psychiatry* 103:309.

Kallmann, F.J. 1953. *Heredity and mental disorder.* New York: W.W. Norton.

Kestenberg, J.S. 1970. The effect on parents of the child's transition into and out of latency. In *Parenthood,* eds., E.J. Anthony and T. Benedek, pp. 289–306. Boston: Little, Brown.

Kidd, K.K.; Prusoff, B.A.; and Cohen, D.J. 1980. Familial pattern of Gilles de la Tourette syndrome. *Arch. Gen. Psychiatry* 37:1336–39.

Kirk, S.; McCarthy, J.J.; and Kirk, W. 1965. *The Illinois test of psycholinguistic abilities (ITPA).* Urbana, Ill.: University of Illinois Press.

Kleeman, J.A. 1966. Genital self-discovery during a boy's second year: a follow-up. *Psychoanal. Study Child.* 21:358–92.

Knobloch, H.; and Pasamanick, B., eds. 1974. *Gesell and Amatruda's developmental diagnosis* 3rd ed. New York: Harper & Row.

Kohlberg, L. 1978. Revisions in theory and practice of moral development. In *New directions in child development: moral development,* ed. W. Damon. San Francisco: Jossey Bass.

Kolvin, I., Humphrey, M., and McNay, A. 1971. Studies in the childhood psychoses. Cognitive factors in childhood psychoses. *Br. J. Psychiatry* 118:415.

Kolvin, I., Ounsted, C.; Humphrey, M., et al. 1971. Studies in the childhood psychoses. The phenomenology of childhood psychoses. *Br. J. Psychiatry.* 118:385.

Kolvin, I., Ounsted, C., and Roth, M. 1971. Studies in the childhood psychoses. Cerebral dysfunction and childhood psychoses. *Br. J. Psychiatry* 118: 407.

Kolvin, I.; Taunch, J.; Currah, J., et al. 1972. Enuresis: a descriptive analysis and a controlled trial. *Dev. Med. Child Psychol.* 14:715–26.

Konopka, G. 1973. Formation of values in the developing person. *Am. J. Orthopsychiatry.* 43:86–96.

Koppitz, E.M. 1968. *Pyschological evaluation of children's human figure drawings.* New York: Grune & Stratton.

Kraus, P.E. 1973. *Yesterday's children: a longitudinal study of children from kindergarten into adult years.* New York: Wiley.

Krumboltz, J, and Krumboltz, H.B. 1972. *Changing childrens' behavior. Behavioral techniques for affective parenting.* Inglewood Cliffs. N.J.: Prentiss-Hall, Inc, pp. 142–158.

Kupietz, S.S.; and Balka, E.B. 1976. Alterations in the vigilance performance of children receiving amitriptyline and methylohanidate pharmacotherapy. *Psychoparmacology* 50(1):29–33.

Leckman, J.F.; Detlor, J.; and Cohen, D.J. 1982. Gilles de la Tourette's syndrome: emerging areas of clinical research. In *Childhood Psychopatho-*

logy and Development. New York: Raven Press. (In Press).

Leckman, J.F.; Detlor, J.; Harcherik, D.F., et al. 1982. Acute and chronic treatment in Tourette's syndrome: Clinical response and effects on plasma and urinary catecholamine metabolites, growth hormone, and blood pressure. (Submitted for publication.)

Lewis, D.O., and Balla, D.A. 1976. *Delinquency and Psychopathology*. New York: Grune & Stratton.

Lewis, M. 1982. *Clinical aspects of child development. An introductory synthesis of developmental concepts and clinical experience*, 2nd ed. Philadelphia: Lea & Febiger.

Lidz, T. 1970. The family as the developmental setting. In *The child and his family*, eds. E.J. Anthony and C. Koupernik, pp. 14–40. New York: Wiley.

Livingston, S.; Paulio, L.L.; and Pruce, I. 1980. Neurological evaluation of the child. In *Comprehensive textbook of psychiatry*, 3rd ed., eds. A.M. Freedman, H.I. Kaplan, and B.J. Sadock, pp. 2461–72. Baltimore: Williams & Wilkins.

Lotter, V. 1974. Factors related to outcome in autistic children. *J. Autism Child. Schizo.* 1:124.

Lourie, R.S. 1971. The first three years of life: an overview of a new frontier of psychiatry. *Am. J. Psychiatry*. 127:1457–63.

Lynn, R.; Gluckin, N.D.; and Kriple, B. 1978. *Learning disabilities: The state of the field*. Social Research Council, New York.

MacCarthy, D. 1974. Communication between children and doctors. *Dev. Med. Child Neurol.* 16: 279–85.

Mahler, M.S. 1968. On the concepts of symbiosis, separation, and individuation. In *On Human symbiosis and the vicissitudes of individuation*, vol. 1, pp. 7–31. New York: International Universities Press.

Mahler, M.S. 1975. *The psychological birth of the human infant: separation and individuation*. New York: Basic books.

Mahler, M.S.; Pine, F; and Bergman, A, eds. 1975. *The psychological birth of the human infant*. New York: Basic Books.

Martin, G.I. 1971. Imipramine pamoate in the treatment of childhood enuresis. *Am. J. Dis. Child.* 122:42.

Matarazzo, J.D. 1978. Heredity and environmental correlates of I.Q. *J. Contin. Ed. Psychiatry.* 39:35.

McDermott, J.F.; and Harrison, S.I. 1972. Psychiatric treatment of the child. Central theories. In *Individual psychotherapy, family, group, and milieu therapy, and pharmacotherapy*. New York: Jason Aronson.

McDonald, P.F. 1965. The psychiatric evaluation of children. *J. Am. Acad. Child Psychiatry* 4:569–612.

Mendlewicz, J., Fieve, R.R.; Rainer, J.D., et al. 1972. Manic-depressive illness: a comparative study of patients with and without a family history. *Br. J. Psychiatry* 120:525.

Mikkelsen, E.J. 1982. Efficacy of neuroleptic medication in pervasive developmental disorders of childhood. *Schizophrenia Bulletin.* 8(2):320–332.

Miller, H. 1975. *Systematic parent training*. Chicago: Research Press.

Minuchin, S. 1974. *Families and family therapy*. Cambridge, Mass.: Harvard University Press.

Minuchin, S.; Baker, L.; Rosman, B.L., et al. 1975. Conceptual model of psychosomatic illness in children. *Arch. Gen. Psychiatry.* 32:1031.

Moerk, E. 1974. Changes in verbal child—mother interactions with increasing language skills of the child. *J. Psycholinguist. Res.* 3:101–16.

Nagera, H. 1964. On arrest in development, fixation, and regression. *Psychoanal. Study Child.* 19:222–39.

Nagera, H. 1970. Children's reactions to the death of important objects: a developmental approach. *Psychoanal. Study Child* 25:360–400.

Napier, A.; and Whitaker, C.A. 1978. *The family crucible*. New York: Harper & Row.

Nelson, K.E. 1977. Aspects of language acquisition and use from 2 to age 20. *J. Am. Acad. Child Psychiatry* 16:554–607.

Neubauer, P.B. 1960. The one-parent child and his oedipal development. *Psychoanal. Study Child* 15:286–309.

Neubauer, P. 1976. *The process of child development*. New York: Jason Aronson.

Newman, L.E.; and Stoller, R.J. 1971. The Oedipal situation in male transsexualism. *Br. J. Med. Psychol.* 44:295–303.

Ornitz, E.M.; and Ritvo, E.R. 1976. The syndrome of autism: a critical review. *Am. J. Psychiatry* 133 (6):609–21.

Ouellette, E. 1977. Adverse effects on offspring of maternal alcohol abuse during pregnancy. *N. Engl. J. Med.* 297:528.

Parke, R.D. 1978. Perspectives on father-infant interaction. In: *The handbook of infant development*, ed. J.D. Osotsky. New York: Wiley.

Pascal, C.R.; and Suttell, B.J. 1951. *The Bender-Gestalt test.* New York: Grune & Stratton.

Paul, R., and Cohen, D.J., 1982. Communication development and its disorders: A psycholinguistic perspective. *Schizophrenia Bulletin.* 8(2):279–293.

Pelham, W.E.; Schnedler, R.W.; Bologna, N.C., et al. 1980. Behavioral and stimulant treatment of hyperactive children: a therapy study with methylphenidate probes in a within-subject design. *J. Appl. Behav. Anal.* 13 (2):221–36.

Piaget, J. 1958. *The growth of logical thinking.* New York: Basic Books.

Prugh, D.G. 1963. Toward an understanding of psychosomatic concepts in relation to illness in children. In *Modern perspectives in child development.* ed., Howells. New York: International Universities Press.

Ritvo, E.R. 1977. Biochemical studies of children with the syndromes of autism, childhood schizophrenia, and related developmental disabilities: a review. *J. Child Psychol. Psychiatry* 18:373.

Robson, K.S.; and Mors, H.A. 1970. Patterns and determinants of maternal attachment. *J. of Pediatr.* 77:976–85.

Rosenthal, D.; and Kety, S., eds. 1968. *The transmission of schizophrenia.* Oxford: Pergamon Press.

Rossi, A.C. 1972. Genetics of learning disabilities. *Behav. Neuropsychiatry* 4 (4–5):2–7.

Rotter, J.B. 1975. Some problems and misconceptions related to the construct of internal versus external control of reinforcement. *J. Consult. Clin. Psychol.* 43:56–67.

Rourke, B. 1978. neuropsychological research in reading retardation: a review. *Dyslexia: An appraisal of current knowledge.* Benton, A. and Pearl, D., eds. New York: Oxford University Press, p. 139.

Rutter, M. 1970. Autistic children: infancy to adulthood. *Semin. Psychiatry* 2:435–50.

Rutter, M. 1971. Normal psychosexual development. *J. Child Psychol. Psychiatry* 11:259–83.

Rutter, M. 1972. Clinical assessment of language disorders in the young child. In *The child with delayed speech*, ed. M Rutter and J.A.M. Martin. Clinics in Developmental Medicine, No. 43. London: SIMP/Heinemann.

Rutter, M. 1976a. Separation, loss and family relationships. In *Child psychiatry*, eds. M. Rutter and L. Hersov. Oxford: Blackwell.

Rutter, M. 1976b. Individual differences. In *Child psychiatry*, eds. M. Rutter and L. Hersov, pp. 3–21. Oxford: Blackwell.

Rutter, M. 1980. Psychosexual development. In *Scientific foundation of developmental psychiatry*, ed. M. Rutter, pp. 322–39. London: Heinemann.

Rutter, M.; and Bax, M. 1972. Normal development of speech and language. In *The child with delayed speech*, ed. M. Rutter and J.A. Martin. Clinics Developmental Medicine, No 43. London: SIMP/Heinemann.

Rutter, M.; Graham, P.; and Yule, W. 1970. *A neurological examination: description*, pp. 27–39. London: SIMP/Heinemann.

Rutter, M.; Quinton, D.; and Yule, B. 1977. *Family pathology and disorder in children.* London: Wiley.

Rutter, M.; and Yule, W. 1975. Specific reading retardation. *J. Child. Psychol. Psychiatry*, 16:181.

Safer, D.J. and Allan, R.P. 1976. *Hyperactive children: diagnosis and management.* Baltimore: University Park.

Sandberg, S.T.; Rutter M.; and Taylor, E. 1978. Hyperkinetic disorder in psychiatric clinic attenders. *Dev. Med. Child Neurol.* 20 (3):279–99.

Sarnoff, C.A. 1976. Ego structure in latency. *Psychoanal. Q.* New York: Jason Aronson. 40:387–414.

Satterfield, J.H.; Cantwell, D.P.; and Satterfield, B.T. 1974. Pathophysiology of the hyperactive child syndrome. *Arch. Gen. Psychiatry* 31 (6):839–44.

Schaefer, C.E. 1976. *Therapeutic use of child's play.* New York: Jason Aronson.

Schaffer, H.R., ed. 1977. *Studies in mother-infant interaction.* London: Academic Press.

Shain, R.J. 1972. *Neurology of childhood: learning disorders.* Baltimore: Williams & Wilkins.

Shouse, M.N.; and Lubar, J.F. 1978. Physiological basis of hyperkinesis treated with methylphenidate. *Pediatrics* 62(3):343–51.

Silver, A.; and Hagin, R. 1975. *Search: a scanning instrument for the identification of potential learning disability: experimental edition.* New York: New York University Medical Center, 1975

Simmons, J.E. 1974. *Psychiatric examination of children.* Philadelphia: Lea & Febiger.

Solomon, S. 1975. Neurological evaluation. In *Comprehensive textbook of psychiatry*, vol. 2, eds. A.M. Freedman, H.I. Kaplan, and B.J. Sadock. Baltimore: Williams & Wilkins.

Sperling, M. 1965. Dynamic considerations and treatment of enuresis. *J. Am. Acad. Child Psychiatry* 4:19–31.

Spring, C.; Greenberg, L.M.; and Yellin, A.M. 1977. Agreement of mothers' and teachers' hyperactivity ratings with scores on drug-sensitive psychological tests. *J. Abnor. Child Psychol.* 5(2):199–204.

Stern, D.N. 1974. Mother and infant at play: the dyadic interaction involving facial, vocal, and gaze behavior. In *The effect of the infant on its caregiver*, eds. M. Lewis and L.A. Rosenblum. New York: Wiley.

Stierlin, H. 1974. Shame and guilt in family relations. *Arch. Gen. Psychiatry* 30:381–89.

Stone, L.J.; Smith, H.T.; and Murphy, L.B. eds. 1973. *The competent infant; research and commentary.* New York: Basic Books.

Sulzbacher, S.I. 1975. The learning-disabled or hyperactive child: diagnosis and treatment. *J.A.M.A.* 234 (9):938–41.

Thomas, A., and Chess, S. eds. 1974. Development in middle childhood. In *Annual progress in child psychiatry and child development*, pp. 172–86. New York: Brunner/Mazel.

Thorndike, R.E. 1973. *Standford-Binet intelligence scale, Form L-M 1972, Norms, Ed.* Boston: Houghton-Mifflin.

Thurston, C.M.; Sobol, M.P.; Swanson, J., et al. 1979. Effects of methylphenidate (Ritalin) on selective attention in hyperactive children. *J. Abnor. Child Psychol.* 7 (4):471–81.

Tseng, W.S.; and McDermott, J.F. 1979. Triaxial family classification. *J. Am Acad. Child Psychiatry* 18:22–43.

Warson, S.R.; Caldwell, M.R.; Warinner, A., et al. 1953. The dynamics of encopresis. Workshop, 1953. *Am. J. Orthopsychiatry* 24:402–15.

Weil, A.P. 1977. Learning disturbances with special consideration of dyslexia. *Issues Child. Ment. Health*, 5:52.

Weiss, B. 1982. Food additives and environmental chemicals as sources of childhood behavior disorders. *J. Am. Acad. Child Psychiatry* 21(2):144–52.

Weiss, G.; and Hectman, L. 1979. The hyperactive child syndrome. *Science* 205:1348–53.

Wender, P.H. 1971. *Minimal brian dysfunction in children.* New York: Wiley-Interscience.

Wender, P H.; Pederson, F.A.; Waldrop, M.F. 1967. A longitudinal study of early social behavior and cognitive development. *Am. J. orthopsychiatry.* 37:691–696

Wender, P.H.; Rosenthal, D; Kety, S.S., et al. 1974. Crossfostering. *Arch. Gen. Psychiatry* 30:121.

Werkman, S.C. 1965. The psychiatric diagnostic interview with children. *Am. J. Orthopsychiatry* 35:764–71.

Whalen, C.K.; Henker, B.; Collins, B.E. et al. 1979. A social ecology of hyperactive boys. Medication effects in structural classroom environments. *J. Appl. Behav. Anal.* 12(1):65–81.

Whalen, C.K.; Henker, B.; and Dotemoto, S. 1980. Methylphenidate and hyperactivity: effects on teacher behaviors. *Science* 1280–82.

Wiig, E.H.; Lapointe, C.; and Semel, E.M. 1977. Relationships among language processing and production abilities of learning disabled adolescents. *J. Learning Disabilities* 10(5):292–99.

Winick, M. 1981. Food and the fetus. *Nat. Hist.* 90:76–81.

Winnicott, D.W. 1965. *The maturational process and the facilitating environment*, pp. 56–93. London: Hogarth.

Winnicott, D.W. 1971. *Therapeutic consultations in child psychiatry.* New York: Basic Books.

Wood, D.R.; Reimherr, F.W.; Wender, P.H., et al. 1976 Diagnosis and treatment of minimal brain dysfunction in adults. *Arch. Gen. Psychol.* 33:1453–60.

Young, J.G.; and Cohen, D.J. 1979. The molecular biology of development. In *Basic handbook of child psychiatry*, ed. J.D. Noshpitz. pp. 22–62. New York: Basic Books.

Young, J.G.; Mikkelsen, E.J.; and Cohen, D.J. 1981. Neurobiological approaches to the treatment of children with severe psychiatric disorders. In *Advances in human psychopharmacology*, vol. 2, pp. 65–98. New York: JAI Press, Inc.

Zucker, K. 1982. Childhood gender disturbance: diagnostic issues. *J. Am Acad. Psychiatry* 21(3):274–80.

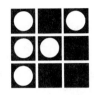

CHAPTER 23

Psychiatric Problems of Adolescence

Robert D. Hunt, M.D.
Donald J. Cohen, M.D.

Adolescence is a particularly turbulent period in one's life. There is often an exaggeration of psychopathology, as well as transient and tentative behavioral experiments, which may eventually determine the adult behavioral pattern. There are special issues in adolescence whose successful mastery have a lasting impact—issues concerning identity formation, sexual feelings, and use of drugs, just to name a few. This chapter provides the physician with the basic understanding concerning the emotional aspects of this transitional period between childhood and adulthood.

EARLY ADOLESCENCE AND PUBERTY

Preadolescence is the developmental phase (approximately ages 11–13 years) which immediately precedes and overlaps with puberty. It is often characterized by increased lability, uncertainty, and unpredictability. Adolescence and puberty are critical organizing phases of psychological and biological development. Rapid bodily changes catapult a child into sexuality, adult appearance, heightened physical strength, energy, and aggressiveness. Strong new impulses and desires can create temporary periods of personality disorganization and family stress (Frank and Cohen, 1979; Hart and Sarnoff, 1971).

In contrast to the phase of latency in which libidinal energies are somewhat more controlled and energy is focused on developing social and academic competencies, puberty brings a state of arousal frequently accompanied by lack of direction. Sexual hormones have direct effects on the brain and mood, in addition to their obvious effects on body morphology and sexual characteristics. This increase in sexual and aggressive feelings occurs concurrent with a qualitative enhancement in cognitive abstract logic and major flux in the child's social world. These simultaneous changes in neuroendocrinology and physique, cognition, emotional attachments, and social focus combine to produce a rapid phase of development and disequilibrium (Freud, 1969).

The industry previously attached to pursuits of learning, hobbies, and friends may fade into deepening introspection, curiosity about the world, and heightened sexual interest. Early adolescence can bring anxiety about separation, autonomy, and decisions, and fear of the power of one's own drives and feelings. Feelings of sexuality, anger, and self-will, accompanied by

---

CASE HISTORY 23–1

David is a 17-year-old, high school dropout. He was brought to his physician by his mother following an arrest for breaking and entering. He had broken into a home with two members of a motorcycle gang, to which he has belonged for about a year. David had behavior problems in school—creating minor distractions in class and being rebellious. His grades were poor, and he quit school in the eleventh grade. He then worked for 3 months as a gardener's assistant for a landscaping company and was fired for missing work and being explosive. He has been unemployed for 5 months. David began using marijuana at age 13 years and rapidly accelerated to a daily consumption of two to four "joints" a day. He drank alcohol frequently on weekends and occasionally experimented with other psychotropic drugs. David has a girlfriend who rides motorcycle with him; their relationship has been stormy. When the criminal charge against David was dismissed on a technicality, his mother decided to bring him to the physician for evaluation. The mother was convinced that David was really a good boy and that underlying depression was making him unable to function properly and feel frustrated. (See appendix at the end of this chapter for further discussion and PEG.)

loss of parental dependency and safety, can be frightening as well as liberating (Blos, 1962, 1971).

Preadolescents often show shorter attention span and may tend to neglect and lose interest in work, hobbies, old friends, and responsibilities. They oscillate between childlike dependency and excessive avoidance of parental involvement. Intrinsic mood changes can produce periods of irritability and depressive infantile behavior, as well as moments of new-found maturity and thoughtfulness (Laufer, 1966).

Family Changes

Sexual symbolism pervades the work and play of preadolescents and is implicit in their curiosity, experimentation, and sharing of romantic and sexual secrets with peers. Heightened embarrassment and privacy may alienate parents and adults. Most early adolescents escape from the family realm into same-sex groups or clubs. Scouts and other organized groups are vehicles for friendship, group learning, and shared adventure. Intense sexual arousal and peer group allegiance often prompts young teenagers to feel alienated from their parents, toward whom they express autonomy, superiority, and boredom.

Alliances within families may change. For example, a father may be uncomfortable about holding or hugging a daughter whose sexual development is becoming obvious. Young adolescents often become modest, shy, more reserved, and self-preoccupied in response to the mental and physical changes facilitated by these hormonal bursts.

Sexual energy of preadolescence reactivates dormant Oedipal issues as intimacy with the opposite sex becomes possible. The emerging teenager often feels the need to break with parents and separate activities and decisions from their sphere of influence. Torn between longings for the old ties of security, closeness, and comfort of middle childhood, but insistent on rebellion, defiance, and assertion to achieve

new autonomy, the young adolescent may experience aspects of mourning. They experience the sadness of losing their childhood and grieve not being able to "go home again" as a little child. Emancipated adolescents may turn their guilt over the forceful breaking of parental ties into hostility against themselves, thereby experiencing a period of anxiety and depression. (Laufer, 1966).

Parents face the difficult task of gradually allowing increasing freedom as teenagers demonstrate competence to care for themselves and exercise judgment outside the home. The gradual process of letting go can easily be subverted into kicking out, giving up, or holding on, depending on the needs of the parent and the maturity of the adolescent. The teenager needs protection and guidance and companionship as well as affirmation of developing competence and increasing freedom. Often behind an adolescent's protest against parental unfairness and statements like, "I don't care what they think," is a lonely pleading to remain important, to be noticed, trusted and even liked by one's parents. At this stage parents and teenagers may benefit from reaffirming their love and importance to each other (Lidz, 1969).

MIDADOLESCENCE

Social Changes

Adolescence reawakens many issues of earlier psychological development as the teenager enters a more complex social environment with heightened impulses. While being more aware of separateness from parents, teenagers continue to need parental reassurance and affection as they seek their role within the world. Sexual desires are reintensified but now the object of these passions is usually a peer, not a parent. Desire for recognition is primarily focused on a teacher, employer, or mentor, rather than a parent. If emergence from the earlier attachments to parents was conflicted, the teenager may be frightened, too eager, or indiscriminate in new attachments (Berman, 1970; Mays, 1971).

The process of "falling in love" is a critical organizing experience for most adolescents (Grinder, 1973). The desire to please a boyfriend or girlfriend—to know and be known personally and sexually—catalyzes the teenager's maturity. Adolescents distinguish between the "purely sexual" and the "romantic, intimate relationship" in which they can share ideals and hopes in the context of love. Teenagers often attempt to do and be their best for their beloved and to live worthy of his or her pride (Nospitz, 1970).

During adolescence, feelings often assume heightened intensity as a youth anguishes over a new-found love. "Will he call?" "Does she like me?" become burning questions of greater emotional intensity. While the initial experience of love and romantic attachment usually begins by sampling a series of brief, intense relationships, it increasingly shifts to focus in depth on one individual for a substantial period.

Identification with an adolescent subculture characterized by its music, the latest dance, and exactly the right clothes enhances the emotional investments outside of the home. The emphasis on peer relations and social acceptance may become almost an obsession. The shift in primacy to the peer group often occurs at the expense of communication with parents and other adults. Collectively, adolescents may flaunt rules and risk danger in groups that strengthen sexual identity and mutual support. Close friendships are much more intense, selective, and intimate. Fantasies and beliefs and ambitions are shared.

The adolescent strives for social acceptance and achievement; success in both areas is a prerequisite for strong self-esteem. When peer group and adult values are relatively compatible, the adolescent learns to utilize competence to gain approval in the adult world. Abilities and accomplishments promote approval that supports confidence, sustained efforts, and concen-

tration. Emerging intellectual powers are as important as physical development in the formation of the inner world of the adolescent (Offer, Marcus, and Offer, 1970).

Cognitive Development

Cognitive growth accompanies and facilitates this stage of biological and social maturation. By midadolescence, cognitive development reaches the stage of formal logic. The teenager develops the ability to think rationally about symbols, concepts, and ideas and to reason abstractly. Gradually, the adolescent learns to reason more abstractly and logically about real and imaginary situations—to think about thoughts, and to evaluate personal and conceptual relationships. They can learn to construct multiple possibilities inherent in a situation, including those not directly observable, and to assume a "hypothetico-deductive" attitude—they understand that a belief or statement is a hypothesis, which is true only if the more concrete notions derivable from it are accurate. The testing of one's intellectual competence often precipitates a battle between parent and teenager as one challenges the validity of parental rules, values, and life style. The adolescent can think about concepts of philosophy, science, and psychology with intellectual maturity and rigor. They also discover subjectivity—the understanding that all experience is really filtered through themselves, whether it originates in the outer world, or in thoughts, dreams, and daydreams.

Teenagers are often serious about religious beliefs, about concepts of truth, fairness, and social justice. Though often lacking in experience and information, they are intrigued by their own developing intellectual sophistication. This cognitive ability becomes the vehicle for redefining a sense of self in the world independent of parents. Clear awareness of past and future, of abilities and interests, enables teenagers to plan meaningfully for future careers and companions (Piaget, 1969).

The rough coincidence in time between the entrance into formal operational thought and the upsurge of instinctual drives allows the preadolescent to create meaning and order to intense drives. Adolescent thought is increasingly oriented toward reality, yet they episodically regress to daydreams and fantasy. As a way of integrating fantasy and reality they select readings and movies about science fiction and romance to bridge imagination and reality. While preadolescents may struggle with abstract and complex principles, they often resort to the familiar use of concrete notions and simple foolproof rules. Not until age 13–16 years do most adolescents achieve the necessary growth of concentration, verbal exactness, and versatility to consistently use formal logic (Flavell, 1965).

Self-Examination

Young adolescents naturally turn their increasing cognitive powers inward. This additional mental sophistication allows a more integrated and clear sense of self, as they place continuing importance on the complex question, Who am I? They reflect a great deal about their bodies, sexual feelings, social relations, and personal successes and failures (Berman, 1970).

Actively striving to understand the many connections between themselves and the environment, they try out different hypotheses about themselves to see whether their accomplishments and the reactions of other people agree with their own images. Though social and romantic relationships are experienced with intense feelings, the healthy adolescent also brings to these relationships considerable reflection and thought. Meaningful distinctions are made between close friends and more casual acquaintances. Older adolescents reflect on their experiences of intimacy, love, and sexuality. They want to know what others think of them. As they test their performance in classroom and work, they develop their own profile of skills and abilities, realizing that they are good at some things and less successful at others. In the healthy adoles-

cent, abilities and self-esteem reinforce each other. Conceiving of themselves as having a personality with specific characteristics of intelligence, interests, preferences, and skills, they begin to frame choices of a future career and companion (Rutter et al., 1976).

The adolescent reflects on differences and similarities between oneself and one's parents in an attempt to clarify personal values. Teenagers acknowledge common beliefs and goals while recognizing differences in personal preferences, style, and abilities which allow them to differentiate from parents. They create an image of how they would like themselves to be and who they hope to become. The ego ideal is often synthesized from experiences with parents, other admired adults, and important peers. If closely linked to their own personalities, the ideal can become an internal guide to self-development. Teenagers also form an idealized image of whom they might love and they project, test and revise this through experiences with boyfriends and girlfriends.

The intensity of these processes led Erikson to emphasize the adolescent's conscious and unconscious efforts to build *ego identity*, and the crisis these endeavors may create for the teenager. However, most teenagers progress through these years as a process of intense but fairly smooth integration. Profound and prolonged periods of depression, psychotic episodes, or destructive antisocial behavior occur in only a small minority of teenagers. Concurrent with overt struggles for independence and separation, healthy adolescents feel considerable respect for and identification with parental life style, values, and even rules (Piaget, 1969; Offer, Marcus, and Offer, 1970; Offer and Offer, 1975).

Values

Adolescents are not merely self-conscious egoists, they are budding philosophers, as well. They apply their new cognitive abilities eagerly to the outside world. From preadolescence onward, many previously accepted rules and values are called into question. This new observant and critical attitude derives from the emerging powers of logic and abstraction, and from learning of new information which seem to contradict preachings and rules. It also stems from the adolescent's own life experience and increasing trust in personal impressions and evaluations. The growing capacity to "decenter" oneself—to see things from another perspective besides one's own—allows more power to compare, generalize, and establish abstract concepts and ideals against which self, family, and society can be measured.

Cognitive growth is also reflected in the moral stances which children take at a certain age. Latency-age children tend to judge actions as good or bad on the basis of their consequences. Older adolescents tend to develop a series of abstract moral principles. Preadolescent moral views reflect thought processes of intermediate sophistication. They understand, as younger children do not, that an individual's intention to help or to please others can be as important as the consequences of an act. Preadolescents tend to see maintenance of family, groups, and national rules as the ultimate criteria of judgment. Older adolescents often adopt a less authoritarian position which tolerates conflicts and diversity based on higher personal principles. For older teenagers loyalty to friends becomes a compelling ideal. This loyalty often extends to a willingness to confront a peer about self-destructive behavior.

LATE ADOLESCENCE

For many older adolescents and young adults, the issues that created internal disequilibrium a few years earlier have now calmed into a more comfortable pattern of behavior reflecting greater mastery and experience. Sexual experience has redefined sexual fantasies and is becoming a familiar and manageable part of one's life. Many older adolescents have established a regular intimate relationship with a special boyfriend or girlfriend. While the specific partner may change a few times during the late teens, the process of striving for intimacy, shared pleasure, and lasting friendships usually reflects more mature personalized attempts at pairing. Earlier desires to simply be accepted or to belong to a group usually become usurped by more discriminate personal alliances. Friendships more accurately reflect shared interests, temperament, and reciprocity and are less dominated by group identity. Older teenagers usually have ties to specific peer groups in which they share achievements, abilities, and activities (Lipsitz, 1979; Offer and Offer, 1975).

Areas of special competence and levels of achievement increasingly define career path. Although the choice of a specific career usually is not complete until adulthood, the general framework of profession or vocation—be it primarily technical or intellectual, skilled or unskilled, interpersonal or mechanical—reflects some dimensions of personality identifiable to the teenager, school, and parents. The process of career selection and preparation, and the attendant competition for academic achievement, is a major task and stress for most teenagers.

The tremendous variability in competence, sophistication, and maturity in social and academic areas reflects the complex dimensions of personality that are becoming organized in this life stage. One teenager prepares to leave home to attend a large university; another chooses a local junior college; a third enters the military; others complete technical, trade, or business school. Many have no defined, marketable skills. The path from late adolescence to adulthood almost always has obstacles and unexpected curves. Some teenagers who achieved high recognition and popularity in high school activities do not easily adapt to the less glamorous pursuit of competence as adults. Many high school scholars are socially "late bloomers"; their sophistication, responsibility, and self-confidence may make them valued leaders, spouses, or friends as they reach adulthood.

Specific beliefs, life styles, and career goals evolve considerably after high school. Yet, fundamental patterns of coping, of relating, and of achieving in specific areas are established by late adolescence and may predict subsequent patterns of adult achievement, intimacy, and enjoyment.

The process of leaving home—as a literal event and as an internal form of self-definition—is a crucial task of late adolescence. Some teenagers escape from an unnourishing or overly controlling home into premature and restrictive marriages. Others exit in anger, leaving home in a storm that may take years to subside. For some, leaving is less conflicted, and home remains a place for "refueling" in a way that does not threaten independence. Separation is much less troubled when one's parents share support and enjoyment of each other. Leaving a parent, or parents, whose life is isolated is more difficult. Teenagers who have established their own competences in social and academic areas and have defined their career goals have prepared a foundation for greater personal independence. Separation usually requires a degree of rebellion on the part of the teenager, or assertion that home is no longer tolerable or is too constricting. This may take the form of conflict over established values, over religious, ethnic, or political identification, or over issues of control and autonomy in selection of friends, curfew hours, regulation of drugs and alcohol, or career choices. Often, once these issues have provided a vehicle for establishing separation, they diminish in significance. These conflicts clarify the extent to which it is mutually tolerable to differentiate, disagree, and separate.

The complex tasks of establishing professional competence in a highly specialized society can prolong the period of training and specialization well into a person's thirties. Graduate education may extend a young person's financial and emotional dependency and complicate the separation process. The selection of life partners is often delayed by the desire to complete a substantial portion of one's training before entering a marriage.

These developmental issues provide the backdrop for many psychiatric concerns of teenagers. The physician can facilitate healthy negotiation of many adolescent issues. He or she must also recognize when a crisis or a teenager's adaptive style is not typical—for example, the adolescent is not simply reflective of the usual emotional stress of adolescent development (Graham and Rutter, 1976).

COUNSELING THE ADOLESCENT

Unlike children, adolescents may decide to contact a physician themselves. The physician may be a teenager's only source of consultation regarding interpersonal or sexual issues, the effects of increasing autonomy on the relationship with parents, or persisting feelings of depression. Sometimes teenagers are brought by others to see a physician for social difficulties including delinquent behavior, promiscuity, or substance abuse. The pediatrician may be continuing previous contact with a child. Some problems which began in earlier childhood, such as developmental delay, learning disability, or hyperactivity may persist into adolescence.

The nature of the physician's relationship with the teenager is often shaped by the type of problem presented and the source of the referral. The lines of accountability for one's work with a teenager may include parents, school, courts, probation officers, or child protective services as well as the patients themselves. Each party may have a different agenda and different ideas about what they want from the physician. Regardless of the specific problem, the physician must consider which of the important participants in the teenager's life are affected by and involved in the issues presented and to whom the physician is accountable. The physician may have a very different relationship with a teenager who is asking privately for birth control pills or for an abortion than with an adolescent referred by the court for school truancy or delinquency. The physician can be caught between conflicting values and loyalties if the teenager is asking for services disapproved of by parents such as birth control and abortion.

When an adolescent is brought in by parents, it is often useful to see the teenager alone before or after a very brief discussion with the parents. This assists in establishing the physician's alliance with the teenager, and underscores the physician's interest in hearing the teenager's view of the problem. With an adolescent the physician may set the stage by saying, "I often talk with teenagers about problems or feelings that make them unhappy and about how they are getting along at home and school. There may be things you would like to tell me that I will keep private." It is usually helpful to ask the adolescent's permission to talk further with parents or others, since if the physician's conversations with parents or teachers are discovered unexpectedly by the teenager, he or she may feel betrayed.

Many teenagers assume that the physician automatically functions as the parents' agent and will immediately attempt to correct, advise, or judge them. Rapport may be established while obtaining a medical history or performing a physical examination or even taking a walk. Later, the physician can ask the teenager more focused questions about events, behavior, and feelings that concern him or her and others. The physician can provide time for crying and experiencing feelings of grief or anger for a teenager seeking a relationship with a trustworthy adult who will not simply tell them to "just try to cheer up and forget about it." Shy or private teenagers may talk more freely out of the office. Having a cup of coffee or taking a walk together may facilitate rapport.

Treatment of an adolescent often involves the family or peers. Concurrent family or group therapy often is a necessary addition to individual counseling (Vick and Kraft, 1973; Rich-

mond, 1974; Abramowitz, 1976; Pasnau et al., 1976; Anderson and Marrone, 1977; Rosenstock and Vincent, 1979).

SEXUAL PROBLEMS OF ADOLESCENCE

The emergence of the bodily changes in adolescence demarcates the transition into adulthood. Powerful feelings of attraction and arousal are evoked. These physical-hormonal changes catalyze a shift in social behavior and in internal self-image. Teenagers' emergent maturity is often experienced as an intensified, renewed link between themselves and their same-sex parent. Whether the teenager is comfortable, hopeful, or dismayed about becoming a man or woman becomes a source of reflection, optimism, or worry. Changes in body images evoke concern about whether one will be attractive, tall or short, have large or small breasts, and be noticed and desired. The changes are often experienced with a mixture of shame and withdrawal during a teenager's entry into sexuality or adulthood (Hart and Sarnoff, 1971; Mays, 1971).

Teenagers frequently encounter physicians in relation to their sexual development and experience. The range of issues presented varies from seeking information about the physiologic aspects of puberty, menstruation, masturbation, ejaculation, or sexual intercourse. Teenagers may request specific contraception or ask about abortion, venereal disease, or highly emotionally charged experiences of seduction, rape, or incest. Even the most mundane aspects of sexuality touch on potentially sensitive aspects of a teenager's internal identity (as "good or bad," desirable or rejectable), and on the social, familial matrix in which he or she lives. The feeling and conduct of one's loving and sexuality become core expressions of the self, and frequently create internal conflict or conflict with parents. For some teenagers, sex and drugs become a battleground for independence, even revenge against parents. In some cases, the teenager presents requests for contraception in clear opposition to parental values and wishes. In other cases the parent drags in a reluctant and embarrassed presexual teenager, saying, "I don't want her to get pregnant." Discrepant wishes between parent and child are an immediate signal to the physician to be thoughtful and carefully consider the interpersonal significance of the request. Rather than being manipulated by either parent or teenager, the physician may choose to identify and discuss the opposing feelings and values presented. There is no simple formula for negotiating this conflict. Neither automatically granting the teenager his or her request, nor insisting on parental agreement and consent seems prudent. The crucial task is to review the meaning of the request with the parties concerned and to clarify its significance within the relationship between teenager and parents. The boundaries of privileged communication are currently being reviewed by many legal authorities and state legislators in effort to define the rights of parents and teenagers. It is helpful for physicians to know the legal constraints in the state in which they practice and to be aware of the underlying values these reflect (Zucker, 1982).

The physician needs to assess the adolescent's competence to make sexual decisions for himself or herself. Does he or she acknowledge the existence of sexual behavior and its possible implications? What level of responsibility can this teenager assume? For example, will a teenager be a more reliable user of the pill than foam or a diaphragm? Is he or she alert to issues of venereal diseases? How will the teenager's sexuality integrate into relationships with parents and peers? If the teenager is acting against parental wishes and values, to what extent is this an angry defiance or a more reasonable difference in values? A teenager who is using sex to get back at parents often may be helped to find other avenues of protest and confrontation that may entail less personal and social risk.

Sex occurring within a context of a close, meaningful—even if temporary—interpersonal relationship with mutual concern for each other's welfare and pleasure can be a positive way of clarifying what is important in choosing and being a lover and spouse.

For some adolescent girls, sexual promiscuity may be an index of distress, helplessness, and lack of self-esteem. Although promiscuity may appear precocious, it is often a pseudoadult sexuality, which aims to satisfy wishes for closeness not received from the parents. This sexual activity may briefly buttress low self-esteem and temporarily relieve loneliness; yet the promiscuous teenager often experiences loss of respect, renewed isolation, and despair. This may be an indication for counseling or psychiatric referral (Schaffer and Pine, 1972).

Contraception

The teenager requesting contraception may raise the physician's concern about parental consent, the type of contraceptive to employ, and the nature of "maturity" of the teenager's sexual activity. A physician cannot assume responsibility for each of these areas, but benevolent interest in them may be of some benefit. The physician may inquire whether the teenager has discussed sexual issues with parents, asking what might happen if they attempted to discuss these. He or she might consider facilitating a joint discussion between parent and teenager. Teenagers often don't know as much as they pretend about facts of sexual anatomy and physiology. The physician or nurse may teach, or refer books following the lead of the adolescent's questions (Zelnik and Kanter, 1980).

It is not the physician's prerogative to judge the legitimacy or advisability of the adolescent's sexual activity. Usually by the time teenagers request contraceptives, they are sexually active. Denial of the contraception seldom limits sexual activity; it merely increases the possibility of pregnancy. It may be useful for the physician to indicate that he or she is available to the adolescent to discuss medical and interpersonal aspects of sexual life.

Frequently teenagers need someone empathetic, experienced, nonjudgmental, and deeply committed to their welfare and development to discuss the management and implications of their love relationships. It may be useful for the physician to inquire whether the adolescent has such a confidant; they may confide in a relative, teacher, or elder. While the physician may become such a counselor, it is important not to presume this role unless it is accepted by the adolescent.

Venereal Disease

Vaginal or penile discomfort from veneral disease or fear of venereal disease can be a source of considerable concern to a teenager. Responses may vary from apparent indifference to exaggerated anxiety about impotence, sterility, or "deserved" punishment for enjoyed pleasure, to feelings of being sexually contaminated, evil, or dirty. Factual clarification of the disease and its treatment may dispel unrealistic fear.

Abortion

In spite of its frequency, abortion evokes profound emotional responses. Pregnant teenagers may be uncertain about whether to seek an abortion and need thoughtful counseling to assist in making this decision. Alternatively, a teenager may have decided to get an abortion but finds herself in conflict with her own values, the preferences of her family, or the desires of the father of the child. Each state has its own rules governing the boundaries of parental consent. The experience of an abortion often evokes worries about control and responsibility for one's own body and destiny, longings about having a baby, concern and moral anguish about inflicting a death, and fear of the pain and the procedure itself. For pregnant teenagers whose feelings, values, and decision may place her in fundamental conflict with parents, boyfriend, or spouse, the decision has tremendous interpersonal and personal implications. For some teenagers the decision to obtain an abortion may be made at the price of alienation from her family or of deep personal feelings of guilt and loss. It is not enough to simply make a rational decision. The process and integration of the complex and frequently ambivalent feelings involved is an important preventative of subsequent depression, guilt, or sexual tension about this act. Reactions to abortion, even if the ultimate decision is clear, may occur months or years after the event (Schaffer and Pine, 1972; Zelnik and Kantor, 1978; McAnarney and Greydanus, 1979).

It is therefore useful for the physician to patiently and without bias assist the adolescent to review her own feelings about each phase of this experience. Did the teenager wish to become pregnant? Was she using contraceptives? What might be the impact on her life of the decision either to have or not to have the child? Does she consider the fetus to be alive, to have a "right" to live, or to be potentially "hurt or killed" by the abortion? How would the act of abortion be viewed in context of her own religious or personal values? What is the opinion of her parents and her partner about the pregnancy? Do they know about it? To what extent can she talk with them about it? How would their knowing of the abortion affect their relationship? Will family and friends support her through this experience? Does she understand the procedure? What plans does she have for future contraception?

It is extremely important for the physician not to impose his or her own values or judgments on this process. Given the press of time, it may be very compelling for physicians to push for a decision—one congruent with their own values and assessment of the situation—and not allow sufficient time and thought for the teenager to reconcile as many facets of this experience as possible before the procedure. It is often useful to refer a candidate for abortion for brief counseling, especially if the patient is having difficulty making a decision, or is likely to feel excessive guilt and ambivalence about the choice, or presents no affect or reflection about a choice of this magnitude. Even when the overt decision is clear, a woman may be expected to feel some sense of depression, loss, and guilt about having an abortion. Often confrontation with these feelings before the procedure will diminish their persistence afterwards. Since many feelings about sexuality, motherhood, even about physicians and surgery, often emerge after the abortion, it may be useful to meet with a teenager to review the process about one month after the procedure (Forrest, Sullivan, and Tietze, 1979; Dreisbach and Kasun, 1981).

Rape

Rape is primarily an experience of violence, violation, and fear rather than being directly sexual. Some victims react with quiet control while others are overwhelmed with fear, anger, and disbelief. Others feel guilt or shame. The need to ventilate feelings of rage and violation must be respected. It is often useful for the patient to have someone familiar with them and/or an experienced rape counselor to be available for support and ventilation shortly after the attack (Brownmiller, 1975; Groth, Burgess, and Holstrom, 1977). As with other traumatic events the impact is not diminished until the victim can relive the experience without profound emotional attachment. Victims often experience exaggerated guilt as though they had precipitated or deserved the abuse even though this may have no rational basis. Homosexual rape may be associated with additional anxiety in someone who is undergoing their first homosexual experience (Symonds, 1976).

Medical aspects of rape management include documentation of abrasions and penetration, evidence of sperm, diagnosis and treatment of possible venereal disease. Specialized rape counseling services including short-term group therapy for victims can often be most helpful (Sadoff, 1976, 1979). Preoccupation with the rape beyond 6 months after the event is often indication for psychiatric referral.

Incest

Incest may have profound impact on the sexual and personal development of a child or teenager. Statistics indicate a *rise* of this phenomenon within our culture. Incest may begin before or during puberty. It is initiated by a trusted older relative. Sexual liaisons most commonly include a girl and her father, stepfather, uncle, or sibling. Occasionally, relations develop between mother or father and son or daughter, older and younger siblings, or other relatives. Incest is rarely a single episode; it is a prolonged liaison which is part of an intense, conflicted, and enmeshed relationship in which boundaries between parent and child have been fractured (Henderson, 1976).

Incest frequently follows a collapse of parental, marital and sexual satisfaction. It occurs in homes marked by other forms of difficulties. In the case of father-daughter incest, often the mother has abdicated her maternal and sexual role and allowed the daughter to assume greater domestic responsibilities. Sometimes with the mother's tacit assent, the daughter may be assigned a sexual relationship with the father. Incestuous fathers are often alcoholic and make their initial overtures while intoxicated. Sometimes fathers are partially disabled, minimally employed, or restricted in their social life. The family is usually enmeshed in problems and isolated prior to the incest (Browning and Boatman, 1977.)

The children are often emotionally deprived prior to the sexual liaison and derive some sense of affection and importance from this special relationship. A combination of special favors or unique power may be offered to reenforce the child's sexual compliance, while physical threats and emotional blackmail may be suggested if the family secret is revealed. Commonly, the sexual relationship is never discussed (Rosenfeld, 1979; Rosenfeld, Nadelson, and Kruger, 1979). The child victim often achieves a sense of special importance and love, and even privileges and power which are exchanged for sexual favors. This aspect of mutual exploitation and manipulation often generates additional guilt. Children frequently feel great shame and embarrassment as, in midadolescence, they become more aware of the deviant and forbidden nature of this relationship. They may blame themselves for compliance and feel added guilt for their partial enjoyment of the sexuality and the favored family position.

The sense of betrayal by a trusted adult is often compounded by a real or covert complicity of the other parent who failed to provide adequate love and protection for the child victim. The child who fails to tell the parents frequently assumes that he or she will be blamed for the event rather than supported and vindicated. As the impact of the incest becomes more apparent, the child often feels profound guilt, identity confusion, and depression. They may develop disgust and avoidance of sexuality; or they resort to promiscuity—an extension of the familial process which suggested that they were only valued for their sexuality.

Subsequent relationships may be fraught with anxieties about trust and abuse. Relationships with the same sex are also frequently conflicted, due to generalization of the resentment for a mother or father who allowed, or even facilitated, this violation and abuse (Lewis and Sarrell, 1969; Borowitz, 1971).

The physician may become aware of incest through secondary manifestations. Depression, anger, defiance, poor and inconsistent performance, promiscuity, running away—all may alert the physician to possible underlying physical or sexual abuse. Careful, but powerful, intervention is needed to halt the abuse and assist the family to reestablish equilibrium. This often requires intensive family treatment and assistance to the victim to resolve intense feelings of anger, guilt, and depression (Weaver, 1979).

Given the complexity and legalities of incest, and the potential for deeply rooted impact on one's subsequent interpersonal and sexual functioning, psychiatric, child protective, and legal assistance is usually mandatory in these cases. Parents also need counseling to reintegrate after open confrontation with incest and sometimes can be assisted to channel their sexuality towards each other.

Homosexuality

Many children have some homosexual experience with peers as a part of adolescent sexual play. This may evoke fears about being "gay" which are usually unjustified. Some children may have a distinctly homosexual orientation from an early age. Homosexual orientation may evolve from early sexual and nonsexual relationships. Early identification with the opposite sex parent or rejection of or by the same sex parent may affect gender identity (Evans, 1969; Kremer and Rifkin, 1969; Siegelman, 1974a, 1974b; Green, 1979).

Children may also be victims of homosexual seduction. Often the targets are attractive children who feel lonely or isolated from their families and are initially courted by an affectionate "protective" adult who offers interest and companionship. For some adolescents, a homosexual experience or preference is a source of profound private and interpersonal conflict. For others homosexuality is accepted quite comfortably as a fact of their life and is not coupled with self-recrimination. However, some gay teenagers who are comfortable with their homosexual orientation may need counseling regarding how to present this to their family. Most teenagers who are in conflict about their sexual identity should be referred for therapy (Saghir et al., 1970; Newman and Stoller, 1971; Siegelman, 1972a, 1972b; Green, 1974).

MEDICAL ILLNESS
IN ADOLESCENCE

Since adolescence is a stage of accelerated bodily change, teenagers are often preoccupied with their appearance and physical development. A boy's increased height and strength and a girl's unfolding beauty are frequently sources of pride and social acceptance and facilitate independence. Physical illness, weakness, or disfigurement are especially threatening during adolescence. The teenager, already prone to feelings of grandiosity and invincibility, may deny the presence of a debilitating illness. Adolescent diabetics may "forget" to take needed insulin injections—or indulge in a binge of sweets— just to see if they "can get away with it." Similarly, asthmatics may "forget" their theophyllin. Considerable embarrassment may be experienced by the teenager with severe acne or dental malalignment requiring braces (Schowalter, 1977).

Younger adolescents have frequent difficulty identifying and expressing feelings, which may impair their talking about it, receiving support, and relieving their resentment. Frequent hospitalizations often mean missing school and important extracurricular activities. For the adolescent, having a chronic or intermittent illness can be stigmatizing and create the hated experience of being different. Emotional or physical illness during adolescence often leads to resentment at having to see a doctor or needing help. The physician may alleviate this by allowing the teenager as much control over his or her activities and treatment as possible. If illness restricts some areas of participation in usual adolescent activities, the physician may suggest other areas for peer involvement. Peer activities with other adolescents experiencing comparable disabilities can enhance self-acceptance and provide emotional support.

Some illnesses have their onset or significant exacerbation during adolescence. The physiologic and emotional changes of puberty may predispose to anorexia nervosa or ulcerative colitis. Anorexia nervosa is of particular interest since its incidence is on the rise, and its etiology suggests roles both for emotional and neurochemical factors.

THE SELF-STARVING
ADOLESCENT:
ANOREXIA NERVOSA

Anorexia nervosa is a disorder of eating which usually has its onset around puberty. Girls are affected about ten times more frequently than boys; sisters of anorectic patients are at higher risk than peers. Profound weight loss may occur as the adolescent retreats from issues of sexuality and independence into preoccupations with weight, food, and dieting. Efforts become directed toward weight loss, including severe restriction of food intake and shifts to low-calorie food. Afflicted teens may resort to self-induced vomiting or the use of laxatives and diuretics; they persist in strenuous exercise in spite of weakness and fatigue. Body image is frequently distorted, and patients are obsessed and preoccupied with striving for thinness and abhorrence of fat. In spite of frequent mirror gazing, they fail to recognize their emaciated condition. Preoccupation with bodily control is evident in food-related behavior. Anorectics may prepare elaborate meals for others, collect recipes, and hoard and hide food inappropriately. They may feel extreme hunger but feel panicked and bloated by eating. They become entrenched in controlling their appetites and impulses, yet frequently feel compelled to indulge in guilt-ridden episodes of bulimia, binges, or gorging massive amounts of food (Burch, 1970b, 1973, 1977; Hsu, Crisp, and Harding, 1979).

Bodily changes subsequent to starvation include bradycardia, hypothermia, hypotension, lanugo hair, amenorrhea, and secondary alterations in hypothalamic-pituitary hormonal regulation and metabolism. The course of the illness is often cyclic with the onset of anorexia following a diet to control obesity which persists until cachexia. Severe weight oscillations may occur over a few months (Halmi, 1980).

Typically, anorectic girls or boys have a prior history of excessive compliance, lack of overt conflict, and inexperience in making choices. They often lack a sense of personal will, direction, or self-definition. The usual passions of adolescence become constrained and smothered by obsessions around food and control. Families become embroiled in efforts to coax or force eating. The dinner table becomes an area for battles over control (Theander, 1970; Cantwell, 1977; Casper and Davis, 1977; Morgan and Russell, 1975).

Treatment

When weight loss is extreme, hospitalization is usually required. Treatment consists of providing consistent rewards for weight gain, family involvement to assist in individuation, and individual or group psychotherapy. Anorectic patients are often quite difficult to treat because they are extremely manipulative and defiant. They frequently avoid the introspection necessary for establishing their own sense of identity by incessantly struggling with staff over issues of autonomy; they may hoard food, vomit, and accuse staff of cruelty and "imprisonment." Behavior modification techniques have been particularly useful in the short-term facilitation of weight gain. While careful supervision with strict limits and rewards for weight gain is necessary during emaciation, dietary control must gradually be returned to the patient before discharge (Minuchin et al., 1974).

Referral for psychotherapy by an experienced clinician is usually essential to recovery. Psychotherapeutic issues often focus on anorectics' experience of themselves and a parent; often they feel they were loved for what they did, not for who they were. Parental feelings of anger and conflict were often denied and expressed covertly—or were so blatantly and violently expressed that the child withdrew. The anorectic

adolescent must be assisted to clarify internal struggles for self-control and fears of autonomy, imperfection, and sexuality. They need to recognize and accept their own impulses, including hunger, and assume responsibility for self-nurturance. Fundamental attitudes about closeness, incorporation, willfulness, dependence, and independence require examination and reintegration. Medications have been tried with questionable results; sedating tricyclic antidepressants (amitriptyline); phenothiazine (Thioridazine); or serotonin antagonist (Cyproheptadine) are occasionally helpful. Increasingly, research supports the presence of physiologic disturbances in neurotransmitters, especially norepinephrine, which modulate appetite (Halmi et al., 1978; Gross et al., 1979; Gerner and Gwirtsman, 1981; Kaye, in press).

Obesity in adolescence often reflects a lack of self-esteem and concerns about social and sex- and Gwirtsman, 1981; Kaye, in press). relieve feelings of boredom, emptiness, and anxiety. Obesity may reflect identification with an overweight parent. In some cases it is a manifestation of hostility towards a controlling, neglectful, rejecting parent. These teenagers often lack a sensitivity to, or may have some disturbance in, their own bodily experience of satiety. Occasionally metabolic disturbances parallel or underline the weight problem. Peer counseling, psychotherapy, behavior modification, and participation in specialized groups for weight control may be useful (Bruch, 1970a, 1971; Knittle, 1971).

THE SUBSTANCE ABUSER

Most adolescents develop the ability to distinguish alcohol and drug use from abuse and restrict use of drugs or alcohol to occasional recreational consumption. They may "get high" at a weekend party, but not during the week or before school. They are able to enjoy themselves and others without chemical assistance; they experience no loss of motivation or direction in school or hobbies. For others, substance use becomes a form of self-medication—a solution for dysphoria. When under stress, when feeling angry, lonely, or depressed—getting high or drunk becomes an escape which thwarts the development of effective mechanisms for handling problems, conflicts, and unhappiness (Miller, 1973).

Some teenagers become habituated or addicted to the use of alcohol or other substances. Such substance abuse is not simply a means of enhancing enjoyment or of diminishing stress; it can become a dominant means of avoiding the pain and struggle of life. Drug use becomes a life style that carries with it the hazards of bodily damage and social deviance. A teenager is more likely to abuse substances if he or she has not developed alternative means of coping and enjoying oneself. Given the important developmental tasks of adolescence—the need to consolidate a sense of identity, to choose interests and companions that fulfill oneself and to establish beginning competence in a career—substance abuse at this age poses a special threat. The developing adolescent brain, somewhat unstabilized through the transformation of puberty, may be pharmacologically more vulnerable to the insult of foreign drugs. Drug use may lead adolescents into a downward cycle: development of competence and school achievement are impeded; deviant and criminal behavior are required to obtain drugs; new anxieties and the absence of meaningful alternatives reinforce drug use (Hauser, 1977; O'Connor, 1977).

Abuse of psychedelic drugs such as LSD, phencyclidine, or psilocybin may precipitate severe disorganization and transient, or occasionally permanent, psychosis. Alcohol and barbiturate abuse is often associated with depression and suicide attempts. Psychostimulants such as amphetamine or cocaine may elicit excitement, aggressive behavior, and psychosis; repeated use is followed by severe depression upon withdrawal.

Substance use or abuse is a frequent source of parent-teenager conflict; contests between the adolescent's need for parental protection and desire for autonomy. Because substance abuse can evoke powerful parental feelings, communication across generations may break down quickly into adversarial stances. In some cases, substance abuse becomes a vehicle of focusing a latent conflict—or of facilitating emotional separation from parents. Although the occasional use of marijuana by adolescents can be as innocent as a social beer, parents may become punitive and rejecting about such behavior.

Treatment

The physician must counsel the family and adolescent without becoming merely another participant in a family dispute. In assessing the impact of substance use or abuse for a teenager, physicians must evaluate not only type, frequency, dosage, and physiologic effects of the substance being used; they must also assess the drug's impact on the adolescent's academic and work performance and peer and family relations. Even drug or alcohol use that is developmentally and biologically benign may become a major source of difficulty if the family's response is extreme.

Peer counseling and group therapy are often more useful than individual psychotherapy for adolescent substance abusers. Peers can assist the abuser to recognize underlying feelings of anger and helplessness which frequently precede indulging. They can effectively confront each other with excuses given for relapse, and provide emotional support at times of vulnerability. Such peer support groups often are experienced by teenagers as a "second family." The mutually caring relationships which evolve may give some purpose to their lives and promote adaptive social skills. The therapeutic task consists not only of relieving the abuse pattern but also of developing constructive skills towards career development and interpersonal intimacy (Rachman, 1971).

Medication may have a role in treating some forms of substance abuse. Disulfiram (Antabuse) is often useful for the impulsive, episodic drinker. Methadone may assist the heroin addict by neutralizing the "high" or euphoric feeling which follows injection. Residential placement may be necessary to obtain behavior control and improve interpersonal relationships (Baker, 1974; Davids and Salvatore, 1976; Marsden, McDermott, and Monor, 1977). Additional aspects of treatment are discussed in Chapters 15 and 16.

DEPRESSION

Disturbances of mood in adolescence may be difficult to identify. Most teenagers experience intense variability of mood as they explore the excitement and disappointment of love, and the successes and frustrations of striving for competence and identity. Some teenagers, however, characteristically exhibit a flatness of affect or overt depression. Persistent boredom, lack of energy, or somatization may be evidence of depression in a teenager. Profound oscillations of mood may occur in early-onset manic-depressive illness (Cytryn and McKnew, 1974).

While many adolescents can clearly describe their own moods, others seem to lack the emotional vocabulary and self-perception to identify their own depression. It is a common error for the physician, parent, or teacher to overlook persistent, serious depression in a teenager because "adolescents are always upset." In fact, low spirits and social withdrawal lasting more than a month, especially when associated with disturbed appetite, troubled sleep, decreased energy, and easy fatigability, are reliable signs of clinical depression. Teenagers may describe themselves as being bored, having nothing to do, feeling worthless or "like a blob." They may feel misunderstood or disliked and hated by their parents. They may complain about aches or headaches or express exaggerated dislike of their body and appearance (Feinstein, 1975).

Recognition of depression is complicated by

the fact that depressed teenagers often show less psychomotor retardation and less persistence of an overtly depressed mood than do adults. Although their mood brightens when they talk with a friend or go to a party, they may rapidly return to a depressive state when alone. Intellectualization may mask depression behind excess cynicism and self-righteous complaints that the world is so unjust and unfair as to not deserve their participation. The relative prominence of subjective distress, somatic complaints, and functional impairment may vary greatly among depressed children and teenagers. Depression may have onset in prepuberty and may be masked by symptoms of hyperactivity, inattention, boredom, or apathy. Loss of interest in school, extra-curricular activities, sports and hobbies, or excessive day dreaming, and self-preoccupation are important signs of depression. However, depressed youngsters frequently reveal their distress, complaining persistently that they feel unloved, bad, unhappy, sad, evil; they often look tearful, angry, or desperate. Yet parents, teachers, and physicians may ignore or dismiss these symptoms as "just a phase."

As discussed in Chapter 10, depression is a major cause of teenage mortality. *Suicide* is the third leading cause of death in adolescence. Many teenagers who commit suicide make attempts or gestures prior to their death. A suicide attempt always requires a careful psychiatric evaluation including the immediate precipitants, the anticipated interpersonal effects, and the social support available to the teenager. In some cases, a suicide attempt is a plea for attention, alliance, or affection from a specific friend or relative. Suicide may represent an identification with a dead relative or friend or be a fantasized method for reunion with an unmourned, deceased parent. While repeated suicide attempts may become a form of social manipulation, more often they are an expression of profound hopelessness, abandonment, emptiness, and anger. The extent of the teenager's support from friends and family affects the immediate risk of a subsequent attempt and the need for hospitalization. Alcohol and substance abuse are frequently associated with teenage depression and suicide attempts. These agents may be unsuccessfully used by an adolescent in an effort to avoid depression; often, however, they may intensify depression, impair judgment, and increase the vulnerability to suicide (Lourie, 1966; Crumley, 1979; Cytryn et al., 1980; Kashani et al., 1981; Carlson, 1981).

Depression in adolescence reduces emotional availability to new experiences and erodes self-esteem by prolonged feelings of guilt and inadequacy (Puig-Antich, 1982a, 1982b).

Some adolescents engage in self-destructive behavior which is dangerous but not intentionally suicidal, such as superficial wrist-cutting, reckless driving, and frequent fights. These symptoms are often suggestive of serious personality disorder. They provide means of stimulus and attention-seeking, and often serve to focus the concern of others on the adolescent's uncontrollable behavior while diverting the adolescent from his own feelings of emptiness, depression, futility. Such a teenager often blames others for difficulties and feels rejected. These behaviors incite conflict within the teenager's family—often leading parents to fight themselves. Peers are often frightened away by repeated episodes of self-destructive behavior— thus leaving the adolescent more isolated and vulnerable (Weinberg et al., 1973; Rabin and Swenson, 1981; Puig-Antich, 1982b). The use of the PEG for assessing depression in a teenager is illustrated in the appendix.

Careful psychiatric evaluation of the teenager, family, and social network is mandatory. In psychotherapy, understanding of the child's life experience may uncover conscious and unconscious sources of depression. Teenagers may need to grieve old or recent losses, increase their abilities to assert and manage their anger, and to clarify and release feelings of guilt or inadequacy. The difficult therapeutic task is to stop the destructive behavior and gradually

facilitate the teenagers' confrontation with their own feelings and impulses. Maintaining a stable relationship with a therapist whom the teenager can experience as having both good and bad qualities is essential for reintegration of the teenager's divided desires. Family conflict is the frequent backdrop of destructive adolescent behavior or personality disorder. Sometimes anger and disappointment towards a spouse may be displaced onto the child—or create an environment of hostile tension with which the teenager identifies—but in which he or she cannot thrive. A residential or hospital setting may be necessary to limit acting out destructive impulses (Masterson, 1967, 1972).

Antidepressant medication has an important role in the treatment of persisting depression, especially if associated with somatic signs such as fatigue, insomnia, and anorexia. Tricyclic antidepressants (imipramine) should be increased gradually from 1 mg/kg daily up to a maximum of about 3 mg/kg/day (for young adults) to 5 mg/kg/day (for children). Divided doses reduce cardiotoxicity, but an ECG should be obtained before increasing the dose to assure that the PR interval is not prolonged beyond 16 seconds, and the QRS segment not increased beyond 130% of baseline (Puig-Antich, 1982c). Blood levels of antidepressants should be obtained if a depressed child or adolescent fails to respond to an appropriate therapeutic dose within 3 weeks (Feinstein and Wolpert, 1973; Lowe et al., 1981).

Bipolar Illness

Mania and manic-depressive illness occur in adolescents, although the onset is usually later. Mania must be distinguished from bursts of normal adolescent exuberance and from the fidgetiness and restlessness of the "hyperactive" or attentionally impaired child or teenager. True mania is characterized by sustained periods, usually several days to weeks, of increased physical activity, decreased sleep, irritability, racing thoughts or flight of ideas, and speech. An increased desire to socialize, coupled with diminished judgment, may lead the teenager to make excessive phone calls, or write numerous letters, party excessively, and be more extroverted than usual. During a manic phase, there may be an increase in sexual activity, promiscuity, and seductiveness. With fading judgment and emerging grandiosity, the manic patient may embark on many projects, spend money, and do or say things which later may·create embarrassment.

Referral for psychiatric evaluation and therapy is mandatory for an adolescent with persisting depression or an episode of mania. Considerable expertise is required for the diagnosis and integration of personal and familial issues in psychotherapy and for the management of medication. In adolescents the distinction between borderline personality disorder, schizophrenia, and manic-depressive psychosis may be difficult. Many adolescents who are hospitalized for an apparent schizophrenic episode are later found to be predominantly experiencing affective swings which often respond to lithium. In evaluating an affectively disturbed adolescent, the patient's emotional development should be reviewed. Were there previous episodes of mania or repeated cycles of depression? Did mood cycles occur according to an intrinsic rhythm or appear as a response to stress, such as the loss of a relationship or a life change? Patients and family tend to "find a reason" or precipitant for mood changes within the normal events of life (Feinstein and Wolpert, 1973).

Psychotherapy can assist the teenager to identify and perhaps avoid precipitants to mood swings, and to acknowledge and integrate sadness and anger in ways that diminish global mood changes. Treatment may also promote a more stable sense of self in spite of mood fluctuations.

Lithium carbonate has been very useful in the treatment and prevention of both adult and adolescent mood changes. Lithium is gradually increased until a therapeutic blood level of 0.8–1.2 mEq/L is obtained. In patients who have severe cyclic affective changes, lithium (0.7–0.9 mEq/L) may be prophylactic. Similarly, lithium is useful in blunting recurrent depressions and may be utilized when an antidepressant might precipitate a manic swing.

THE ANXIOUS ADOLESCENT

Many adolescents experience diffuse anxiety or fears in response to separation, meeting strangers, or not reaching expectations of performance. Adolescent anxiety often has its roots in childhood experience. Whereas the stimulus for anxiety is often less specific in younger children, it usually becomes more focused in adolescence. Anxiety is a common feature of many major psychiatric disorders, such as phobias, depression, or psychosis, but is not usually diagnosed separately in these contexts (Compton, 1972; Yorke and Weisberg, 1976; May, 1977).

Clinical anxiety in adolescence may have many roots. Some teenagers experience generalized anxiety that is not focused on a specific worry, fear, or situation (in contrast to separation or stranger anxiety) and has no traumatic precipitant. Some adolescents may still harbor childhood fears of harm from burglars, kidnappers, animals, or machines, or a fear of the dark. More commonly adolescents experience performance anxiety as their apprehension focuses on school, exams, deadlines, or papers and talks. Teenagers experience considerable insecurity about the future. A sense of personal futility may derive from excessive concern about their eventual economic security or possible political or military dangers. As teenagers become concerned with peer acceptance, considerable anxiety may be evoked by actual social or heterosexual experiences or may center on vague concern about "being popular" or being accepted by a specific peer group. Anxiety may precipitate somatic symptoms, such as a "lump in the throat," shortness of breath, nausea, or may lead to nightmares, insomnia, or enuresis. Traveling, sleeping away from home, and driving a car may become limited. Anxious children may be perfectionistic, obsessive, approval-seeking, restless, and "nervous," but anxiety may be a major symptom in children with varied personality difficulties, including antisocial disorders.

Counseling or behavioral therapy may be effective in acute, focused, or phobic anxiety. Tricyclic antidepressants, especially imipramine, may be useful in blunting phobic or panic anxiety reactions. Referral for psychiatric evaluation and psychotherapy is indicated when the anxiety is intense, vague, generalized, or interferes with social or academic functioning. Specialized therapeutic expertise may be needed to clarify the personal meaning and precipitants of the anxiety and its relationship to family conflict and life history.

Several specific forms of anxiety—related to separation, emancipation, performance inhibition, and identity consolidation—will be discussed in more detail later and are described in Chapter 11.

SEPARATION ANXIETY

Some teenagers feel extreme homesickness and discomfort approaching panic when they are away from home. They may become sad, depressed, tearful, anxious, or nauseated; they may develop vomiting, headaches, or dizziness while anticipating or experiencing separation. They may present a series of somatic complaints to physicians who, unless they ask, may fail to link these responses to a change in life circumstances. Yet, these children are asymptomatic when not threatened with separation. Onset of symptoms may be in early childhood when the child leaves home to go to school. Symptoms may wax or wane during adolescence. In severe form, separation anxiety can lead to school refusal, social isolation, and may result in multiple physical examinations and medical procedures. Whether the onset is in childhood or adolescence, these individuals are often demanding, intrusive, and in need of constant attention;

they tend to be preoccupied with reunion fantasies. Separation anxiety characteristically develops in conscientious, conforming youths from close-knit families. Onset may follow a loss, death, move, or other life stress.

EXTREME SHYNESS

Excessive shyness even after prolonged exposure to strangers is manifested by staying at home and actively avoiding strangers. Overly shy teenagers are primarily embarrassed, timid, and unaggressive, rather than angry or fundamentally uncommunicative. Although they are able to separate from parents without prominent anxiety, they have extreme difficulty with involvement with strangers and are overly inhibited in social situations, such as school. This difficulty can impair socialization and peer relationships and lead to school refusal. Academic performance and self-esteem may be diminished, eventually precipitating truancy and depression. For some children, stranger anxiety is episodic, while for others, it is continuous.

Physician counseling may be useful in helping the adolescent to function independently and help clarify the fears of loneliness, rejection, or incompetence that frequently mobilize this anxiety. Behavioral techniques may support a teenager's increasing experience of independence. Psychiatric referral is indicated if the anxiety persists for greater than 6 months or interferes with social, career, or academic adjustment away from home. Insight-oriented psychotherapy may be useful to an adolescent whose fear of separation derives from ambivalent feelings towards parents from whom the adolescent may paradoxically seek both independence and perpetual supervision.

Disguised hostility may be overtly expressed as excessive concern for a parent's welfare and consequent inability to differentiate and separate. Family therapy is often useful in identifying subtle familial expectations of eternal loyalty and dependency. Parents may engender guilt and fear in a teenager who is attempting appropriate separation and autonomy. The therapist can assist parents to care for each other, to develop interests and friendship beyond their children, and eventually give genuine permission and support to their teenagers efforts at independence.

Medication (tricyclic antidepressants) may be useful if separation anxiety is a manifestation of more pervasive depression. Panic anxiety attacks may also respond to tricyclics, to propranolol, or clonidine. Individuals who are withdrawn, anxious, rejection-sensitive, or have paranoid anxiety and depression may respond best to monoamine inhibitors (MAOs) such as phenelzine sulfate (Nardil).

EMANCIPATION DISORDER

Upon leaving home, some older adolescents and young adults experience symptoms of internal conflict over the independence which they overtly desire. They may have difficulty making decisions and be very dependent on peers or parents for advice and support. Others respond to this transition by oppositionally rejecting parental support and values—or by vacillating between extremes. Transient appetite, sleep, or other somatic difficulties may accompany anxiety or depression associated with this new adjustment. Separation anxiety reflects the conscious desire to reunite; emancipation anxiety follows the choice to separate.

Physician support can greatly assist newly emancipated teenagers to establish themselves securely outside the home, to care for themselves, and to maintain contact with an older, experienced adult. Only if the adolescent has continued difficulties with this separation or if intense identity issues arise is psychiatric referral necessary. Peer group therapy may support this transition outside the home. Individual insight-oriented therapy may clarify and diminish guilt regarding emancipation. Family therapy may be

beneficial if the parents can first resolve their feelings of loss or blame attendant to the teenager's separation. Medications may have a role comparable to that described for separation anxiety.

THE PASSIVE LONER: UNSOCIALIZED, UNAGGRESSIVE CONDUCT DISORDER

Some adolescents show no depth of interpersonal attachment and have little capacity for appropriate guilt. Relating to others through manipulation, they can be friendly and ingratiating when they expect benefit and then ignore the same person when there is no potential gain. They are detached, and have no stable relationships or bonds; they lack friends and personal loyalties. Though usually not violent or aggressive, they may lie brazenly, steal, cheat, and feel remorse and anxiety only when they are caught and stand in danger of punishment. They are usually seclusive, lonesome, withdrawn, and apathetic; they may daydream excessively and avoid tasks or assignments requiring sustained effort or concentration (McConville and Boag, 1973; Gelfand, 1978).

While usually less violent than the individuals described in the subsequent sections, they may be arrested for stealing, forgery, gambling, or substance abuse. Depression, discouragement, drug abuse, and suicide attempts may follow in the wake of social isolation, characterized by lack of attachment, direction, and integrity. Some of these individuals later may commit isolated acts of extreme violence. These teenagers frequently come from chaotic, nonnurturing homes or from institutional settings where they failed to form primary attachments.

Therapy is difficult due to their lack of subjective attachment and motivation. Intensive and prolonged group confrontation and support is sometimes useful. For such adolescents, the conflicting needs to be cared for and comforted and to gain autonomy and self-esteem may be usefully explored by the primary physician. Psychiatric consultation for the teenager and family may be helpful in dealing with underlying feelings of depression and poor judgment, and may assist the teenager to achieve greater self-esteem and autonomy. Often such teenagers need a primary relationship as a springboard for achieving self-confidence and thoughtfulness, but are extremely limited in their capacity for involvement.

ACADEMIC OR WORK INHIBITION

Individuals who have previously performed adequately at school or work may temporarily become unproductive and ineffective due to anxiety about exams, papers, performance, or work tasks. They may experience inability to concentrate, to organize their efforts; they may procrastinate or fail to complete tasks which are ordinarily within their level of competence. This dysfunction most often occurs during a period of internal reorganization or stress—such as while making a career choice or taking college entrance exams, completing major school or work assignments. There may be associated anxiety and transient reactive depression. The difficulty is usually temporary and can frequently be alleviated by physician counseling which clarifies the nature of the distress and its symbolic significance. Psychiatric referral is indicated if this lack of productivity persists or is associated with more generalized depressive symptoms or cognitive disorganization. Underlying feelings of guilt may attend either the teenager's perception of having failed to fulfill parental and personal expectations or paradoxically, having exceeded fulfillment of these expectations. A teenager may feel that he or she has disappointed his or her parents, or alternatively, surpassed them in certain areas. If an adolescent's values and aspirations are markedly discrepant from those held by the parents, he or she may feel "at a loss," empty, or confused while embarking on a new direction. Particularly if parents condemn or feel intimidated by the adolescent's life choices and life style, the youth confronts a difficult task of integrating personal desires with heritage. He or she may face a major conflict in identity consolidation.

VIOLENCE AND AGGRESSION

Unsocialized Aggressive Conduct Disorder

Teenagers with conduct or behavior disorders may have impaired ability to modulate aggression, form attachments, and consolidate personal values. Some teenagers with aggressive behavior lack empathy, respect, and attachment to others. Alienated from peers as well as from adults, they may bully and torment peers and become hostile, defiant, and abusive with adults. Their antisocial behavior may include destruction of property, vandalism, persistent lying, stealing, truancy, physical violence, and cruelty. Difficulties at home, school, and in the community may arise in areas of sexuality, violence, and substance abuse. These individuals frequently lack the ability for sustained closeness with others and usually have not developed vocational skills for self-support. They may give and receive physical abuse at home and from peers, and they are almost always in trouble with school and legal authorities. They often come from fractured homes characterized by parental abuse, rejection, inconsistent harsh discipline, or similar parental antisocial behavior. Boys from lower socioeconomic environments are at highest risk. The prognosis is poor for those adolescents who show impoverished attachment and disregard for others, little self-control and direction, and few social skills (Evans, 1966; Wardrop, 1967; Lewis and Balla, 1976). As adults they may experience many of the difficulties described in Chapters 17 and 4.

Referral for individual or intensive group therapy may be usefully combined with placement in a residential school, which has clearly defined rules and behavioral consequences. Often extreme social isolation requires intensive long-term psychotherapy for the teenager to form an important relationship through which to internalize socially acceptable values.

Frequently these teenagers lack genuine empathy for others. Inexperienced at discriminating their own feelings, they often are unable to imagine the emotional consequences of their actions on others. Their own lives are often fraught with anxiety, loss, and deprivation. Frequently these teenagers were raised by inconsistent, emotionally unavailable, excessively strict or negligent parents. Physical abuse and violence are frequent components of these adolescents' life histories.

Other medical and psychiatric disorders may underlie the behavior of some antisocial adolescents. Seizure disorders have been noted in increased frequency among children and adolescents who have committed homicide (Lewis, 1978). Psychosis and schizophrenia have been evident in a disproportionate percentage of severely antisocial adolescents. Depression may be a treatable substrate for violent or antisocial behavior in others. Thus, "character disorder" is not the sole determinant of antisocial behavior.

Socialized Aggressive Conduct Disorder

Other adolescents exhibit antisocial, violent, criminal, or risk-taking behavior as part of their group identity. As members of a gang or club, they may share dangerous initiation and leadership rites which confirm intense loyalties to the group members and their values. In quest of adventure, power, acceptance, or protection, they may fight other gangs, seek revenge, or steal money, property, and drugs. Group loyalties often supercede and conflict with familial ties and with academic pursuits. Truancy, arrest, and injury are common. Many gang members come

from dysfunctional, impoverished families with absent or alcoholic fathers. While some individuals later become adult criminals, many achieve an adaptive social adjustment spurred by their ability to form meaningful attachments. Therapy aimed at redirection of group goals and activities or integration of the individual into groups with socially productive goals may be beneficial (Richmond, 1974).

The evaluation of teenagers who are aggressive, violent, or destructive requires assessment of many dimensions of their personalities and their social interactions. Such behavior reflects social isolation and lack of group values; for others, delinquent behavior is part of a group identity. Intense attachment to a group or gang may be an attempt to compensate for a lack of family involvement. For a few teenagers antisocial behavior represents an identification with deviant familial values. Other teenagers are violent or destructive as an expression of severe depression, anger, or inadequate cortical inhibition of impulses—such as may occur in some children with hyperactivity or seizure disorders. For some teenagers, violence occurs in context of psychosis or substance abuse (Jenkins, 1973; Lewis et al., 1979).

IDENTITY DISORDERS

Identity disorders are manifested by intensive subjective distress regarding issues such as long-term goals, career choices, values, and personal loyalties—choices that reflect and consolidate a sense of personal identity. This inability to decide and pursue a commitment—the ambivalent attraction to incompatible alternatives in friends, life style, religious or moral values—indicates a lack of coherent identity. Such an individual's self-view may be markedly discrepant from the impression others have of him or her. The teenager may experience anxiety and depression regarding these internal issues, which intensifies self-doubt and despair about the future. He or she may resort to impulsive experimentation in life style or vacillate between widely divergent roles, or may become oppositional and negativistic in an effort to achieve a sense of independence but remain unable to direct that freedom toward meaningful, self-defined goals. Identity diffusion may occur as such adolescents attempt to establish themselves apart from familial values; or it may arise later as they question earlier life decisions. Achieving a sense of integrated identity is more complex if there is great discrepancy between rigidly held parental, peer, and personal values; identity formation is more difficult and hazardous if the teenager faces the possibility of extreme parental rejection if he or she chooses values which differ from those of parents. The process is compounded by the increasing range of options and life in today's pluralistic society. Chronic failure to resolve these issues may result in inability to complete or enjoy tasks, failure to achieve academic or career goals, and frequent shifts in interests or personal relationships. While it is an appropriate focus of adolescence to struggle with issues of identity—selection of career and companion, values, and life style—referral for psychiatric evaluation is indicated if the teenager is unable to make any choices, becomes depressed, and remains confused about himself or herself (Hauser, 1976).

THE NEGATIVISTIC, DEFIANT TEENAGER: OPPOSITIONAL DISORDER

Some children and teenagers exhibit a pattern of oppositional or negativistic behavior directed toward parents, teachers, or peers without concomitant antisocial behavior. They are continuously argumentative, unresponsive to reasonable persuasion, provocative, stubborn, actively or passively resistive, dawdling, or belligerent, in spite of clear expectations, limits, and discipline. This pervasive opposition to authority persists regardless of self-interest, reason or the personality of the authority. The teenager's passive-aggressive or resistive style provokes anger and rejection from caretakers and authorities. School difficulties and academic underachievement often follow resistance to external demands. Onset may be at any stage of childhood after age 2 years. This diagnosis only applies to individuals whose oppositional behavior reflects a personality style that continues for years and is directed against various authority figures. It does not describe a teenager who becomes angry at a parent for several months during specific conflicts about curfew, limits, or values. Oppositional teenagers exhibit less antisocial behavior than those with aggressive conduct disorders, but this behavior pattern may coexist with other psychiatric disorders. Treatment of the oppositional adolescent is difficult because the physician or therapist may be seen as simply another authority to be resisted. An alliance must be formed with the teenager that gradually acknowledges the difficulties created by this belligerence (Anthony, 1976; Gilpin, 1976).

SUMMARY

Each life stage builds upon past experience while adding new arenas and tasks for development. In prepuberty children often experience a reflective withdrawal from parental intimacy and from previously defined values. Concern about bodily development and appearance, about sexuality and popularity predominate during early adolescence. Propelled by hormones into a burst of physical and emotional change further buttressed by the emerging capacity for formal logic, teenagers integrates another level of identity formation. They think about their own personality and values in comparison to those of their parents. In late adolescence, the developmental tasks become those of establishing a career direction which reflects actual abilities and interests, forming meaningful and potentially sexual relationships, and beginning the exodus from home.

The phenotype or clinical manifestation of many childhood psychiatric disorders evolve with the child's development and may be altered by environmental influences. For example, attentionally impaired children frequently become less motorically hyperactive and fidgety in late adolescence and young adulthood, but frustration due to inadequate academic performance and lack of job skills may increase their potential for antisocial behavior. The increased physical strength and aggressiveness of adolescence frequently creates increased problems for the families of intellectually impaired and autistic children. A temper tantrum consisting of kicking and throwing in a 3-year-old is much easier to control than the same behavior in a 16-year-old. These adolescents' sexual desires may be untempered by social skills or controls. The ubiquitous teenage desire to have friends and be accepted by a peer group may make adolescence a time of poignant, lonely disappointment for retarded teenagers. New life concerns often bring adolescents to physicians. Issues related to bodily functioning, sexual relations, veneral disease, pregnancy, contraception, and abortion are encountered by physicians in their dealings with teenagers.

Affective disturbance may emerge in childhood and adolescence as a reaction to loss or failure, and as symptom of inadequate emotional nurturance and support. Depression may be manifested by diminished functioning in academic or social arenas, coupled with a loss of interest in past pleasures and achievements or by increasing somatic complaints. Antisocial behavior more often emerges in adolescents who have underlying organic disturbance, who lack self-esteem, or who have not developed sufficient internalized controls, values, and competencies. This behavior, especially when performed in social isolation, may reflect an inadequate personality or defective superego. Substance abuse when employed as a means of avoiding unpleasant feelings or difficult tasks, may be a symptom of masked depression and eventually

deplete the adolescent of his or her energies and direction. Less severe disorders such as anxiety about separation, socialization, and emancipation concern many adolescents. These concerns may present as pervasive opposition in some teenagers, work inhibition in others, or as frustration in identity formation. Physician counseling can often be effective for these individuals unless symptoms persist or generalize.

The ability of the physician to form a trusting relationship with adolescents and parents of varying ages is a prerequisite to evaluating emotional disturbance within the child or family. The relationship not only facilitates the disclosure of emotionally significant information, but it is often the healing vehicle of treatment. Psychiatric treatment may be necessary since some adolescents are inexperienced and resistant in forming relationships, especially with adults. They need time and interest to begin to share their own view of themselves and their lives. Group and family therapy may be useful adjuncts or alternatives to individual sessions. Medications have increasingly precise benefit in the treatment of selected teenage disorders.

Referral

Referral to or consultation with a psychiatrist may provide information and clarification and new techniques for the primary physician in evaluating and counseling patients. While many problems of children's physical or emotional adjustment and of parenting can be handled by physician counseling, sometimes psychiatric help is needed in managing difficult situations. Referral of a teenager or family for direct psychiatric evaluation may be indicated by the severity or persistence of symptoms in spite of counseling. Some families or adolescents may be reluctant to discuss very personal issues with a physician whom they know in a medical or social context. Psychiatric referral may be introduced as a means of offering focused attention to, and providing relief from, the pain experienced by family and youth. Frequently, parents need reassurance that psychiatric evaluation is not a sign of their failure, and does not imply that they or their child are "crazy" or incompetent. It is the psychiatrist's role to function as an ally of the family and the physician—to assist in the task of the teenagers ultimately achieving responsible independence and self-esteem.

The adolescent needs thoughtful preparation for psychiatric consultation. Parents and physician may lose credibility if a child or teenager is brought to a psychiatrist under pretense. Referral should be presented in a manner that links the psychiatrist with the youth's own desires for happiness, competence, friendship, and diminished conflict. A child should be told that he or she will have the opportunity to talk, perhaps to play or tell stories; a teenager should know that he or she may take walks with the psychiatrist, share some sport or craft activities,

or eventually participate in group or family sessions. These experiences will ultimately help him or her feel and function better. Although the objectives are serious, the process is often enjoyable and should not be presented as an ordeal. Professionals, child, and family should all appreciate the boundaries of confidentiality that are expected as they seek consultation.

The physician who can recognize psychiatric problems of children and who is able to provide effective counseling or prepare a family for referral, contributes a special service to patients. In an era of fragmented, mobile families with diminished ties to church and community, the physician is frequently called on to be the adviser to both mind and body. A relationship of reciprocal communication and trust between family physician and psychiatrist can assist the physician to provide comprehensive patient care.

APPENDIX: CASE HISTORY—THE YOUTHFUL BURGLAR

David seemed to be somewhat relieved to talk with the physician, who approached him in a nonjudgmental, inquiring way. David readily admitted to the physician that he had felt depressed, frustrated, guilty, and worried that he did not seem to enjoy much of anything. He admitted privately that, although the criminal charges were dismissed, he had, in fact, participated in several break-ins, selling stolen property and using money primarily to buy marijuana and liquor.

He also admitted having had practically no sexual interest for the past several months (which contributed to the stormy relationship with his girlfriend), had trouble sleeping through the night with "bad dreams" and pessimistic thoughts, and a loss of appetite with weight loss of about 5–10 pounds in the last 6 months.

On the basis of his talks with David, his family and school, the following additional information was obtained.

Family history

David is the oldest of two boys. His parents separated when David was 10 years old—due to father's alcoholism. David and his brother live with mother; David sees his father about every third weekend.

His father, age 42, an auto mechanic, had learning difficulties in elementary school and was frequently disciplined for being disruptive in class. He finished high school. He began binge drinking in late adolescence. This is his second marriage. He has been argumentative and episodically violent, but has been sober since joining AA 3 years ago; he is angered by his son's substance abuse and delinquent behavior.

Mother, age 37, a secretary, graduated from high school and business school. Married at 19 years; worked since David was 6 months old. She had two episodes of depression requiring medication and psychotherapy: first was shortly after David's birth; the second occurred after the divorce.

Birth and development

David was born full-term; his birthweight was 3.1 kg; labor and delivery were unremarkable. As an infant he was irritable and colicky, but slept and ate well. As a toddler he was overactive and very willful—but easily frustrated. In elementary school David was described as aggressive, inattentive, easily distracted, and prone to temper tantrums. A specific reading disability was defined in third grade. David made poor academic progress in spite of special education assistance. The pattern of restlessness, inability to concentrate, and academic delay continued. In junior high school an added dimension of social isolation was observed. David seemed unhappy, discouraged and withdrawn.

Medical history

Allergies exist but do not currently need treatment. At age 14, David had a seizure after head trauma. EEG 1 month after and again 1 year later were normal; no medication; no personality change noted. Fracture of left humerus in street fight 8 months ago. His present physical condition is healthy and unremarkable.

Mental status

Appearance is of a tough boy with a sad face who is nervous and restless. Speech is punctuated, brief, guarded. His mood is unhappy and depressed. He says he occasionally enjoys himself, but rapidly returns to depression. David was worried and remorseful about his recent crimes. He has about average intelligence, but is not interested in reading or studying. He exhibits some judgment and insight: David seems aware that his drinking and marijuana use are connected to his generally depressed mood. He still feels sad about his distant relationship with his father; at other times professes no interest in "seeing the bum."

Evaluation

David's hyperactivity and learning disability may have contributed to his depression through his repeated failures at school. Other contributants to depression include: the loss of his father, at age 10 years through divorce; the subsequent infrequent visits; the mother's history of depression and unavailability to David during infancy and following the separation. David's depressed mood and low self-esteem appear to underlie his social isolation in junior high school and his drug dependence in high school.

Diagnosis

1. Biological dimension: None

2. Personal dimension: Depressive syndrome (probably major affective disorder); substance abuse; attention deficit disorder; socialized aggressive conduct disorder

3. Environmental dimension: Social isolation and antisocial, maladaptive peers

Treatment

The family physician saw David several times and developed a cautious but continuing relationship with him. David came willingly, talked about his uncertainty about what to do with his life and his despair about "whether he could make it." He agreed to go to a few AA meetings—which he didn't like—but diminished his alcohol-drug abuse. Because his mood continued to be depressed, the physician referred David to a psychiatrist, who prescribed an antidepressant, saw him individually for three months and placed David in group therapy with peers. The group had a strong "no drug or alcohol" contract reinforced by a buddy system. David became less depressed and less reliant on drugs and has not been involved in any criminal behavior. His peer group changed during the course of treatment as David selected friends who were more ambitious. He is now considering a training program to learn truck maintenance and repair.

PATIENT EVALUATION GRID			
	CONTEXTS		
DIMENSIONS	**CURRENT** (Current States)	**RECENT** (Recent Events and Changes)	**BACKGROUND** (Culture, Traits, Constitution)
BIOLOGICAL	Healthy	Fracture of left humerus in street fight—8 mo ago	Allergies: house dust, pollen seizure after head trauma EEG normal, no medication
PERSONAL	Moody, sullen, depressed, joyless, appears tough but sad ADD with hyperactivity	Marijuana 2–4 joints a day for 3 yrs Alcohol—frequently drunk on weekends Weight loss (5–10 lbs)—6 mo Decreased appetite —4 mo Difficulty sleeping through night—6 mo Decreased sexual interest—6 mo	Infant—irritable, colicky Toddler— overactive, willful Elementary school— agressive, inattentive, low frustration tolerance, specific learning disability High School—loner, awkward, drug use
ENVIRONMENTAL	Family: Lives with mother (secretary) who brought him to physician Father, mechanic, parents separated 5 yrs School and Work: Unemployed—5 mo Peers: Girlfriend— 5 mo. stormy relationship	Family: Father in hospital with cirrhosis School and work: Arrested for break-in with 3 friends—3 mo ago worked briefly. Unemployed—5 mo Peers: Joined motorcycle gang 1 yr ago Loner in high school	Family: Father reformed alcoholic LD, ADD, parents separated—age 10 yr; Mother, secretary, depressive episodes School and work: Special classes for learning disabled; poor grades, poor study habits: dropped out of school—11th grade Peer: No close friends
Demographic data: 17-year-old single high school dropout			

RECOMMENDED READINGS

Berlin, I. 1976. *Bibliography of child psychiatry.* New York: Human Science Press. This is a guide to references by topic in child and adolescent psychiatry.

Eissler, R.S.; Freud, A.; Kris, M., et al. 1977. *Psychoanalytic assessment: the diagnostic profile.* New Haven, Conn.: Yale University Press. This is an introduction to psychoanalytic assessment and formulation in children.

Freud, A. 1965. *Normality and pathology in childhood.* New York: International Universities Press. This is the classic description of psychoanalytic concepts of normal and pathologic libidinal and ego development.

Masterson, J.F. 1967. *The psychiatric dilemma of adolescence.* London: Little, Brown & Co. This is an excellent description of emotional transitions and problems of teenagers.

Nicholi, A. 1978. *The Harvard guide to modern psychiatry.* Cambridge, Mass.: Harvard University Press. Here is a brief overview and reference for clinical psychiatrists.

Nospitz, J.D. 1979. *Basic handbook of child psychiatry,* 4 vols. New York: Harper & Row. These four volumes are an excellent reference text in child psychiatry.

Quay, H.; and Werry, J. 1972. *Psychopathological disorders of children.* New York: John Wiley & Sons. This is a description of psychiatric symptoms and diagnoses of childhood.

Schulterbrandt, J.G.; and Raskin, A. 1977. *Depression in childhood: diagnosis, treatment, and conceptual models.* New York: Raven Press. This is a recent review of the diagnosis and treatment of depression in children and adolescents.

REFERENCES

Abramowitz, C.V. 1976. The effectiveness of group psychotherapy with children. *Arch. Gen. Psychiatry* 33:320.

Anderson, N.; and Marrone, R.T. 1977. Group therapy for emotionally disturbed children: a key to effective education. *Am. J. Orthopsychiatry* 47:12.

Anthony, E.J.; D.C. Gilpin, eds. 1976. The genesis of oppositional child: Is the black child at a greater risk? In *Three clinical faces of childhood.* New York: Spectrum.

Barker, P. 1974. *The residential psychiatric treatment of children.* New York: John Wiley & Sons.

Berman, S. 1970. Alienation: an essential process of the psychology of adolescence. *J. Am. Acad. Child Psychiatry* 9:233–50.

Blos, P. 1962. *On adolescence.* New York: Free Press of Glencoe.

Blos, P. 1971. The child analyst looks at the young adolescent. *Daedalus* 100:961–78.

Borowitz, G. 1971. Character disorder in childhood and adolescence: some considerations of the effects of sexual stimulation in infancy and childhood. *Adolesc. Psychiatry* 1:343.

Browning, D.; and Boatman, B. 1977. Incest: children at risk. *Am. J. Psychiatry* 134:69.

Brownmiller, S. 1975. *Against our will: men, women, and rape.* New York: Simon & Schuster.

Bruch, H. 1970a. Juvenile obesity: its course and outcome. *Int. Psychiatry Clin.* 7(1):231–54.

Bruch, H. 1970b. Changing approaches to anorexia nervosa. *Int. Psychiatry Clin.* 7(1):3–24.

Bruch, H. 1971. Obesity in adolescence. In *Modern perspectives in adolescent psychiatry;* vol. 4, ed. J.B. Howells, pp. 244–73. Edinburgh: Oliver and Boyd.

Bruch, H. 1973. *Eating disorders: obesity, anorexia nervosa, and the person within.* New York: Basic Books.

Bruch, H. 1977. Anorexia nervosa. *Adolesc. Psychiatry* 5:293.

Cantwell, D. 1977. Anorexia nervosa, and affective disorder? *Arch. Gen. Psychiatry* 34:1087.

Carlson, G.A. 1981. The phenomenology of adolescent depression. *Adolesc. Psychiatry* 9:411–21.

Casper, R.; and Davis, J. 1977. On the course of anorexia nervosa. *Am. J. Psychiatry* 134:974.

Compton, A. 1972. A study of the psychoanalytic theory of anxiety. *J. Am. Psychoanal. Assoc.* 20:3.

Crumley, F.E. 1979. Adolescent suicide attempts. *J.A.M.A* 241:2404–2407.

Cytryn, L.; and McKnew, D.H., Jr. 1974. Proposed classification of childhood depression. In *Annual progress in child psychiatry and child development: 1973,* S. Chess, ed. Pp. 419–432. New York: Brunner Mazel.

Cytryn, L.; McKnew, D.H.; Bunney, W.E. 1980. Diagnosis of depression in children: A reassessment. *Am. J. Psychiatry* 137:22–25.

Davids, A.; and Salvatore, P.D. 1974. Residential treatment of disturbed children and adequacy of their subsequent adjustment: a follow-up study. *Am. J. Orthopsychiatry* 46:62.

Dreisbach, P.B., and Kasun, J.R. 1981. Teenage pregnancy (letter). *N. Engl. J. Med.* 304:121.

Evans, J. 1966. Analytic group therapy with delinquents. *Adolescence* 1:2.

Evans, R. 1969. Childhood parental relations of homosexual men. *J. Consult. Clin. Psychol.* 39:140.

Feinstein, S. 1975. Adolescent depression. In *Depression and Human existence*. Boston: Little, Brown & Co.

Feinstein, S.; and Wolpert, E. 1973. Juvenile manic-depressive illness. *J. Am. Acad. Child Psychiatry* 12:123.

Flavell, J.H. 1963. *The developmental psychology of Jean Piaget,* pp. 150–63. New York: Van Norstrand.

Frank, R.A.; and Cohen, D.J. 1979. Psychosocial concomitants of biological maturation in preadolescence. *Am. J. Psychiatry* 136:12.

Freud, Anna. 1969. Adolescence as a developmental disturbance. *Adolescence: psychosocial perspectives.* S.G. Caplan and S. Levovici, eds. NY: Basic Books.

Forrest, J.D.; Sullivan, E.; and Tietze, C. 1979. Abortion in the United States, 1977–1978. *Fam. Plann. Perspect.* 11:329–41.

Gelfand, D. M. 1978. Social withdrawal and negative emotional states: behavior therapy. In *Handbook of treatment of mental disorders in childhood and adolescence*. Englewood Cliffs, N.J. Prentice-Hall.

Gerner, R.H.; and Gwirtsman, H.E. 1981. Abnormalities of dexamethasone suppression test and urinary MHPS in anorexia nervosa. *Am. J. Psychiatry.* 138(5):650–53.

Gilpin, D.C. 1976. Psychotherapy of the oppositional child. In *Three clinical faces of childhood,* eds. Anthony E.J., and Gilpin D.C. New York: Spectrum.

Graham, P.; and Rutter, M. 1976. Adolescent disorders. In *Child psychiatry*, eds. M. Rutter and L. Hersov, pp. 407–27. Oxford: Blackwell.

Green, R. 1974. *Sexual identity conflict in children and adults.* New York: Basic Books.

Green, R. 1979. Childhood cross-gender behavior and subsequent sexual preference. *Am. J Psychiatry* 136:106–08.

Grinder, R.E. 1973. *Adolescence.* New York: John Wiley & Sons.

Gross, H.A.; Lake, C.R.; Ebert, M.H., et al. 1979. Catecholamine metabolism in primary anorexia nervosa. *J. Clin. Edocrinol. metab.* 49:805–09.

Groth, A.N.; Burgess, A.W.; and Holmstrom, L.L. 1977. Rape: power, anger and sexuality. *Am. J. Psychiatry* 134:1239.

Halmi, K.A.; Dekirmenjian, H.; Davis, J.M., et al. 1978. Catecholamine metabolism in anorexia nervosa. *Arch. Gen. Psychiatry* 35:459–60.

Halmi, K.A. 1980. Eating disorders. In *Comprehensive textbook of psychiatry*, 3rd ed., eds. A.M. Freedman, H.I. Kaplan, and B.J. Sadock, pp. 2598–2604. Baltimore: Williams & Williams.

Hart, M.; and Sarnoff, C.A. 1971. The impact of the monarch: a study of two stages of organization. *J. Am. Acad. Child Psychiatry* 10:257–71.

Hauser, S.T. 1976. Self-image complexity and identity formation in adolescence. *J. Youth Adol.* 5: 161–78.

Henderson, D.J., ed. 1976. Incest. In *The sexual experience*. Baltimore: Williams & Williams.

Hsu, L.K.G., Crisp, A.; and Harding, B. 1979. Outcome of anorexia nervosa. *Lancet* 1:61–65.

Jenkins, R.L. 1973. *Behavior disorders of childhood and adolescence.* Springfield, Ill: Charles C. Thomas.

Kashani, J.H.; Husain, A.; Shekim, W.O.; et al. 1981. Current perspectives on childhood depression: An overview. *Am. J. Psychiatry* 138:143–153.

Kaye, W.H.; Ebert, M.H.; Gold, P., et al. (In press.) *CNS neurotransmitter function in anorexia nervosa.*

Knittle, J.L. 1971. Childhood obesity. *Bull. N. Y. Acad. Med.* 47:579–89.

Kremer, M.; and Rifkin, A. 1969. The early development of homosexuality: a study of adolescent lesbians. *Am. J. Psychiatry* 126:91.

Laufer, M. 1966. Object loss and mourning during adolescence. *Psychoanal. Study Child* 21:269–93.

Lewis, M.; and Sarrel, P.M. 1969. Some psychological aspects of seduction, incest, and rape in childhood. *J. Am. Acad. Child Psychiatry* 8:606–19.

Lewis, D.O.; and Balla, D.A. 1976a. Psychiatric and

sociological viewpoints: changing perspectives and emphases. In *Delinquency and psychopathology,* eds. D.O. Lewis and D.A. Balla, pp. 7–18. New York: Grune & Stratton.

Lewis, D.O.; and Balla, D.A. 1976b. *Delinquency and psychopathology.* New York: Grune & Stratton.

Lewis, D.O.; Shanok, S.S.; Pincus, J.H.; et al. 1979. Violent juvenile delinquents: Psychiatric, neurological, psychological and abuse factors. *J. Am Acad. Child. Psychiatry* 18:307–319.

Lidz, T. 1970. The family as the developmental setting. In *The child and his family*, eds. E.J. Anthony and C. Koupernik, pp. 19–40. New York: John Wiley & Sons.

Lipsitz, J.S. 1979. Adolescent development. *Child Today* 8:2–7.

Lourie, R.S. 1966. Clinical studies of attempted suicide in childhood. *Clinical Proceedings of the Children's Hospital* 22:163–173.

Lowe, T.L.; Cohen, D.J.; Detlor, J., et al. Stimulant medications precipitate Tourette syndrome. *J.A.M.A.* 247:1729–1731.

Marsden, G.; Mcdermott, J.F.; and Monor, D. 1977. Selection of children for residential treatment. *J. Am. Acad. Child Psychiatry* 16:427.

Masterson, J.F. 1967. *The psychiatric dilemma of adolescence.* New York: Little, Brown & Co.

Masterson, J.F. 1972. *Treatment of the borderline adolescent: a developmental approach.* New York: John Wiley and Son, Inc.

May, R. 1977. *The meaning of anxiety.* New York: W.W. Norton.

Mays, J.B. 1971. The adolescent as a social being. In *Modern perspectives in adolescent psychiatry* vol 4 ed., J.G. Howells, pp. 126–51. Edinburgh: Oliver and Boyd.

McAnarney, E.R.; and Greydanus, D.E. 1979. Adolescent pregnancy: a multifaceted problem. *Pediatr. Rev.* 1:123–26.

McConville, B.J.; and Boag, L. 1973. Dropouts without drugs: a study of prolonged withdrawing reactions in younger adolescents. *J. Am. Acad. Child Psychiatry* 12:333.

Miller, D. 1973. The drug-dependent adolescent. *Adolesc. Psychiatry* 2:70

Minuchin, S.; Rosman, B.L.; and Baker, L. 1978. *Psychosomatic families: anorexia nervosa in context.* Cambridge: Harvard University Press.

Morgan, H.G.; and Russell, G.F.M. 1975. Value of family background and clinical features as predictors of long-term outcome in anorexia nervosa: four year follow-up study of 41 patients. *Psychol. Med.* 5:355–71.

Nospitz, J.D. 1970. Certain cultural and familial factors contributing to adolescent alienation. *J. Am. Acad. Child Psychiatry* 9:216–23.

O'Connor, J. 1977. Normal and problem drinking among children. *J. Child Psychol. Psychiatry* 18:229–84.

Offer, D.; Marcus, D.; and Offer, J.L. 1970. A longitudinal study of normal adolescent boys. *Am. J. Psychiatry* 126:917–24.

Offer, D.; and Offer, J. 1975. *From teenage to young manhood: a psychological study.* New York: Basic Books.

Pasnau, R.D.; Meyer, M.; Davis, L.J., et al. 1976. Coordinated group psychotherapy of children and parents. *Int. J. Group Psychother.* 26:1.

Piaget, J. 1969. The intellectual development of the adolescent. In *Adolescence: psychosocial perspectives,* eds. G. Caplan and S. Lebovici, pp. 22–26. New York: Basic Books.

Puig-Antich, J. 1982a. The use of RDC criteria for major depressive disorder in children and adolecents *Am. Acad. Child Psychiatry* 21(3):291–93.

Puig-Antich, J. 1982b. Major depression and conduct disorder in prepuberty. *J. Am. Acad. of Child Psychiatry* 21(2):118–28.

Puig-Antich, J. 1982c. Psychobiological correlates of major depressive disorder in children and adolescents. In *Psychiatry, 1982, Annual Review,* ed. L. Grinspoon. Washington, D.C.: American Psychiatric Press, Inc.

Rabin, P.L., and Swenson, B.R. 1981. Teenage suicide and parental divorce. *N. Engl. J. Med.* 304:1048.

Rachman, A.W. 1971. Encounter techniques in analytic group psychotherapy with adolescents. *Int. J. Group Psychother.* 21:319.

Richmond, L. 1974. Observations on private practice and community clinic adolescent psychotherapy groups. *Group Proc.* 6:57.

Rosenfeld, A. 1979. Incest among female patients. *Am. J. Psychiatry* 136:791.

Rosenfeld, A.; Nadelson, C.; and Kruger, M. 1979. Fantasy and reality in patient reports of incest. *J. Clin. Psychiatry.* 40:159.

Rosenstock, H.A.; and Vincent, K.R. 1979. Parental involvement as a requisite for successful adolescent therapy. *J. Clin. Psychol.* 40:132.

Rutter, M.; Graham, P.; Chadwick, O.; et al. 1976. Adolescent turmoil: Fact or fiction? *J. Child. Psychol. Psychiatry* 17:33–36.

Sadoff, R.L. 1976. Sex and the law. In *The sexual experience.* Baltimore: Williams and Williams.

Sadoff, R.L. 1979. Criminal sexual behavior. *Med. Aspects. Hum. Sex.* 13:53.

Saghir, M.; Robins, E.; Walbran, B., et al. 1970. Homosexuality: psychiatric disorders and disability in the male homosexual. *Am. J. Psychiatry* 126:1079.

Schaffer, C.; and Pine, F. 1972. Pregnancy, abortion, and the developmental tasks of adolescence. *J. Am. Acad. Child Psychiatry* 11:511–36.

Schowalter, J. 1977. Psychological reactions to physical illness. *J. Am. Acad. Child. Psychiatry* 16:500.

Siegelman, M. 1972a. Adjustment of male homosexuals and heterosexuals. *Arch. Sex. Behav.* 2:9.

Siegelman, M. 1972b. Adjustment of homosexual and heterosexual women. *Br. J. Psychiatry* 120:477.

Siegelman, M. 1974a. Parental background of male homosexuals and heterosexuals. *Arch. Sex. Behav.* 3:3.

Siegelman, M. 1974b. Parental background of homosexuals and heterosexuals. *Arch. Sex. Behav.* 3:3.

Symonds, M. 1976. The rape victim: psychological patterns of response. *Am. J. Psychoanal* 36:27.

Theander, S. 1970. Anorexia nervosa: a psychiatric investigation of 94 female patients. *Acta Med. Psychiatry Scand.* (suppl.) pp. 214–228.

Vick, J.; and Draft, I. A. 1973. Creative activities. In *Group therapy for the adolescent.* New York: Jason Aronson.

Wardrop, K.R.H. 1967. Delinquent teenage types. *Br. J. Criminal.* 7:371–80.

Weaver, B.M. 1979. Incest: detection and assessment. *Psychiatric News.* 14:12.

Weinberg, W.; Rutman, J.; Sullivan, L.; et al. 1973. The ten symptoms of childhood depression and the characteristic behavior for each symptom. *J. Pediatrics.* 83:1072–81.

Yorke, C.; and Weisberg, S. 1976. A developmental view of anxiety. *Psychoanal. Study Child* 31:107.

Zelnik, M.; and Kantner, J.S. 1978. First pregnancies to women aged 15–19: 1976 and 1971. *Fam. Plann. Perspect.* 10:11.

Zelnik, M.; and Kantner, J.S. 1980. Sexual activity, contraceptive use and pregnancy among metropolitan area teenagers, 1971–1979. *Fam. Plann. Perspect.* 12:230.

Zucker, K. 1982. Childhood gender disturbance: Diagnostic issues. *J. Acad. Child. Psychiatry* 21(3): 274–280.

Appendix

DSM-III Classification Axis I–V

All official DSM-III codes and terms are included in ICD-9-CM. However, in order to differentiate those DSM-III categories that use the same ICD-9-CM codes, unofficial non-ICD-9-CM codes are provided in parentheses for use when greater specificity is necessary.

The long dashes indicate the need for a fifth-digit subtype or other qualifying term.

AXES I AND II: CATEGORIES AND CODES

Disorders Usually First Evident in Infancy, Childhood or Adolescence

---

Mental Retardation (Code in fifth digit: 1 = with other behavioral symptoms [requiring attention or treatment and that are not part of another disorder], 0 = without other behavioral symptoms.)

317.0(x)	Mild Mental Retardation, _____
318.0(x)	Moderate Mental Retardation, _____
318.1(x)	Severe Mental Retardation, _____
318.2(x)	Profound Mental Retardation, _____
319.0(x)	Unspecified Mental Retardation, _____

Attention Deficit Disorder

314.01	with Hyperactivity
314.00	without Hyperactivity
314.80	Residual Type

Conduct Disorder

312.00	Undersocialized, Aggressive

Source: The American Psychiatric Association, Diagnostic and Statistical Manual of Mental Disorders, Third Edition, Washington, D.C., APA 1980. Reprinted by permission.

312.10	Undersocialized, Nonaggressive
312.23	Socialized, Aggressive
312.21	Socialized, Nonaggressive
312.90	Atypical

Anxiety Disorders of Childhood or Adolescence

309.21	Separation Anxiety Disorder
313.21	Avoidant Disorder of Childhood or Adolescence
313.00	Overanxious Disorder

Other Disorders of Infancy, Childhood, or Adolescence

313.89	Reactive Attachment Disorder of Infancy
313.22	Schizoid Disorder of Childhood or Adolescence
313.23	Elective Mutism
313.81	Oppositional Disorder
313.82	Identity Disorder

Eating Disorders

307.10	Anorexia Nervosa
307.51	Bulimia
307.52	Pica
307.53	Rumination Disorder of Infancy
307.50	Atypical Eating Disorder

Stereotyped Movement Disorders

307.21	Transient Tic Disorder
307.22	Chronic Motor Tic Disorder
307.23	Tourette's Disorder
307.20	Atypical Tic Disorder

307.30   Atypical Stereotyped Movement Disorder

Other Disorders with Physical Manifestations

307.00   Stuttering

307.60   Functional Enuresis

307.70   Functional Encopresis

307.46   Sleepwalking Disorder

307.46   Sleep Terror Disorder (307.49)

Pervasive Developmental Disorders   Code in fifth digit: 0 = Full Syndrome Present, 1 = Residual State.

299.0x   Infantile Autism, _____

299.9x   Childhood Onset Pervasive Developmental Disorder, _____

299.8x   Atypical, _____

Specific developmental disorders
Note: These are coded on Axis II.

315.00   Developmental Reading Disorder

315.10   Developmental Arithmetic Disorder

315.31   Developmental Language Disorder

315.39   Developmental Articulation Disorder

315.50   Mixed Specific Developmental Disorder

315.90   Atypical Specific Developmental Disorder

Organic Mental Disorders

Section 1. Organic Mental Disorders whose etiology or pathophysiological process is listed below (taken from the mental disorders section of ICD-9-CM).

Dementias Arising in the Senium and Presenium
Primary Degenerative Dementia, Senile Onset,

290.30   with Delirium

290.20   with Delusions

290.21   with Depression

290.00   Uncomplicated

Code in fifth digit:
1 = with Delirium, 2 = with Delusions, 3 = with Depression, 0 = Uncomplicated.

290.1x   Primary Degenerative Dementia, Presenile Onset, _____

290.4x   Multi-infarct Dementia, _____

Substance-induced

ALCOHOL

303.00   Intoxication

291.40   Idiosyncratic Intoxication

291.80   Withdrawal

291.00   Withdrawal Delirium

291.30   Hallucinosis

291.10   Amnestic Disorder

Code severity of Dementia in fifth digit: 1 = Mild, 2 = Moderate, 3 = Severe, 0 = Unspecified.

291.2x   Dementia Associated with Alcoholism, _____

BARBITURATE OR SIMILARLY ACTING SEDATIVE OR HYPNOTIC

305.40   Intoxication (327.00)

292.00   Withdrawal (327.01)

292.00   Withdrawal Delirium (327.02)

292.83   Amnestic Disorder (327.04)

OPIOID

305.50   Intoxication (327.10)

292.00   Withdrawal (327.11)

COCAINE

305.60   Intoxication (327.20)

AMPHETAMINE OR SIMILARLY ACTING SYMPATHOMIMETIC

305.70   Intoxication (327.30)

292.81   Delirium (327.32)

292.11   Delusional Disorder (327.35)

292.00   Withdrawal (327.31)

PHENCYCLIDINE (PCP) OR SIMILARLY ACTING ARYLCYCLOHEXYLAMINE

305.90   Intoxication (327.40)

292.81   Delirium (327.42)

292.90   Mixed Organic Mental Disorder (327.49)

HALLUCINOGEN

305.30   Hallucinosis (327.56)

292.11   Delusional Disorder (327.55)

292.84   Affective Disorder (327.57)

CANNABIS

305.20   Intoxication (327.60)

292.11   Delusional Disorder (327.65)

TOBACCO

292.00   Withdrawal (327.71)

CAFFEINE

305.90   Intoxication (327.80)

OTHER OR UNSPECIFIED SUBSTANCE

305.90   Intoxication (327.90)

292.00   Withdrawal (327.91)

292.81   Delirium (327.92)

292.82   Dementia (327.93)

292.83   Amnestic Disorder (327.94)

292.11   Delusional Disorder (327.95)

292.12 Hallucinosis (327.96)
292.84 Affective Disorder (327.97)
292.89 Personality Disorder (327.98)
292.90 Atypical or Mixed Organic Mental Disorder (327.99)

Section 2. Organic Brain Syndromes whose etiology or pathophysiological process is either noted as an additional diagnosis from outside the mental disorders section of ICD-9-CM or is unknown.

293.00 Delirium
294.10 Dementia
294.00 Amnestic Syndrome
293.81 Organic Delusional Syndrome
293.82 Organic Hallucinosis
293.83 Organic Affective Syndrome
310.10 Organic Personality Syndrome
294.80 Atypical or Mixed Organic Brain Syndrome

Substance Use Disorders

Code in fifth digit: 1 = Continuous, 2 = Episodic, 3 = in Remission, 0 = Unspecified

305.0x Alcohol Abuse, _____
303.9x Alcohol Dependence (Alcoholism), _____
305.4x Barbiturate or similarly acting sedative or hypnotic Abuse,
304.1x Barbiturate or similarly acting sedative or hypnotic Dependence, _____
305.5x Opioid Abuse, _____
304.0x Opioid Dependence, _____
305.6x Cocaine Abuse, _____
305.7x Amphetamine or similarly acting sympathomimetic Abuse, _____
304.4x Amphetamine or similarly acting sympathomimetic Dependence, _____
305.9x Phencyclidine (PCP) or similarly acting arylcyclohexylamine Abuse, _____ (328.4x)
305.3x Hallucinogen Abuse, _____
305.2x Cannabis Abuse, _____
304.3x Cannabis Dependence, _____
305.1x Tobacco Dependence, _____
305.9x Other, mixed or unspecified Substance Abuse, _____
304.6x Other Specified Substance Dependence,_____
304.9x Unspecified Substance Dependence, _____
304.7x Dependence on Combination of Opiod and other Nonalcoholic Substance, _____

304.8x Dependence on Combination of Substances, excluding opioids and alcohol, _____

Schizophrenic Disorders

Code in fifth digit: 1 = Subchronic, 2 = Chronic, 3 = Subchronic with Acute Exacerbation, 4 = Chronic with Acute Exacerbation, 5 = in Remission, 0 = Unspecified.

SCHIZOPHRENIA
295.1x Disorganized, _____
295.2x Catatonic, _____
295.3x Paranoid, _____
295.9x Undifferentiated, _____
295.6x Residual, _____

Paranoid Disorders

297.10 Paranoia
297.30 Shared Paranoid Disorder
298.30 Acute Paranoid Disorder
297.90 Atypical Paranoid Disorder

Psychotic Disorders Not Elsewhere Classified

295.40 Schizophreniform Disorder
298.80 Brief Reactive Psychosis
295.70 Schizoaffective Disorder
298.90 Atypical Psychosis

Neurotic Disorders

These are included in Affective, Anxiety, Somatoform, Dissociative, and Psychosexual Disorders. In order to facilitate the identification of the categories that in DSM-II were grouped together in the class of Neuroses, the DSM-II terms are included separately in parentheses after the corresponding categories. These DSM-II terms are included in ICD-9-CM and therefore are acceptable as alternatives to the recommended DSM-III terms that precede them.

Affective Disorders

Major Affective Disorders Code Major Depressive Episode in fifth digit: 6 = in Remission, 4 = with Psychotic Features (the unofficial non-ICD-9-CM fifth digit 7 may be used instead to indicate that the psychotic features are mood-incongruent), 3 = with Melancholia, 2 = without Melancholia, 0 = Unspecified.

Code Manic Episode in fifth digit: 6 = in Remission, 4 = with Psychotic Features (the unofficial non-ICD-9-CM fifth digit 7 may be used instead to indicate that the psychotic features are mood-incongruent), 2 = without Psychotic Features, 0 = Unspecified.

BIPOLAR DISORDER
296.6x Mixed, _____
296.4x Manic, _____
296.5x Depressed, _____

MAJOR DEPRESSION
296.2x Single Episode, _____
296.3x Recurrent, _____

Other Specific Affective Disorders
301.13 Cyclothymic Disorder
300.40 Dysthymic Disorder (or Depressive Neurosis)

Atypical Affective Disorders
296.70 Atypical Bipolar Disorder
296.82 Atypical Depression

Anxiety Disorders

PHOBIC DISORDERS (OR PHOBIC NEUROSES)
300.21 Agoraphobia with Panic Attacks
300.22 Agoraphobia without Panic Attacks
300.23 Social Phobia
300.29 Simple Phobia

ANXIETY STATES (OR ANXIETY NEUROSES)
300.01 Panic Disorder
300.02 Generalized Anxiety Disorder
300.30 Obsessive Compulsive Disorder (or Obsessive Compulsive Neurosis)

POST-TRAUMATIC STRESS DISORDER
308.30 Acute
309.81 Chronic or Delayed
300.00 Atypical Anxiety Disorder

Somatoform Disorders

300.81 Somatization Disorder
300.11 Conversion Disorder (or Hysterical Neurosis, Conversion Type)
307.80 Psychogenic Pain Disorder
300.70 Hypochondriasis (or Hypochondriacal Neurosis)
300.70 Atypical Somatoform Disorder (300.71)

Dissociative Disorders (or Hysterical Neuroses, Dissociative Type)

300.12 Psychogenic Amnesia
300.13 Psychogenic Fugue
300.14 Multiple Personality

300.60 Depersonalization Disorder (or Depersonalization Neurosis)
300.15 Atypical Dissociative Disorder

Psychosexual Disorders

Gender Identity Disorders Indicate sexual history in the fifth digit of Transsexualism code: 1 = Asexual, 2 = Homosexual, 3 = Heterosexual, 0 = Unspecified.
302.5x Transsexualism, _____
302.60 Gender Identity Disorder of Childhood
302.85 Atypical Gender Identity Disorder

Paraphilias
302.81 Fetishism
302.30 Transvestism
302.10 Zoophilia
302.20 Pedophilia
302.40 Exhibitionism
302.82 Voyeurism
302.83 Sexual Masochism
302.84 Sexual Sadism
302.90 Atypical Paraphilia

Psychosexual Dysfunctions
302.71 Inhibited Sexual Desire
302.72 Inhibited Sexual Excitement
302.73 Inhibited Female Orgasm
302.74 Inhibited Male Orgasm
302.75 Premature Ejaculation
302.76 Functional Dyspareunia
302.51 Functional Vaginismus
302.70 Atypical Psychosexual Dysfunction

Other Psychosexual Disorders
302.00 Ego-dystonic Homosexuality
302.89 Psychosexual Disorder not elsewhere classified

Factitious Disorders

300.16 Factitious Disorder with Psychological Symptoms
301.51 Chronic Factitious Disorder with Physical Symptoms
300.19 Atypical Factitious Disorder with Physical Symptoms

Disorders of Impulse Control Not Elsewhere Classified

312.31 Pathological Gambling
312.32 Kleptomania
312.33 Pyromania
312.34 Intermittent Explosive Disorder

312.35 Isolated Explosive Disorder
312.39 Atypical Impulse Control Disorder

Adjustment Disorder

309.00 with Depressed Mood
309.24 with Anxious Mood
309.28 with Mixed Emotional Features
309.30 with Disturbance of Conduct
309.40 with Mixed Disturbance of Emotions and Conduct
309.23 with Work (or Academic) Inhibition
309.83 with Withdrawal
309.90 with Atypical Features

Psychological Factors Affecting Physical Condition

Specify physical condition on Axis III.
316.00 Psychological Factors Affecting Physical Condition

PERSONALITY DISORDERS
Note: These are coded on Axis II.
301.00 Paranoid
301.20 Schizoid
301.22 Schizotypal
301.50 Histrionic
301.81 Narcissistic
301.70 Antisocial
301.83 Borderline
301.82 Avoidant
301.60 Dependent
301.40 Compulsive
301.84 Passive-Aggressive
301.89 Atypical, Mixed or other Personality Disorder

V Codes for Conditions Not Attributable to a Mental Disorder That Are a Focus of Attention or Treatment

V65.20 Malingering
V62.89 Borderline Intellectual Functioning (V62.88)
V71.01 Adult Antisocial Behavior
V71.02 Childhood or Adolescent Antisocial Behavior
V62.30 Academic Problem
V62.20 Occupational Problem
V62.82 Uncomplicated Bereavement
V15.81 Noncompliance with Medical Treatment
V62.89 Phase of Life Problem or Other Life Circumstance Problem

V61.10 Marital Problem
V61.20 Parent-Child Problem
V61.80 Other Specified Family Circumstances
V62.81 Other Interpersonal Problem

Additional Codes

300.90 Unspecified Mental Disorder (Nonpsychotic)
V71.09 No Diagnosis or Condition on Axis I
799.90 Diagnosis or Condition Deferred on Axis I

V71.09 No Diagnosis on Axis II
799.90 Diagnosis Deferred on Axis II

AXIS III: PHYSICAL DISORDERS OR CONDITIONS

Axis III permits the clinician to indicate any current physical disorder or condition that is potentially relevant to the understanding or management of the client. These are the conditions exclusive of the "mental disorders section" of ICD-9-CM. (The 9th edition of the International Classification of Diseases.) In some instances the condition may be etiologically significant; in other instances the physical disorder is important to the overall management of the client. In yet other instances, the clinician may wish to note the presence of other significant associated physical assessment findings, such as "soft neurological signs." Multiple diagnoses are permitted on this axis.

AXIS IV: SEVERITY OF PSYCHOSOCIAL STRESSORS

Code	Term	Adult Examples	Child or Adolescent Examples
1	None	No apparent psychosocial stressor	No apparent psychosocial stressor
2	Minimal	Minor violation of the law; small bank loan	Vacation with family
3	Mild	Argument with neighbor; change in work hours	Change in schoolteacher; new school year

4	Moderate	New career; death of close friend; pregnancy	Chronic parental fighting; change to new school; illness of close relative; birth of sibling
5	Severe	Serious illness in self or family; major financial loss; marital separation; birth of child	Death of peer; divorce of parents; arrest; hospitalization; persistent and harsh parental discipline
6	Extreme	Death of close relative; divorce	Death of parent or sibling; repeated physical or sexual abuse
7	Catastrophic	Concentration camp experience; devastating natural disaster	Multiple family deaths
0	Unspecified	No information, or not applicable	No information, or not applicable

AXIS V: HIGHEST LEVEL OF ADAPTIVE FUNCTIONING PAST YEAR

Levels	Adult Examples	Child or Adolescent Examples
1 SUPERIOR Unusually effective functioning in social relations, occupational functioning, and use of leisure time.	Single parent living in deteriorating neighborhood takes excellent care of children and home, has warm relations with friends, and finds time for pursuit of hobby.	A 12-year-old girl gets superior grades in school, is extremely popular among her peers, and excels in many sports. She does all of this with apparent ease and comfort.
2 VERY GOOD Better than average functioning in social relations, occupational functioning, and use of leisure time.	A 65-year-old retired widower does some volunteer work, often sees old friends, and pursues hobbies.	An adolescent boy gets excellent grades, works part-time, has several close friends, and plays banjo in a jazz band. He admits to some distress in "keeping up with everything."
3 GOOD No more than slight impairment in either social or occupational functioning.	A woman with many friends functions extremely well at a difficult job, but says "the strain is too much."	An 8-year-old boy does well in school, has several friends, but bullies younger children.
4 FAIR Moderate impairment in either social relations or occupational functioning, *or* some impairment in both.	A lawyer has trouble carrying through assignments; has several acquaintances, but hardly any close friends.	A 10-year-old girl does poorly in school, but has adequate peer and family relations.
5 POOR Marked impairment in either social relations or occupational functioning, *or* moderate impairment in both.	A man with one or two friends has trouble keeping a job for more than a few weeks.	A 14-year-old boy almost fails in school and has trouble getting along with his peers.
6 VERY POOR Marked impairment in both social relations and occupational functioning.	A woman is unable to do any of her housework and has violent outbursts toward family and neighbors.	A 6-year-old girl needs special help in all subjects and has virtually no peer relationships.
7 GROSSLY IMPAIRED Gross impairment in virtually all areas of functioning.	An elderly man needs supervision to maintain minimal personal hygiene and is usually incoherent.	A 4-year-old boy needs constant restraint to avoid hurting himself and is almost totally lacking in skills.
0 UNSPECIFIED	No information.	No information.

Index

Abortion
adolescents and, 458–459
suicide and, 148
Abscesses
drug dependence and, 271,
272
organic brain syndromes and,
96, 97
Abstraction, in mental status
examination, 18
Acidosis, and organic brain
syndromes, 96
Acromegaly, and sexual
dysfunctions, 328
Acute intermittent porphyria (AIP)
differential diagnosis of
depression, 71
disordered thinking, 74
mood alterations, 68
psychosis, 76
drugs and
barbiturates, 393
chloral hydrate, 394
symptoms of
catatonia, 66
psychiatric, 65, 75–76
Acute organic brain sydrome,
87–88
causes of, 96
diagnosis of, 94–95
Addison's disease
depression and, 70
mood alterations and, 68
organic brain syndromes and,
96
Adjustment disorders, and referral
for psychotherapy, 370
Adjustment reaction. See
Situational disturbance
syndrome
Adolescence, 449–476
academic inhibition in, 469
aggression in, 469–470
alcoholism in, 253
anorexia nervosa in, 461–462
anxiety in, 466–467

cognitive development in,
452–453
counseling during, 455–456
defiance in, 471
delinquency in, 27, 29, 473–476
depression in, 464–466
diabetes in, 356
ego identity in, 453
emancipation disorder in,
468–469
extreme shyness in, 467–468
family changes in, 451
identity disorders in, 470–471
medical illness in, 461
passive loners in, 468–469
referral in, 472–473
self-examination in, 453
sexuality in, 451, 452
sexual problems in
abortion, 458–459
contraception, 457–458
homosexuality, 460
incest, 459–460
rape, 459
venereal disease, 458
social changes in, 451–452
stages of
early (puberty), 450–451
late, 454–455
middle, 451–454
substance abuse in, 462–464
suicide in, 143–144, 464–465
values and, 453–454
violence in, 469–470
work inhibition in, 469
Adrenal disorders, and mood
alterations, 68, 69–70
Adrenocorticotrophic hormones
(ACTH)
depression and, 70, 127
mood alterations and, 68, 70
Affect, in mental status
examination, 18–19
Affective disorders, 123–137
atypical, 128
major, 124

signs and symptoms of
anxiety, 162
compulsions, 163
depression, 130
obsessions, 163
sexual dysfunction, 322
violence, 304
"Affective escalation," 178
Affectivity, in families, 24
Age, and suicide, 143–144
Aggression
in adolescents, 469–470
alcoholism and, 240, 248
See also Violence
Aging, and families, 26, 30
See also Elderly
Agoraphobia, 163
antidepressants and, 165
psychotherapy and, 165
Akathisia, and antipsychotic
medications, 387
Alcohol
antianxiety drugs and, 392
medical problems and
organic brain syndromes,
92–93
subdural hematoma, 77
prenatal development and, 411
psychological problems and
anxiety, 72, 73, 161, 162
depression, 70, 127
disordered thinking, 74
mood alterations, 68
paranoia, 66
violence, 301–302
Alcohol abstinence syndromes,
232–235
Alcoholic blackout, 231–232
Alcoholic dementia, 97, 223, 251
Alcoholic hallucinosis, 236, 240
Alcoholic paranoia, 236, 240
Alcoholic psychosis, 223, 236, 240
Alcoholics Anonymous, 237, 249
Alcoholism, 221–258
acute, 231, 232–236
adolescent, 253

Alcoholism *(Cont.)*
  aggression and, 240, 248
  appearance and, 16
  case history of, 222, 257–258
  central nervous system and, 231
  classifications of
    Diagnostic and Statistical
      Manual, 223, 226
    International Statistical, 223,
      226
    National Council on
      Alcoholism, 223
  craving in, 239
  defensive postures in, 237–239
  definition of, 223
  diagnostic criteria for, 224, 225
  drug abuse and, 228
  epidemiologic problems and,
    228–229
  family and, 252–254
  Jellinek's phases of, 226–228
  legal issues of, 255–256
  mental status examination and,
    237
  neuropsychological deficits
    and, 239, 251–252
  PEG for, 258
  predisposition to
    gender, 230
    genetics, 229–230, 411
    personality factors, 230–231
  prognostic indicators in, 248
  psychologic symptoms of,
    239–240, 241–247
  referral for, 254–255
  social problems and, 228–229
  subacute stage of, 236–237
  suicide and, 240
  treatment of
    aversion therapy, 249
    conditioning therapy, 249
    drug therapy, 233–234, 235,
      249–250
    individualizing, 248
    lithium therapy, 250
    psychological therapies, 249
    self-help support systems,
      249
Alcohol withdrawal
  delirium tremens and, 105, 108,
    233, 236
  seizures and, 233
  treatment of, 233–234, 235
Aldomet. *See* Methyldopa
Alkalosis, and organic brain
    syndromes, 96
Altruistic suicide, 142

Alzheimer's senile dementia, and
    organic brain syndromes,
    94, 97
American Association of Sex
    Educators, Counselors and
    Therapists (AASECT), 331
Amitriptyline, 388–389
  anorexia nervosa and, 462
  anxiety and, 165
  depression and, 125, 131–133
  narcotic withdrawal and, 288
Amnesia, and remote memory, 17
Amobarbital, 202, 393
"Amotivational syndrome," 278
Amphetamines
  abuse of, 275
  ADD children and, 433, 434
  anxiety and, 72, 73, 161, 162
  depression and, 369
  disordered thinking and, 74
  MAO inhibitors and, 390
  mood alterations and, 68
  paranoia and, 66, 77
  psychosis and, 77, 106
  schizophrenia and, 116
  withdrawal from, 283
Amytal. *See* Amobarbital
Analgesics
  for narcotic-dependent patients,
    285–286
  organic brain syndromes and,
    96
  psychosis and, 105
  See also Narcotic analgesics
Analytically oriented
    psychotherapy, 375
Anemia
  alcoholism and, 232
  dementia and, 88
  depression and, 67
  drug abuse and, 272
  mood alterations and, 68
  organic brain syndromes and,
    96
  psychiatric dysfunctions with, 65
Angiitis, and drug dependence,
    272, 275
Anileridine, methadone
    equivalent of, 287
"Anniversary reactions," 61
Anomic suicide, 142
Anorexia nervosa, 27, 461–462
Antabuse. *See* Disulfiram
Antemetics, and migraines, 181
Antianxiety agents, 391–392
  headaches and, 182
  side effects of, 392

Anticholinergics
  antidote for, 95
  delirium and, 78
  disordered thinking and, 74
  organic brain syndromes and,
    96
  paranoia and, 66
  psychosis and, 105, 106, 107
Antidepressant drug therapy,
    131–134
  electroconvulsive therapy
    (ECT), 134
  lithium, 133–134, 390–391
  MAO inhibitors, 133, 389–390
  tricyclics, 131–133, 388–389
Antidepressants, 387–391
  adolescents and, 465
  anxiety and, 164, 165
  chronic illness and, 344, 351
  depressive syndrome and, 130
  hemodialysis and, 353–354
  narcotic withdrawal and, 288
  psychosis and, 106
  psychotherapy and, 372
  schizophrenia and, 117
  suicide and, 152
Antihistamines
  anxiety and, 164
  psychosis and, 106
Antihypertensive drugs
  depression and, 126, 344
  suicide and, 152
Antimalarial drugs, and psychosis,
    105
Antiparkinsonism drugs, and
    psychosis, 106
Antipsychotic medication, 117,
    384–387
  dosage, 385–387
  drug-disease interactions, 387
  drug-drug interactions, 387
  guidelines for, 386
  toxicity of, 387
  types of
    butyrophenone, 385
    phenothiazines, 385
Antisocial personality disorder
  case history of, 50
  dysfunctional response to, 50
  intervention for, 50–51
  problem of, 50
  recognition of, 49–50
  violence and, 301, 305
Antispasmodics, and delirium, 78
Anxiety, 159–168
  in adolescence, 466–467
  case history of, 160, 167–168

differential diagnosis of, 161–164
evaluation of, 161
headaches and, 181
major affective disorders and, 162
management of
  antidepressants, 165
  benzodiazepines, 164–165, 391–392
  beta-blocking agents, 165
  environmental manipulation, 166
  neuroleptics, 164, 165
  psychotherapies, 165–166
PEG for, 161, 168
physical disorders and
  cardiac conditions, 72–73
  drugs, 162
  endocrine disorders, 72, 161–162
  organic brain syndromes, 89–90, 162
  respiratory conditions, 72
referral for, 166
schizophrenia and, 162
separation, 467
with somatic complaints, 59–64
stress reactions and, 61, 163–164
surgery and, 164
theories of, 160
Anxiety disorders, 161
  generalized, 162, 165
  obsessive-compulsive, 162–163, 165, 166
  panic, 162, 165
  phobic, 163, 165, 166
  posttraumatic stress, 163–164
Aphasia, 16, 419–421
Appearance, in mental status examination, 16
Arteritis, and drug abuse, 272
Arthritis, 172, 272
Asthma
  anxiety and, 72–73
  disulfiram or DDC and, 250
  family and, 27
  psychiatric dysfunctions with, 65
  as psychosomatic disorder, 172
Atavin. *See* Lorazepam
Atropine, 273
Attention
  in mental status examination, 17–18
  in organic brain syndromes, 86

Attention deficit disorder (ADD), 430–434
Atypical affective disorders, 128
Autism, childhood, 417–418, 419
Autoimmune disease, 116
Aversion therapy, and alcoholism, 249
Avoidant personality. *See* Schizoid personality disorder

Background context (in PEG), 4, 6–7
Bacteremia, 272
Barbiturates, 393–394
  abuse of, 273–275
  alcoholism and, 228
  alcohol withdrawal and, 234, 235
  antianxiety drugs and, 392
  antisocial personality and, 50
  anxiety and, 73, 161, 162, 164, 369
  narcotics and, 273
  paranoia and, 66
  side effects of, 393–394
  suicide and, 393
  tricyclics and, 389
  violence and, 299
  withdrawal from, 274–275, 283, 290–292
Basilar artery migraine, 180
Behavioral therapy, 166
Behavioral toxicity, 277
Behavior changes, 62
Behavior modification, 330, 375, 419
Benadryl. *See* Diphenhydramine
Bender–Gestalt test, 405–406
Benzodiazepines, 391–392, 393
  anxiety and, 72, 162, 164–165, 391–392
  depression and, 127, 129
  elderly and, 165
  insomnia and, 393
  medical problems and
    alcohol withdrawal, 234
    headaches, 182
    hemodialysis, 353
    organic brain syndromes, 97, 165
  psychosis and, 107
  psychotherapy and, 372
  side effects of, 392
  violence and, 299
  withdrawal from, 283

Benztropine
  psychosis and, 107
  sedatives and, 299
Benztropine mesylate, 387
Bereavement, 7, 8
  See also Grief reaction
Beta-blocking agents, anxiety and, 164, 165
Biofeedback, 181, 376
Biological amines, and depression, 125–126
Biological components (in PEG), 4, 6, 7, 8, 13
Bipolar disorder of major affective disorder, 128
Bipolar illness. *See* Affective disorders; Manic-depressive illness
Blacks, suicide among, 145, 148
Blindness
  diabetes and, 356, 357
  drug dependence and, 272
Blood alcohol tests, 255–256
Blood disorders, psychiatric dysfunctions with, 65
Bone marrow depression, and drug abuse, 272
Borderline personality disorder
  case history of, 52
  intervention for, 51–52
  problem of, 51
  recognition of, 51
  violence and, 301
Brain tumor
  disordered thinking and, 74
  manic-depressive illness and, 91
  paranoia and, 66
  personality changes and, 6, 92
  seizures and, 77
Brief psychiatric rating scale (BPRS), 241–243
Briquet's syndrome, 183, 196–197
Bromides
  paranoia and, 66
  psychosis and, 105
"Burn-out syndrome," 278
Burns, and drug dependence, 271
Butorphanol, 286
Butyrophenones, 384, 385
  alcohol withdrawal and, 234
  psychotherapy and, 372
  schizophrenia and, 117

Caffeine
  anxiety and, 72, 73
  migraines and, 180
  prenatal development and, 411

Cancer, 357–362
  diagnosis of, 357–359
  unproven treatments of, 360
Cancer patients, 357–362
  case histories of, 358, 361
  counseling of, 360–361
  death and dying and, 360
  depression in, 67, 69, 126, 127,
    359
  grief in, 359
  informing of, 64, 358–359
  mood alterations in, 68
  organic brain syndromes in,
    360
  physical reactions of, 361–362
  psychological reactions to
    treatment, 359
  side effects and, 359
Cannabis sativa, 278
Carcinoid syndrome, and anxiety,
    72, 162
Cardiac arrhythmia
  alcoholism and, 232
  anxiety and, 72
  drug abuse and, 272, 275
  medications and
    lithium, 391
    tricyclic antidepressants, 388,
      389
Cardiac conditions
  alcoholism and, 232
  anxiety and, 72–73
  medications and
    chloral hydrate, 394
    lithium, 134
    tricyclic antidepressants, 389
Cardiovascular disease
  drug abuse and, 272
  medications and
    haloperidol, 387
    tricyclic antidepressants, 389
  psychiatric dysfunctions with,
    65
Catapres. See Clonidine
"Catastrophic reaction," 87, 162
Catatonia
  medical disease and, 66
  psychosis and, 106
Catecholamine theory of
    depression, 125
Central anticholinergic syndrome
    (CAS), 106, 107, 108
Central nervous system (CNS),
    and personality, 38, 39
Central nervous system disorders
  alcoholism and, 231
  anxiety and, 73

Cerebral embolism, and organic
    brain syndromes, 97
Cerebral hemorrhage, and
    organic brain syndromes,
    97
Cerebral sclerosis, and organic
    brain syndromes, 97
Cerebral thrombosis, 97
Cerebrovascular disease,
    psychiatric dysfunction
    with, 65
Certification, emergency, 308
Cheilitis, and drug dependence,
    271, 275
Chemotherapy, side effects of, 359
Child development, 410–417
  infancy, 411–412
  middle childhood, 421–422
  prenatal, 410–411
  preschoolers,
    413–414   toddlers,
    412–413
Children, 399–441
  academic performance of, 408
  antisocial personality and,
    49–50, 432
  attention deficit disorder in,
    430–434
  delinquency in, 27, 29
  diagnosis of, 409–410
  disruptive behavior in, 400, 401
  emotional maturity of, 401, 407
  evaluation of
    family sessions, 405
    interviewing the child,
      404–405
    psychological testing,
      405–406, 440
    talking with parents, 402–403
    talking with school
      personnel, 404
  as evolutionary family task,
    24–25
  fantasies of, 404–405, 421–422
  formulation of data on, 406–409
  hyperactivity in, 426, 430–434
  independence of, 25–26
  indications for counseling,
    409–410
  integration and, 25
  learning disabilities of, 404,
    429–430, 436–439
  medical problems and
    asthma, 27
    chronic illness, 425–426
    colic, 27

  diabetes, 27, 355–356
  encopresis, 428
  enuresis, 426–428
  failure to thrive, 24
  hospitalization, 424–425
  obesity, 27
  Tourette syndrome, 434–436
  nurturance of, 25
  PEG and, 407, 438–439
  personality development of,
    38–39, 416, 432
  physical abuse of, 24, 27, 422
  psychiatric problems in
    aphasia, 419–421
    autism, 417–418, 419
    pandevelopmental delay and
      organicity, 417
    schizophrenia, 418–419
    stuttering, 421
  psychotherapy and, 433
  referral of, 410
  school avoidance by, 428–429
  self-esteem of, 404–405
  separation and, 25, 412
  sex education of, 31
  sexuality in, 414–417, 421
  socialization of, 25, 28, 412
  suicide by, 144
  traumatic events and, 409
Chloral hydrate, 394
  alcohol withdrawal and, 234
  anxiety and, 369
  narcotic withdrawal and,
    288
Chlordiazepoxide, 392
  alcohol withdrawal and, 235
  anxiety and, 164, 165
  depression and, 71, 127
  dosage of, 392
  side effects of, 392
  violence and, 299
Chloropromazine, 385
  dosage of, 386
  methadone substitution and,
    288
  psychosis and, 107
  schizophrenia and, 117
  side effects of, 384, 385, 387
Chronic illness, 339–362
  in adolescents, 461
  behavioral responses to
    compliance, 343–344,
      348–349, 354–355
    dependency, 342–343
    depression, 344
    pain, 344–346
    sexual dysfunction, 346

caregiver-patient interactions in, 340–341
case histories of
  adjustment to severe complications, 357
  adolescent diabetes, 356
  cancer, 358, 361
  dependent personality, 341, 343
  drug dependence, 345
  hemodialysis, 348–353
  obsessive-compulsive personality, 342
  paranoia, 353
  patient compliance, 348, 349
  patient denial, 358
  sexual dysfunction, 346
in children, 425–426
examples of
  cancer, 357–362
  diabetes, 354–357
  hemodialysis, 346–354
Chronic organic brain syndrome, 88
  causes of, 97
  diagnosis of, 94–95
Cinetidine, and benzodiazepines, 392
Cirrhosis
  alcoholism and, 232
  drug abuse and, 272
Classic migraine, 179
Clonidine
  adolescents and, 468
  anxiety and, 73
  migraines and, 181
  Tourette syndrome and, 435
Clorazepate, and anxiety, 164
Cluster headache, 180
Cocaine
  abuse of, 275
  anxiety and, 72, 73
  disordered thinking and, 74
  mood alterations and, 68
  paranoia and, 66, 77
  psychosis and, 77, 106
Codeine
  abuse of, 271
  methadone equivalent of, 287
Cogentin. *See* Benztropine mesylate
Cognitive processes, 17–18
  abstraction, 18
  attention, 17–18
  comprehension, 17–18
  concentration, 17–18
  content of thought, 18

judgment, 18
  memory, 17
  orientation, 17
  perceptions, 18
Cognitive styles, and personality, 39
Coincidental medical-surgical disorders, 42
Colds, and mood alterations, 68, 71
Colic, and family, 27
Colitis, ulcerative, 27, 172, 198
Communication
  by children, 25
  in family, 24
  in mental status examination, 16–17
  in sexual relationship, 329
Compensation neurosis, 200–201
Comprehension
  in mental status examination, 17–18
  in organic brain syndromes, 85
Compulsive personality disorder
  anxiety disorder vs., 163
  case history of, 45
  dysfunctional response to, 45
  intervention for, 45
  problem of, 44–45
  recognition of, 44
Concentration, in mental status examination, 17–18
Concussion, and organic brain syndromes, 96
Conditioning therapy, and alcoholism, 249
Conflict
  personality development and, 38
  psychotherapy and, 370
Confusion
  medical illnesses with, 73–78
  organic brain syndromes and, 75
Congenital expressive aphasia, 420
Consciousness, levels of, 16
Contraception
  adolescents and, 457–458
  sexual dysfunctions and, 328
Contraceptives, and depression, 127
Conversion disorder, 192–194
  catatonia and, 66
  diagnosis of, 193–194
  diagnostic criteria for, 194
  referral for, 202

social-communication model of, 192–193
  traditional model of, 192
Conversion headache, 182–184
Coping styles, 407
Coronary artery disease
  etiologic factors in, 67
  psychiatric dysfunctions with, 65
Coronary patient
  case history of, 4, 11–13
  reactions of, 13, 63
Couples therapy, 376
Creatine phosphokinase (CPK), and schizophrenia, 115
Creutzfeldt–Jakob disease, 97
Current context (in PEG), 4, 5–6, 8
Cushing's disease
  depression and, 70
  mood alterations with, 68, 70
  organic brain syndromes and, 96
  suicide and, 141
Cushing's syndrome
  depression and, 127
  mood alterations with, 68, 70
  psychosis and, 106
Cyclothymic disorder, 128
Cyclothymic leveler. *See* Lithium
Cyproheptadine, and migraines, 181

Death
  cancer patients and, 360
  families and, 30
Decongestants, and psychosis, 106
Defense mechanisms, 7
  anxiety and, 160
  endocrine system, 173
Deficiencies, and organic brain syndromes, 96
Degenerative diseases
  hysteria and, 201
  organic brain syndromes and, 97
Dehydration, and alcoholism, 232
Delinquency, 27, 29, 473–476
Delirium
  age and, 91
  diagnosis of, 94–95
  diagnostic criteria for, 88
  disordered thinking and, 74
  drug abuse and, 272
  paranoia and, 66
  See also Organic brain syndromes

Delirium tremens, 105, 108, 233, 236
Delusional headache, 182–184
Delusions, 73
    in manic-depressive illness, 91
    in mental status examination, 18
    in organic brain syndromes, 86
    in schizophrenia, 91–92
Dementia
    alcohol and, 236, 251
    diabetes and, 70
    diagnosis of, 94–95
    diagnostic criteria for, 89
    physician handling of patients with, 64
    signs and symptoms of
        appearance, 16
        depression, 67
        hysteria, 16
        orientation, 17
        paranoia, 66
    See also Organic brain syndromes
Demyelinating disorders, psychiatric dysfunctions with, 65
Denial of defect, 87
Dependency, 267, 342–343
Dependent personality disorder
    chronic illness and, 341
    dysfunctional response to, 44
    intervention for, 44
    problem of, 44
    recognition of, 43
Depression, 123–137
    in adolescence, 464–466
    "anniversary reactions," 61
    antidepressant drug therapy for
        electroconvulsive therapy, 134
        lithium, 133–134, 390–391
        MAO inhibitors, 133, 389–390
        tricyclics, 131–133, 388–389
    biological events and, 8
    case history of, 124, 135–137
    diagnosis of, 67–71, 126–128
    environmental therapy for, 134–135
    etiologic theories of
        biological, 125–126
        psychological, 125
    genetics and, 411
    Hamilton psychiatric rating scale for, 244–247
    "ideopathic," 128

management of
    grief and situational adjustment reaction, 129–130
    hospitalization, 129
    in major affective disorders, 130
    medical disease, toxins, or drugs, 130
    masked, 59
    PCP and, 278
    PEG for, 136
    physical illness and
        cancer, 359
        chronic illness, 344, 351, 359
        diabetes mellitus, 70, 127
        drugs, 70–71, 126, 127, 130
        endocrine disorders, 69–70, 126, 127
        infectious diseases, 71
        organic brain syndromes, 90
        systemic diseases, 71
    sexual dysfunction and, 321, 322
    signs and symptoms of
        appearance, 16
        attention, 18
        catatonia, 66
        comprehension, 18
        concentration, 18
        disordered thinking, 73, 74–75
        hallucinations, 73
        headaches, 181
        hysteria, 66
        with somatic complaints, 59–64
        stress reactions, 61
        suicide and, 60–61, 124, 129, 130, 131, 141
Depressive neurosis, 128
Depressive syndrome, 124–125
    diagnostic criteria for, 127
    differential diagnostic categories for, 128
    evaluation of, 126–128
    headaches and, 182
    psychotherapy and, 130–131
    violence and, 301
Dermatitis, and drug dependence, 271
Desipramine
    depression and, 125, 126, 131, 132
    side effects of, 389
Detoxification, 283
    from barbiturates, 283, 290–292

methods of
    clonidine hydrochloride, 289–290
    methadone substitution, 283, 286–289
    from sedatives, 283, 290–292
Developmental tests, 405–406, 440
Dextroamphetamine
    abuse of, 275
    Tourette syndrome and, 435
Diabetes, 27, 354–357
    age of onset and, 355–356
    case histories of, 356, 357
    compliance and, 354–355
    complications of, 356–357
    etiologic factors in, 67
    hypoglycemia and, 355
    impotence and, 322
    medication and
        disulfiram or DDC, 250
        lithium, 391
    mood alterations and, 68
    obesity and, 355
    psychiatric disorders and, 70
    sexual dysfunctions and, 322, 356
Diabetic ketoacidosis, and catatonia, 66
Diagnostic and Statistical Manual (DSM-III), 42, 223, 226
Diazepam, 392
    abuse of, 274–275
    alcohol withdrawal and, 235
    anxiety and, 164, 165
    compulsive personality disorders and, 45
    depression and, 71, 127, 129
    dosage of, 392
    organic brain syndromes and, 97
    PCP and, 277
    psychosis and, 107
    side effects of, 392
    violence and, 299
Diethyldithiocarbamate (DDC), 250
Digitalis, and organic brain syndromes, 96
Digit span, 18
Dihydroindolenes, 384
Dilandanum, methadone equivalent of, 286
Dilantin. See Diphenylhydantoin
Dilaudid. See Dilandanum
Dimethoryphenylethylamine (DMPE), 115

Dimethyltryptamine (DMT), 275–276
Diphenhydramine
    antipsychotic side effects and, 387
    narcotic withdrawal and, 288
Diphenylhydantoin, 50
Disease
    approach to, 4
    mood alterations and, 68
    organic vs. functional, 58
    psychiatric dysfunctions with, 65
    role of family system deficiencies in, 28
    See also Chronic illness; Infectious diseases; Physical disorders
Disordered thinking
    medical illness with, 73–78
    organic brain syndromes and, 74–75
Dissociation
    catatonia and, 66
    remote memory and, 17
Disulfiram, 249–250, 464
Disulfiram-ethanol reaction (DER), 249, 250
Diuretics
    depression and, 71
    lithium and, 391
    mood alterations and, 68
DOM, dependence on, 275–276
Dopamine, and schizophrenia, 116
Doriden. *See* Glutethimide
Doxepin, and narcotic withdrawal, 288
Draw-a-Person (DAP) test, 406
Drug abuse, 267, 462–464
Drug dependence, 265–293
    case histories of, 266, 292–293, 345
    chronic pain and, 344–346
    definition of, 266
    etiology of
        availability, 267–268
        pharmacologic disturbance, 268
        psychological deficit, 268
        social factors, 268
        socioeconomic factors, 268
    evaluation of
        drug history, 269
        laboratory tests, 279
        physical examination, 270–271

psychological status, 270
    social situation, 269–270
family and, 280–281
medical complications of, 272
PEG for, 293
referral for, 281–282
treatment of
    counseling, 282–283
    detoxification, 283, 286–292
    methadone maintenance, 284–285, 286–289
    narcotic antagonists, 285
    outpatient programs, 284
    panic management, 285–286
    rapid withdrawal with clonidine hydrochloride, 289–290
    therapeutic communities, 283–284
types of
    hallucinogens, 275–276
    marijuana, 278–279
    narcotics, 271–273
    phencyclidine, 276–278
    sedatives, 273–275
    stimulants, 275
Drug history, 269
Drug-induced states, 18
Drug misuse, 266–267
Drug reactions, toxic, 65
Drugs
    anxiety and, 73, 161, 162
    behavior-altering, 67
    catatonia and, 66
    definition of, 266
    depression and, 70–71, 126, 127, 130
    illegal, 266
    medical problems and
        alcoholism, 228
        headaches, 180–181, 182
        organic brain syndromes, 92–93, 96
    mood alterations and, 68
    paranoia and, 66
    psychosis and, 77–78, 105–106
    See also Medication; Psychotropic medication
Drug use, 266
Dysarthria, 16
Dyskinesia
    antipsychotic medications and, 67, 117, 386
    neuroleptics and, 165
Dyspnea, 60, 73
Dysthymic disorder, 128

Edema
    drug dependence and, 271, 272
    lithium and, 391
Education, and suicide, 147
    See also Special education
Egoistic suicide, 142
Ejaculatory incompetence, 324–325
Ejaculatory inhibitions, 324–325
Elavil. *See* Amitriptyline
Elderly
    disordered thinking in, 74
    families and, 30
    organic brain syndromes and, 84
    subdural hematoma and, 77
Electroconvulsive therapy (ECT), 67
    depression and, 134
    suicide and, 152
Electrolyte levels
    alcoholism and, 232
    psychosis and, 106
    suicide and, 152
Emancipation disorder, 468
Emergency certification, 308
Emotional reactions
    catastrophic, 87
    in organic brain syndromes, 86, 87
"Empty nest," 26
Encephalitis, 63
    case history of, 64
    catatonia and, 66
    depression and, 71
    disordered thinking and, 74, 76
    manic-depressive illness and, 91
    mood alterations and, 68
    organic brain syndromes and, 96, 97
    psychosis and, 76, 106
Encephalopathies
    organic brain syndromes and, 96
    psychiatric dysfunctions with, 65
Encopresis, 428
Endocarditis, and drug dependence, 272
Endocrine disorders
    anxiety and, 72, 161–162
    depression and, 69–70, 126, 127
    mood alterations and, 68, 69
    organic brain syndromes and, 96
    paranoia and, 66

Endocrine disorders (*Cont.*)
  psychiatric dysfunctions with,
    65, 66
  psychosis and, 106
  psychosomatic disorders and,
    172–177
  sexual dysfunctions and, 328
Endometriosis, and sexual
    dysfunctions, 328
Endorphins
  affective disorders and, 126
  drug dependence and, 268
  pain and, 178
Enkephalins
  drug dependence and, 268
  pain and, 178
Enuresis, 426–428
Environmental interaction (in
    PEG), 4, 6, 7, 13
  See also Families
Environmental manipulation,
    166
Epidural hematoma, and organic
    brain syndromes, 96
Epilepsy
  alcoholism and, 233
  anxiety and, 72, 73
  disordered thinking and, 74
  disulfiram or DDC and, 250
  manic-depressive illness and,
    91
  narcotic withdrawal and, 273
  organic brain syndromes and,
    96, 97
  paranoia and, 66
  psychiatric symptoms with, 65
  psychosis and, 76–77, 106
  violence and, 301, 307–308
Epinephrine
  sedatives and, 299
  tricyclics and, 389
Episodic dyscontrol syndrome,
    medication for, 50
Erectile problems, 321–322
Ergotamine tartrate, and
    migraines, 180
Estrogen replacement therapy,
    and sexual dysfunctions,
    328
Ethchlorvynol
  depression and, 71
  efficacy of, 394
Ethnic groups, and suicide,
    145–146
Ethyl alcohol, and psychosis, 105
  See also Alcohol; Alcoholic
    psychosis

Evaluation
  mental status examination in,
    15–19
  use of PEG in, 4–13
Evolutionary family tasks, 24–26
  children, 24–25
  independence, 25–26
  integration, 25
  nurturance and separation, 25
  socialization, 25
Extrapyramidal side effects (EPS),
    385, 387

Factitious illness, 199, 200
Families, 21–32
  adolescents and, 451
  aging and, 26, 30
  alcoholism and, 229–230, 238,
    252–254
  cancer and, 360–361
  counseling of, 360–361
  death and, 30
  drug dependence and, 280–281
  illness and, 22, 26–30
  levels of intergenerational
    transmission in, 32
  personality assessment and, 41
  psychosomatic conditions and,
    26–27
  response to illness, 29–30
  schizophrenia and, 116
  violence and, 301, 306
  See also Parents
Family boundaries, 23–24
Family counseling, 376, 405,
    467–468
Family evaluation, 21–32
Family health, 30–31
Family health care, 31–32
Family history, and suicide, 146
Family pathology, 27, 29
Family systems, 23–26
  affectivity in, 24
  boundaries in, 23–24
  communication in, 24
  evolutionary family tasks in,
    24–26
  leadership in, 23
Fetal alcohol syndrome (FAS),
    253–254, 410
Fibrosing myopathies, and drug
    dependence, 272
Fixation, 401
Fluorescent Treponema antibody
    (FTA) test, 279
Fluphenazine, and schizophrenia,
    117

Flurazepam
  anxiety and, 164
  depression and, 129
  dosage of, 393
  insomnia and, 393
  narcotic withdrawal and,
    288–289
Friedreich's ataxia, and organic
    brain syndromes, 97
Frigidity. *See* Orgasmic
    dysfunctions, female
Functional disease, 58
Functional psychosis, 107

Gallbladder disease, and hysteria,
    66
Gastritis
  alcoholism and, 232
  chloral hydrate and, 394
Gastrointestinal complications
  alcoholism and, 232
  drug abuse and, 272
Generalized anxiety disorder, 162,
    165
Genetics
  alcoholism and, 229–230
  psychiatric problems and, 411
  schizophrenia and, 114–115,
    410–411
Genitourinary complications, and
    drug abuse, 272
Genotype, 401–402
Geriatric medicine, 30
Glaucoma, and tricyclic
    antidepressants, 389
"Glove anesthesia," 193
Glutethimide
  abuse of, 273–275
  barbiturate withdrawal and, 291
  depression and, 71
  drug dependence and, 273
  efficacy of, 394
Granulomas, drug dependence
    and, 272
Grief reaction
  depression and, 129–130, 359
  psychosomatic disorders and,
    176
Group therapy, 376
Guanethidine, and tricyclics, 389

Habits, patient, 7
Haldol. *See* Haloperidol
Hallucinations, 73
  alcoholism and, 236
  medical illness and, 74
  in mental status examination, 18

in organic brain syndromes, 86
in schizophrenia, 73, 91
suicide and, 150
Hallucinogens
dependence on, 275–276
disordered thinking and, 74
paranoia and, 66
psychosis and, 105, 106, 108
suicide and, 106
Haloperidol, 384, 385
ADD children and, 434
anxiety and, 165
dosage of, 386
EPS of, 385, 387
mania and, 133, 391
psychosis and, 107, 353
schizophrenia and, 117
Tourette syndrome and, 435
violence and, 299
Hamilton psychiatric rating scale
for depression, 244–247
Headaches, 177–186
case history of, 172, 185–186
classification of
combined, 182
delusional, 182–183
muscle contraction, 181–182
posttraumatic, 183–184
vascular migraine, 179–181
vasomotor reaction, 182
pain and, 177–178
treatment of
biofeedback training, 181,
182
pharmacotherapy, 180–181,
182
psychotherapy, 181, 182
stress reduction, 181, 182
Health care, family, 30–32
Health screening, 31
Heart disease
disulfiram or DDC and, 250
PEG and, 8
Heart failure
depression and, 67
disordered thinking and, 74, 75
mood alterations and, 68
organic brain syndromes and,
96
Heavy metal poisoning, 96, 97
Hematologic disorders, and mood
alterations, 68
Hematopoietic complications, and
drug dependence, 272
Hemiplegic migraine, 180
Hemodialysis, 346–354
case histories of, 348–353

compliance in, 348–351
depression and, 351
at home, 349–350
organic brain syndromes and,
352
paranoia and, 352
psychosis and, 352
psychotropic medications and,
353–354
quality of life and, 347
schizophrenia and, 352–353
sex and, 350–351
suicide and, 351–352
treatment milieu of, 347–348
violence and, 352
Hemoglobinopathies, psychiatric
dysfunctions with, 65
Hepatic disease
drug abuse and, 272
medication and:
antianxiety drugs, 392
chloral hydrate, 394
disulfiram or DDC, 250
psychiatric symptoms and, 62
Hepatic failure
depression and, 67
drug abuse and, 272
medications and:
antianxiety drugs, 392
disulfiram or DDC, 250
mood alterations and, 68
Hepatitis
alcoholism and, 232
depression and, 71, 126, 127
drug abuse and, 272
mood alterations and, 68
psychiatric dysfunctions with,
65
suicide and, 71
Heroin
alcoholism and, 228
methadone equivalent of, 286
violence and, 301, 303
withdrawal from, 273, 283, 284
Hirschsprung's disease, 428
Histrionic personality disorder
case history of, 46
diagnostic criteria for, 196
dysfunctional response to, 46
hysteria and, 195–196
intervention for, 46–47
problem of, 46
recognition of, 45–46
violence and, 301, 305
Home hemodialysis, 349–350
Homosexuality, 460
Hospices, 30

Huntington's chorea
organic brain syndromes and,
97
paranoia and, 66
suicide and, 141
Hydralazine, and suicide, 152
Hydrocephalus
dementia and, 88
organic brain syndromes and,
96, 97
Hyperactivity, 426, 430–434
Hypercalcemia
catatonia and, 66
depression and, 127
organic brain syndromes and,
96
Hyperinsulinism
anxiety and, 72
psychosis and, 106
Hyperparathyroidism
anxiety and, 72
depression and, 126, 127
mood alterations and, 68
organic brain syndromes and,
96
Hypertension
alcoholism and, 232
anxiety and, 73
drug abuse and, 272
as psychosomatic disorder,
172
Hyperthyroidism
anxiety and, 72, 162
depression and, 69
organic brain syndromes and,
96
suicide and, 69
Hyperventilation, and medical
illness, 72
Hypnotherapy, and hysteria,
202
Hypnotics. *See* Sedative-hypnotic
compounds
Hypochondria, and suicide, 150
Hypochondriacal headache,
182–184
Hypochondriasis, 183, 198–199
Hypoglycemia
alcoholism and, 232
anxiety and, 72, 162
diabetes and, 355
organic brain syndromes and,
96
psychiatric symptoms and, 70
Hypokalemia
alcohol withdrawal and, 233
depression and, 71

Hypomagnesia
    alcohol withdrawal and, 233
    organic brain syndromes and,
        96
Hypomania, 16
Hyponatremia, and organic brain
    syndromes, 95, 96
Hypoparathyroidism
    anxiety and, 72
    mood alterations and, 68
    organic brain syndromes and,
        96
Hypotension
    drug abuse and, 272
    MAO inhibitors and, 390
    tricyclics and, 388, 389
Hypothalamic syndromes, and
    mood alterations, 68
Hypothyroidism
    dementia and, 88
    depression and, 69, 127
    lithium and, 134, 391
    mood alterations and, 69
    organic brain syndromes and,
        96
    psychosis and, 69
    suicide and, 141
Hypovolemia, and organic brain
    syndromes, 96
Hysteria, 189–204
    case history of, 190, 203–204
    factitious illness, 199
    genetics and, 411
    historical note on, 190–192
    histrionic personality, 45–47,
        195–196
    hypochondriasis, 183, 198–199
    malingering, 200
    management of, 201–202
    medical disease and, 65–66
    narcotic withdrawal and, 273
    psychogenic pain disorder,
        194–195
    referral for, 202
    somatization disorder, 196–197
    suicide and, 65
    types of
        compensation neurosis,
            200–201
        conversion disorder,
            192–194
"Hysterical" personality. See
    Histrionic personality
    disorder

Identity disorders, 470–471
Ideopathic depression, 128

Illinois Test of Psycholinguistic
    Ability (ITBA), 406
Illness
    factitious, 199
    families and, 22, 26–30
    family response to, 29–30
    parenthood and, 29–30
    patient reaction to, 13,
        63–64
    personality and, 43
    See also Chronic illness;
        Physical disorders
Illusions, in mental status
    examination, 18
Imipramine, 388–389
    ADD children and, 434
    adolescents and, 465, 467
    anxiety and, 165
    depression and, 125, 126,
        131–133, 465
    enuresis and, 427
Immediate memory, 17, 93–94
Immunoglobulin levels, and
    schizophrenia, 116
Impotence, 321–322
Incest, 24, 459–460
Independence, as evolutionary
    family task, 25
Inderal. See Propranolol
Indoleamine theory of affective
    disorders, 125
Infant development, 411–412
Infection
    alcoholism and, 232
    disordered thinking and, 74, 75,
        76
    psychosis and, 76
Infectious diseases
    depression and, 71
    disordered thinking and, 74
    mood alterations and, 68
    organic brain syndromes and,
        97
    paranoia and, 66
    psychiatric dysfunctions with,
        65, 66
    suicide and, 71
Influenza
    depression and, 71, 127
    mood alterations and, 68
Informed consent, and blood
    alcohol tests, 256
Inherent medical-surgical
    disorders, 42
Insight-orientated psychotherapy,
    165–166, 375
Insomnia, and suicide, 150

Integration, as evolutionary family
    task, 25
Intensive psychotherapy, 165–166
International Statistical
    Classification of Diseases,
    223, 226
Intracranial neoplasm, psychiatric
    symptoms with, 65
Ismelin. See Guanethidine
Isoniazid, 250

Jaundice
    drug dependence and, 271
    tricyclics and, 388
Jejunitis, and alcoholism, 232
Judgment, in mental status
    examination, 18, 94

Klinefelter's syndrome
    mood alterations and, 68
    paranoia and, 66
Korsakoff's psychosis, 97, 98,
    223

Laetrile, 360
Latency, 421
Laudanum, methadone equivalent
    of, 287
Leadership, in families, 23
Learning disabilities, 404,
    429–430, 436–439
Learning theory
    anxiety and, 160
    suicide and, 142
Leritine. See Anileridine
Leukocytosis, and lithium, 134
Levarterenol, and tricyclics, 389
Levodopa
    MAO inhibitors and, 390
    paranoia and, 66
    psychosis and, 106
    schizophrenia and, 116
Levo-Dromoran. See Levorphanol
Levorphanol, methadone
    equivalent of, 287
Librium. See Chlordiazepoxide
Life change events, 210
Life-style changes, 6
Lithium, 390–391
    adolescents and, 466
    alcoholism and, 250
    depression and, 133–134
    episodic dyscontrol syndrome
        and, 50
    migraines and, 181
    psychotherapy and, 372
    side effects of, 134, 390–391

Long-suffering, self-sacrificing
personality type
case history of, 53
dysfunctional response to, 53
intervention for, 53
problem of, 53
recognition of, 53
Lorazepam, and insomnia, 393
LSD
anxiety and, 162
dependence on, 275–276
psychosis and, 77, 106
Lymphoma, and depression, 69

Major affective disorder, 124
anxiety and, 162
compulsions and, 163
depression in, 130
obsessions and, 163
Major depression of major
affective disorders, 128
Malingering, 200
Mania
depression and, 71, 90–91
diagnosis of, 62, 71
lithium and, 133
organic brain disorder and,
90–91
signs and symptoms of
attention, 18
comprehension, 18
concentration, 18
delusions, 18, 73
hallucinations, 73
paranoia, 66
speech, 16
theories of, 125–126
Manic-depressive illness, 124
in adolescents, 465–466
catatonia and, 66
delusions and, 91
genetics and, 411
hyperactivity and, 91
organic brain syndromes and,
90–91
organic factors in, 67
suicide and, 141
tricyclics and, 389, 391
violence and, 301, 304
Manic syndrome, 125
Marijuana
alcoholism and, 228
dependence on, 278–279
paranoia and, 66
psychosis and, 106
Marital status, and suicide, 144
Marriage counseling, 376

MDA, dependence on, 275–276
Medical history, and PEG, 8
Medical illness. *See* Chronic
illness; Physical disorders
Medical-surgical disorders
coincidental, 42
inherent, 42
Medicare, 30
Medication
depression and, 71
mood alterations and, 71
organic brain syndromes and,
96
patient reaction to, 63
psychotherapy and, 369,
372–373
schizophrenia and, 117
violence and, 299
See also Drugs; Psychotropic
medications
Mellaril. *See* Thioridazine
Memory
immediate, 17, 93–94
recent, 17, 85, 93
remote, 17, 85, 93
Meningitis
alcoholism and, 232
drug dependence and, 272
hysteria and, 66
organic brain syndromes and,
96, 97
Menopause, and sexual
dysfunction, 328
Menstrual irregularities, and drug
dependence, 272
Mental disorders. *See* Psychiatric
disorders
Mental retardation
in children, 417
judgment and, 18
violence and, 301, 306
Mental status examination,
15–19
affect, 18–19
alcoholism and, 237
appearance, 16
cognitive processes, 17–18
level of consciousness, 16
mood, 18–19
movement, 16–17
organic brain syndromes and,
93–94
speech, 16–17
Meperidine
abuse of, 271
MAO inhibitors and, 133, 390
methadone equivalent of, 287

Meprobamate
anxiety and, 391
barbiturate withdrawal and, 291
depression and, 71
Mescaline
catatonia and, 66
dependence on, 275–276
psychosis and, 77
Metabolic disorders
organic brain syndromes and, 96
psychiatric symptoms and, 66
Metaraminol, and MAO inhibitors,
390
Methadone
abuse of, 271–272
hemodialysis and, 354
withdrawal from, 273
Methadone maintenance, 284–285
Methadone substitution, 286–289,
464
Methamphetamine abuse, 275
Methaqualone abuse, 273–275
Methyldopa
depression and, 71, 127, 344
mood alterations and, 68
suicide and, 152
Methylphenidate
abuse of, 275
ADD children and, 433, 434
tricyclics and, 389
Methyprylon, efficacy of, 394
Methysergide, and migraines, 181
Microinfarcts, and drug
dependence, 272
Middle-life crises, 26
Migraines, vascular
personality traits and, 180
situational factors and, 180, 181
treatment of
biofeedback training, 181
pharmacotherapy, 180–181
psychotherapy, 181
stress reduction, 181
types of
basilar artery, 180
classic, 179
cluster headache, 180
common, 179–180
hemiplegic, 180
ophthalmoplegic, 180
Miltown. *See* Meprobamate
Minimal brain dysfunction (MBD),
430
Minnesota Multiphasic Personality
Inventory (MMPI), 41–42
Monoamine-oxidase (MAO)
inhibitors, 389–390

Monoamine-oxidase (*Cont.*)
   adolescents and, 468
   anxiety and, 165
   depression and, 125, 131, 133
   migraines and, 181
   paranoia and, 66
   psychosis and, 106
   psychoterapy and, 372
   side effects of, 389–390
   suicide and, 152
   tyramine and, 389–390
Mononucleosis
   depression and, 127
   psychiatric dysfunctions with, 65
Mood, in mental status
     examination, 18
Mood changes, 6, 62
   endocrine disorders and, 69–70
   medical illnesses with, 68
   in organic brain syndromes, 86
Morphine
   abuse of, 271–272
   methadone equivalent of, 286
   withdrawal from, 273
Movement, in mental status
     examination, 16
Multiple sclerosis
   hysteria and, 201
   organic brain syndromes and, 97
Munchausen's syndrome, 199
Muscle contraction headache,
     181–182
Muscle relaxants, and headaches,
     182
Myeletis, and drug dependence,
     272
Myocardial infarction
   asymptomatic, 8
   disordered thinking and, 74, 75
   lithium and, 391
   organic brain syndromes and,
     99–101
Myocarditis, and drug abuse, 272

Nalbuphine, 286
Naltrexone, 285
Narcissistic personality disorder
   dysfunctional response to, 48
   intervention for, 48
   problem of, 48
   recognition of, 48
Narcoanalysis, 202
Narcotic analgesics
   delirium and, 78
   disordered thinking and, 74
   hemodialysis and, 354
   mood alterations and, 68

Narcotic antagonists, 285
Narcotics, 271–273
   anxiety and, 73, 161, 162
   depression and, 344
   hemodialysis and, 354
   methadone maintenance and,
     284–285
   overdose of, 272–273
   pain management and,
     285–286, 344–346
   symptoms of intoxication,
     271–272
   withdrawal from, 273, 283,
     286–289
Nardil. *See* Phenelzine
Nasal septum, and drug abuse,
     271, 275
National Council on Alcoholism,
     223, 225
Native Americans
   alcoholism among, 228
   suicide among, 145
Nembutal. *See* Pentobarbital
Neoplasia, 65, 152
Nephritic conditions, 250
Nephrotic syndrome, and drug
     dependence, 272
Nervous headache, 181–182
Neurodermatitis, 172
Neuroleptic drugs
   ADD children and, 434
   anxiety and, 164, 165
   psychosis and, 106, 107, 108
   schizophrenia and, 117
   side effects of, 165
Neurologic disorders
   catatonia and, 66
   drug dependence and, 272
   organic brain syndromes and,
     96, 97
   paranoia and, 66
   psychosis and, 76–77
Neuronal hyperexcitability, 233
Neuroses
   family system deficiencies and,
     28
   organic brain syndromes and, 92
   types of
     compensation, 200
     depressive, 128
     obsessive-compulsive, 92,
       162–163
Neurosyphilis, tertiary, 58
Neurotic disorders, and referral
     for psychotherapy, 370
Neurotransmitters
   depression and, 126

pain and, 178
   schizophrenia and, 116
Noludar. *See* Methyprylon
Norepinephrine
   anorexia nervosa and, 462
   depression and, 125, 131, 133
Nortriptyline, and cardiovascular
     disease, 389
Nubain. *See* Nalbuphine
Nursing homes, 30
Nurturance, as evolutionary family
     task, 25

Obesity
   in adolescence, 462
   diabetes and, 355
   family and, 27
Object constancy, 413
Obsessive-compulsive disorders,
     162–163
   organic brain syndromes and,
     92
   psychotherapy and, 165–166
Obsessive-compulsive personality,
     38, 342
Occupation, and suicide, 146
Ophthalmoplegic migraine, 180
Opiates, and prenatal
     development, 411
Opiate withdrawal
   anxiety and, 72, 73
   clonidine hydrochloride and,
     283, 289–290
   convulsions and, 273
Opium alkaloids, methadone
     equivalent of, 287
Organic brain syndromes,
     83–101
   cancer and, 360
   case history of, 84, 99–101
   causes of, 96, 97
   cell death in, 84–85, 88
   criteria for referral, 99
   diagnosis of
     basic evaluation procedure,
       95
     criteria for delirium, 88
     criteria for dementia, 89
     specific, 94–95
   differential diagnosis of
     alcohol abuse, 92–93
     anxiety, 89–90
     depression, 90–91
     drug abuse, 92–93
     mania, 90–91
     obsessive-compulsive
       disorders, 92

personality disorders, 92
schizophrenia, 91–92
elderly and, 74–75, 84
hemodialysis and, 352
management of, 98–99
medication and
    antipsychotic drugs, 386–387
    lithium, 391
    sedatives, 95, 97
    tranquilizers, 97
PEG and, 99–101
rapidity of onset of, 87–88
reversibility of, 88, 95–98
signs and symptoms of
    anxiety, 162, 164
    cognitive processes, 17, 85,
        92, 94
    confusion, 75, 87
    delusions, 18, 86, 91–92
    emotional reactions, 86, 87
    judgment, 18, 87, 94
    memory, 17, 85, 92, 93–94
    mood changes, 86
    orientation, 17, 74, 75, 85, 92
    paranoia, 86
    personality change, 87
types of
    acute, 87–88, 94–95, 96
    chronic, 88, 94–95, 97
violence and, 301, 306–307
Organic disease, 58
Organic solvents, and psychosis,
    105
Orgasmic dysfunctions
    female, 322–324
    male, 324–325
Orientation
    in mental status examination, 17
    in organic brain syndromes, 85
Osteomyelitis, and drug
    dependence, 272
Oxazepam
    anxiety and, 164
    insomnia and, 393
Oxycodone, and hemodialysis,
    354

Pain
    chronic illness and, 344–346
    drug dependence and, 344–346
    headache and, 177–178
    psychogenic pain disorder,
        194–195
Pancreatitis
    alcoholism and, 232
    drug dependence and, 272
Panic disorder, 162, 165

Paraldehyde
    alcohol withdrawal and, 234,
        235
    disulfiram or DDC and, 250
Paranoia
    alcoholic, 236
    drug abuse and, 275, 276
    hemodialysis and, 352, 353
    medical disease and, 66
Paranoid personality disorder
    case history of, 47
    intervention for, 47–48
    problem of, 47
    recognition of, 47
    violence and, 301, 305–306
Parathyroid adenoma, and
    catatonia, 66
Paregoric, methadone equivalent
    of, 287
Parents
    in evaluation of child's
        psychiatric problems,
        402–403
    incest and, 459–460
    See also Families
Parkinsonism
    antipsychotic medications and,
        387
    paranoia and, 66
Parkinson's disease, and organic
    brain syndromes, 97
Parnate. *See* Tranylcypromine
Paroxysmal tachycardia, and
    anxiety, 72
Passive-aggressive personality
    disorder, 301, 305
Pathologic intoxication, 236
Pathophysiology, 67
Patient care
    in medicine, 4
    in psychiatry, 4
    PEG and, 8
    See also Chronic illness
Patient Evaluation Grid (PEG)
    aim of, 8–9
    application to patient care
        planning, 8
    case histories using
        adolescent psychiatric
            problems, 475–476
        alcoholism, 258
        anxiety, 167–168
        child psychiatric problems,
            438–439
        coronary patient, 4, 11–13
        depression, 135–137
        drug dependence, 293

headaches, 185–186
hysteria, 203–204
organic brain syndromes,
    99–101
psychosis, 110–111
schizophrenia, 119–120
sexual dysfunction, 333–334
situational disturbance
    syndrome, 217–218
suicide, 154–155
children and, 407
contexts in
    background, 4, 6–7
    current, 4, 5–6, 8
    recent, 4, 6, 8
dimensions of
    biological, 4, 6, 7, 8, 13
    environmental, 4, 6, 7, 13
    personal, 4, 6, 7, 13
evaluation and, 5
example of, 12
management plans from, 8
medical history and, 8
model for, 5
organization of, 4–7
use of, 7–9, 99–101
value of, 9, 13
Patients
    coronary, 11–13
    death rates among, 65
    environmental interaction with,
        4, 6 7
    habits of, 7
    informing of, 63–64
    medical history of, 8
    personal attributes of, 4, 6,
        7, 13
    personality type of, 7
    psychological state of, 6
    psychosomatic disorders and,
        174–177
    reaction to illness, 13, 63–64
    recent changes of, 6
    recent events of, 6
    referral for psychotherapy,
        370–372, 377–380
    sick role and, 173–174
    See also Chronic illness; Stress
Pellagra
    catatonia and, 66
    organic brain syndromes and,
        96
Pemoline, and ADD children,
    434
Penicillamine, and Wilson's
    disease, 75
Pentazocine, 96, 286

Pentobarbital, 393
  alcohol withdrawal and, 234,
    235
  barbiturate withdrawal and,
    283, 290–292
Pentopon. *See* Opium alkaloids
Perceptions, in mental status
    examination, 18
Permissive theory of affective
    disorders, 125
Perphenazine, 384, 385
  anxiety and, 164, 165
  dosage of, 386, 387
  EPS of, 387
  psychosis and, 107
  schizophrenia and, 117
Personal attributes (in PEG), 4, 6,
    7, 13
Personality
  alcoholism and, 230–231
  avoidant, 48–49
  hysterical, 45–47
  illness and, 43
  obsessive-compulsive, 38
  sick role and, 173–174
  stress and, 43
  Type A, 44, 67
  Type B, 67
Personality assessment, 39–42
  asking questions, 40–41
  case history of, 40
  listening, 40
  observation, 39–40
  observations of family, friends,
    and staff, 41
  psychological testing, 41–42
Personality change, 6, 87
Personality development, 38–39,
    416, 432
  conflict and, 38
  cognitive styles and, 39
  constitutional endowment and,
    38–39
Personality disorders, 42–54
  definition of, 42
  general management
    considerations for, 53–54
  genetics and, 411
  judgment and, 18
  organic brain syndromes and, 92
  referral for psychotherapy and,
    370
  types of
    antisocial, 49–51
    borderline, 51–52
    compulsive, 44–45
    dependent, 43–44

histrionic, 45–47
long-suffering, self-sacrificing
    type, 52–53
narcissistic, 48
paranoid, 47–48
schizoid, 48–49
violence and, 301, 304–306
Personality traits, 43, 180, 182
Personality types, 7, 39–54
  recognition of, 39–42
  sick role expectations and, 13
Pertofrane. *See* Desipramine
Phencyclidine (PCP), 276–278
  anxiety and, 162
  catatonia and, 66
  disordered thinking and, 74
  overdose of, 277–278
  paranoia and, 66
  psychosis and, 78, 105–106, 108
  sedatives and, 299
  signs of intoxication, 276–277
  violence and, 301, 302–303
Phenelzine, 389–390
  adolescents and, 468
  anxiety and, 165
  depression and, 133
Phenobarbital, and barbiturate
    withdrawal, 283
Phenothiazines, 384, 385
  ADD children and, 434
  alcohol withdrawal and, 234
  anorexia nervosa and, 462
  anticholinergic psychosis and,
    106
  anxiety and, 165
  catatonia and, 66
  delirium and, 78
  disordered thinking and, 74
  PCP and, 277
  psychosis and, 353
  psychotherapy and, 372
  schizophrenia and, 117
  side effects of, 387
  Tourette syndrome and, 435
  tricyclics and, 389
Phenotype, 401–402
Phenylbutazol, and tricyclics, 389
Phenylephrine
  MAO inhibitors and, 390
  tricyclics and, 389
Phenytoin
  alcohol withdrawal and, 234
  disulfiram or DDC and, 250
  paranoia and, 66
  tricyclics and, 389
Pheochromocytoma, and anxiety,
    72, 162

Phobic disorders
  psychotherapy for, 165–166
  types of
    agoraphobia, 163, 165
    simple phobia, 163, 165
    social phobia, 163, 165
Phosphate, organic, and organic
    brain syndromes, 96
Photomyoclonus, 233
Physical disorders
  anxiety and, 71–73, 164
  depression and, 67, 69–71, 130
  diagnosis of, 58, 67–78
  differential diagnosis of
    anxiety, 71–73
    confusion, 73–78
    depression, 67, 69–71
    disordered thinking, 73–78
    mood changes, 68
    psychosis, 73–78, 106
  patient reaction to, 63–64
  psychiatric disorders and,
    58–59, 62–64, 67–78
  with psychiatric symptoms
    catatonia, 66
    hysteria, 65–66
    other symptoms, 66–67
    paranoia, 66
  suicide and, 148–149
  underdiagnosis of, 62, 65
  See also Biological components;
    Chronic illness
Physostigmine, and
    anticholinergic drugs, 95,
    106, 107
Pick's disease, and organic brain
    syndromes, 97
Piloerection, and drug
    dependence, 271
Pimozide, and Tourette syndrome,
    435
Pituitary adeuomas, and sexual
    dysfunctions, 328
Pituitary disorders, and mood
    alterations, 68, 69–70
Pituitary syndromes, and mood
    alterations, 68
Placebos, 195
Placidyl. *See* Ethchlorvynol
Pneumonia
  alcoholism and, 232
  delirium and, 94
  disordered thinking and, 74, 75
  drug dependence and, 272
  psychiatric dysfunctions with, 65
Polyarteritis nodosa, and organic
    brain syndromes, 96

Posttraumatic headache, 183–184
Posttraumatic stress disorders,
    163–164
Prazepam, and anxiety, 164
Pregnancy
    barbiturates and, 393–394
    benzodiazepines and, 392
    effect of on child development,
        411
    lithium and, 391
    suicide and, 148
Premature ejaculation, 324, 330
Prenatal development, 410–411
Preschoolers, 413–414, 417–421
Prolixin. *See* Fluphenazine
Propanediol carbamates, 391
Propoxyphene, and hemodialysis,
    354
Propranolol
    adolescents and, 468
    alcohol withdrawal and, 234
    depression and, 71, 127
    migraines and, 181
    mood alterations and, 68
    organic brain syndromes and, 96
    tachycardias and, 133
Pseudodementia, 90
Psychalgia, 183
Psychedelic drugs
    dependence on, 275–276
    psychosis and, 77–78
Psychiatric disorders
    characteristics of, 62
    diagnosis of, 58–59, 61–64
    physical disorders and
        acute intermittent porphyria,
            65, 66, 68, 75–76
        cardiac conditions, 65, 72–73
        central nervous system
            disorders, 73
        diabetes mellitus, 67, 68, 70
        drugs, 66–68, 70–71, 73, 74,
            77–78
        endocrine disorders, 68–70,
            72
        infectious diseases, 65, 66, 68,
            71, 74, 76
        neurologic disorders, 74,
            76–77
        organic brain syndromes,
            74–75
        respiratory conditions, 72–73
        systemic diseases, 68, 71
        systemic lupus
            erythematosus, 65, 66, 68,
            70, 76
        Wilson's disease, 65, 68, 75

somatic complaints with, 59–64
    suicide and, 147
Psychiatric symptoms, 65–67
    catatonia, 66
    hysteria, 65–66
    other symptoms, 66–67
    paranoia, 66
Psychiatry, patient care in, 4
"Psychic numbing," 163
Psychoanalysis, 375–376
Psychoanalytic theory of anxiety,
    160
Psychobiological drives, and
        personality development, 38
"Psychogenic" headache, 181–182
Psychogenic pain disorder,
    194–195, 196
Psychological testing, and
        personality assessment,
        41–42
Psychopaths. *See* Antisocial
        personality disorder
Psychophysiologic symptom, 172
Psychosexual development, and
        personality, 39
Psychosis, 91, 103–111
    alcoholic, 223, 236
    case history of, 104, 110
    chronic, 109
    clinical evaluation of, 104–105
    disulfiram or DDC and, 250
    drug abuse and, 275, 276, 278
    etiology of
        drug use, 105–106
        functional psychosis, 107
        general metabolic illness, 106
    family and, 27
    functional, 107
    hemodialysis and, 352
    management of, 107, 108
    PEG for, 111
    physical illness and
        AIP, 76
        drugs, 77–78
        hypothyroidism, 69
        infections, 76
        neurologic disorders, 76–77
        organic brain syndromes,
            74–75
        SLE, 76
        Wilson's disease, 75
    psychotropic medications and,
        353, 384–387
    referral for, 107–109
    schizophrenia and, 91, 108
    signs and symptoms of, 16, 18,
        91

Psychosocial management, 8
Psychosomatic disorders, 172–177
    of children, 423–436
    of endocrine system, 173
    evaluation of, 174–177
    family and, 26–27
    patients and, 174–177
    physician's response to, 177
    sick role and, 173–174
    See also Headaches
Psychotherapist, selection of,
    376–377
Psychotherapy, 367–380
    alcoholism and, 249
    anxiety and, 165–166
    depression and, 130–131
    drug dependence and, 282–283
    evaluation for
        discussion with patient,
            370–372
        indications, 368–370
        referral conditions, 370
    headaches and, 181, 182
    medication and, 369, 372–373
    referral for
        conditions of, 370
        financial considerations in,
            379–380
        immediate, 372–373
        patient reaction to, 379
        primary physician's role in,
            377–378
        timing of, 373–374
    schizophrenia and, 117–118
    types of
        analytically oriented, 375
        behavioral, 166
        behavior modification, 375
        biofeedback, 376
        brief, 374
        couples, 376
        family, 376
        gestalt, 374
        group, 376
        intensive, 165–166, 374
        long-term, 74
        psychoanalysis, 375–376
        supportive, 165, 375
Psychotomimetics, and anxiety,
    162
Psychotropic medications,
    383–394
    antianxiety
        benzodiazepines, 392
        drug-disease interactions, 392
        drug-drug interactions, 392
        toxicity, 392

Psychotropic medications (*Cont.*)
  antidepressant
    lithium carbonate, 390–391
    MAO inhibitors, 389–390
    tricyclics, 388–389
  antipsychotic
    butyrophenone, 385
    dosage, 385–387
    drug-disease interactions, 287
    drug-drug interactions, 387
    phenothiazines, 385
    toxicity, 387
  hemodialysis and, 353–354
  psychotherapy and, 372–373
  sedatives
    alternatives, 394
    barbiturates, 393–394
    benzodiazepines, 393
Puberty, 450–451
  See also Adolescence
Pulmonary disorders
  anxiety and, 72, 73
  drug dependence and, 272
  medication and
    antianxiety drugs, 392
    barbiturates, 393
  organic brain syndromes and,
    96
  psychiatric dysfunctions with,
    65
Pulmonary edema, and drug
    dependence, 272
Pulmonary embolism, and
    disordered thinking, 74, 75
Pulmonary fibrosis, and drug
    dependence, 272

Quinidine
  organic brain syndromes and,
    96
  psychosis and, 105
  tricyclics and, 389

Rabies
  depression and, 71
  mood alterations and, 68
Race, and suicide, 145
Radiotherapy, side effects of, 359
Rape, in adolescence, 459
Recent context (in PEG), 4, 6, 8
Recent memory, 17, 85, 93
Regression, 401
Relaxation therapies, and
    headaches, 182
Religion, and suicide, 142,
    147–148
Remote memory, 17, 85, 93

REM rebound, and alcoholism,
    233
Renal disease
  chloral hydrate and, 394
  lithium and, 134, 391
  psychiatric symptoms and, 62
  See also Hemodialysis
Renal failure
  depression and, 67, 69
  mood alterations and, 68
Reproductive system, and drug
    dependence, 272
Reserpine
  depression and, 71, 127, 130,
    344
  mood alterations and, 68
  suicide and, 152
Respiratory conditions, and
    anxiety, 72–73
Restoil. *See* Temaylpam
Retirement, 26
Rhabdomyolysis, and drug
    dependence, 272
Rheumatic heart disease,
    psychiatric dysfunctions
    with, 65
Ritalin. *See* Methylphenidate
Rubella, and prenatal
    development, 411

St. Louis encephalitis
  depression and, 71
  mood alterations and, 68
Schilder's disease, and organic
    brain syndromes, 97
Schizoaffective psychosis, 107, 114
Schizoid personality disorder
  case history of, 49
  dysfunctional responses to, 49
  intervention for, 49
  problem of, 49
  recognition of, 48–49
Schizophrenia, 107, 113–120
  case history of, 114, 119
  childhood, 418–419
  definition of, 115
  diagnostic criteria for, 115
  etiologic theories of
    autoimmune and infectious
      agents, 116
    biochemical, 115
    central neurotransmitters,
      116
    family studies, 116
    genetic, 114–115, 410–411
    psychological studies, 116
    socioeconomic class, 116

family system deficiencies and,
    28
  hospitalization for, 118
  management of, 116–118
    biological dimension, 117
    environmental dimension,
      118
    personal dimension, 117–118
  medical problems and
    brain tumors, 77
    hemodialysis, 352–353
    organic brain syndromes,
      91–92
  medication for, 117
  organic factors in, 67
  PEG for, 120
  psychosis and, 91, 108
  psychotherapy for, 117–118
  referral for, 118
  sexual dysfunction and, 322
  suicide and, 141
  symptoms of, 114, 115
  in twins, 115
  violence and, 301, 303–304
Secobarbital, 393
  alcohol withdrawal and, 234,
    235
  barbiturate withdrawal and, 290
Seconal. *See* Secobarbital
Sedative-hypnotic compounds,
    273–275, 392–394
  alcoholism and, 228
  anxiety and, 72, 73
  depression and, 70, 344
  mood alterations and, 68
  organic brain syndromes and,
    95, 97
  overdose of, 274
  psychosis and, 105, 108, 109
  types of
    alternatives, 394
    barbiturates, 393–394
    benzodiazepines, 393
  violence and, 299
  withdrawal from, 234, 274–275,
    283, 290–292
Seizure disorders
  hysteria and, 201
  psychiatric dysfunctions with,
    65
  psychosis and, 106
  tricyclics and, 388–389
Seizures
  alcohol withdrawal and, 233
  anxiety and, 72, 162
  brain tumor and, 77
  drug abuse and, 272

"hysterical," 193
  psychiatric symptoms with, 65
  psychosis and, 76–77
Separation, as evolutionary family
    task, 25
Separation anxiety, 467
Sepsis, and disordered thinking, 74
Sequential Multiple Analyzer
    (SMA 12/60), 279
Serax. *See* Oxazepam
Serotonin, and depression, 125,
    131, 133
Serotonin theory of affective
    disorders, 125
Serynlan. *See* Phencyclidine
Sex
  alcoholism and, 230
  hemodialysis and, 350–351
  suicide and, 144
Sex behavior, 312
Sex counseling, 328–329
Sex education, 31, 328–329
Sex therapy, 312–313, 330, 331
Sexual Attitude Restructuring
    (SAR) programs, 331
Sexual aversion
  female, 317–318
  male, 319–320
Sexual drive, 312
Sexual dysfunctions, 311–334
  case history of, 312, 333–334
  chronic illness and, 346, 356
  classification of, 315–316
  diabetes and, 356
  diagnosis of
    excitement phase
      dysfunctions, 320–322
    female desire phase
      dysfunctions, 316–318, 328
    female orgasmic phase
      dysfunctions, 322–324
    male desire phase
      dysfunctions, 318–320
    male orgasmic phase
      dysfunctions, 324–325
    vaginismus, 320, 326–327
  distractability and, 321
  lubrication and, 320–321
  medical conditions and, 314
  PEG for, 334
  prevention of, 331–332
  referral for, 330–331
  treatment of
    appropriate reading, 329
    attitude changes, 329–330
    behavior modification, 330
    communication, 329

impact of contraception, 328
  problem clarification, 327
  self-help, 329
  sex education and
    counseling, 328–329
  treatment of physical causes,
    328
Sexual functioning
  basic principles of, 312–313
  physiologic change in, 313
Sexual history, 315
Sexuality, 313–314, 414–417
  adolescent, 451, 452, 456–460
  childhood, 414–417, 421
Sexual orientation, 312
Sexual response, 312, 313–314
Shyness, extreme, 467–468
Sinsimmela, 278
Situational disturbance syndrome,
    208
  case histories of, 208, 214, 215,
    217–218
  diagnosis of, 208
  management of, 212–213
  recognition of, 208–212
  referral for, 213–214
Skeletal system, and drug
    dependence, 272
Sleep remedies, OTC
  delirium and, 78
  psychiatric symptoms with, 74,
    78
Smoking
  alcoholism and, 228
  antianxiety drugs and, 329
  prenatal development and, 411
Social-communication theory, and
    conversion disorder, 193
Socialization, 25, 28
Social phobia, 163, 165
Socioeconomic class
  drug dependence and, 268
  schizophrenia and, 116
  suicide and, 148
Sociopaths. *See* Antisocial
    personality disorder
"Somatic displacement," 176
Somatization disorder, 183,
    196–197
Special education, 419, 433
"Spectatoring," 313, 329
Speech
  autistic, 417–418
  content of, 16–17
  explosive, 16
  in mental status examination,
    16–17

Stadol. *See* Butorphanol
Stelazine. *See* Trifluoperazine
Steroids
  catatonia and, 66
  depression and, 70, 127
  mood alterations and, 68, 70
  organic brain syndromes and,
    96
  paranoia and, 66
  psychosis and, 105
  SLE and, 76
  suicide and, 152
Stimulants
  abuse of, 275
  ADD children and, 433–434
  anxiety and, 72, 73, 162
  psychosis and, 106
  withdrawal from, 275, 283
STP, dependence on, 275–276
Stress, 207–218
  case histories of, 208, 214, 215,
    217–218
  endocrine system and, 173
  headaches and, 181–182
  life change events and, 210
  mitigating factors in, 209
  personality and, 43
  psychosomatic disorders and,
    176–177
  reactions to, 61, 67, 176–177
  reduction of, 181, 182, 212–213
  symptoms of, 209
  traumatic, 163–164
Stuttering, 421
Subarachoid hemorrhage, and
    paranoia, 66
Subdural hematoma
  diagnosis of, 88
  disordered thinking and, 74
  organic brain syndromes and,
    96, 97
  paranoia and, 66
  psychiatric symptoms and, 77
Substance abuse
  in adolescence, 462–464
  antisocial personality and, 50
  definition of, 223
  See also Alcoholism
Substance dependence, 223, 226
  See also Drug dependence
Suicide, 139–155
  adolescents and, 143–144,
    464–465
  alcoholism and, 240
  case history of, 140, 154–155
  child-rearing practices and, 142
  children and, 144

Suicide (*Cont.*)
    correlates to
        abortion, 148
        accident proneness, 150
        age, 143–144
        command hallucinations, 150
        crisis event, 150
        day of week, 148
        education, 147
        ethnic group, 145–146
        family history, 146
        hypochondria, 150
        insomnia, 150
        location, 146
        marital status, 144
        method, 146–147
        occupation, 146
        physical illness, 148–149
        pregnancy, 148
        previous attempts, 149
        psychiatric illness, 147
        psychological correlates, 149
        race, 145
        religion, 147–148
        sex, 144
        socioeconomic factors, 148
        surgery, 148
    depression and, 60–61, 124,
        129, 130, 131, 141, 464–465
    hallucinogens and, 106
    hemodialysis and, 351–352
    homicide and, 142
    hyperthyroidism and, 69
    hysteria and, 65
    incidence of, 140
    infectious diseases and, 71
    learning theory and, 142
    management of
        antidepressants, 152
        electroconvulsive therapy,
            152
        hospitalization, 151
        social support, 152–153
    PEG for, 155
    religion and, 142, 147–148
    theories on, 141–148
    types of
        altruistic, 142
        anomic, 142
        egoistic, 142
Suicide equivalents, 150
Supportive psychotherapy, 165,
    375
Surgery, and suicide, 148
"Survivor guilt," 163
Sympathomimetics, and anxiety,
    72, 73

Symptoms
    ability to function and, 176
    personal meaning of, 176
Syphilis
    diagnosis of, 71
    manic-depressive illness and,
        91
    mood alterations and, 68, 71
    organic brain syndromes and,
        97
    treatment of, 98
Systemic diseases
    depression and, 71
    mood alterations and, 68
Systemic lupus erythematosis
    (SLE)
    depression and, 71
    disordered thinking and, 74
    hysteria and, 201
    mood alterations and, 68, 70
    organic brain syndromes and,
        96
    psychiatric symptoms with, 65,
        70, 76
    psychosis and, 76

Tachyarrythmias, and anxiety, 72
Tagamet. *See* Cinetidine
Takayashu's syndrome, and
    hysteria, 66
Talwin. *See* Pentazocine
Taraxeine, and schizophrenia, 115
Teenagers. *See* Adolescence
Temaylpam, and insomnia, 393
Tension headache, 181
Terminal illness
    depression and, 69
    family and, 30
Testicular atrophy, and sexual
    dysfunction, 328
Tetanus, and drug dependence,
    272
Tetracyclics, and psychotherapy,
    372
Tetracycline, and prenatal
    development, 411
Tetrahydrocannabinol (THC), 276,
    278–279
Thalidomide, and prenatal
    development, 411
Thematic Apperception Test
    (TAT), 406
Theophylline, and anxiety, 73
Therapeutic communities,
    283–284
Thiazide diuretics, and lithium,
    391

Thioridazine, 384, 385
    ADD children and, 434
    anorexia nervosa and, 462
    dosage of, 386
    schizophrenia and, 117
    side effects of, 385, 387
    violence and, 299
Thiothixene, and schizophrenia,
    117
Thioxanthine, 117, 384
Thorazine. *See* Chlorpromazine
Thought
    contents of, 18
    disordered, 73–78
Thrombocytopenia, and
    alcoholism, 232
Thrombophlebitis, and drug
    dependence, 271, 272
Thyroid disease
    anxiety and, 72
    depression and, 67
    mood alterations and, 68, 69
    organic brain syndromes and,
        96
    psychiatric dysfunctions with,
        65
    psychosis and, 106
Thyrotoxicosis, 172
Tobacco. *See* Smoking
Toddlers, 412–413
Tofranil. *See* Imipramine
Tourette syndrome
    in children, 434–436
    compulsions and, 163
    genetics and, 411
    haloperidol and, 385
    obsessions and, 163
    speech and, 16
Toxins
    depression and, 130
    organic brain syndromes and,
        96, 97
    psychosis and, 105
Tranquilizers
    abuse of, 273–275
    depression and, 129, 344
    hemodialysis and, 353
    organic brain syndromes and,
        96, 97
    psychotherapy and, 372
Transverse myelitis, and drug
    dependence, 272
Tranylcypromine, 133, 389–390
Tremor, and alcoholism, 233
Tricyclic antidepressants,
    388–389
    ADD children and, 434

adolescents and, 465, 467, 468
anorexia nervosa and, 462
anxiety and, 165
delirium and, 78
depression and, 125, 126, 131–133
disordered thinking and, 74
dosage and schedule of, 132–133, 388
hemodialysis and, 354
maintenance of, 133
narcotic withdrawal and, 288
overdoses of, 388
paranoia and, 66
precautions for, 33
psychosis and, 106
psychotherapy and, 372
side effects of, 131, 388–389
suicide and, 152
withdrawal of, 133
Trifluoperazine, and schizophrenia, 117
Trilafon. *See* Perphenazine
Tuberculosis
alcoholism and, 232
drug dependence and, 272
Two-disease theory of depression, 125–126
Type A personality, 44, 67
Type B personality, 67
Typhoid
depression and, 71
mood alterations and, 68

Typhus
depression and, 71
mood alterations and, 68
Tyramine, and MAO inhibitors, 389–390

Ulcers
alcoholism and, 232
drug dependence and, 271
duodenal, 172
peptic, 232
Unipolar depression, 124
Uremia, and organic brain syndromes, 96

Vaginismus, 320, 326–327, 330
Vaginitis, 326, 328
Valium. *See* Diazepam
Vascular disorders, 65, 96, 97
Vascular migraines, 179–181
Vasomotor reaction headache, 182
"Vasomotor rhinitis," 182
Venereal diseases, 65, 458
Violence, 295–308
in adolescents, 469–470
case history of, 296
differential diagnosis of
affective disorders, 304
alcohol intoxication, 301–302
family violence, 306
heroin, 303
mental retardation, 306
organic brain syndromes, 306–307

personality disorders, 304–306
phencyclidine, 302–303
schizophrenia, 303–304
temporal lobe epilepsy, 307–308
emergency certification and, 308
evaluation of, 299–301
hemodialysis and, 352
medication and, 299
restraints and, 298–299
safety precautions and, 297–298
See also Aggression
Viral infections, and depression, 67
Visualization techniques, 360
Vitamin B_{12} deficiency
dementia and, 88
disordered thinking and, 74
organic brain syndromes and, 96

Wernicke-Korsakoff syndrome, 236, 251–252
Wilson's disease, 58
depression and, 71
disordered thinking and, 74
mood alterations and, 68
organic brain syndromes and, 96, 97
psychiatric symptoms with, 65
psychotic symptoms and, 75